HUMAN BRAIN FUNCTION

Richard S. J. Frackowiak

Karl J. Friston

Christopher D. Frith

Raymond J. Dolan

Wellcome Department of Cognitive Neurology
Institute of Neurology
University College London
London, United Kingdom

John C. Mazziotta

Division of Brain Mapping
Department of Neurology
UCLA School of Medicine
Reed Neurological Center
Los Angeles, California

Academic Press

SAN DIEGO   LONDON   BOSTON   NEW YORK   SYDNEY   TOKYO   TORONTO

Copyright © 1997 by ACADEMIC PRESS

Academic Press
a division of Harcourt Brace & Company
525 B Street, Suite 1900, San Diego, California 92101-4495, USA
http://www.apnet.com

Academic Press Limited
24-28 Oval Road, London NW1 7DX, UK
http://www.hbuk.co.uk/ap/

Library of Congress Cataloging-in-Publication Data

Human brain function / edited by Richard S. J. Frackowiak.
        p.   cm.
    Includes bibliographical references and index.
      ISBN 0-12-264840-4 (alk. paper)
      1. Neuropsychology.   2. Brain mapping.   3. Cognition.   4. Brain-
    -Imaging.   I. Frackowiak, Richard S. J.
      [DNLM: 1. Brain--physiology.   2. Brain Mapping.   3. Cognition-
    -physiology.   4. Diagnostic Imaging.   WL 300 H9182 1997]
    QP360.H863   1997
    612.8'2--dc21
    DNLM/DLC
    for Library of Congress   97-17952
                                                                        CIP

PRINTED IN CANADA
    98   99   00   01   02   FR   9   8   7   6   5   4   3   2

To our families and loved ones;
to our students, fellows, teachers and collaborators;
and to the memory of Sir Henry Wellcome, philanthropist.

CONTENTS

AUTHORS

PREFACE

Is it timely to propose a book about our present knowledge of the functional organization of the human brain? This volume represents an explicit answer to that question. Since the time of Gall, science has attempted to collect more accurate details about how our perception, cognition, and action are mediated by brain function. The clinico-anatomical method, with its more modern version, clinical neuropsychology, has provided much information that has been complemented by classical psychological studies in normal people. Nevertheless, throughout this century an underlying tension has existed between those who espoused a pure localisationist approach and those to whom functional integration has been a guiding principle. It is no exaggeration to say that the arrival of noninvasive brain monitoring techniques, especially those that show the anatomy of the living brain, has revolutionized the field. The investigation of relationships between brain function and brain anatomy in normal subjects is now a reality whereas as little as two decades ago it was a mere twinkle in the eye of researchers. Though revolutionary, the new methods have not created a new science. The older and traditional methods have generated a body of knowledge that informs and structures current investigation. In the perceptual field, discoveries made on the basis of data from single-cell recordings in primates serve to generate testable hypotheses in humans. The correlation of dysfunction with sites of brain lesions provides a framework for investigating networks that mediate complex higher function. It is a decade since the new imaging methods were introduced and we think it, therefore, timely to take stock.

This book is not encyclopaedic in concept or scope. It is written by members of a multidisciplinary collaborative group of scientists who have worked together for a number of years using functional imaging as an experimental method. Functional imaging is often regarded as "big science"—implying considerable capital expenditure and investment in human resources, on a scale equivalent to that of a large particle physics laboratory. The term "big science," slightly pejorative in the view of some, is meant to contrast such activity with that of individual scientists thinking and discovering things in isolation and with limited resources. There is no doubt that in this sense functional imaging is big science. However, this century has seen many major advances that have come about from this way of working. The magnificent achievements of CERN in particle physics and the collaborative (if encyclopaedic) mathematical work of the Bourbaki Group stand as shining examples amongst many others. This book, therefore, presents a coherent view, if not an all embracing one. To those that do not see their work cited we apologize. Our idea is to convey certain concepts and definitive data. This is an unfair process, as definitive data frequently follow preliminary studies by others. However, considerations of space, coherence, and intelligibility have dictated this course of action.

Two colleagues external to the Wellcome Department of Cognitive Neurology's Functional Imaging Laboratory (FIL) were invited to join us in this endeavour. First was Dr. John Mazziotta, from UCLA, because of his pioneering contributions, with his colleagues, to the problem of bridging our understanding derived from noninvasive techniques with those achieved at the cellular or molecular levels. His group entered into transatlantic collaboration with us in 1991, developing much needed methods for effective registration of images within and between modalities, whilst we took on the problem of standardising statistical analyses and experimental design. Much has happened since those enabling days, and the field has reached a large degree of methodological consensus as a result of this division of labour in the early stages. Dr. Keith Worsley, from McGill University, Montreal, has collaborated extensively with us on the development of techniques incorporated into the system of statistical parametric mapping (SPM). The recent proposal of unified equations that allow assessment of the significance of change of brain activity on the basis of magnitude and extent is the last in a series of innovative developments over the past five years.

Science progresses through developments, methods, and advances in concepts. This book is, therefore, organized into three parts. The first part addresses methods principally from a conceptual perspective and is geared towards those who wish to understand how experiments are constructed and the ensuing data interpreted. These chapters can be read by the mathematically illiterate and include many illustrative biological examples. The second part deals with those areas that have been the prime objects of our studies. Input systems, including vision and aspects of somatosensory function, are dealt with first. Following this, there is a description of work on the normal motor system and on patients with brain lesions who have shown functional recovery. Cognition is addressed by focusing on language, memory, higher cognitive function, and neuromodulation using pharmacological agents. We conclude with a third section of three chapters that looks to the future. The first examines ways and means of integrating information from the behavioural level down to the synapse. The second introduces functional magnetic resonance imaging and the new methodological problems and opportunities that this technique provides. The third is pure fantasy and put up as a straw man to draw criticism and provoke discussion. Readers will undoubtedly note that much of the biological information described in this book has been obtained using perfusion mapping with positron emission tomography (PET). This apparent bias is attributable to the fact that the functional magnetic resonance (fMRI) technique is still young. In the case of the conceptually and technically simpler PET, 10 years of development were required before novel and biologically meaningful information began to accrue. Functional MRI with the brain oxygen level dependent technique has existed for half that time, and considerable progress is now being made to optimise the technique as a neuroscientific tool. In this final section we hope to convey the anticipation and excitement of what awaits us.

The Medical Research Council, through its support of the Neuroscience Group at the Cyclotron Unit in Hammersmith Hospital between 1988 and 1994, facilitated the laying down of much of the groundwork. The support was unstinting and we are extremely grateful for it. During this period most of us began working together and formed the collaborations that have led to this volume and the foundation of the FIL. The Wellcome Trust provided us with the best possible facilities and environment for continuing this work from 1994. The occupation of new laboratories at the Institute of Neurology, University College London, in 1995 also provided us with the opportunity to develop fMRI for promoting our program of neuroscience research. University College London has provided new collaborations with a large community of cognitive neuroscientists that augur well for the future. For these various opportunities we are grateful, and we express this gratitude with this volume.

Finally, our thanks go to Academic Press, in particular, Jasna Markovac and Graham Lees, who have put this volume to bed; to all our students, fellows, and associates at the FIL; and to Graham Lewington and his staff, Terry Morris, Nicki Roffe, and their staff for contributing in multitudinous ways to the generation of this volume.*

London 1997

* All the programs necessary for image analysis that are dealt with in this book can be downloaded free from http://www.fil.ion.ucl.ac.uk/spm.

PART ONE

PRINCIPLES AND METHODS

CHAPTER ONE

LINKING BRAIN AND BEHAVIOUR

In this book we shall review what has been learned about human brain function from the application of brain imaging techniques. It is about 10 years since the first of these studies started to appear in the literature, but the impact on neuroscience has been considerable. Brain imaging techniques developed at just the right time to fill the gap between direct studies of brain function at the physiological level and studies of psychological processes at the cognitive level, which are, of course, indirect studies of brain function. This first chapter will describe the various techniques that were used to study relationships between brain and behaviour before the new imaging techniques were available. It is from these studies that the scientific framework within which brain imaging has been able to flourish was developed.

I. BRAIN AND BEHAVIOUR—CROSSING SCIENTIFIC BOUNDARIES

It is very useful to treat reality as if it was organised in a series of layers [1]. At the bottom layer we have subatomic particles such as quarks and positrons characterised by properties such as spin and charm. Higher up there are elements and molecules such as water with properties like density and viscosity. Higher still there are cells with "vital" properties and above them are organisms with intentions and consciousness. Scientific disciplines such as physics or psychology usually apply to one specific level, but most scientists believe that, in principle, there is a continuous chain of interlocking theories running from the lowest to the highest levels of description. Structures at higher levels are made up of entities belonging to lower levels. A reductionist account requires that everything that happens at one level can be explained in terms of entities in the level below, but there is an equally viable expansionist account in which events at a lower level can be explained in terms of higher level entities.

There are two fundamental break points in this hierarchy of levels. The first occurs between nonliving and living things. The problem of how life emerged from inert matter was a major preoccupation in the 18th and 19th centuries [2], but was essentially solved by Darwin's theory of evolution. The second break point occurs when we reach a level where organisms have minds. A major preoccupation of late 20th century science is how consciousness and a sense of self can emerge from the physical matter of brains. This problem is addressed by disciplines such as neuropsychology in which the relationship between mind and brain is studied directly. The intractability of the problem is often blamed on Descartes who made such a clear distinction between physical entities (atoms, neurons) that are extended in space and mental entities (memories, beliefs) that are not. However, Descartes also made clear that much of the activity of the brain is not to do with mind work. He made a sharp distinction between actions that can be explained in mechanical terms (all actions of animals and many actions of humans) and that subset of human actions that require the postulation of a mind. *"Two different principles of our movements are to be distinguished, the one entirely mechanical or corporeal... the other, incorporeal"* (The Passions of the Soul, 1637). Actions which he considered to derive from the mind included expert action (based on knowledge) and the creative use of language to express thoughts. Today we might add to this list actions based on beliefs and say that all these are actions determined by particular kinds of mental representations or propositions. We believe that the distinction made by Descartes continues to be useful. We shall call the problem of explaining "mechanical" actions and perceptions the brain–behaviour problem and the problem of explaining actions and perceptions derived from mental entities the brain–mind problem.

The work the brain does in controlling movements or responding differently to one face than another (to take two of many possible examples) is an example of the brain–behaviour problem. Such work does not involve crossing levels between the mental and the physical. We can make machines that can perform such tasks with a considerable degree of skill. Such machines are the descendants of the automata with which Descartes was familiar. In these cases the problem is to explain how the brain uses information about the environment (past and present) coded as neural signals in order to generate appropriate behaviour. The solution to such problems depends on specifying the mechanisms by which neurons modulate the passage of signals through the brain. This requires that we can write down algorithms or equations that specify the way in which signals are transformed, in other words a computational level of description. Nearly all of animal neuropsychology and much of human neuropsychology is concerned with the brain–behaviour problem. Most of the chapters in this book will be concerned with the brain–behaviour problem.

The brain–mind problem is essentially concerned with consciousness. How can neural signals in the brain lead to the experience of being me, of feeling happy, of enjoying the blue of the sky? No one has yet answered these questions, but we are beginning to learn a lot about the patterns of brain activity associated with particular states of consciousness (see Chapter 14 on higher cognitive functions). In the present chapter we shall largely be concerned with techniques for studying the brain–behaviour problem.

II. MODELS OF BRAIN FUNCTION

The brain is essentially a device for processing information about the environment (past, present, and future) coded as neural signals. The brain uses this information in the form of patterns of neural firing to generate the actions most likely to achieve the organism's goals. David Marr has provided a popular framework for discussing information processing in the brain [3]. He suggests that most processes can be described in terms of the transformation from one form of information (the input) into another (the output). There are three levels at which these processes can be discussed. At the top level there is computational theory. This level is concerned with the goal of the process and the strategy by which this goal is achieved. At the middle level there are codes and algorithms. This level is concerned with the nature of the codes and of the algorithms by which the transformation from one code to another is achieved. At the bottom level there is the implementation of the process in terms of interactions between neurons. The first two levels are in the cognitive domain of discourse, while the bottom level concerns neurophysiology.

Evidence about processes at the top or computational level will come largely from studies of behaviour (*e.g.*, reaction times and errors) and sometimes from introspection. For example, the many visual illusions in which there is a discrepancy between reality and experience give us clues about underlying computational processes. At the middle level, the development of theories about the nature of the codes and the processing algorithms must be constrained equally by evidence from behaviour and neurophysiology. The relationship between these algorithms and their implementation (the bottom level) lies at the heart of the problem of how to map the cognitive onto the physical.

A. Functional Segregation and Integration

How does the brain solve problems? We could conceive of the brain as a black box which transformed input into output and we might assume that any particular transformation was achieved by some action of the brain *"as a whole"* [4]. This idea is almost certainly wrong. An alternative is provided by the principle of functional segregation. This implies that the brain consists of a great many modules that process information more or less independently of each other [5]. It seems likely that it will be easier to discover how one of these modules works than to explain the functioning of the brain as a whole.

The initial evidence for functional segregation in the human brain came from two sources, neuropsychology and anatomy. First, there was Broca's [6] demonstration that a circumscribed brain lesion could cause a specific disorder of language while other cognitive functions remained intact. This observation leads to two claims: first that language is a function that can be damaged separately from other cognitive processes and second that this function is localisable. This claim was elaborated by Wernicke [7] and by Lichtheim [8] who proposed that there were a number of separable and localisable subcomponents of language. These included centres for *"auditory word representations"* and for *"motor word representations."* In addition Lichtheim speculated on how information might flow between these centres.

Meanwhile, Korbinian Brodmann [9] was engaged in the prodigious task of showing that the cortex of the human brain could be mapped into 52 discrete areas on the basis of cytoarchitectonics; the structure of cells and the characteristic arrangement of these cells into layers. The assumption is that if areas of the brain have different anatomical structures, then they must also have different functions. However, the reverse need not be true. A single

"Brodmann area" is unlikely to subserve the same function throughout even if there is no obvious difference in cytoarchitecture.

For the first half of the 20th century this evidence for functional segregation was considered discredited and was largely ignored. However, with the advent of powerful new methods of data collection such as direct stimulation and recording from the cortex [10] and the rise of cognitive neuropsychology [11], functional segregation has again become the dominant framework for thinking about how the brain works (see Chapter 9). There are now demonstrations that many different psychological functions can be discretely impaired by brain lesions [12]. Furthermore Brodmann's anatomical claims have been confirmed and refined [13].

As is so often the case, after the empirical demonstration has been achieved a number of powerful intellectual arguments have been put forward to show that we should expect functional segregation on purely theoretical grounds.

First, there is the argument from evolution [14,15]. The brain is an enormously complex system that has been "designed" by evolution. In other words this system has developed through a series of very small, random changes. If the brain functioned as a single, heavily interconnecting entity, then a small change on one part would require balancing changes throughout the system. In these circumstances it is very unlikely that any small change is going to produce an improvement in the functioning of the system as a whole. However, if the brain contains a number of relatively independent modules then a small change in one module will hardly affect the functioning of the other modules and improvement of local functioning is more likely to occur. On the basis of this argument a modular brain will evolve more rapidly and be more successful than one that works by mass action.

Second, there is the argument from economy [16]. Representation of environmental features like contours depends upon mechanisms such as lateral inhibition which require interactions between neurons concerned with particular subfeatures (*e.g.*, orientation). Such interactions depend upon connections between neurons. These connections will be achieved more economically if the relevant neurons are grouped together. Thus, neurons are likely to be grouped in terms of what they code for, *i.e.*, their function.

Third, there is the argument from complexity [17]. It is possible to derive a measure of the complexity of systems like the brain that consist of a large number of heavily interconnected units. Simulations show that this measure of neural complexity is low for systems that are composed either of completely independent parts (maximum segregation) or of parts that show completely homogeneous behaviour (maximum integration, mass action). Neural complexity is highest for systems that conjoin local specialisation with global integration. This result emphasises that although functional segregation is an important principal of brain design, we must also consider functional integration. Brain function also depends on the interactions between the modules.

A question remains as to the size of these functionally specialised areas. Data from patients with lesions can suggest areas spanning hundreds of millimetres and millions of nerve cells. In contrast the columns and hypercolumns discovered by recording from single cells are less than 1 mm in size and contain thousands of cells. These differences do not simply reflect precision of measurement. The organisation of the brain is self-similar. In other words, at whatever scale we choose to study the relation between structure and function, we will see segregation. However, what appears to be a homogenous patch at one scale will be seen to consist of segregated areas at a higher level of magnification.

B. The Popularity of Neural Networks

The success of neural networks as models of brain function [18] does not imply a return to fashion of mass action. Within the modules defined by functional segregation there is, by definition, heavy interconnection between all the components. The behaviour of a module is therefore appropriately modeled in terms of a neural network. However, it is critical for the success of the system as a whole that when the weights in one module are adjusted, this does not alter the functioning of other modules.

In summary, the brain should be considered as a device for processing neural signals that code for properties of the environment that are of evolutionary, social, and personal significance to the individual. In particular it is a device for detecting changes in the environment and responding appropriately on the basis of preexisting goals. To this end the brain represents and transforms information about the environment and about its own state. The brain contains of a large number of modules that specialise in different kinds of information.

III. PROBLEMS OF MEASUREMENT

One of the most direct methods for studying brain function involves applying a carefully controlled stimulus to an organism and observing the response. For example, we might ask the question, how does the brain discriminate wavelength? There are many ways to approach this problem. (1) The activity of a single cell is recorded while different wavelengths are projected onto the retina. Cells can be identified that respond to certain changes in wavelength, but not to others. (2) An animal (or human) is trained to press a button to one wavelength, but not to another. We can then measure the smallest difference in wavelength the animal (or human) can detect. (3) We can show someone two wavelengths and ask, "can you see any difference between them?" and thus measure the smallest difference in colour that can be detected. In each case we are studying a rather low level aspect of brain function that Descartes would certainly have considered capable of mechanical explanation. However, in method 3 we rely on the subject to tell us what he is experiencing. In other words we are using his phenomenological consciousness as an instrument for observing the consequences of brain function. In practice, it is extremely convenient to ask people to describe their experiences. Indeed, most clinical investigations start by asking patients to tell us about their problems. This approach works well as long as we remember that our data are being filtered through someone's mind. There are two fundamental reasons why this dependence upon introspection will sometimes fail us.

A. The Cognitive Unconscious

The first is simply that there are many types of brain activity that do not give rise to anything that is available to introspection. For instance, it has been proposed that we are never aware of cognitive processes, but only the results of cognitive processes [19]. If we are trying to think of a word beginning with "A" then we are frequently unaware of anything happening until an appropriate word suddenly pops into our mind. However, there are almost certainly many results of cognitive processes that are not available to introspection either. This possibility is revealed dramatically by certain neurological cases (see Section D for more detail). Milner and Goodale [20] have described a patient with a severe deficit in her perception of shape. She can see vague areas of light and shade, but cannot report the orientation of a line. Nevertheless, if asked to grasp an object or "post a letter" through a slot she will orient her hand appropriately before contacting the object. Clearly she is gaining information about orientation which can guide her behaviour, but this information is not available to introspection (see also the phenomenon of "blind sight"). Ingenious experiments show that these two types of visual information are also present independently in people with intact brains with the neural signals that guide movements being unavailable to introspection [21]. What this example shows is that data collected via introspection may give a different story from data collected via behaviour. Many of the apparent discrepancies between animal and human studies (*e.g.*, hippocampal lesions causing amnesia in humans, but having little effect on certain memory tests in animals) can be traced to the fact that many human studies depend upon introspection ("do you recall the address I gave you a few moments ago?"), while all animal studies depend upon behaviour [22].

The arch-behaviourist, Skinner tried to get round this problem by calling the results of introspection *"verbal behaviour"* [23]. However, the data obtained from introspection will be qualitatively different depending on whether the experimenter treats it as a verbal report or as verbal behaviour. The verbal report is "about" something; it has a content and has the potential to be untrue. Behaviour, whether verbal or otherwise, is not about anything; it is something we observe. We may misinterpret it, but it is neither true nor untrue. It simply happens. In nearly all cases it is very convenient to assume that what subjects tell us is true. It is far more difficult to interpret behaviour.

B. The Mechanisms of Introspection

The second case where introspection may fail occurs when the mechanism of introspection has itself been damaged. We are making a distinction here between the content, what we introspect about, sensations, desires, *etc.*, and the mechanism that acts on this content enabling us to know and report on sensations, desires, *etc.* Clearly there is, in a sense, a trivial reason for introspection failing when we are unable to report what we feel. Someone who has lost the power of speech or whose muscles are paralysed may still be able to introspect, but cannot tell us what he feels. Of course he may recover and then be able to tell us what it was like when he was paralysed. However, there exists in principle the more striking case where the ability to introspect has been lost or has always been abnormal. Such a patient might still be able to speak, but he would not be able to tell us how he felt. Indeed, he would not understand the question. The best he might do is produce a stereotyped, automatic response, "I feel fine." With such a case the clinical interview effectively fails. We have the immensely difficult task of inferring what the patient is experiencing from his behaviour. Do such cases exist? The obvious possibilities are severe dementia, confusional states, certain extreme phases of schizophrenia, and, more controversially, autism. As yet there have been few systematic studies of what happens when introspection fails [24].

There is no body of scientific evidence to help us understand such cases. Their state is captured by the lay person's crude metaphor, "the lights are on, but there is no one at home." This metaphor shows us that by using introspection we are entering the realm of the deep problems associated with the self and the mind and how they emerge from the brain. The metaphor emphasises the strong, but misleading feeling that consciousness is like having a little man in our heads that observes the results of brain work.

IV. TECHNIQUES LINKING BRAIN AND BEHAVIOUR

In the rest of this chapter we shall avoid, as far as possible, consideration of the brain–mind problem. We shall concentrate instead on how we have learned about the links between brain and mental processes in humans using the various techniques that were available before the development of brain imaging methodology.

There are two ways by which we can investigate relations between brain and behaviour. These are determined by whether we choose brain or behaviour as the dependent variable. First, we can modify the brain and study the effects on behaviour. Studies of patients with lesions fall into this category with the major restriction that the nature of the lesion cannot be chosen to suit some experimental design; the lesion results from either "an accident of nature" or the requirements of neurosurgery in a brain that is already to some degree abnormal. Stimulation with intracortical electrodes is another technique with rather similar restrictions. We can also modify brain function by giving people drugs.

Second, we can manipulate behaviour (or experience) and study the effect on brain activity. This has been done by measuring electrical (or magnetic) activity from scalp electrodes or intracortical electrodes. The new imaging techniques based on cerebral blood flow are also in this class.

These two classes of technique have special problems stemming from the fact that we never have perfect control over the independent variable. The precise location of the relevant area of damaged brain will always be in doubt. Even in experimental studies with animals this problem can arise. For example, there were many studies of the effects of hippocampal lesions that had to be reinterpreted when it was shown that incidental damage to adjacent tissue (in particular the parahippocampal gyrus) had major behavioural effects [25]. There are also the problems associated with secondary damage to distant areas that are consequent upon the lesion and the reallocation of function that may underlie recovery of function.

Similar problems arise when behaviour is the independent variable. For example, an apparent modulation of brain activity due to selective attention to tones could have resulted from movements of the animal's head relative to the source of sound.

A. Experimental Psychology

In introductory textbooks the brain is often described as the "organ of thought" or the "organ that controls our behaviour." Given such characterisations, the scientific study of thinking and behaviour (*i.e.*, psychology) provides fundamental information about how the brain works, even though that organ may never be mentioned in such studies.

The simple observation that we do not see in the ultraviolet range or hear the cries of bats tells us something about the restrictions in the range of information coded for in the human brain. The Weber–Fechner law [26], that just noticeable differences in perception are proportional to the intensity of the signal, tells us something about the form of the neural transduction of signals in sensory pathways. Much of contemporary psychology is concerned with specifying as accurately as possible the nature of particular psychological processes at a cognitive level. The success of this programme depends upon the assumption that processes that are relatively independent of each other can be identified (*i.e.*, functional segregation). In this section we shall give examples of just a few of the various techniques that have been developed.

1. Dual Task Interference

One way to identify cognitive modules is to ask people to do two things at once. If someone can do two things at once without compromising performance of either task then we can infer that the processes underlying the two tasks function independently. This methodology has been used extensively in the study of working memory. First, studies using dual-task methodology give support to the idea that working memory includes a number of independent, modality specific components [27]. Verbal working memory (*e.g.*, remembering a telephone number for a short time) is impaired if we have to articulate (*i.e.*, say "blah blah blah blah") continuously while trying to remember the material. Visuo-spatial working memory (remembering a complex pattern of lines) is not impaired by concurrent articulation. In contrast, producing a pattern of key presses will interfere with visuo-spatial working memory, but not verbal working memory. These results are evidence that verbal working memory and visuo-spatial memory depend upon independent cognitive modules.

It is also possible to identify independent components within the verbal working memory system: a speech based rehearsal system (the "inner voice") and a temporary auditory store (the "inner ear"). Together these form the "articulatory loop." By subvocal rehearsal of material in the auditory store is continuously refreshed. Thus it is possible to keep verbal material in working memory almost indefinitely even though the auditory store has a very short life. Having to articulate interferes with the inner voice, while hearing irrelevant speech interferes with the inner ear.

2. The Sternberg Paradigm

The logic of the dual-task paradigm is essentially the same as that applied to experimental designs in which the distinction is made between main effects and interactions. Two factors are said to interact if the difference in effects between levels of one of the factors is influenced by the level of the other factor (Fig. 1A). In the dual task paradigm such an interaction is present if the performance of task A is altered by the requirement to perform task B at the same time. In other words, the presence of interference is equivalent to an interaction. Sternberg [28] applied the same logic to different processes occurring within the same task. Most tasks can plausibly be divided into stages such as input, processing and output. One of the tasks studied by Sternberg involved a search through working memory. Subjects were given a list of target letters to remember (*e.g.*, A H L). They were then shown a random sequence of letters and asked to indicate whether each letter was in the target list or not. In such a task there are very few errors and performance can be

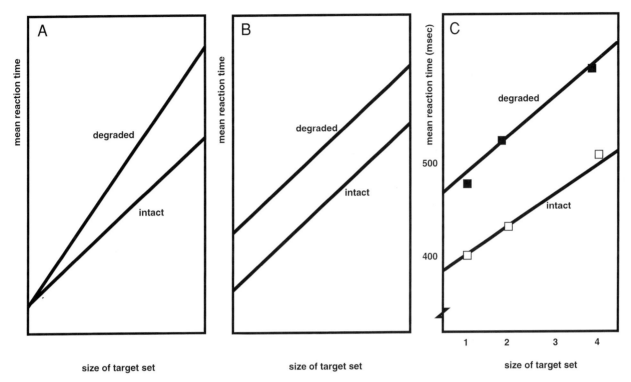

FIGURE 1 The Sternberg paradigm. Subjects see a sequence of letters and have to respond to specified targets. In the example shown two stages of this task are considered: (1) the letter currently presented is decoded and (2) the letter is compared with the letters in a set of target letters. In the experiment two factors are manipulated: (1) the letters are presented in intact or degraded form and (2) the number of targets in the set are varied. (A) An interaction between the quality of the stimulus and the set size such that quality has a greater effect with larger set sizes. This implies that encoding and comparison are not separable. (B) An additive effect: the effect of quality is the same with different set sizes. In this case encoding and comparison are separable. (C) The results of the experiment are shown (from Sternberg (28)). Encoding and comparison are clearly separable (redrawn from Sternberg (28)).

measured in terms of response time. This task can be divided into at least three stages between a letter being presented and a response being made:

a. perceive and identify the letter,
b. decide whether it is in the target list,
c. make a response.

If these stages are truly independent and sequential, then altering the difficulty of one stage should not affect the time spent on another stage (see Fig. 1B). In other words, the effects of difficulty at each stage should be additive. The problem is that we cannot measure directly the time spent at each stage separately, but only the sum of all stages. However, we can alter the difficulty of each stage separately and observe the effect on performance. Stage (b) can be made more difficult by increasing the number of items in the list. Indeed there is a linear relationship between response time to correctly detect a target and the number of items in the list. Stage (a) can be made more difficult by degrading the appearance of the letters in some way (adding noise, reducing exposure time, *etc.*). When both these manipulations are applied in the same experiment it is found that the effects are additive: degrading the letters increases response time by the same amount however many letters there are in the target list (see Fig. 1C). In other words, there is a (main) effect of both manipulations, but no interaction between them. On the basis of these purely behavioural data we can conclude that the perception of letters (stage a) depends upon a cognitive module that functions independently of the processes involved when searching through a list of items held in working memory.

3. Integral Stimulus Dimensions

The same strategy can be used to show evidence for independent processes within the perceptual stage. Any fairly complex stimulus (such as a rectangle) varies along a number of dimensions (such as width, height, shape, and size). Garner [29] has shown that some pairs of dimensions are "integral" while others are "nonintegral." Height and width are integral because variation in one of these dimensions affects our perception of the other. It is easier to judge the height of a series of rectangles if the widths remain constant than it is if the widths vary. In contrast, size and shape are nonintegral. Our ability to judge the shapes of rectangles does not become more difficult if they vary in size (Fig. 2). In the terms we have been using in the previous sections, height and width are perceptual dimensions which interact, while size and shape are perceptually independent. The implication is that size and shape are coded for independently in the brain while height and width are not. These dimensions have to be extracted from codes for size and shape in which both height and width are involved.

4. Pop Out

This is another technique for revealing independent stimulus dimensions. In most cases, if we are presented with a page full of stimuli and have to find a target then we will have to search through the stimuli. The more background stimuli there are then the longer it will take to find the target. However, in some circumstances the target just "pops out" immediately, however many background stimuli there are [30]. This happens if the target is a blue X among red Xs or a blue O among blue Xs. Pop out does not occur if we have to find a red O from a mixture of blue Os and red Xs (Fig. 3). The case of pop out suggests that colour (and shape) are coded independently of position in space since these targets can be found without attending to their position in space. The case where pop out does not occur suggests that the perception of the conjunction of colour and shape interacts with the position of the object in space.

In this section we have illustrated some of the techniques used by experimental psychologists to characterise and isolate some of the processes underlying memory and perception. The presumption is that cognitive processes that can be isolated on the basis of behavioural measures will also be isolated at the physiological level. The truth of this assumption is currently being examined through brain imaging studies.

B. Electrophysiology

Electroencephalography (EEG) is a technique in which we measure the electrical activity of the brain and observe how this changes in association with

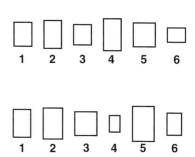

FIGURE 2 Integral and nonintegral dimensions. In the first row the height of the rectangles varies randomly, while all but one are the same width. The odd-one-out (5) is difficult to detect. In the second row the area of the rectangles varies randomly, while all, but one are the same shape. The odd-one-out (3) is easy to detect. Size and area are separable dimensions, while height and width are not (after Garner (29)).

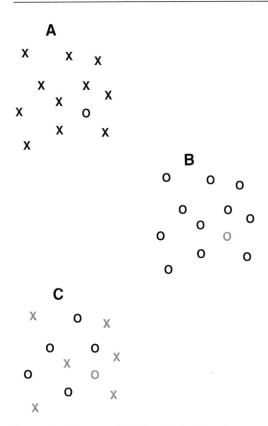

Figure 3 Pop-out. (A) The O stands out among the Xs. (B) The the gray O stands out among the black Os. The target in (C) is defined by the conjunction of shape and color. The grey O does not stand out from among the black Os and grey Xs (after Treisman (30)).

stimuli, responses, or mental states such as attention. The joy of EEG is that it has very high temporal resolution which is in the order of a few milliseconds. The drawback of these signals is that it is difficult to discover precisely where in the brain they are coming from. In the vast majority of studies the electrical activity is recorded from electrodes attached to the scalp. The spatial resolution of these signals is particularly poor for activity occurring deep within the brain and thus far from any of the electrodes. In addition, little is known about the relationship between the signal recorded at the scalp and the activity in individual neurons or groups of neurons that gives rise to this signal. In these circumstances the major successes that have been achieved using EEG concern the delineation of brain activity associated with specific cognitive processes and the measurement of precisely when this activity occurs. We shall briefly discuss two components of the event related potential (ERP), the N100 and the N400, that have been intensively studied.

1. ERPs and Attention

Immediately after an auditory stimulus, such as a tone, there is a transient change of brain activity. This response can be revealed by time-locked averaging. Stimuli in different modalities are associated with different patterns of activity. The early components (~0–10 msec for auditory stimuli) of this activity are generated in the brain stem, while later components (~10–200 msec) probably arise in primary sensory cortex. There are even later components which may arise from a number of widely distributed sources. The form of the early components is almost entirely determined by the nature of the eliciting stimulus (*e.g.*, intensity). Later components depend upon the specific information processing operations recruited by the stimuli. However, the form of the later components can also be altered by the prior state of the subject even though the stimuli presented in the two states are physically identical. In particular, the N100 component of the auditory evoked potential (a negative deflection occurring approximately 100 msec after the eliciting stimulus) is altered by whether or not the subject is attending to the stimulus [31]. In the most commonly used design a series of tones is presented fairly rapidly (~200 msec interstimulus interval) to the left and the right ear. The subject is asked to attend to one ear in order to detect target tones that differ slightly from nontarget tones in pitch or intensity. Tones in the attended ear elicit larger N100 responses than tones in the unattended ear (Fig. 4). This effect of attention is not limited to activity at 100 msec but extends from about 50 to 500 msec. This is an example of a "top–down" effect. The attentive state of the subject, usually brought about by instructions from the experimenter, has modulated the response of the brain to an auditory stimulus. This is an example of a mental state modifying physiology. The timing of this modulation is believed to have important implications for theories of attention at the cognitive level. There is a long standing controversy between proponents of early and late effects of attention. One party believes that the effects of attention apply before any detailed analysis of the stimulus (*e.g.*, semantic aspects) have occurred. The early occurrence of the N100 and the evidence that the source of this signal is in primary auditory cortex provide support for this position. This example is telling us something about functional integration in the brain. Activity in a brain area concerned with the early stages of auditory analysis is modulated by top–down signals from regions concerned with the direction of attention.

2. ERPs and Context

The N400 is a late negative component of the ERP which occurs anywhere between 300 and 600 msec after the stimulus that elicits it. This compo-

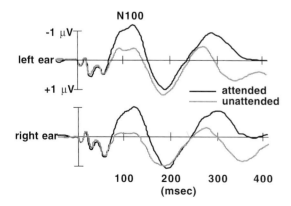

FIGURE 4 N100. The subjects heard sequences of tones in both the left and the right ear and had to detect targets in the specified ear. There is a large negative going wave (N100) approximately 100 msec after a tone in the attended ear (redrawn from Hillyard (31)).

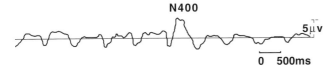

FIGURE 5   N400. A negative going wave (N400) occurs about 400 msec after the presentation of a word that is anomalous in terms of the context in which it occurs (redrawn from Kutas and Van Petten (32)).

nent is robustly evoked by the last word of a sentence (presented visually or aurally) when this word is unexpected in the context of the sentence [32]. It is possible to vary systematically the degree to which the last word of the sentence is expected by altering the "textual constraint" exerted by the sentence (Fig. 5). The magnitude of the N400 response is linearly related to the textual constraint. This is another example of functional integration whereby expectations alter the response of brain regions to incoming stimuli. However, the source of the N400 ERP component remains unknown and may well be multiple. If sentences are presented in the visual modality the N400 has a predominantly centro-parietal distribution, while in the auditory modality the distribution is more frontal. At the cognitive level the expectations about the last word built up by the rest of the sentence could relate to a number of different features including what the word might mean (semantics), what the word might sound like (phonology), and what the word might look like (orthography). To some extent these features can be altered independently of one another. Thus, the word at the end of a sentence might have the sound we expected, but not the meaning. There is evidence that there are subcomponents of the associated ERP which reflect these different aspects of the word, suggesting that aspects are processed at different times and in different brain regions [33].

In these examples we have illustrated how electrophysiological measures can reveal the timing and, to a lesser extent, the location of brain activity associated with discrete cognitive processes. These techniques are particularly suited to showing how the response of the brain to stimuli is modified by preexisting mental states.

C. Psychopharmacology

By administering a centrally active drug it is possible to alter brain states and observe the effects on mental state and on behaviour. During the past decade there has been a proliferation of drugs which target particular neurotransmitter systems (*e.g.*, the dopamine system) or even receptors within a neurotransmitter system (*e.g.*, the D2 dopamine receptor). One fond hope is that particular neurotransmitter systems are involved with particular cognitive processes. Certainly different drugs are associated with different profiles of behaviour change, but it has proved very difficult to characterise these profiles in terms of specific cognitive processes.

The cholinergic system has received more attention than most, in part because of a report that in Alzheimer's disease severity of damage to the cholinergic system is correlated with the degree of memory impairment [34]. Administering an anti-cholinergic drug such as scopolamine to healthy volunteers causes marked impairments of memory. However, not all aspects of memory are equally impaired. Short-term memory is unaffected and only certain aspects of long-term memory are impaired. In particular it is the acquisition of new material into episodic memory that suffers [35]. In some respects the volunteers resemble patients with amnesia (having a specific memory impairment) rather than dementia (having a memory impairment in the context of a more general cognitive impairment). At first sight these results suggest a nice mapping between a circumscribed cognitive impairment and a single neurotransmitter system. Unfortunately other results show that this simple idea is not sustainable. First, treatment with benzodiazepenes (*e.g.*, diazepam) produces an identical pattern of memory impairments even though a completely different neurotransmitter system (GABA) is involved [36]. Second, anti-cholinergics can also impair performance in situations that have no episodic memory component. These include complex reaction time tasks [37] and procedural learning [38] and dual-task paradigms [39]. We would speculate that the memory problems associated with anti-cholinergic treatment might be a secondary consequence of impairments in various elaborative processes that improve memory acquisition, but the nature of these processes remains obscure.

There are good reasons why a single neurotransmitter system might not be associated with a single cognitive process. Even when we use a drug which targets a specific neurotransmitter system we cannot prevent its effects from occurring throughout the brain. While a neurotransmitter might be involved in the same specific mechanism (*e.g.*, increasing signal to noise ratio) throughout the brain, its cognitive effects will vary with its location. For this reason a drug is likely to have multiple effects. Brain imaging provides, for the first time, a technique for identifying where a drug is having its effect on cognition. Using this technique it may still be possible to relate particular neurotransmitter systems to particular classes of cognitive component.

D. Lesion Studies

A major theme of this book is that the study of people with brain abnormalities can inform our understanding of normal cognitive function. Those who have argued against this position have used the metaphor of the television set that has been attacked with an axe. By studying the behaviour of your set after it has been randomly damaged in this way, they ask, how would it be possible to infer the normal function of its various components. Gregory [40] has articulated the problem very precisely: *"In a serial system the various identifiable elements of the output are not separately represented by the discrete parts of the system.... The removal, or activation, of a single stage in a series might have almost any effect on the output of a machine, and so presumably also for the brain..."* (p. 321). The key word in this criticism is "serial." If, as seems most likely, the brain is not a serial system, but a collection of many modules which function in parallel and with a great deal of independence, then it *is* possible to discover the function of at least some of its components on the basis of circumscribed damage.

1. The Independence of Short-Term Memory and Long-Term Memory

Early theoretical accounts of memory suggested that there was an important distinction between short-term memory (minutes) and long-term memory (hours, days, years), but assumed that material was passed through the short-term store into long-term memory. However, in the early 1970s a series of patients were described by Elizabeth Warrington and her colleagues who had a severe and specific impairment with short-term memory and no impairment of long-term memory [41]. One of these cases is JB. JB had a meningioma removed from the temporo-parietal region of her left hemisphere when she was in her 20s. Some 20 years later she still has a severe deficit of short-term memory for spoken words. She cannot remember a string of random letters or numbers longer than about two items. In spite of this handicap she has no problem with producing or understanding speech and her long-term memory is perfectly normal. Furthermore her span for strings of letters or numbers presented visually is normal. Because her short-term memory deficit is so circumscribed she has no difficulty with her responsible job as a medical secretary. Practical problems arise for her only when she is given a telephone number or a long and unusual name over the telephone.

JB has a specific problem with short-term storage of verbal material (words, numbers, letters) presented through the auditory modality. This phonological store seems to be located in the left inferior parietal region of the brain. What this and similar cases suggest is that there are different short-term stores for different kinds of material and that long-term memory can function independently of these short-term stores.

2. Describing and Reaching

There are many different syndromes associated with brain damage in which information seems available for the control of behaviour, that is not accessible to consciousness. A particularly striking example is provided by certain neurological cases with damage to the posterior parts of the temporal lobe. These patients can still see in the sense of distinguishing light and shade, but can no longer recognise objects from their shape. This loss of shape awareness applies even to low level aspects like the orientation of a line. One such patient is unable to adjust a stick so that it lines up with a narrow slot. Her performance on this task is hardly better than chance. However, if she is asked to push her hand through a slot she can perform this task perfectly well (Fig. 6) and adjusts her hand to the appropriate orientation before it reaches the slot [20]. Clearly information about the orientation of the slot is available to control reaching movements of the hand, but this information is not available to consciousness. In addition information about the shapes of objects is not available to permit recognition of the identity of objects. Patients have also been reported who have precisely the opposite problem. These patients have lesions in the parietal lobe. They can easily tell you what the orientation of a slot is, but cannot orient their hand appropriately when pushing it through the slot. They can readily distinguish between a square and a rectangle from the lengths of its sides, but they cannot use this information to choose the appropriate distance between thumb and finger when picking up such objects.

In these cases it appears that the same information (about orientation) is available to describe or identify an object, but is not available to control reaching (or *vice-versa*). However, it is possible that this information is in different forms. In order to reach for something, information about orientation or distance or size must be in egocentric coordinates that relate directly to our own current position relative to the object or, more particularly, relate to the position of the limb that is going to do the reaching. In contrast, in order to describe or recognise an object we need information concerning its

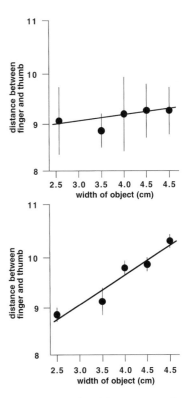

Figure 6 Visual-form agnosia. (Top) Data from an experiment in which the patient indicated the width of objects in terms of the distance between finger and thumb. Performance is very variable (large error bars) and there is no significant relationship between the width of the objects and the width indicated by the patient. (Bottom) Data in which the same patient reached for the same objects. In this case the width between finger and thumb prior to grasping is tightly constrained (small error bars) and is closely related to the width of the objects (redrawn from Goodale and Milner (20)).

shape, such as size, orientation, and distance, in terms which are independent of our current position or the current position of the object (*e.g.*, object centred coordinates). If this account is correct, then it is not that the brain damage has prevented access to consciousness of information that still exists, rather it is that the intact region that controls reaching contains information that never has access to consciousness, even in the undamaged brain. In this case it should be possible to demonstrate the existence of this "unconscious" control of action in normal volunteers.

In one such experiment subjects look at a screen on which there is a target surrounded by a frame. In certain circumstances it is possible to make the subject report that the target has moved when, in fact, it was the frame that moved. However, if the subject is asked to point to the target rather than report its position, then no error occurs [21]. This example shows that there is a separation between the information that the subject reports and the information that is used to control his pointing response. This latter information is not conscious. We have here a further example of how studies of the effects of lesions can demonstrate functional segregation. However, in addition, we have evidence suggesting that only a subset of brain regions may be associated with conscious experience. A classification of brain regions along this dimension would be an important step towards understanding the relationship between brain and consciousness.

3. Capgras' Syndrome

A similar dissociation can be observed in a disorder which lies in the psychiatric domain. A patient with Capgras' syndrome believes that a member of his immediate family (*e.g.*, his wife) has been replaced by a double. This symptom is rare, but can be found in both psychiatric cases (*e.g.*, schizophrenia) and in patients with a clear cut organic disorder (*e.g.*, Alzheimer's disease). Similar disorders are also reported in which the patient believes that, for example, his house has been replaced by a duplicate. When asked to explain the reason for these strange beliefs, patients often report that the person (or the house) looks slightly different from usual, but they have some difficulty specifying what these differences are. In the past such symptoms were explained in psychodynamic terms. However, in recent years explanations have been proposed in terms of loss of access to certain types of information about faces [42]. As we shall see, such explanations have many parallels with our discussion in the previous section about the distinction between reaching for and identifying objects.

Lesions in posterior regions of the brain can sometimes lead to a disorder of face perception known as prosopagnosia. This disorder has been studied in some detail and its cognitive basis is well described although there is still argument about the precise location of the lesion or lesions that are necessary and/or sufficient to produce it. A patient with prosopagnosia can no longer recognise familiar faces [43]. He can usually distinguish one face from another, but he no longer knows whose face it is. However, he is still able to recognise who the person is from other cues. He does not recognise his wife's face, but, as soon as she speaks or moves, he knows her. It appears that the perceptual appearance of a face no longer provides the necessary information for identifying that face. However, in a number of cases it has been shown that information about the identity of the face is controlling his behaviour even though the patient remains unaware of this. For example a patient can identify which faces are familiar even though he cannot say who they are. In one study, it was shown that patients could be primed by the identity of a face even though they were unaware of this identity. Thus, a photograph of Princess Diana would be unrecognised, but the subsequent recognition of the name PRINCE CHARLES (presented in written form) would be faster. It has also been observed that patients will show autonomic responses to familiar faces even though they do not recognise them. These results suggest that different kinds of information about identity are available when looking at faces. One kind of information leads to conscious identification of the face, while other kinds do not. This distinction is analogous to the one we have just drawn between reaching for and identifying objects. In prosopagnosia the information that permits conscious identification of faces is no longer available. What kind of information is available in the intact channel? The answer is still unclear, but it seems plausible that aspects such as familiarity and emotional responses might be included.

How can this account help us understand Capgras' syndrome? The interesting suggestion has been made that Capgras' syndrome is the mirror of prosopagnosia [42]. The conscious channel by which faces are identified is intact, but the unconscious channel which brings a sense of familiarity and an emotional response is no longer transmitting. The patient is confronted with a person who clearly looks like his wife, but who does not elicit in him either a sense of familiarity or the usual emotional response. There is clearly something different about this person. If the patient has also developed a psychotic tendency to accept bizarre beliefs and detect conspiracies, then he might conclude that his wife had been replaced by another.

Just as in the case of reaching for or identifying objects, in the case of face perception also, results from the study of pathological groups are highly revealing. In both cases the results strongly suggest that there are many parallel and independent pathways involved in our interactions with the world. Some of these pathways are accessible by consciousness, others are not.

V. CONCLUSIONS

We have discussed a number of different techniques for studying the relationship between behaviour/mental activity and brain function. It is important to remember that the different techniques we have described for investigating the relationships between brain and behaviour are complementary. They are not in competition. It is obviously a useful validation if the same result is obtained by different techniques. For example, one of our early brain imaging studies [44] confirmed the suggestion from experimental psychology that verbal working memory consisted of two independent components. However, it is actually more informative if different techniques give different results and thereby increase knowledge. Understanding the source of these differences will considerably enhance our understanding of brain/behaviour relationships. We have listed in the Appendix some of the differences that might occur and we have suggested how they might be interpreted.

Results from all these disciplines suggest that at both the physiological and the cognitive level it is extremely useful to characterise the brain as a system that is segregated. Information from the outside world is sampled, coded as neural signals, and processed into many parallel streams that are subsequently integrated in order to generate appropriate and coherent behaviour. This characterisation of the brain/behaviour problem suggests that there are four fundamental questions that the new brain imaging techniques, used alongside older techniques can begin to answer.

1. What is the vocabulary of neural codes in the brain? It should be possible to provide a list of the various kinds of features or submodalities (colour, pitch, fearfulness, *etc.*) that are coded for in the brain. Behavioural studies of normal volunteers can reveal independent features and processes, but studies of the behavioural effects of brain damage (or perturbations caused by drugs or psychosis) will also be informative. We assume that these codes are associated with specialised processing modules.

2. Where are these codes represented? If the features and submodalities associated with the specialised modules can be identified then it should also be possible to identify circumscribed brain regions associated with these modules. It is to these regions that the neural codes referring to these features will be transmitted. Such information comes from studies of patients with circumscribed brain lesions and from functional brain imaging.

3. How are the various modules linked together? By definition the connections between modules are far less dense than the connections within modules. Functional segregation arises precisely because every module is not connected directly to every other module. We can therefore ask questions about which modules are directly connected (and in contrast, which are not) and also about the timing of the flow of signals from one module to another. Information about the topology of these connections comes from neuroanatomy and functional brain imaging (functional connectivity). Information about timing comes from electrophysiology.

4. What are the mechanisms by which one neural code is transformed into another? Clues about the underlying algorithms can be obtained from behavioural studies. Understanding the exact mechanisms probably requires knowledge of interactions at the level of single cells or cell assemblies.

These are all questions about the links between mental activity and brain function. But they can no longer be dismissed as ill-posed questions. With a combination of the new brain imaging techniques and the cognitive approach these are questions that will be answered.

APPENDIX

In this chapter we have considered a number of different techniques for studying the relationships between brain activity and behaviour. In most cases the results from these different techniques should give similar answers. However, the techniques are not all measuring the same variables and the answers they give will not always be identical. Indeed, when robust differences are observed between the techniques this will be of considerable interest. In this appendix we list the kinds of difference that might arise and suggest how they might be interpreted.

1. Brain Imaging and Lesions

Brain imaging: Area A is reliably activated during performance of task X.

Lesion: Damage to area A does not affect performance of task X.

Conclusion: Area A is not necessary for performance of task X. Subjects are engaging cognitive processes that are not necessary for performance of the task. Engaging these processes may be automatic and involuntary or may constitute a deliberate strategy due to boredom or ignorance.

Hypothesis: Elimination of activity in area A (by a secondary task) will not affect performance of task X.

Brain imaging: Area A is not activated during performance of task X.
Lesion: Damage to area A impairs performance of task X.
Conclusion 1: Damage is to fibres of passage.
Conclusion 2: The necessary activity in area A lasts only a short time (msec).
Conclusion 3: Activation is too weak or area is too small to generate a detectable signal.
Test: EEG and/or postmortem neuroanatomy.

2. Brain Imaging and ERPs

Brain imaging: Area A is not activated by task X.
ERP: Area A is activated by task X.
Conclusion: Task X increases neural synchrony, but not total activity.

Brain imaging: Area A is activated by task X.
ERP: Area A is not activated by task X.
Conclusion: The neurons activated during task X are not synchronised in time and/or lined up in space.

3. Brain Imaging and Behaviour

Brain imaging: Manipulation of difficulty, time, *etc.* has no effect on brain activity.
Behaviour: Manipulation of difficulty, time, *etc.*, increases errors and/or reaction time.
Conclusion: Brain is working at full capacity. Increasing difficulty can only increase errors or time taken.

Brain imaging: Increasing difficulty increases brain activity.
Behaviour: Increasing difficulty has no effect on errors, *etc.*
Conclusion: Increased brain activity can cope with increased difficulty without producing errors.

References

1. J. Kim. The nonreductivist's trouble with mental causation. *In* "Supervenience and Mind: Selected Philosophical Essays" (J. Kim, Ed.). Cambridge Univ. Press, Cambridge, 1993.
2. M. W. Shelley. "Frankenstein: Or, the Modern Prometheus." J. M. Dent, London, 1818.
3. D. Marr. "Vision." Freeman, San Francisco, 1982.
4. K. S. Lashley. "Brain Mechanisms and Intelligence." Univ. of Chicago Press, Chicago, 1929.
5. S. Zeki. "A Vision of the Brain." Blackwells, Oxford, 1993.
6. P. Broca. Remarques sur le siège de la faculté du langage articulé, suives d'une observation d'aphemie. *Bul. Mém. Soc. Anat. Paris* **2,** 330–357 (1861).
7. C. Wernicke. "Der Aphasische Symptomenkomplex." Coh & Weigart, Breslau, 1874.
8. L. Lichtheim. On aphasia. *Brain* **7,** 433–484 (1885).
9. K. Brodmann. "Vergleichende Localisationslehre der Grosshirnrinde," 2nd ed. Barth, Leipzig, 1909.

10. W. Penfield and L. Roberts. "Speech and Brain Mechanisms." Princeton Univ. Press, Princeton, NJ, 1959.

11. T. Shallice. "From Neuropsychology to Mental Structure." Cambridge Univ. Press, Cambridge, UK, 1988.

12. R. A. McCarthy and E. K. Warrington. "Cognitive Neuropsychology." Academic Press, London, 1990.

13. M. Petrides and D. N. Pandya. Comparative architectonic analysis of the human and the macaque frontal cortex. *In* "Handbook of Neuropsychology" (F. Boller and J. Grafman, Eds.), Vol. 9, pp. 17–58. Elsevier, Amsterdam, 1994.

14. D. Marr. Early processing of visual information. *Phil. Trans. R. Soc. London B,* **275,** 483–524 (1976).

15. H. A. Simon. "The Sciences of the Artificial." MIT Press, Cambridge, MA, 1969.

16. A. Cowey. Sensory and non-sensory disorders in man and monkey. *Phil. Trans. R. Soc. London B.* **298,** 3–13 (1982).

17. G. Tononi, O. Sporns, and G. Edelman. A measure for brain complexity: Relating functional segregation and integration in the nervous system. *Proc. Natl. Acad. Sci. USA* **91,** 5033–5037 (1994).

18. J. L. McClelland and D. E. Rumelhart. "Parallel Distributed Processing." MIT Press, Cambridge, MA, 1986.

19. R. E. Nisbett and T. D. Wilson. Telling more than we can know: Verbal reports on mental processes. *Psychol. Rev.* **84,** 231–259 (1977).

20. M. A. Goodale and A. D. Milner. Separate visual pathways for perception and action. *Trends Neurosci.* **15,** 20–25 (1992).

21. B. Bridgeman. Conscious *vs* unconscious processes: The case of vision. *Theory Psychol.* **2,** 73–88 (1992).

22. S. D. Iversen. Brain lesions and memory in animals. *In* "The Physiological Basis of Memory" (J. A. Deutsch, Ed.), pp. 305–364. Academic Press, New York, 1973.

23. B. F. Skinner. "Verbal behavior." Appleton–Century–Crofts, New York, 1957.

24. R. T. Hurlburt. "Sampling Normal and Schizophrenic Inner Experience." Plenum, New York, 1990.

25. D. Gaffan and E. A. Murray. Monkeys (Macaca fascicularis) with rhinal cortex ablations succeed in object discrimination learning despite 24-hr intertrial intervals and fail at hatching to sample despite double sample presentations. *Behav. Neurosci.* **106,** 30–38 (1992).

26. J. P. Guilford. "Psychometric Methods," 2nd ed. McGraw-Hill, New York, 1954.

27. A. Baddeley. "Working Memory." Oxford Univ. Press, Oxford, UK, 1986.

28. S. Sternberg. Memory-scanning: Mental processes revealed by reaction time experiments. *Am. Sci.* **57,** 421–457 (1969).

29. W. R. Garner. "The Processing of Information and Structure." Erlbaum, Potomac, 1974.

30. A. M. Treisman. Features and objects: The 14th Bartlett Memorial Lecture. *Q. J. Exp. Psychol.* **40A,** 201–237, 1988.

31. S. A. Hillyard, G. R. Mangun, M. G. Woldorff, and S. J. Luck. Neural systems mediating selective attnetion. *In* "The Cognitive Neurosciences" (M. S. Gazzaniga, ed.), pp. 665–682. MIT Press, Cambridge, MA, 1995.

32. M. Kutas and C. Van Petten. Event-related brain potential studies of language. *In* "Advances in Psychophysiology" (P. K. Ackles, J. R. Jennings, & M. G. H. Coles, Eds.), pp. 139–187. JAI Press, Greenwich, CT, 1988.

33. J. F. Connolly and N. A. Phillips. Event-related potential components reflect phonological and semantic processing of the terminal word of spoken sentences. *J. Cognit. Neurosci.* **6,** 256–266 (1994).

34. E. K. Perry, B. E. Tomlinson, G. Blessed, K. Bergmann, P. H. Gibson, and R. H. Perry. Correlation of cholinergic abnormalities with senile plaques and mental test scores in senile dementia. *Br. Med. J.* **2,** 1457–1459 (1978).

35. M. D. Kopelman and T. H. Corn. Cholinergic "blockade" as a model for cholinergic depletion. *Brain* **111,** 1079–1110 (1988).

36. G. C. Preston, P. Broks, M. Traub, C. Ward, P. Poppleton, and S. M. Stahl. Effects of lorazepam on memory, attention and sedation in man. *Psychopharmacology* **95,** 208–215 (1988).

37. P. Broks, G. C. Preston, M. Traub, P. Poppleton, C. Ward, and S. M. Stahl. Modelling dementia: Effects of scopolamine on memory and attention. *Neuropsychologia* **26,** 685–700 (1988).

38. C. D. Frith, M. A. McGinty, I. Gergel, and T. J. Crow. The effects of scopolamine and clonidine upon the performance and learning of a new motor skill. *Psychopharmacology* **98,** 120–125 (1989).

39. J. M. Rusted. Dissociative effects of scopolamine on working memory in healthy young volunteers. *Psychopharmacology* **96,** 487–492 (1988).

40. R. L. Gregory. The brain as an engineering problem. *In* "Current Problems in Animal Behaviour" (W. H. Thorpe and O. L. Zangwill, eds.). Cambridge Univ. Press, Cambridge, UK, 1961.

41. E. K. Warrington, V. Logue and R. T. C. Pratt. The anatomical localisation of selective impairment of auditory verbal short-term memory. *Neuropsychologia* **9,** 377–387 (1971).

42. H. D. Ellis and A. W. Young. Accounting for delusional misidentifications. *Br. J. Psychiatry* **157,** 239–248 (1990).

43. A. W. Young and E. H. F. De Haan. Face recognition and awareness after brain injury. *In* "The Neuropsychology of Consciousness" (A. D. Milner and M. D. Rugg, Eds.), pp. 69–90. Academic Press, London, 1992.

44. E. Paulesu, C. D. Frith, and R. S. J. Frackowiak. The neural correlates of the verbal component of working memory. *Nature* **362,** 342–344 (1993).

CHAPTER TWO

ANALYSING BRAIN IMAGES: PRINCIPLES AND OVERVIEW

I. INTRODUCTION

This chapter provides an overview and background for subsequent chapters that describe, in detail, some of the different approaches to characterising and analysing brain activation studies. This chapter is meant to underscore the following point, although we may take for granted that the results of functional neuroimaging studies can facilitate our understanding of how the brain works, the converse is also true. Our understanding of the brain's functional organisation constrains and informs the way in which functional neuroimaging data are analysed and, consequently, affects the ensuing results. In what follows we review some fundamental ideas about brain organisation and how these ideas relate to different approaches to data analysis. The aim of this chapter is to introduce various techniques that have been developed, or adapted, for analysing functional imaging data and to place them in some broad context. The theoretical foundations and procedural nature of the techniques are then described in subsequent chapters.

The first half of this chapter focuses on principles of brain organisation and their relation to the analytic techniques available. We will make a distinction between *functional integration* and *functional segregation* at a theoretical level and a corresponding distinction between *multivariate* and *univariate* analyses at a procedural level (univariate means pertaining to one variable). The multivariate analyses considered here include eigenimage analysis, multidimensional scaling, multivariate analysis of covariance (MANCOVA), and canonical variates analysis (CVA). The univariate approaches are collectively brought under the heading of statistical parametric mapping. The second half of this chapter considers stages of data analysis that are required to implement the above. These stages include realignment, spatial normalisation, smoothing, statistical analysis, and, when appropriate, statistical inference. Many of the techniques described here start off with the general linear model and a short introduction to the general linear model is included at the end of this introductory chapter.

II. PRINCIPLES OF FUNCTIONAL ORGANISATION AND IMPLICATIONS FOR IMAGING

A. Specialisation or Integration?

The brain appears to adhere to two fundamental principles of functional organisation, functional integration and functional segregation, with the integration within and among functionally segregated areas mediated by functional or effective connectivity. The characterisation of functional segregation, integration, and connectivity is an important endeavour in many areas of neuroscience, not least in imaging neuroscience.

The distinction between functional segregation and integration relates to the distinction between *localisationism* and *[dis]connectionism* that dominated thinking about cortical function in the 19th century. Since the early anatomic theories of Gall, the identification of a particular brain region with a specific function has become a central theme in neuroscience. However, functional localisation *per se* was not easy to demonstrate in a compelling way: For example, a meeting that took place on the morning of August 4th, 1881, addressed the difficulties of attributing function to a cortical area, given the dependence of cerebral activity on underlying connections [1]. This meeting was entitled *"Localisation of Function in the Cortex Cerebri."* Goltz [2], although accepting the results of electrical stimulation in dog and monkey cortex, considered the excitation method inconclusive, in that movements elicited might have originated in related pathways, or current could have spread to distant centres. In short the excitation method could not be used to infer functional localisation because localisationism discounted interactions, or functional integration, among different brain areas. It was proposed that lesion studies could supplement excitation experiments; ironically, it was observations on patients with brain lesions [3] some years later that led to the concept of disconnection syndromes and the refutation of localisationism as a complete or sufficient explanation of cortical organisation. Functional localisation and functional segregation are used here to refer to different concepts. Functional localisation implies that a function can be localised in a cortical area, whereas segregation suggests that a cortical area is specialised for some aspects of perceptual or motor processing, and that this specialisation is anatomically segregated in the cortex. The cortical infrastructure supporting a single function may then involve many specialised areas whose union is mediated by the functional integration among them. In this view functional segregation is meaningful only in the context of functional integration and *vice versa.*

The cerebral excitation paradigm of the mid-19th century is, in a way, still employed today. With modern methods excitation is usually elicited by asking subjects to perform different tasks and the neuronal responses are measured with functional imaging. Despite advances over the past century, the central issue remains unresolved. Are the physiological changes elicited by sensorimotor or cognitive challenges best characterised by the activation of functionally segregated areas, or are they better described in terms of the behaviour of anatomically distributed, but functionally integrated systems. The position that we have adopted is to simply acknowledge that both perspectives are valid and that the description of, and inferences about, brain activations can proceed at both levels.

What then are the implications for analysing and interpreting brain activation experiments? There are two basic approaches that are predicated on the distinction between functional integration and segregation presented above. The first set of approaches is based on correlated physiological dynamics in different parts of the brain and deals with distributed brain systems. These approaches are inherently multivariate in nature. The second depends on detecting focal differences using a functional segregation or specialisation view of the brain.

The first set of approaches to analysis includes *eigenimage analysis* and *multidimensional scaling*. These are useful ways of characterising distributed neurophysiological changes in a parsimonious and sometimes revealing fashion. They are closely related to each other (mathematically speaking) but have different and interesting interpretations in relation to functional imaging data. Neither eigenimage analysis nor multidimensional scaling can be used to make statistical inferences about what is observed (*i.e.*, estimate the significance of results obtained in terms of a *P* value). The second approach, considered under the heading of functional integration, is *MANCOVA* with CVA. Like eigenimage analysis, CVA characterises brain responses in terms of anatomically distributed profiles or spatial modes. Unlike any of the techniques mentioned so far, MANCOVA provides for statistical inference about the responses, where this inference is about the entire brain (*i.e.*, it has no regional specificity). To address the significance of regionally specific effects one turns, finally, to *statistical parametric mapping*. Statistical parametric mapping is an approach that is predicated on functional segregation or specialisation and is used to characterise physiology in terms of regionally specific responses. It does this characterisation by treating each voxel separately (*i.e.*, it is a univariate approach) and by performing voxel-wise statistical analyses in parallel, creating an image of a statistic or "significance." The next two sections review the concepts of functional integration and segregation, as they relate to functional imaging, and describe more fully the multivariate and univariate techniques mentioned above.

B. Functional Integration and Connectivity

Functional integration is mediated by the interactions between functionally segregated areas. One way of characterising these interactions is in terms of functional or effective connectivity. In the analysis of neuroimaging time series functional connectivity has been defined as the temporal correlations between spatially remote neurophysiological events [4]. The alternative is to refer explicitly to effective connectivity (*i.e.*, the influence one neuronal system exerts over another) [5]. These concepts were developed in the analysis of separable spike trains obtained from multiunit electrode recordings [6–9]. Functional connectivity is simply a statement about the observed correlations; it does not provide any direct insight into how these correlations are mediated. For example, at the level of multiunit microelectrode recordings, correlations can result from stimulus-locked transients, evoked by a common afferent input, or reflect stimulus-induced oscillations, phasic coupling of neural assemblies, mediated by synaptic connections [7]. To examine the integration within a distributed system, defined by functional connectivity, one turns to effective connectivity. Effective connectivity is closer to the intuitive notion of a connection. In electrophysiology there is a close relationship between effective connectivity and synaptic efficacy: *"It is useful to describe the effective connectivity with a connectivity matrix of effective synaptic weights"* [7]. It has also been proposed that *"the [electrophysiological] notion of effective connectivity should be understood as the experiment and time dependent, simplest possible circuit diagram that would replicate the observed timing relationships between the recorded neurons"* [9].

Although functional and effective connectivity can be invoked at a conceptual level in both neuroimaging and electrophysiology, they differ fundamentally at a practical level. This is because the time scales and nature of the neurophysiological measurements are very different (seconds vs milliseconds and haemodynamic vs spike trains). In electrophysiology it is often necessary to remove the confounding effects of stimulus-locked transients (that introduce correlations not causally mediated by direct neural interactions) in order to reveal the underlying connectivity. The confounding effect of stimulus-evoked transients is less problematic in neuroimaging because the promulgation of dynamics from primary sensory areas onwards is mediated by neuronal connections (usually reciprocal and interconnecting). However, it should be remembered that functional connectivity is not necessarily due to effective connectivity and, where it is, effective influences may be indirect (*e.g.*, polysynaptic relays through multiple areas).

C. Functional Connectivity at Different Spatio-Temporal Scales

Clearly there is an enormous difference between correlations in regional cerebral blood flow (rCBF) measured over seconds and the fast phasic dynamics that mediate neural interactions on a time scale of milliseconds. The purpose of this section is to suggest that there is a relationship between functional connectivity at a large-scale physiological level and at a neural level. Functional connectivity between two areas (in terms of functional imaging) implies that their pool activity goes up and down together. Is it reasonable to suppose that two regions with high pool activity will share a significant number of neurons whose dynamic interactions occur within a time frame of milliseconds? We suggest that it is. There are two lines of evidence in support of a relationship between fast dynamic interactions and slower variations in pool activity: (i) Aertsen and Preissl [9] have investigated the behaviour of artificial networks, analytically and using simulations. They concluded that short-term effective connectivity varies strongly with, or is modulated by, pool activity. Pool activity was defined as the product of the number of neurons and their mean firing rate. The mechanism is simple; the efficacy of subthreshold EPSPs (excitatory postsynaptic potentials) for establishing dynamic interactions is a function of postsynaptic depolarisation, which in turn depends on tonic background activity. (ii) The second line of evidence is experimental and demonstrates that the presence of fast interactions is associated with intermediate or long-term correlations between distant neurons. Nelson *et al.* [10] have characterised effective connections between neurons, or small groups of neurons, in BA 17 and BA 18 of cat extrastriate cortex. By cross-correlating activity they demonstrated that the most likely temporal relationship between spikes was a synchronous one. Furthermore, the cross-correlograms segregated into three nonoverlapping groups with modal widths of 3, 30, and 400 msec. The short-term correlation structures (3 and 30 msec) were almost always associated with the intermediate (400 msec) correlations. These observations suggest an interaction between short-term (<100 msec) and intermediate (100–1000 msec) correlations. In summary, the idea is that coactivated regions will have increased (correlated) perfusion and neuronal pool activity. Higher background discharge rates augment postsynaptic depolarisation and susceptibility to fast dynamic interactions at a neural level, both within and between the regions coactivated. This susceptibility may facilitate functional and effective connectivity at a neural level.

D. Eigenimage Analysis and Functional Connectivity

A powerful use of functional connectivity is in the characterisation of distributed brain systems. Usually pair-wise functional connectivity between any two points in the brain is not as interesting as patterns of correlations that obtain on considering all correlations together. Important patterns can be identified as follows. The functional connectivity (covariance) matrix, obtained from a time series of images, is subject to principal component analysis (PCA) or singular value decomposition (SVD). The resulting eigenimages (principal components or spatial modes) each correspond to a spatial pattern or distributed system, comprising regions that are jointly implicated by virtue of their functional interactions. This analysis of neuroimaging time series is predicated on established techniques in electrophysiology (both EEG and multiunit recordings). For example, in an analysis of multichannel EEG data the underlying spatial modes that best characterise the observed spatiotemporal dynamics are identified with a Karhunen Loeve expansion [11]. Commonly, this expansion is in terms of eigenvectors of a covariance matrix associated with a time series. The spatial modes are then identical to the principal components identified with a PCA. SVD is a related technique [12] that has been used with the Karhunen Loeve expansion to identify spatial modes in multiunit electrode recordings [13]. Having identified important spatial modes their functional role can be inferred on the basis of their expression over time or over different brain states. Note that this sort of analysis is entirely data-led and does not refer to any model or hypothesis.

E. Multidimensional Scaling and Functional Connectivity

In imaging neuroscience, functional mapping usually implies mapping function into an anatomical space, for example, using statistical parametric mapping to identify activation foci, or characterisation of distributed changes with spatial modes or eigenimages as described in the previous section. This section introduces a complementary approach, namely mapping anatomy into a functional space. The basic idea here is to construct a space where functional connectivity is used to define the proximity of two anatomical areas. In Chapter 6 a simple variant of multidimensional scaling (principal coordinates analysis) is described that uses functional connectivity as a metric (or measure of distance). This scaling transformation maps anatomy into a functional space. The topography, or proximity relationships, in this space embody the functional connectivity among brain regions. The higher the functional connectivity the closer the regions. Like eigenimage analysis the technique represents a descriptive characterisation of anatomically distributed changes in the brain that reveals the structure of cortico-cortical interactions in terms of functional connectivity and, in fact, uses the same mathematics to do so. This form of multidimensional scaling can be regarded as equivalent to eigenimage analysis but looked at from a different point of view.

F. MANCOVA–CVA and Eigenimage Analysis

Neither eigenimage analysis nor multidimensional scaling are statistical techniques in the sense that they do not have an explicit statistical model that allows for statistical inference. MANCOVA, on the other hand, uses the general linear model (an important linear equation that is described more fully below and in subsequent chapters; see Chapter 4) to make inferences about distributed activation effects. The nature of these effects can be characterised using an eigenimage analysis or a CVA. MANCOVA is a multivariate technique. In other words, it considers as one observation all the voxels in a single scan. The importance of this multivariate approach is that the effects due to activations, confounding effects, and error effects are assessed statistically, in terms of both effects at each voxel and interactions among voxels. The price paid for adopting a multivariate approach is that one cannot make statistical inferences about regionally specific changes. This is because the inference pertains to all the components (voxels) of the multivariate variable (not a particular voxel or set of voxels). In functional imaging there is a caveat to the application of MANCOVA. Generally speaking MANCOVA requires the number of observations (*i.e.*, scans) to be greater than the number of components of the multivariate observation (*i.e.*, voxels). Clearly this is not the case for most functional imaging studies. The number of components is therefore reduced by using eigenimages as opposed to voxels. This works because the number of eigenimages is always less than or equal to the number of scans.

In general, multivariate analyses are implemented in two steps. First the significance of the hypothesised effect is assessed in an omnibus sense in terms of a *P* value and then the nature of this response is characterised. CVA is one way of doing this. The canonical images obtained with CVA are similar to eigenimages but use both the activation and the error effects. Intuitively these approaches can be understood as finding the eigenimages that capture the effects of interest and simultaneously avoid patterns due to error.

This concludes a brief review of multivariate techniques that take explicit account of interactions among brain regions or voxels. In general the effects elicited by experimental design are described in terms of spatial modes (*i.e.*, eigenimages or canonical images) that are single, anatomically distributed patterns. We now turn to functional segregation and univariate approaches that describe neurophysiological effects in terms of a number of regionally specific changes whose significance can be assessed independently of changes elsewhere in the brain.

III. FUNCTIONAL SEGREGATION AND STATISTICAL PARAMETRIC MAPPING

A. Functional Segregation and Specialisation

The functional role played by any component (*e.g.*, a neuron) of a connected system (*e.g.*, the brain) is largely defined by its connections. Certain patterns of cortical projections are so common that they could amount to rules of cortical connectivity. *"These rules revolve around one, apparently, overriding strategy that the cerebral cortex uses—that of functional segregation"* [14]. Functional segregation demands that cells with common functional properties be grouped together. This architectural constraint in turn necessitates both convergence and divergence of cortical connections. Extrinsic connections between cortical regions are not continuous but occur in patches or clusters. This patchiness has, in some instances, a clear relationship to functional segregation. For example, V2 has a distinctive cytochrome oxidase architecture, consisting of thick stripes, thin stripes, and interstripes. When recordings are made in V2, directionally selective (but not wavelength or colour selective) cells are found exclusively in the thick stripes. Retrograde (*i.e.*, backwards) labeling of cells in V5 is limited to these thick stripes. All the available physiological evidence suggests that V5 is a functionally homogeneous area that is specialised for visual motion. Evidence of this nature supports the notion that patchy connectivity is the anatomical infrastructure that mediates functional segregation and specialisation (see Zeki [14] for a full discussion). If it is the case that neurons in a given cortical area share a common responsiveness (by virtue of their extrinsic connectivity) to some sensorimotor or cognitive attribute, then this functional segregation is also an anatomical one. Challenging a subject with the appropriate sensorimotor attribute or cognitive process should lead to activity changes in, and only in, the area of interest. This is the model upon which a search for regionally specific effects is based.

B. Statistical Parametric Mapping and Regionally Specific Effects

Functional mapping studies are usually analysed with some form of statistical parametric mapping. Statistical parametric mapping refers to the construction of spatially extended statistical processes to test hypotheses about regionally specific effects. Statistical parametric maps (SPMs) are image processes with voxel values that are, under the null hypothesis, distributed according to a known probability density function (usually Gaussian).

The success of statistical parametric mapping is largely due to the simplicity of the idea. Namely, one analyses each and every voxel using any standard (univariate) statistical test. The resulting statistical parameters are assembled into an image—the SPM. SPMs are interpreted as spatially extended statistical processes by referring to the probabilistic behaviour of stationary Gaussian fields [15]. Stationary fields model both the univariate probabilistic characteristics of an SPM and any stationary spatial covariance structure (stationary means not a function of position). "Unlikely" excursions of the SPM are interpreted as regionally specific effects, attributable to a sensorimotor or cognitive process that has been manipulated experimentally. This characterisation of physiological responses appeals to functional segregation as the underlying model of brain function. One could regard all applications of statistical parametric mapping as testing some variant of the functional segregation hypothesis.

The ideas behind statistical parametric mapping are, of course, not new. Statistical parametric mapping represents the convergence of two earlier ideas: change distribution analysis and significance probability mapping. Change distribution analysis was a voxel-based assessment of neurophysiological changes developed by the St. Louis group for PET activation studies [16]. The essential difference between change score maps and SPMs is that the former simply reflect the size of the activation, whereas SPMs are images of the statistical reliability or significance of the effect. Significance probability mapping was developed in the analysis of multichannel EEG data and involves the construction of interpolated pseudomaps of a statistical parameter. Unlike pseudomaps in electrophysiology SPMs are well behaved in the sense that they are stationary (due to the fact that neuroimaging samples uniformly and that the point spread function is stationary). This well-behaved aspect of SPMs (under the null hypothesis) meant that theoretical advances could be made to a point where this analytical area is now a rapidly growing and exciting part of applied spatial statistics. This development has occurred in the context of the theory of Gaussian fields [17–20], in particular the theory of level-crossings [17] and differential topology [18].

C. Statistical Parametric Mapping—Implementation and Applications

Statistical parametric mapping is a framework, subsuming the general linear model and the theory of Gaussian fields, that allows for a diverse interrogation of functional imaging data. The same ideas and implementation can accommodate approaches that range from simple unpaired t tests to multifactorial ANCOVA. The experimental design and the model used to test for specific neurophysiological responses are embodied in a mathematical structure called the *design matrix*. The nature and role of the design matrix is described more fully below and in subsequent chapters. The approach adopted in our version of statistical parametric mapping partitions the design matrix according to whether the effect is interesting (*e.g.*, an activation) or not (*e.g.*, a nuisance effect like global activity). These effects can reflect factor levels (using indicator-type variables to denote the presence of a particular cognitive component) or can be continuous functions (a covariate, like reaction time).

The contribution of each effect (*i.e.*, each column of the design matrix modeling the various response components) to the observed physiological responses is estimated using the general linear model and standard least squares. These estimated contributions are known as parameter estimates and can be as simple as the mean activity associated with a particular condition or as complicated as an interaction term in a multifactorial experiment. Regionally specific effects are framed in terms of differences among these parameter estimates (*e.g.*, an activation effect) and are specified using linear compounds or contrasts. The significance of each contrast is assessed with a statistic whose distribution has Student's t distribution under the null hypothesis. For each contrast or difference in parameter estimates, a t statistic is computed (in parallel) for each and every voxel to form a SPM$\{t\}$. For convenience the SPM$\{t\}$ is transformed to a Gaussian field or SPM$\{Z\}$. Statistical inferences are then made about local excursions of the SPM$\{Z\}$ above a specified threshold, using distributional approximations from the theory of Gaussian fields. These distributions pertain to simple characterisations of the "blobs" of activation; namely, their maximal value and their spatial extent (or both). The resulting P values can be considered corrected for the volume of brain tested. By specifying different contrasts one can test for a variety of effects. These effects generally fall into one of three broad categories.

1. Cognitive and Sensorimotor Subtraction

The tenet of this approach is that the difference between two tasks can be formulated as a separable cognitive or sensorimotor component and that the regionally specific differences in brain activity identify the corresponding functionally specialised area. Early applications of subtraction range from the functional anatomy of word processing [21] to functional specialisation in extrastriate cortex [22]. The latter studies involved presenting visual stimuli with and without some specific sensory attribute (*e.g.*, colour, motion, *etc.*). The areas highlighted by subtraction were identified with homologous areas in monkeys that showed selective electrophysiological responses to equivalent visual stimuli.

2. Parametric Designs

The premise is that regional physiology will vary systematically with the degree of cognitive or sensorimotor processing. Examples of this approach include the experiments of Grafton *et al.* [23] who demonstrated significant correlations between rCBF and the performance of a visually guided motor tracking task. On the sensory side Price *et al.* [24] demonstrated a remarkable linear relationship between perfusion in periauditory regions and frequency of aural word presentation. Significantly this correlation was not observed in Wernicke's area, where perfusion appeared to correlate, not with the discriminative attributes of the stimulus, but with the presence or absence of semantic content.

3. Factorial Designs

At its simplest an interaction represents a change in a change. Interactions are associated with factorial designs where two or more factors are combined in the same experiment. The effect of one factor, on the effect of the other, is assessed by the interaction term. Factorial designs have a wide range of applications. An early application in neuroimaging examined physiological adaptation and plasticity [25] during motor performance by assessing time by condition interactions [26]. Psychopharmacological activation studies are examples of factorial design [27]. In these studies subjects perform a series of baseline-activation pairs before and after being given a drug. The interaction term reflects the modulatory drug effect on the task-dependent activation [28]. We will expand on the role of factorial designs in the context of cognitive science and additive factors logic in a later chapter (see Chapters 8 and 16).

In summary the applications of statistical parametric mapping have been introduced using a framework of activation studies that distinguishes between subtractive (categorical), parametric (dimensional), and factorial (interaction) designs. Subtractive designs are well established and powerful devices in functional mapping but are predicated on possibly untenable assumptions about the relationship between brain dynamics and the functional processes that ensue. Parametric approaches avoid many of the shortcomings of "cognitive subtraction" by testing for nonlinear but systematic relationships between neurophysiology and sensorimotor, psychophysical, pharmacologic, or cognitive parameters. The fundamental difference between subtractive and parametric approaches lies in treating a cognitive process not as a categorical invariant but as a dimension or attribute that can be expressed to a greater or lesser extent. It is anticipated that parametric designs will find an increasing role in psychological and psychophysical activation experiments. Finally, factorial experiments provide a rich way of assessing the affect of one manipulation on the effects of another and incidently allow one to test some of the assumptions implicit in cognitive subtraction.

Having established some of the theoretical precedents, and placed the approaches considered here in a general context, we will now review a series of data transformations that are required to implement data analysis at a practical or operational level.

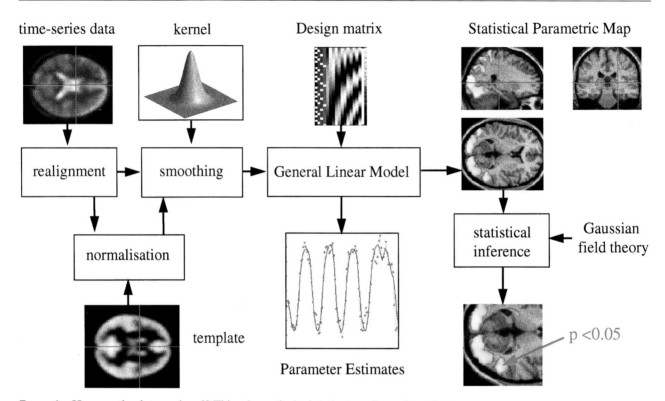

FIGURE 1 How are the data analysed? This schematic depicts the transformations that start with the imaging time series and end with a statistical parametric map (SPM). SPMs can be thought of as "X-rays" of the significance of an effect. Voxel-based analyses require the data to be in the same anatomical space: This is effected by realigning the data [in fMRI it is usually necessary to remove signal components, that are correlated with displacements that remain after realignment]. After realignment the images are subject to nonlinear warping so that they match a template that already conforms to a standard space [29]. After smoothing, the general linear model [31] is employed to perform the appropriate univariate test at each and every voxel. The test statistics that ensue (usually t or F statistics) constitute the SPM. The final stage is to make statistical inferences on the basis of the SPM and characterise the responses observed using the fitted responses or parameter estimates. If one knew where to look beforehand then this inference could be based on the value of the statistic without correction. If, however, one did not predict an anatomical site *a priori*, then a correction for the multiple dependent comparisons performed has to be made. These corrections are usually made using distributional approximations from the theory of Gaussian fields [15,17–20].

IV. THE OPERATIONAL COMPONENTS OF FUNCTIONAL IMAGING DATA ANALYSIS

The following represents a summary of the stages required for an analysis of PET and fMRI activation studies (see also Fig. 1). With regard to fMRI we are concerned principally with the analysis of fast techniques (*e.g.*, echo-planar imaging [EPI]) that provide volumetric data (by multislice acquisition). Slower fMRI techniques, with an interscan interval that is greater than the haemodynamic response time (about 6 to 8 sec), can be treated in the same way as PET data because temporal autocorrelations due to the haemodynamic response function or introduced by temporal smoothing do not have to be considered. The stages of analysis include (i) *realignment*, (ii) *spatial normalisation*, (iii) *spatial smoothing*, (iv) *voxel-wise statistical analysis* using the general linear model (for fast fMRI we have to use an extended model that accommodates temporal smoothing and autocorrelations over time), and (v) *statistical inference* based on the spatial extent and maxima of thresholded activation foci that ensue (using the theory of random Gaussian fields).

A. Realignment

Movement-related variance components in PET and fMRI time series represent one of the most serious confounds of analysis. For PET this stage involves estimating movement relative to the first scan (using a least squares analysis that obtains after linearising the problem with a first order Taylor series) and realigning the scans post hoc using these estimates. Removing movement-related effects from fMRI time series is not as simple as it may seem at first glance. This is because movement in earlier scans can affect the signal in subsequent scans (due to differential spin-excitation histories). The procedure we have adopted is to estimate head movements as for PET data. These estimates are then used to (i) realign the images and (ii) perform a mathematical adjustment to remove movement-related components that persist after simple realignment. The adjustment procedure is based on a moving average-autoregression model of spin-excitation history effects. The latter components can be prominent and are specific to the way the fMRI signal is acquired.

B. Spatial Normalisation

Clearly, to implement voxel-based analysis of imaging data, data from different subjects must derive from homologous parts of the brain. Spatial transformations are therefore applied that move and "warp" the images such that they all conform (approximately) to some idealized or standard brain. This normalisation facilitates intersubject averaging and the reporting of results in a conventional way even if intersubject averaging is not used. The transformation of an image into a standard anatomical space, usually that described in the atlas of Talairach and Tournoux [29] as proposed by Fox *et al.* [30], corresponds to spatial normalisation. For PET the normalising transformations can be computed on the basis of the PET data themselves or on the basis of coregistered high resolution anatomical MRI scans. If the T_2^*-weighted fMRI data are of sufficiently good quality it is possible to normalise these directly.

C. Spatial Smoothing

Smoothing (convolving the data with a smoothing kernel) has several important objectives. First, it generally increases signal relative to noise. The neurophysiological effects of interest are produced by haemodynamic changes that are expressed over spatial scales of several millimetres, whereas noise usually has higher spatial frequencies. For PET the spatial frequency structure of noise is determined by the reconstruction process used to create the images. In fMRI the noise can (to a first approximation) be regarded as independent for each voxel and has therefore very high spatial frequency components. Second, convolving with a Gaussian (or other) kernel conditions the data in the sense that the data conform more closely to a Gaussian field model. This is important if one wants to use the theory of Gaussian fields to make statistical inferences about (*i.e.*, assign *P* values to) the ensuing regionally specific effects. The requirement that the data be a good lattice representation of a Gaussian field includes (i) that the autocorrelation function be twice differentiable and (ii) that the spatial correlations be stationary. Both these requirements are assured (approximately) after smoothing. The final reason for smoothing is specific to intersubject averaging. It ensures that haemodynamic changes from subject to subject are assessed on a spatial scale at which homologies in functional anatomy are typically expressed. For example, at a scale of 100 μm it is highly unlikely that (even with perfect spatial normalisation) the functional anatomy and organisation of the middle frontal gyri in two subjects will show meaningful homologies. However, at an anatomical scale of 8 mm they do, as evidenced by the success of multisubject PET activation studies. In other words, a mapping of function onto anatomy may be meaningful only at a resolution that is not confounded by microscopic and macroscopic organisational details that are unique to a given individual.

D. Statistical Analysis

This stage corresponds to modeling the data in order to partition observed neurophysiological responses into components of interest, confounds of no interest and an error term. This partitioning is effected using the general linear model to estimate the components in terms of parameters associated with the design matrix (see below).

The analysis of regionally specific effects uses the general linear model to assess differences among parameter estimates (specified by a contrast) in a univariate sense, by referring to the error variance. This assessment is in terms of a *t* value for each and every voxel (*i.e.*, a SPM{*t*}). The SPM{*t*} is transformed to the unit normal distribution to give a Gaussian field or SPM{*Z*}. For fast fMRI data there is a caveat. In order to maximise signal components one can smooth in time. The autocovariances in the error terms that result from this smoothing require analysis by an extended general linear model that takes account of such autocorrelations or serial correlations.

E. Statistical Inference

Statistical inference can proceed at a number of levels. If one has employed a MANCOVA–CVA approach then a single *P* value obtains (based on Wilk's Lambda or a related statistic) that compares the variance–covariance accounted for by effects of interest relative to error. This single *P* value tells one nothing about regionally specific effects. Statistical inference about specific regional changes requires statistical parametric mapping. With an anatomically constrained hypothesis about effects in a particular brain region *a priori* the *Z* value in that region in the SPM{*Z*} can be used to test the hypothesis. With an anatomically "open" hypothesis (*i.e.*, a null hypothesis that there is no effect anywhere in the brain), a correction for multiple nonindependent comparisons is required. It is at this point that the theory of Gaussian fields provides a way of computing a corrected *P* value.

The SPM{*Z*} of the previous section is subject to standard procedures developed for statistical parametric mapping using the theory of Gaussian fields. These procedures give *P* values that pertain to different levels of inference; these levels of inference can be in terms of (i) the number of activated regions (*i.e.*, number of clusters above some height and volume thresholds), (ii) the number of activated voxels (*i.e.*, volume) comprising a particular region, and (iii) the *P* value for each voxel within that region. These *P* values are corrected for the multiple nonindependent comparisons implicit in an analysis. These results [the SPM{*Z*} and associated *P* values] are the endpoint of analysis.

V. THE GENERAL LINEAR MODEL

Many of the above techniques depend, at some level, on the general linear model. This section introduces the general linear model and terms that will be adopted in subsequent chapters. The general linear model is simply an equation that relates what one observes, to what one expected to see, by expressing the observations (*response variable*) as a linear combination of expected components (or *explanatory variables*) and some residual error. The general linear model comes in a number of guises, for example multiple linear regression, analysis of covariance or a simple *t* test. The general linear model for a response variable x_{ij} such as regional CBF at voxel $j = 1, \ldots, J$ is

$$x_{ij} = g_{i1}\beta_{1j} + g_{i2}\beta_{2j} + \cdots g_{iK}\beta_{Kj} + e_{ij}, \tag{1}$$

where $i = 1, \ldots, I$ indexes the observation (*e.g.*, scan). The general linear model assumes the errors (e_{ij}) are independent and identically distributed normally [$N(0, \sigma_j^2)$]. For example, in activation studies this means assuming an equal error variance (σ_j^2) across conditions and subjects (but not from one voxel or brain structure to the next). β_{kj} are K unknown parameters for each voxel j that represent the relative contribution of each of the explanatory variables.

The coefficients g_{ik} are explanatory variables relating to the conditions under which the observation (scan) i was made. These coefficients can be of two sorts: (i) a covariate (*e.g.*, global CBF, time, plasma prolactin level, *etc.*) in which case Eq. (1) is a familiar multivariate regression model or (ii) indicator-type or dummy variables, taking integer values to indicate the level of a factor (*e.g.*, condition, subject, drug, *etc.*) under which the response variable (*e.g.*, perfusion) is measured. Mathematically speaking, there is no distinction between these two kinds of variables but we make a distinction here for didactic reasons. Equation (1) can be written in matrix form as a multivariate general linear model:

$$\mathbf{X} = \mathbf{G}\boldsymbol{\beta} + \mathbf{e}. \tag{2}$$

Here **X** is a perfusion data matrix with elements x_{ij}. **X** has a column for each voxel j and one row for each scan. The matrix **G** is composed of the coefficients g_{ik} and is the design matrix. The design matrix has one row for every scan and one column for every effect (factor or covariate) in the model. $\boldsymbol{\beta} = [\boldsymbol{\beta}_1|\boldsymbol{\beta}_2|, \ldots, \boldsymbol{\beta}_J]$ is the parameter matrix where $\boldsymbol{\beta}_j$ is a column vector of parameters for voxel j. **e** is a matrix of normally distributed error terms. It may be noted that Eq. (2) does not have a constant term. The constant term can be explicitly removed by mean correcting the data matrix or implicitly by adding a column of ones to **G**. Here and throughout we will assume the data **X** are mean corrected unless otherwise stated. Least squares estimates of $\boldsymbol{\beta}$, say **b**, satisfy the normal equations [31],

$$\mathbf{G}^T\mathbf{G}\mathbf{b} = \mathbf{G}^T\mathbf{X},$$

if **G** is of full rank then $\mathbf{G}^T\mathbf{G}$ is invertible and the least squares estimates are given uniquely by

$$\mathbf{b} = (\mathbf{G}^T\mathbf{G})^{-1}\mathbf{G}^T\mathbf{X},$$

where

$$E\{\mathbf{b}_j\} = \boldsymbol{\beta}_j \text{ and } \mathrm{Var}\{\mathbf{b}_j\} = \sigma_j^2(\mathbf{G}^T\mathbf{G})^{-1}. \tag{3}$$

If the errors are normally distributed then the least squares estimates are also the maximum likelihood estimates and are themselves normally distributed [32]. $E\{\mathbf{b}_j\}$ is simply the expectation or average of the parameter estimates. $\mathrm{Var}\{\mathbf{b}_j\}$ is the variance–covariance matrix for the parameter estimates corresponding to the jth voxel. These equations can be used to implement a vast range of statistical analyses. The issue is therefore not so much the mathematics but the formulation of a design matrix (**G**) appropriate to the study design and inferences that are sought.

The design matrix can contain both covariates and indicator variables reflecting the experimental design. Each column of **G** has an associated unknown parameter in the vectors $\boldsymbol{\beta}_j$. Some of these parameters will be of interest [*e.g.*, the effect of particular sensorimotor or cognitive condition or the regression coefficient of rCBF (the response variable) on reaction time (covariate)]. The remaining parameters will be of no interest and pertain to confounding effects (*e.g.*, the effect of being a particular subject or the regression slope of voxel activity on global activity). Confounding is used to denote an uninteresting effect that could confound the estimation of interesting effects (*e.g.*, the confounding effect of global changes on regional activations).

The general linear model and associated parameter estimation have a central role in nearly everything that follows and forms the starting point for most of the statistical procedures considered in this book.

VI. SUMMARY

This chapter has reviewed the basic distinction between approaches inspired by functional integration (eigenimage analysis, multidimensional scaling, and MANCOVA–CVA) and those predicated on functional segregation (statistical parametric mapping). Functional integration is mediated by anatomical, functional, and effective connections. In imaging neuroscience these concepts form the basis for characterising patterns of correlations using eigenimages, singular images, or canonical images (*i.e.*, spatial modes). These spatial modes describe distributed systems. Functional segregation and specialisation speak to regionally specific aspects of functional organisation and require a different approach to characterising brain responses. Statistical parametric mapping provides for many ways in which to make inferences about functional segregation. Three important classes of experimental design used in this endeavour are subtractive, parametric, and factorial. Each of these is a particular instance of the general linear model and can be framed in terms of an SPM{Z}. Statistical inferences about the resulting SPM{Z} are made using distributional approximations from the theory of Gaussian fields.

The two basic approaches to data analysis can be contrasted in a number of ways. SPMs rely on functional segregation as a conceptual model, eigenimage analyses and related approaches (*e.g.*, CVA) address the integration of distributed changes in terms of systems. The characterisation of changes with a SPM is in terms of (multiple) activation foci that are identified following thresholding. The equivalent characterisation with eigenimage analyses is in terms of spatially extended anatomical profiles (spatial modes). SPM is a statistical procedure that permits statistical inferences about regionally specific findings (*e.g.*, the probability of finding an activation focus by chance). Approaches based on eigenvalue solutions are mathematical devices that simply orthogonalise the variance–covariance and make no comment on the significance of the resulting spatial modes (although a set of canonical images can be said to characterise a significant effect if MANCOVA is used to make an inference about these effects beforehand).

The second half of this chapter reviewed the necessary steps employed in implementing these analyses. This set of data transformations can be broadly classed as spatial transformations (*i.e.*, realignment, spatial normalisation, and smoothing) and statistical transformations (*i.e.*, eigenimage analysis of the adjusted data or the construction of SPMs). Statistical inference is usually based on SPMs and can either be made about a specific region or about regionally specific effects in a specified brain volume. In the latter case a corrected *P* value is required that protects against false positives. This correction is achieved using the theory of Gaussian fields.

A. The Ensuing Chapters on Data Analysis and Characterisation

The next chapter deals with spatial transformations and subsequent chapters deal in a more formal way with the techniques introduced above, covering first univariate approaches and then multivariate approaches. These chapters discuss (i) statistical models in the context of the general linear model, (ii) statistical inference in the context of the theory of Gaussian fields, and (iii) eigenimage analysis and multivariate analyses based on the general linear model. The next chapter addresses functional integration from a different perspective and introduces effective connectivity and related models (*e.g.*, structural equation modeling and nonlinear extensions). It complements the previous chapter about characterising distributed brain responses, but frames the characterisation explicitly in terms of connections or influences among brain regions. The following chapter returns to the different kinds of experimental design that have been employed in elucidating functional anatomy. It focuses on parametric and factorial designs to illustrate how modern brain activation experiments can (i) address some fundamental issues about functional organisation and (ii) call for revisions of some of our basic assumptions. The order in which these chapters are presented reflects the ontology of their development and application. The vast majority of imaging research is predicated on some form of statistical parametric mapping so that a greater emphasis has been placed on these techniques.

References

1. C. G. Phillips, S. Zeki, and H. B. Barlow. Localization of function in the cerebral cortex. Past, present and future. *Brain* **107,** 327–361 (1984).

2. F. Goltz. *In* "Transactions of the 7th International Medical Congress" (W. MacCormac, Ed.), Vol. I, pp. 218–228. Kolkmann, London, 1881.

3. J. R. Absher and D. F Benson. Disconnection syndrome: An overview of Geschwind's contributions. *Neurology* **43,** 862–867 (1993).

4. K. J. Friston, C. D. Frith, P. F. Liddle, and R. S. J. Frackowiak. Functional connectivity: The principal component analysis of large (PET) data sets. *J. Cereb. Blood Flow Metab.* **13,** 5–14 (1993a).

5. K. J. Friston, C. D. Frith, and R. S. J. Frackowiak. Time-dependent changes in effective connectivity measured with PET. *Hum. Brain Mapping* **1,** 69–80 (1993b).

6. G. L. Gerstein and D. H. Lerkel. Simultaneously recorded trains of action potentials: Analysis and functional interpretation. *Science* **164,** 828–830 (1969).

7. G. L. Gerstein, P. Bedenbaugh, and A. M. H. J. Aertsen. Neuronal assemblies IEEE. *Trans. Biomed. Eng.* **36,** 4–14 (1989).

8. P. M. Gochin, E. K. Miller, C. G. Gross, and G. L. Gerstein. Functional interactions among neurons in inferior temporal cortex of the awake macaque. *Exp. Brain Res.* **84,** 505–516 (1991).

9. A. Aertsen and H. Preissl. Dynamics of activity and connectivity in physiological neuronal networks. *In* "Non Linear Dynamics and Neuronal Networks" (H. G. Schuster Publishers Inc., Ed.), pp. 281–302. H. G. Schuster, New York, 1991.

10. J. I. Nelson, P. A. Salin, N. M. J. Munk, M. Arzi, and J. Bullier. Spational and temporal coherence in cortico-cortical connections: A cross-correlation study in areas 17 and 18 in the cat. *Visual Neurosci.* **9,** 21–37 (1992).

11. R. Friedrich, A. Fuchs, and H. Haken. Modelling of spatio-temporal EEG patterns. *In* "Mathematical Approaches to Brain Functioning Diagnostics" (I. Dvorak and A. V. Holden, Eds.). Manchester Univ. Press, New York, 1991.

12. G. H. Golub and C. F Van Loan. *In* "Matrix Computations," 2nd ed., pp. 241–248. Johns Hopkins Univ. Press, Baltimore and London, 1991.

13. G. Mayer-Kress, C. Barczys, and W. Freeman. Attractor reconstruction from event-related multi-electrode EEG data. *In* "Mathematical Approaches to Brain Functioning Diagnostics" (I. Dvorak and A. V. Holden, Eds.). Manchester Univ. Press, New York, 1991.

14. S. Zeki. The motion pathways of the visual cortex. *In* "Vision: Coding and Efficiency" (C. Blakemore, Ed.), pp. 321–345. Cambridge Univ. Press, UK, 1990.

15. R. J. Adler. *In* "The Geometry of Random Fields." Wiley, New York, 1981.

16. P. T. Fox and M. A. Mintun. Non-invasive functional brain mapping by change distribution analysis of averaged PET images of H15O2 tissue activity. *J. Nuclear Med.* **30,** 141–149 (1989).

17. K. J. Friston, C. D. Frith, P. F. Liddle, and R. S. J. Frackowiak. Comparing functional (PET) images: The assessment of significant change. *J. Cereb. Blood Flow Metab.* **11,** 690–699 (1991).

18. K. J. Worsley, A. C. Evans, S. Marrett, and P. Neelin. A three-dimensional statistical analysis for rCBF activation studies in human brain. *J. Cereb. Blood. Flow Metab.* **12,** 900–918 (1992).

19. K. J. Worsley. Local maxima and the expected Euler characteristic of excursion sets of χ^2, F and t fields. *Adv. Appl. Prob.* **26,** 13–42 (1994)

20. K. J. Friston, K. J. Worsley, R. S. J. Frackowiak, J. C. Mazziotta, and A. C. Evans, Assessing the significance of focal activations using their spatial extent. *Hum. Brain Mapping* **1,** 214–220 (1994).

21. S. E. Petersen, P. T. Fox, M. I. Posner, M. Mintun, and M. E. Raichle. Positron emission tomographic studies of the processing of single words. *J. Cog. Neurosci* **1,** 153–170 (1989).

22. C. J. Lueck, S. Zeki, K. J. Friston, N. O. Deiber, P. Cope, V. J. Cunningham, A. A. Lammertsma, C. Kennard, and R. S. J. Frackowiak. The colour centre in the cerebral cortex of man. *Nature* **340,** 386–389 (1989).

23. S. Grafton, J. Mazziotta, S. Presty, K. J. Friston, R. S. J. Frackowiak, and M.

Phelps. Functional anatomy of human procedural learning determined with regional cerebral blood flow and PET. *J. Neurosci.* **12,** 2542–2548 (1992).

24. C. Price, R. J. S. Wise, S. Ramsay, K. J. Friston, D. Howard, K. Patterson, and R. S. J. Frackowiak. Regional response differences within the human auditory cortex when listening to words. *Neurosci. Lett.* **146,** 179–182 (1992).

25. P. F. C. Gilbert and W. T. Thach. Purkinje cell activity during motor learning. *Brain Res.* **128,** 309–328 (1977).

26. K. J. Friston, C. Frith, R. E. Passingham, P. F. Liddle, and R. S. J. Frackowiak. Motor practice and neurophysiological adaptation in the cerebellum: A positron tomography study. *Proc. R. Soc. London B* **248,** 223–228 (1992a).

27. K. J. Friston, P. Grasby, C. Bench, C. Frith, P. Cowen, P. Little, R. S. J. Frackowiak, and R. Dolan. Measuring the neuromodulatory effects of drugs in man with positron tomography. *Neurosci. Lett.* **141,** 106–110 (1992b).

28. P. Grasby, K. J. Friston, C. Bench, P. Cowen, C. Frith, P. Liddle, R. S. J. Frackowiak, and R. Dolan. Effects of 5-HT1A partial agonist buspirone on regional cerebral blood flow in man. *Psychopharmacology* **108,** 380–386 (1992).

29. P. Talairach and J. Tournoux. "A Stereotactic Coplanar Atlas of the Human Brain." Thieme, Stuttgart, 1988.

30. P. T. Fox, J. S. Perlmutter, and M. E. Raichle. A stereotactic method of anatomical localization for positron emission tomography. *J. Comput. Assist. Tomogr.* **9,** 141–153 (1985)

31. C. Chatfield and A. J. Collins. "Introduction to Multivariate Analysis," p. 189–210. Chapman and Hall, London, 1980.

CHAPTER THREE

SPATIAL TRANSFORMATION OF IMAGES

I. INTRODUCTION

This chapter describes how to identify the spatial and intensity transformations that map one image onto another. A general technique that implements nonlinear spatial (stereotactic) normalisation and image realignment is presented. This technique minimises the sum of squares between two images following nonlinear spatial deformations and scaling of the voxel (intensity) values. The spatial transformations are obtained using a few iterations of a Gauss–Newton-like optimisation algorithm. The technique can be applied in any number of dimensions. Various applications are considered, both to illustrate the nature of the approach and to speculate on potential applications in the future.

Spatial transformations are important in many aspects of image analysis. For example, in activation studies the realignment of a time series of scans from the same subject (correcting for movement) is necessary for voxel-based analyses of time dependent changes. Intersubject averaging requires that images be transformed into some standard sterotactic space. Anatomical variability and structural changes due to pathology can be framed in terms of the transformations required to map the abnormal onto the normal. The interpretation of functional mapping studies often refers to some notion of normal anatomical variability [1]. This variability embodies neuroanatomical information of a probabilistic nature that is the focus of some important new brain mapping initiatives. All these fields of enquiry depend on a spatial mapping of images from one space to another. How are these transformations identified?

Spatial transformations can be broadly divided into *label-based* and *non-label-based*. Label-based techniques identify homologous spatial structures, features, or landmarks in two images and find the transformations that best superpose the labeled points. These transformations can be linear [2] or non-linear (*e.g.*, thin plate splines [3]). Non-label-based approaches identify a spatial transformation that minimises some index of the difference between an object and a reference image, where both are treated as unlabeled continuous processes. Again these can be linear (*e.g.*, principal axes [4], image realignment

[5–7]) or nonlinear (*e.g.*, plastic transformation [8,9] with some interesting developments using neural nets [10]).

Without any constraints it is of course possible to transform any image such that it matches another exactly. The issue is therefore less about the nature of the transformation and more about defining constraints under which a transformation is effected. The validity of a transformation can usually be reduced to the validity of these constraints. The first tenet of the general approach described here is that the constraints are explicit, reasonable, and operationally specified. The reliability of label-based approaches is limited by the reproducibility of labeling. The second key aspect of our approach is therefore that it is non-label-based and automatic. In short, we have developed and describe an efficient, automatic, and multidimensional nonlinear spatial transformation technique (where rigid body and affine transformations were considered as special linear cases of this more general approach). This method is implemented in the software used for statistical parametric mapping known as *SPM96*.

II. THE UNDERLYING PRINCIPLES

We can consider an image as a scalar field. For example, for every point $\mathbf{x}$ (where $\mathbf{x}$ is a vector representing a point in space), the image $\mathbf{f}$ would have a value $f(\mathbf{x})$. For the proposed techniques to work we need to assume that images are good lattice representations of continuously differentiable deterministic scalar functions.

We begin by assuming that the difference between two images (say $\mathbf{f}$ and $\mathbf{g}$) can be attributed only to misalignment or differences in the shape and size of the brain. This spatial discrepancy between images is characterised by a vector function of position $\mathbf{h}(\mathbf{x}, \gamma)$, where γ is a set of parameters that define the transformation. This difference between the voxel intensities of two images can be expressed as

$$ug(\mathbf{x}) = f(\mathbf{h}(\mathbf{x}, \gamma)) + e(\mathbf{x}), \tag{1}$$

where u is a simple scaling (more general intensity transformations will be discussed later) and $e(\mathbf{x})$ is some error scalar function. For simplicity this error term will be omitted in subsequent expressions. The next step is to linearise Eq. (1) so that $\mathbf{h}(\mathbf{x}, \gamma)$ has explicit least squares solutions. This can be effected by low order approximations and by imposing some constraints on the form of $\mathbf{h}(\mathbf{x}, \gamma)$. The constraints are that $\mathbf{h}(\mathbf{x}, \gamma)$ can only change slowly with location, meaning that the spatial transformation is smooth and that local contiguity relationships are preserved. Stronger constraints can be imposed on $\mathbf{h}(\mathbf{x}, \gamma)$. For example, in realigning scans from the same individual $\mathbf{h}(\mathbf{x}, \gamma)$ would represent a rigid-body transformation with six parameters, but it would still be smooth. The objective now is to linearise $\mathbf{h}(\mathbf{x}, \gamma)$ so that linear algebra can be used to solve the transformations. Using the above constraints this linearisation can be achieved as follows:

$$ug(\mathbf{x}) \simeq f\left(\mathbf{x} + \sum g_k \mathbf{b}_k(\mathbf{x})\right).$$

Now, if $\mathbf{f}$ is smooth we can expand the right-hand side of this equation using Taylor's theorem, where, ignoring high order terms,

$$f(\mathbf{x} + q_k \mathbf{b}_k(\mathbf{x})) \simeq f(\mathbf{x}) + \sum q_k \frac{\partial f(\mathbf{x})}{\partial q_k}.$$

Note that $\partial f(\mathbf{h}(\mathbf{x}))/\partial q_k = \mathbf{b}_k(x) \nabla f(\mathbf{x})$. Combining these equations we get

$$ug(\mathbf{x}) \simeq f(\mathbf{x}) + \sum q_k \frac{\partial f(\mathbf{x})}{\partial q_k}.$$

This can be expressed in matrix notation as

$$\left(\mathbf{g} - \frac{\partial \mathbf{f}}{\partial \mathbf{q}}\right)\binom{u}{\mathbf{q}} \simeq \mathbf{f}, \tag{2}$$

where $(u \quad \mathbf{q}^T)^T$ is a vector of the unknown coefficients. $\mathbf{g}$ and $\mathbf{f}$ are column vectors with one element per voxel. $\partial \mathbf{f}/\partial \mathbf{q}$ is a matrix with a row for each voxel position and a column for each spatial coefficient q_k. The elements of $\partial \mathbf{f}/\partial \mathbf{q}$ reflect the small change in voxel value associated with each component of the spatial distortion.

The above matrix equation can be solved by

$$\binom{u}{\mathbf{q}} \simeq \left(\left(\mathbf{g} - \frac{\partial f}{\partial q}\right)^T \left(\mathbf{g} - \frac{\partial f}{\partial q}\right)\right)^{-1} \left(\mathbf{g} - \frac{\partial f}{\partial q}\right)^T \mathbf{f}.$$

This solution for $\mathbf{q}$ can then be used to carry out the spatial transformation that maps $f(\mathbf{x})$ onto $g(\mathbf{x})$ given that $\mathbf{h}(\mathbf{x}) = \mathbf{x} + \sum q_k \mathbf{b}_k(\mathbf{x})$.

The above linear approximation works best when the amount of movement required is small relative to the smoothness of the images. To accommodate this limitation, images are normally convolved with a Gaussian kernel before matching. In practise these equations are solved iteratively using a scheme like the following:

1. Assign initial estimates for u and $\mathbf{q}$.
2. Set $f'(\mathbf{x}) = f(\mathbf{x} + \sum q_k \mathbf{b}_k(\mathbf{x}))$.
3. Compute $(\mathbf{g} - \partial \mathbf{f}'/\partial \mathbf{q})^T(\mathbf{g} - \partial \mathbf{f}'/\partial \mathbf{q})$ and $(\mathbf{g} - \partial \mathbf{f}'/\partial \mathbf{q})^T \mathbf{f}'$.
4. Solve this set of simultaneous equations for u and $\mathbf{q}'$.
5. Set $\mathbf{q} = \mathbf{q} + \mathbf{q}'$.
6. Repeat steps 2–5 for a fixed number of iterations, or until convergence.

III. THE AFFINE TRANSFORMATION

One of the simplest and well defined of spatial transformations is the affine transformation. For each point (x_0, y_0, z_0) in an image, a mapping can be defined into the coordinates of another space. This is simply expressed:

$$x_1 = m_{11}x_0 + m_{12}y_0 + m_{13}z_0 + m_{14}$$
$$y_1 = m_{21}x_0 + m_{22}y_0 + m_{23}z_0 + m_{24}$$
$$z_1 = m_{31}x_0 + m_{32}y_0 + m_{33}z_0 + m_{34}.$$

This mapping is often expressed in matrix form:

$$\begin{pmatrix} x_1 \\ y_1 \\ z_1 \\ 1 \end{pmatrix} = \begin{pmatrix} m_{11} & m_{12} & m_{13} & m_{14} \\ m_{21} & m_{22} & m_{23} & m_{24} \\ m_{31} & m_{32} & m_{33} & m_{34} \\ 0 & 0 & 0 & 1 \end{pmatrix} \begin{pmatrix} x_0 \\ y_0 \\ z_0 \\ 1 \end{pmatrix}.$$

It is possible to combine a number of different affine transformations together by multiplying the matrixes to form a single matrix. Image realignment or coregistration require a rigid body transformation that is simply a more constrained form of the general affine transformation. In three dimensions a rigid body transformation can be defined by six parameters. These parameters are, typically, three translations (shifts) and three rotations about orthogonal axes. A matrix which implements the translation is:

$$\begin{pmatrix} 1 & 0 & 0 & x_{trans} \\ 0 & 1 & 0 & y_{trans} \\ 0 & 0 & 1 & z_{trans} \\ 0 & 0 & 0 & 1 \end{pmatrix}.$$

Matrixes that carry out rotations (Θ, Φ, and Ω—in radians) about the x, y, and z axes, respectively, are:

$$\begin{pmatrix} 1 & 0 & 0 & 0 \\ 0 & \cos(\Theta) & \sin(\Theta) & 0 \\ 0 & -\sin(\Theta) & \cos(\Theta) & 0 \\ 0 & 0 & 0 & 1 \end{pmatrix}, \begin{pmatrix} \cos(\Phi) & 0 & \sin(\Phi) & 0 \\ 0 & 1 & 0 & 0 \\ -\sin(\Phi) & 0 & \cos(\Phi) & 0 \\ 0 & 0 & 0 & 1 \end{pmatrix},$$

$$\text{and } \begin{pmatrix} \cos(\Omega) & \sin(\Omega) & 0 & 0 \\ -\sin(\Omega) & \cos(\Omega) & 0 & 0 \\ 0 & 0 & 1 & 0 \\ 0 & 0 & 0 & 1 \end{pmatrix}.$$

The order in which the operations are performed is important. For example, a rotation about the x axis of $\pi/2$ radians followed by an equivalent rotation about the y axis would produce a very different result if the order of the operations was reversed.

A. Determining the Optimum Affine Transformation to Match Two Images

There are many possible ways of parameterising an affine transformation. However, the simplest parameters to use are the elements of the affine transformation matrix ($q_1 = a_{11}$, $q_2 = a_{21}$, $q_4 = a_{12}$, etc.). If we assume that two images to be registered are similar in appearance, then the optimum transformation can be determined by iteratively solving (for u and $\mathbf{q}$)

$$(\mathbf{A})(u \quad q_1 \quad q_2 \quad \dots)^{\mathrm{T}} = \mathbf{f},$$

where $\mathbf{f}$ is the object image (treated as a column vector) and matrix $\mathbf{A}$ consists of

$$\left(\mathbf{g} \quad \frac{\partial \mathbf{f}}{\partial m_{11}} \quad \frac{\partial \mathbf{f}}{\partial m_{21}} \quad \frac{\partial \mathbf{f}}{\partial m_{31}} \quad \frac{\partial \mathbf{f}}{\partial m_{12}} \quad \frac{\partial \mathbf{f}}{\partial m_{22}} \quad \dots \quad \frac{\partial \mathbf{f}}{\partial m_{34}} \right).$$

Here $\mathbf{g}$ is the template image and $\partial \mathbf{f}/\partial m_{..}$ are column vectors containing the derivative of image $\mathbf{f}$ with respect to each parameter. It is possible to compute these derivatives numerically by resampling the image $\mathbf{f}$ after slightly changing the parameters. However, a better way of computing **A** is by

$$\left(\mathbf{g} \quad \mathrm{diag}(\mathbf{x}) \left(\frac{\partial \mathbf{f}}{\partial \mathbf{x}} \ \frac{\partial \mathbf{f}}{\partial \mathbf{y}} \ \frac{\partial \mathbf{f}}{\partial \mathbf{z}} \right) \quad \mathrm{diag}(\mathbf{y}) \left(\frac{\partial \mathbf{f}}{\partial \mathbf{x}} \ \frac{\partial \mathbf{f}}{\partial \mathbf{y}} \ \frac{\partial \mathbf{f}}{\partial \mathbf{z}} \right) \quad \mathrm{diag}(\mathbf{z}) \left(\frac{\partial \mathbf{f}}{\partial \mathbf{x}} \ \frac{\partial \mathbf{f}}{\partial \mathbf{y}} \ \frac{\partial \mathbf{f}}{\partial \mathbf{z}} \right) \right)$$

where **x**, **y**, and **z** are column vectors containing the coordinates of the voxels of **g**, and $\partial \mathbf{f}/\partial \mathbf{x}$, $\partial \mathbf{f}/\partial \mathbf{y}$, and $\partial \mathbf{f}/\partial \mathbf{z}$ are column vectors of the gradient components of image **f**. $\mathrm{diag}(\mathbf{x})$ is the operation of generating a sparse matrix containing the elements of **x** along its diagonal. One would never actually construct $\mathrm{diag}(\mathbf{x})$ but emulate the required matrix operation with the equivalent element by element operations. The unknown parameters (u and **q**) are solved for by computing $(\mathbf{A}^T\mathbf{A})^{-1}\mathbf{A}^T\mathbf{f}$, and the values of **q** are subtracted from the current estimates of the affine transform. This process is repeated (until convergence or a fixed number of iterations), resampling the image **f** on each iteration according to the latest parameter estimates.

Determining this 12-parameter transformation is relatively robust and is suitable as a first pass approach for spatial normalisation. However, a rigid body transformation would be more appropriate for image realignment. We can impose the constraints of a rigid body transformation by reparameterising the affine transformation. If we define the elements of the transformation matrix by a function of the six rigid body transformation parameters (**t**), we can make a simple modification to the technique described here that will constrain our transformations. For each iteration, it is possible to compute a matrix **D** (either numerically, or algebraically), which will rotate the partial derivatives into the new parameter space:

$$\mathbf{D} = \begin{pmatrix} 1 & 0 & 0 & 0 & 0 & 0 & 0 \\ 0 & \dfrac{\partial m_{11}}{\partial t_1} & \dfrac{\partial m_{11}}{\partial t_2} & \dfrac{\partial m_{11}}{\partial t_3} & \dfrac{\partial m_{11}}{\partial t_4} & \dfrac{\partial m_{11}}{\partial t_5} & \dfrac{\partial m_{11}}{\partial t_6} \\ 0 & \dfrac{\partial m_{12}}{\partial t_1} & \dfrac{\partial m_{12}}{\partial t_2} & \dfrac{\partial m_{12}}{\partial t_4} & \dfrac{\partial m_{12}}{\partial t_4} & \dfrac{\partial m_{12}}{\partial t_5} & \dfrac{\partial m_{12}}{\partial t_6} \\ \vdots & \vdots & \vdots & \vdots & \vdots & \vdots & \vdots \\ 0 & \dfrac{\partial m_{34}}{\partial t_1} & \dfrac{\partial m_{34}}{\partial t_2} & \dfrac{\partial m_{34}}{\partial t_3} & \dfrac{\partial m_{34}}{\partial t_4} & \dfrac{\partial m_{34}}{\partial t_5} & \dfrac{\partial m_{34}}{\partial t_6} \end{pmatrix}.$$

Rather than computing $(\mathbf{A}^T\mathbf{A})^{-1}\mathbf{A}^T\mathbf{f}$, we now compute:

$$(\mathbf{D}^T(\mathbf{A}^T\mathbf{A})\mathbf{D})^{-1}\mathbf{D}^T(\mathbf{A}^T\mathbf{f}).$$

The results of this calculation tell us how much the reparameterised estimates should be changed. This approach works extremely well for the correction of subject movement during a series of scans. Typically, only five iterations of the algorithm are required before convergence is reached (for images smoothed with an 8-mm FWHM Gaussian kernel). This application is important because it removes variance from time series that would otherwise be attributed to error (and hence decreased sensitivity) or to evoked effects (*i.e.*, movement artifacts). Although important in PET studies, these effects can seriously confound the analysis of fMRI studies, where the slightest subvoxel movement can profoundly affect the signal. Our experience with this approach to fMRI realignment shows that movements on a scale of 10–100 μm can be detected and that this degree of movement can produce quite substantial changes in observed signal [11]. In fMRI there is a further movement-related component of signal variance that sometimes needs removal after realignment. This component is due to movement-dependent changes in spin-excitation history and will be discussed in Chapter 18.

B. Between Modality Registration

We have covered image realignment within the same modality. Now we discuss the coregistration of images of the same subject—but from different modalities. This section also introduces image segmentation as a prelude to solving coregistration problems. The algorithm described above will not perform well in coregistering (say) a T_1 MRI with a PET image, because there is not enough similarity between the two images. However, with some preprocessing of the MR image, coregistration becomes possible. We can do this by first partitioning the MR image and then recombining the partitions such that they emulate a PET image.

1. Image Segmentation

Healthy brain tissue can generally be classified into three broad tissue types on the basis of an MR image. These are grey matter (GM), white matter (WM), and cerebro-spinal fluid (CSF). This classification can be performed manually on a good quality T_1 image, simply by selecting suitable image intensity ranges that encompass most of the voxel intensities of a particular tissue type. However, this manual selection of thresholds is highly subjective, and manual editing of the resultant images is required to remove the scalp.

Many workers have used clustering algorithms to partition MR images into different tissue types, either using images acquired from a single MR sequence or combining information from two or more registered images acquired using different sequences (*e.g.*, T_1 and T_2). The approach we have adopted here is a modified version of one of these clustering algorithms. The clustering algorithm of choice is the maximum likelihood "Mixture Model" algorithm described in Hartigan [12].

We assume that the MR image (or images) consists of a few distinct tissue types (clusters) from which every voxel has been drawn. The intensities of voxels belonging to each of these clusters form a multivariate normal distribution that can be described by a mean vector, a covariance matrix, and the number of voxels belonging to the distribution.

In addition, we have approximate knowledge of the spatial distributions of these clusters, in the form of probability images (provided by the Montreal Neurological Institute [13–15]) that have been derived from MR images of many subjects. The original images were segmented into binary images of GM, WM, and CSF, and all normalized into the same space using a nine-parameter (three translations, three rotations, and three orthogonal zooms) affine transformation. The probability images are the means of these binary images, so they contain values between zero and one. These images represent the *a priori* probability of a voxel being either GM, WM, or CSF after an image has been normalised to a template of the same space as these images using a nine-parameter affine transformation.

We describe here a simplified version of the algorithm as it would be applied to a single image. We begin by determining a suitable mapping between the space of the MR image (**a**), and that of the probability images (**B**, where each column is a probability image). In practice, we use a 12-parameter affine transformation that allows simple "on-the-fly" sampling of the probability images into the space of the image we wish to partition (however, the algorithm does generate a slightly better classification if a nonlinear transformation is used). Generally, we use six or seven clusters: one each for GM, WM, and CSF, two or three clusters to account for scalp, eyes, *etc.*, and a background cluster.

Since we have no probability maps for scalp and background, we estimate them by subtracting $\mathbf{b}_{GM}$, $\mathbf{b}_{WM}$, and $\mathbf{b}_{CSF}$ from a map of all ones, and divide the results equally between the remaining clusters. We then assign initial probabilities for each of the M voxels being drawn from each cluster (**P**). These probabilities are based upon the *a priori* probabilities. The following steps (1 to 6) are repeated until convergence (or a prespecified number of iterations) is reached.

1. Compute the number of voxels belonging to each of the K clusters (**g**) as

$$g_k = \sum_{m=1}^{M} p_{mk}.$$

2. Mean voxel intensities for each cluster (**x**) are computed. This step effectively produces a weighted mean of the image voxels, where the weights are the current belonging probability estimates:

$$x_k = \frac{\sum_{m=1}^{M} p_{mk} a_m}{g_k}.$$

3. Then the variance of each cluster (**c**) is computed in a similar way to the mean:

$$c_k = \frac{\sum_{m=1}^{M} p_{mk}(a_m - x_k)}{g_k}.$$

Now that we have all the parameters that describe the current estimates of the distributions, we have to recalculate the belonging probabilities (P).

4. Compute the probability density functions for the clusters at each voxel:

$$r_{mk} = g_k(2c^k)^{-1/2} \exp\left(\frac{-(a_m - x_k)^2}{2c_k}\right).$$

5. Then use the *a priori* information (**B**) (this is the only deviation from the pure Mixture Model algorithm):

$$q_{mk} = \frac{r_{mk} b_{mk}}{\sum_{i=1}^{M} b_{ik}}.$$

6. And finally normalise the probabilities so that they integrate to unity at each voxel:

$$p_{mk} = \frac{q_{mk}}{\sum_{i=1}^{M} q_{mi}}.$$

With each iteration of the algorithm, the parameters describing the distributions (**x**, **c**, and **g**) move towards a better fit to the data. Conversely, the belonging probabilities (**P**) change slightly to reflect the new distributions. The parameters that describe the clusters that have corresponding *a priori* probability images tend to converge more rapidly than those for the other clusters—a fact that is partly due to the better starting estimates. The final values of **P** are in the range of zero to one, although most values tend to stabilise very close to one of the two extremes.

Strictly speaking, the assumption that multinormal distributions should be used to model MRI intensities is not quite correct. After Fourier reconstruction, the moduli of the complex pixel values are taken, thus rendering positive any potentially negative values. Where the cluster variances are of comparable magnitude to the cluster means, the distribution deviates significantly from normal. This is only really apparent for the background, where the true mean voxel intensity is zero. The algorithm is suitably modified to account for the discrepancy between the model and reality. For the background cluster, the value of x is set to zero before the variance c is computed. Assuming that the true mean should be zero, this is an appropriate modification.

The model assumes that each voxel contains tissue from only one of the underlying clusters. There are a few voxels which lie on the interface between different tissue types. These voxels contain a mixture of different tissues (an effect that is most obvious with T_1 segmentation at the interface between WM and CSF, where the voxels are misclassified as GM). These partial volume effects can be reduced by using very high resolution images. The greatest problem which the technique faces is image nonuniformity. The current algorithm assumes that the voxel values for GM (for example) have the same intensity distribution throughout the image. The nonstationary nature of MR image intensities from some scanners can lead to a significant amount of tissue misclassification. In those cases, a preliminary normalisation of images to correct for inhomogeneities due to scanner hardware effects should be performed.

2. Coregistration

Despite the problems mentioned above, the algorithm is reliable enough to partition images for use with PET (blood flow or FDG) to MRI coregistration. By assigning the GM segment a value of one, WM a value of about 0.3, and CSF a value of about 0.1, it is possible (with smoothing) to generate an image that resembles a PET image. It is then possible to apply any within-modality coregistration algorithm to determine the rigid body transformation that best matches a subject's PET and MR images. Alternatively, the image segments themselves can be used for coregistration by solving directly (and simultaneously) for the above coefficients (*i.e.*, fitting spatially a transformed PET image to a linear combination of the image segments). This procedure involves solving the following equation for **q** (where **f** and **g** refer to the tissue probabilities—**P**—derived above):

$$\left(\mathbf{g}_{\text{GM}} \quad \mathbf{g}_{\text{WM}} \quad \mathbf{g}_{\text{CSF}} \quad \frac{\partial \mathbf{f}}{\partial a_{11}} \quad \frac{\partial \mathbf{f}}{\partial a_{21}} \quad \cdots \right) \begin{pmatrix} u_{\text{GM}} \\ u_{\text{WM}} \\ u_{\text{CSF}} \\ q_1 \\ q_2 \\ \vdots \end{pmatrix} = \mathbf{f}.$$

It may be desirable to register a T_2 MR image with a T_1 image from one subject. Grey and white matter components can be segmented from each of these images. It should then be possible to register simultaneously the WM and GM segments from two images. This coregistration would involve iteratively solving the following sets of equations for $\mathbf{q}$:

$$\begin{pmatrix} \mathbf{g}_{GM} & 0 & \dfrac{\partial \mathbf{f}_{GM}}{\partial \mathbf{a}_{11}} & \dfrac{\partial \mathbf{f}_{GM}}{\partial \mathbf{a}_{21}} & \cdots \\[2ex] 0 & \mathbf{g}_{WM} & \dfrac{\partial \mathbf{f}_{WM}}{\partial \mathbf{a}_{11}} & \dfrac{\partial \mathbf{f}_{WM}}{\partial \mathbf{a}_{21}} & \cdots \end{pmatrix} \begin{pmatrix} u_{GM} \\ u_{WM} \\ q_1 \\ q_2 \\ \vdots \end{pmatrix} = \begin{pmatrix} \mathbf{f}_{GM} \\ \mathbf{f}_{WM} \end{pmatrix}.$$

Alternatively, since the values of $\mathbf{u}$ should all be approximately one, similar results should be obtained by solving

$$\begin{pmatrix} \dfrac{\partial \mathbf{f}_{GM}}{\partial \mathbf{a}_{11}} & \dfrac{\partial \mathbf{f}_{GM}}{\partial \mathbf{a}_{21}} & \cdots \\[2ex] \dfrac{\partial \mathbf{f}_{WM}}{\partial \mathbf{a}_{11}} & \dfrac{\partial \mathbf{f}_{WM}}{\partial \mathbf{a}_{21}} & \cdots \end{pmatrix} \begin{pmatrix} q_1 \\ q_2 \\ \vdots \end{pmatrix} = \begin{pmatrix} \mathbf{f}_{GM} - \mathbf{g}_{GM} \\ \mathbf{f}_{WM} - \mathbf{g}_{WM} \end{pmatrix}.$$

IV. NONLINEAR SPATIAL NORMALISATION

In this section we consider the general problem of spatial or stereotaxic transformation. Intersubject averaging of PET activation studies requires that all images be mapped into some standard space. We [8] suggested that this mapping can be effected by "matching" an individual's image with an ideal reference image, model, or template, where the template conforms to the standard space in question. The first step of spatial normalization is to determine the optimal affine transformation that will map a brain image ($\mathbf{f}$) to the template ($\mathbf{g}$). The method we use for this step is described above. Following the affine component, we need to correct for gross nonlinear differences between the shapes of the two brains. Without suitable constraints, this nonlinear correction would be very ill posed. The constraints we impose upon the defomations are that they should be smooth. Smoothness is achieved by forcing the deformations to consist of a linear combination of predefined smooth spatial basis functions. These basis functions can be thought of as smooth functions of, or profiles in, space that are (usually) chosen to be independent or orthogonal. The basis functions of choice for our implementation are the lowest frequency basis functions for the three-dimensional discrete cosine transform (DCT) (Fig. 1). Figure 2 illustrates how these deformation fields are applied.

Here we introduce the basic idea of how the coefficients for each basis function are computed. The technique assumes that a template image ($\mathbf{g}$) can be approximated by a scaled (by factor u) and spatially deformed version of the object image ($\mathbf{f}$). The best approximation for the deformation field is assumed to be that which minimises the sum of squares of the differences between $\mathbf{f}$ and $\mathbf{g}$. By constraining the deformations to consist of a linear combination of smooth basis images ($\mathbf{B}$, where each column is an image), the deformations themselves are forced to be smooth. Improvements to

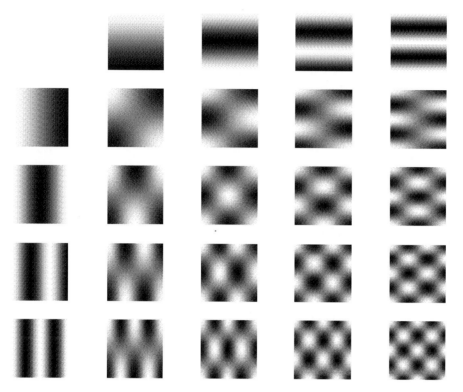

FIGURE 1 The lowest frequency basis images for a two-dimensional discrete cosine transform.

the estimation of the distortion field are made by iteratively computing $(\mathbf{A}^T\mathbf{A})^{-1}\mathbf{A}^T\mathbf{f}$, in order to determine the values of the vector $(\mathbf{t_x} \quad \mathbf{t_y} \quad u)^T$, where $\mathbf{t_x}$ and $\mathbf{t_y}$ are the required increments to the parameters for the (two-dimensional) deformation field $(\mathbf{Bt})$. The matrix $\mathbf{A}$ consists of $(\mathrm{diag}(\partial\mathbf{f}/\partial x)\mathbf{B} \quad \mathrm{diag}(\partial\mathbf{f}/\partial y)\mathbf{B} \quad \mathbf{g})$, where $\partial\mathbf{f}/\partial x$ and $\partial\mathbf{f}/\partial y$ are the numerical partial derivatives of the image $\mathbf{f}$. After each iteration, the image is regenerated by resampling from the original (using linear interpolation) according to the latest parameter estimates.

$\mathbf{A}$ is typically very large, so $\mathbf{A}^T\mathbf{A}$ and $\mathbf{A}^T\mathbf{f}$ need to be calculated on the fly in order to reduce computational memory requirements. Even so, the straightforward computation of these matrices is extremely time consuming. However, there are some "tricks" that enable this computation to be speeded up by several orders of magnitude. When the lowest frequency components of a two-dimensional DCT are used for the matrix of basis functions $(\mathbf{B})$, this matrix can be generated from the *Kronecker tensor product* of matrixes $\mathbf{B_x}$ and $\mathbf{B_Y}$ (where matrixes $\mathbf{B_x}$ and $\mathbf{B_Y}$ each perform one dimensional DCTs). This operation is usually denoted by $\mathbf{B} = \mathbf{B_Y} \otimes \mathbf{B_X}$ and expands to

$$\mathbf{B} = \begin{pmatrix} b_{Y11}\mathbf{B_X} & b_{Y12}\mathbf{B_X} & b_{Y13}\mathbf{B_X} & \ldots \\ b_{Y21}\mathbf{B_X} & b_{Y22}\mathbf{B_X} & b_{Y23}\mathbf{B_X} & \ldots \\ b_{Y31}\mathbf{B_X} & b_{Y32}\mathbf{B_X} & b_{Y33}\mathbf{B_X} & \ldots \\ \vdots & \vdots & \vdots & \ddots \end{pmatrix}.$$

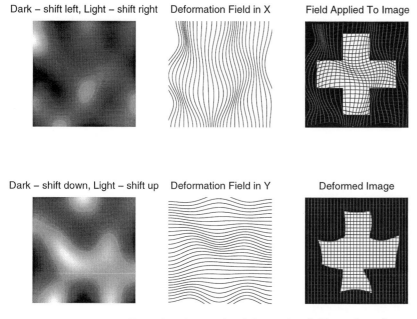

Dark – shift left, Light – shift right   Deformation Field in X   Field Applied To Image

Dark – shift down, Light – shift up   Deformation Field in Y   Deformed Image

FIGURE 2 For the two-dimensional case, the deformation field consists of two scalar fields. One for deformations in x, and the other for deformations in y. The images on the left show the deformation fields as a linear combination of the basis images. The center column shows them in a more intuitive sense. The deformation field is applied by overlaying it on the object image, and resampling (right).

There are many useful properties of Kronecker products that enable programmers to develop fast algorithms for operations that can be expressed in the correct form. The computation of $\mathbf{A}^T\mathbf{A}$ and $\mathbf{A}^T\mathbf{f}$ in the current implementation of spatial normalisation in *SPM96* is one such example.

When computing the parameters for a three-dimensional spatial normalisation, the matrix $\mathbf{A}$ may have about 376 columns. One column would be the template image, and there would be three blocks of columns for deformations in $\mathbf{x}$, $\mathbf{y}$, and $\mathbf{z}$. These 125 column blocks contain the basis images for the $5 \times 5 \times 5$ lowest frequency components of a three-dimensional DCT. An optimisation of this sort with 376 unknowns will not normally find a good solution. However, since the nonlinear deformations deviate only slightly from the affine, the algorithm is provided with good starting estimates, and a reasonable solution is found after only about five iterations (each iteration takes approximately 20 sec on a Sun SPARC 20).

There is no claim that this approach can register every sulcus of one brain to the exact location of another. For one reason, there is no one-to-one mapping between the highly variable structures of different brains. Additionally, the allowed deformations are constrained to be of low frequency, and so high resolution sulcus to sulcus matching cannot be achieved. The introduction of higher spatial frequency basis functions allows for potentially more accurate estimation of deformations. However, this accuracy is at the expense of slowing the algorithm and making it less stable. Part of the stability problem is that there is nothing to constrain the deformation fields to have a unique one to one correspondence from one space to the other. The use of smooth basis functions only reduces the likelihood of this constraint being broken

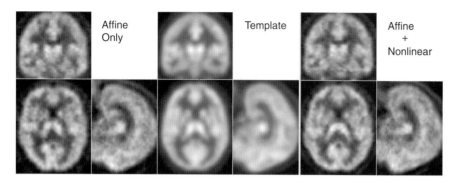

FIGURE 3 An example of nonlinear normalisation performed on a PET image. (Left) Affine transformation only. (Center) The template. (Right) The PET image after affine and nonlinear normalisation. The differences between the image on the left and that on the right are subtle. The most obvious improvement is in the shape of the frontal lobes.

(which occurs when the gradients of the deformation field are less than -1). As it stands, the method does ensure that each point in the space of the template maps to only one point in the space of the object image. However, the reverse is not true, and it is possible for the algorithm to produce deformation fields that loop back on themselves (Fig. 3).

A. Matching One Image to a Linear Combination of Templates

Another idea is that a given image can be matched not to one reference image, but to a series of images that all conform to the same space. The idea here is that (ignoring the spatial differences) any given image can be expressed as a linear combination of a set of reference images. For example these reference images might include different modalities (*e.g.*, PET, SPECT, [18F] DOPA, [18F] deoxyglucose, T_1-weighted MRI, T_2^*-weighted MRI, *etc.*) or different anatomical tissues (*e.g.*, grey matter, white matter, and CSF segmented from the same T_1-weighted MRI) or different anatomical regions (*e.g.*, cortical grey matter, subcortical grey matter, cerebellum, *etc.*) or finally any combination of the above. Any given image, irrespective of its modality could be approximated with a function of these images. Let the series of R reference images be denoted by $\mathbf{g}_R(\mathbf{x})$; then Eq. (2) becomes

$$(\mathbf{g}_1 \quad \mathbf{g}_2 \quad \cdots \quad \mathbf{g}_R \quad -\partial \mathbf{f}/\partial \mathbf{q})(u_1 \quad u_2 \quad \cdots \quad u_R \quad \mathbf{q})^T. \tag{3}$$

V. INTENSITY TRANSFORMATIONS

A related extension to the above approach involves matching the image $\mathbf{f}$ to a linear combination of functions of $\mathbf{g}$. For example in Eq. (3) above $\mathbf{g}_1$ could represent $\mathbf{g}^i$.

More generally one could solve

$$(c_0\{\mathbf{g}\} \quad c_1\{\mathbf{g}\} \quad \cdots \quad c_R\{\mathbf{g}\} - \partial \mathbf{f}/\partial \mathbf{q})(u_1 \quad u_2 \quad \cdots \quad u_R)^T \simeq \mathbf{f},$$

where the intensity transformation

$$c\{\mathbf{g}\} = u_1 c_0\{\mathbf{g}\} + u_2 c_1\{\mathbf{g}\} + \cdots + u_R c_R\{\mathbf{g}\} \tag{4}$$

is solved simultaneously with the spatial transformation. This extension speaks to a very general formulation of the spatial normalisation problem that explicitly embodies both an intensity and a spatial transformation:

$$c\{g(\mathbf{x})\} = f(\mathbf{h}(\mathbf{x}, \gamma)) + e(\mathbf{x}). \tag{5}$$

Note that Eq. (1) is a special case of this general equality where $c\{g(\mathbf{x})\} = ug(\mathbf{x})$. This formulation acknowledges that the differences between two images ($\mathbf{f}$ and $\mathbf{g}$) have two components. The first component is due to voxel value or intensity differences when two images are in perfect anatomical register. These differences may be artifactual (*e.g.*, different resolutions, or different methods of rCBF parameter estimation used for PET) or real (*e.g.*, reduced perfusion due to brain lesions, differences in global activity, or experimentally induced physiological activations). To model these intensity differences we assume that there is some function $c\{\bullet\}$ that transforms voxel values from one image to those of another (assuming perfect anatomical congruence). The second difference between two images is due to misalignment or differences in the shape and size of the brains. This spatial discrepancy between two scans is characterised by a vector function of position $\mathbf{h}(\mathbf{x}, \gamma)$. In short, Eq. (5) expresses the conjecture that two images can be approximated by applying an *intensity transformation* $c\{\bullet\}$ to one and a *spatial transformation* $\mathbf{h}(\mathbf{x}, \gamma)$ to the other.

Spatial dependence in the form of an intensity transformation can be modeled by simply expanding the coefficient u_i in Eq. (4) in terms of spatial basis functions (*e.g.*, **B**). For further details and application of this general approach see Friston *et al.* [11].

VI. APPLICATIONS

The applications of spatial transformations are numerous. Applications can be classified according to the goal of the transformation. The objectives of most transformations fall under three general headings:

   i. Reducing differences of a specific sort to facilitate comparison among images,
   ii. Characterisation of differences in spatial topography,
   iii. Image restoration and segmentation.

The examples above have focused on the first class of applications in the sense that image realignment and normalisation is usually done as a prelude to comparison among scans. The second class of applications asks "what are the important modes of anatomical (topographic) variation?" or "what are the anatomical differences between one set of scans and another?" The answers to both these questions depend on a complete specification of the spatial topography of each image. We have proposed that this specification could be in terms of the spatial distortion required to map an arbitrary image onto some reference [11]. For example, the topography of an image can be characterised in terms of coefficients corresponding to spatial basis functions. This simple list of coefficients, taken together with the reference image, is a complete specification of the topography of the original image (down to the resolution imposed by the basis functions). The importance of this observation is that anatomical topography can be characterised by a multivariate measure (the coefficients) and subjected to conventional multivariate statistics.

Important examples of this characterisation could include the normal modes of anatomical variability defined on a series of MRI scans from normal subjects. The exciting concept here is that once normal modes of anatomical variation are established they can then be used as the basis functions in the transformations. The charm of this "bootstrapping" is in constraining the transformations to lie in the space of normal anatomical variability. This capability would increase the face validity of the transformation and probably reduce the number of basis functions considerably. These modes are simply defined by singular value decompositions (SVD) of the spatial transformations (or the coefficients of the spatial basis functions).

A. Issues of Validity

The criteria for "good" spatial transformations can be framed in terms of validity, reliability, and computational efficiency. The validity of a particular transformation device is not easy to define or measure and indeed varies with the application. For example a rigid body transformation may be perfectly valid for realignment but not for spatial normalization of an arbitrary brain into a standard stereotactic space. Generally the types of validity that are important in spatial transformations can be divided into (i) *Face validity,* established by demonstrating the transformation does what it is supposed to, and (ii) *Construct validity,* assessed by comparison with other techniques or constructs. In functional mapping face validity is a complex issue. At first glance, face validity might be equated with the coregistration of anatomical homologues in two images. This would be complete and appropriate if the biological question referred to structural differences or modes of variation. In other circumstances, however, this definition of face validity is not appropriate. For example, the purpose of spatial normalisation (either within or between subjects) in functional mapping studies is to maximise the sensitivity to neurophysiological change elicited by experimental manipulation of sensorimotor or cognitive state. In this case a better definition of a valid normalisation is that which maximizes condition-dependent effects with respect to error (and if relevant, intersubject) effects. This aim will probably be effected when functional anatomy is congruent. This may or may not be the same as registering structural anatomy.

VII. SUMMARY

Prior to any statistical analysis within SPM, it is important that all the functional images (PET or fMRI) from each subject are aligned together. This step is performed by determining a rigid body transformation for each of the images which registers them to the first in the series. This step is a within modality procedure, and results in an optimisation of the parameters by minimising the residual sum of squares.

Often, it is desirable to register a structural image to the functional image series. Again this is a rigid body registration, but because the structural image is acquired in a different modality to the functional images, the registration cannot simply be performed by minimising the residual sum of squares. Within SPM, these between modality registrations are performed by first partitioning the images into CSF and grey and white matter and simultaneously registering the partitions together.

Images from several subjects can be analysed together by first normalising them all to the same space. In order to facilitate reporting of significant activations by their location within a standard coordinate system, this space is usually that described by Talairach and Tournoux [16]. Brains vary in shape and size so more parameters are needed to describe the spatial transformations. The spatial normalisation usually begins by determining the optimum 12-parameter affine transformation to register the brain with a template image. The template image is of the same modality as the image to be registered, so the optimisation is simply done by minimising the residual sum of squares. This 12-parameter transformation corrects for the variation in position and size of the image, before more subtle differences are corrected by a nonlinear registration. In order to reduce the number of parameters to be fitted, only smoothly varying deformations are corrected by the nonlinear registration. These deformations are modeled by a linear combination of smooth basis functions, and a fast optimization method has been developed to determine the best coefficients for each of the basis functions. Once the transformation parameters have been determined from one image, they can be applied to any other image which is in register with it.

References

1. H. Steinmetz and R. J. Seitz. Functional anatomy of language processing: Neuroimaging and the problem of individual variability. *Neuropsychologia* **29,** 1149–1160 (1991).
2. C. A. Pelizzari, G. T. Y. Chen, D. R. Spelbring, R. R. Weichselbaum, and C. T. Chen. Accurate three-dimensional registration of CT, PET and MR images of the brain. *J. Comput. Assist. Tomogr.* **13,** 20–26 (1988).
3. F. L. Bookstein. Principal warps: Thin-plate splines and the decomposition of deformations. *IEEE Trans. Pattern Anal. Machine Intelligence* **11,** 567–585 (1989).
4. N. M. Alpert, J. F. Bradshaw, D. Kennedy, and J. A. Coreia. The principal axis transformation—A method for image registration. *J. Nuclear Med.* **31,** 1717–1722 (1990).
5. R. P. Woods, S. R. Cherry, and J. C. Mazziotta. Rapid automated algorithm for aligning and reslicing PET images. *J. Comput. Assist. Tomogr.* **16,** 620–633 (1992).
6. D. L. Collins, P. Neeling, T. M. Peters, and A. C. Evans. Automatic 3D intersubject registration of MR volumetric data in standardized taliarach space. *J. Comput. Assist. Tomogr.* **18,** 192–205 (1994).
7. N. Lange. Some computational and statistical tools for paired comparisons of digital images. *Statist. Methods Med. Res.* **3,** 23–40 (1994).
8. K. J. Friston, C. D. Frith, P. F. Liddle, and R. S. J. Frackowiak. Plastic transformation of PET images. *J. Comput. Assist. Tomogr.* **15,** 634–639 (1991).
9. D. L. Collins, T. M. Peters, and A. C. Evans. "An Automated 3D Non-linear Image Deformation Procedure for Determination of Gross Morphometric Variability in Human Brain," pp. 180–190. Proceedings of Conference on Visualisation in Biomedical Computing, 1994.
10. Y. Kosugi, M. Sase, H. Kuwatani, N. Kinoshita, T. Momose, J. Nishikawa, and T. Watanabe. Neural network mapping for nonlinear stereotactic normalisation of brain MR images. *J. Comput. Assist. Tomogr.* **17,** 455–460 (1993).
11. K. J. Friston, J. Ashburner, C. D. Frith, J.-B. Poline, J. D. Heather, and R. S. J. Frackowiak. Spatial registration and normalization of images. *Hum. Brain Mapping* **2,** 165–189 (1995).
12. J. A. Hartigan. "Clustering Algorithms," pp. 113–129. Wiley, New York, 1975.
13. A. C. Evans, D. L. Collins, and B. Milner. An MRI-based stereotactic atlas from 250 young normal subjects. *Soc. Neurosci. Abstr.* **18,** 408 (1992).

14. A. C. Evans, D. L. Collins, S. R. Mills, E. D. Brown, R. L. Kelly, and T. M. Peters. 3D statistical neuroanatomical models from 305 MRI volumes. *In* "Proceedings, IEEE-Nuclear Science Symposium and Medical Imaging Conference," IEEE Inc., Piscataway, New Jersey, pp. 1813–1817. 1993.

15. A. C. Evans, M. Kamber, D. L. Collins, and D. Macdonald. An MRI-based probabilistic atlas of neuroanatomy. *In* "Magnetic Resonance Scanning and Epilepsy" (S. Shorvon, D. Fish, F. Andermann, G. M. Bydder, and H. Stefan, Eds.), NATO ASI Series A, Life Sciences, Vol. 264, pp. 263–274. Plenum, New York, 1994.

16. J. Talairach and P. Tournoux. "Coplanar Stereotaxic Atlas of the Human Brain." Thieme Medical, New York, 1988.

CHAPTER FOUR

CHARACTERISING BRAIN IMAGES WITH THE GENERAL LINEAR MODEL

I. INTRODUCTION

In the absence of prior anatomical hypotheses regarding the physical location of a particular function, the statistical analysis of functional mapping experiments must proceed by assessing the acquired data for evidence of an experimentally induced effect at every intracerebral voxel individually and simultaneously.

After reconstruction, realignment, stereotactic normalisation, and (possibly) smoothing, the data are ready for statistical analysis. This involves two steps. First, statistics indicating evidence against a null hypothesis of no effect at each voxel are computed. This procedure results in an "image" of statistics. Second, this statistic image must be assessed, reliably locating voxels where an effect is exhibited whilst controlling the probability of false positives. In this chapter we shall address the former topic.

Current methods for assessing the data at each voxel are predominantly parametric: specific forms of probability distribution are assumed for the data and hypotheses are specified in terms of models assumed for the (unknown) parameters of these distributions. The parameters are estimated, and a statistic reflecting evidence against the null hypothesis is formed. Statistics with known null distribution are used, such that the probability (under the null hypothesis) of obtaining a statistic as or more extreme than that observed can be computed. This is hypothesis testing in the classical parametric sense. The majority of the statistical models used are special cases of the general linear model.

SPM has become an acronym for the entire process of voxel based analysis of functional mapping experiments, for the software package implementing these processes, and for a statistic image (statistical parametric map). To avoid confusion we shall take SPM to refer to the software package.

II. THE GENERAL LINEAR MODEL

Before turning to the specifics of PET and fMRI, consider the general linear model. In what follows, an understanding of basic matrix algebra and the statistical concepts of hypothesis testing are required. Healy [1] presents a brief summary of matrix methods relevant to statistics. The statistically naive are directed towards Mould's excellent *Introductory Medical Statistics* [2], while the more mathematically experienced will find Chatfield's *Statistics for Technology* [3] useful. Draper and Smith [4] give a good exposition of matrix methods for the general linear model and go on to describe regression analysis in general. The definitive tome for practical statistical experimental design is Winer *et al.* [5].

A. The General Linear Model—Introduction

Suppose we are to conduct an experiment during which we will measure a *response variable* (such as regional cerebral blood flow (rCBF) at a particular voxel) Y_j, where $j = 1, \ldots, J$ indexes the observation. In statistical parlance, Y_j is a random variable, conventionally denoted by a capital letter.[1] Suppose also that for each observation we have a set of $L(L < J)$ *explanatory* variables (each measured without error) denoted by x_{jl}, where $l = 1, \ldots, L$ indexes the explanatory variables. The explanatory variables may be continuous (or sometimes discrete) covariates, functions of covariates, or they may be dummy variables indicating the levels of an experimental factor.

A *general linear model* explains the variation in Y_j in terms of a linear combination of the explanatory variables, plus an error term:

$$Y_j = x_{j1}\beta_1 + \cdots + x_{jl}\beta_l + \cdots + x_{jL}\beta_L + \epsilon_j. \tag{1}$$

Here the β_l are (unknown) parameters, corresponding to each of the L explanatory variables. The errors ϵ_j are assumed to be independent and identically normally distributed with zero mean and variance σ^2, written $\epsilon_j \overset{iid}{\sim} \mathcal{N}(0, \sigma^2)$. General linear models with other error distributions are generalised linear models, for which the acronym GLM is usually reserved. The use of the general linear model is also widely known as regression analysis.

1. Examples

Many classical parametric statistical procedures are special cases of the general linear model. The simplest example is linear regression, where only one continuous explanatory variable x_{1j} is measured for each observation. The model is usually written as

$$Y_j = \mu + x_{1j}\beta_1 + \epsilon_j, \tag{2}$$

where the unknown parameter μ is the Y "intercept," the expected value of Y at $x_1 = 0$. β_1 is the (unknown) regression slope. Here, $\epsilon_j \overset{iid}{\sim} \mathcal{N}(0, \sigma^2)$. This can be rewritten as a general linear model by the use of a dummy explanatory

---

[1] We talk of *random variables*, and of observations prior to their measurement, because classical (frequentist) statistics is concerned with what could have occurred in an experiment. Once the observations have been made, they are known, the residuals are known, and there is no randomness.

variable, an indicator variable x_{j1} whose values are all one:

$$Y_j = x_{1j}\mu + x_{2j}\beta_2 + \epsilon_j. \tag{3}$$

Similarly the two-sample t test: Suppose Y_{1j} and Y_{2j} are two independent groups of random variables; the two-sample t test assumes $Y_{qj} \overset{iid}{\sim} \mathcal{N}(\mu_q, \sigma^2)$, for $q = 1, 2$, and assesses the null hypothesis $\mathcal{H}:\mu_1 = \mu_2$. The standard statistical way of writing the model is

$$Y_{qj} = \mu_q + \epsilon_{qj}. \tag{4}$$

The q subscript on the μ_q indicates that there are two *levels* to the group *effect*, μ_1 and μ_2. Here, $\epsilon_{qj} \overset{iid}{\sim} \mathcal{N}(0, \sigma^2)$. This can be rewritten in the form of the general linear model using two dummy variables x_{1qj} and x_{2qj} as

$$Y_{qj} = x_{1qj}\mu_1 + x_{2qj}\mu_2 + \epsilon_{qj}, \tag{5}$$

which is of the form of Eq. (1) on reindexing for jq. Here x_{1qj} indicates that observation Y_{qj} is from the first group, taking the value 1 when $q = 1$ and 0 when $q = 2$. Similarly, $x_{2qj} = \begin{cases} 0 & \text{if } q = 1 \\ 1 & \text{if } q = 2 \end{cases}$.

B. Matrix Formulation

The general linear model can be succinctly expressed using matrix notation. Consider writing out Eq. (1) in full, for each observation j, giving a set of simultaneous equations,

$$Y_1 = x_{11}\beta_1 + \cdots + x_{1l}\beta_l + \cdots + x_{1L}\beta_L + \epsilon_1$$
$$\vdots = \vdots$$
$$Y_j = x_{j1}\beta_1 + \cdots + x_{jl}\beta_l + \cdots + x_{jL}\beta_L + \epsilon_j$$
$$\vdots = \vdots$$
$$Y_J = x_{J1}\beta_1 + \cdots + x_{Jl}\beta_l + \cdots + x_{JL}\beta_L + \epsilon_J,$$

which are equivalent to

$$\begin{pmatrix} Y_1 \\ \vdots \\ Y_j \\ \vdots \\ Y_J \end{pmatrix} = \begin{pmatrix} x_{11} & \cdots & x_{1l} & \cdots & x_{1L} \\ \vdots & & \vdots & & \vdots \\ x_{j1} & \cdots & x_{jl} & \cdots & x_{jL} \\ \vdots & & \vdots & & \vdots \\ x_{J1} & \cdots & x_{Jl} & \cdots & x_{JL} \end{pmatrix} \begin{pmatrix} \beta_1 \\ \vdots \\ \beta_j \\ \vdots \\ \beta_J \end{pmatrix} + \begin{pmatrix} \epsilon_1 \\ \vdots \\ \epsilon_j \\ \vdots \\ \epsilon_J \end{pmatrix},$$

of the form $\mathbf{Y} = X\boldsymbol{\beta} + \boldsymbol{\epsilon}$ for $\mathbf{Y}$ the column vector of observations, $\boldsymbol{\epsilon}$ the column vector of error terms, and $\boldsymbol{\beta}$ the column vector of parameters; $\boldsymbol{\beta} = [\beta_1 \cdots \beta_l \cdots \beta_J]^\top$. The $J \times L$ matrix X is the *design matrix*. This has one row per observation and one column per model parameter.

C. Estimation

Once an experiment has been completed, we have observations of the random variables Y_j, which we denote by y_j. Assuming that no two observations are equal and have identical explanatory variables, the number of parameters L is (usually) less than the number of observations J, and the simultaneous equations implied by the general linear model (with $\mathbf{\epsilon} = \mathbf{0}$) cannot be solved. Therefore, some method of estimating parameters that "best fit" the data is required. This is achieved by *least squares.*

Denote a set of parameter estimates by $\tilde{\mathbf{\beta}} = (\tilde{\beta}_1, \dots, \tilde{\beta}_L)^\top$. These parameters lead to *fitted values* $\tilde{\mathbf{Y}} = (\tilde{Y}_1, \dots, \tilde{Y}_J)^\top = X\tilde{\mathbf{\beta}}$, giving residual errors $\mathbf{e} = (e_1, \dots, e_J)^\top = \mathbf{Y} - \tilde{\mathbf{Y}} = \mathbf{Y} - X\tilde{\mathbf{\beta}}$. The *residual sum of squares* $S = \sum_{j=1}^{J} e_j^2 = \mathbf{e}^\top\mathbf{e}$ is the sum of the square differences between the actual and fitted values and thus measures the fit of the model with these parameter estimates.[2] The *least squares* estimates are the parameter estimates $\hat{\mathbf{\beta}}$ which minimise the residual sum of squares. In full:

$$S = \sum_{j=1}^{J} (Y_j - x_{j1}\tilde{\beta}_1 - \cdots - x_{jL}\tilde{\beta}_L)^2.$$

This is minimised when

$$\frac{\partial S}{\partial \tilde{\beta}_l} = 2 \sum_{j=1}^{J} (-x_{jl})(Y_j - x_{j1}\tilde{\beta}_1 - \cdots - x_{jL}\tilde{\beta}_L) = 0.$$

This equation is simply the jth row of $X^\top\mathbf{Y} = (X^\top X)\tilde{\mathbf{\beta}}$. Thus, the least squares estimates, denoted by $\hat{\mathbf{\beta}}$, satisfy the *normal equations*:

$$X^\top\mathbf{Y} = (X^\top X)\hat{\mathbf{\beta}}. \tag{6}$$

The least squares estimates are the *maximum likelihood estimates* (if the model is correct and the errors are normal) and are the *best linear unbiased estimates.*[3] That is, of all linear parameter estimates consisting of linear combinations of the observed data whose expectation is the true value of the parameters, the least squares estimates have the minimum variance.

If $(X^\top X)$ is invertible, which it is if and only if the design matrix X is of full rank, then the least squares estimates are

$$\hat{\mathbf{\beta}} = (X^\top X)^{-1} X^\top \mathbf{Y}. \tag{7}$$

D. Overdetermined Models

If X is not of full rank (it has linearly dependent columns), then the model is overdetermined. There are infinitely many parameter sets describing the same model. Correspondingly, there are infinitely many least squares estimates $\hat{\mathbf{\beta}}$ satisfying the normal equations.

---

[2] $\mathbf{e}^\top\mathbf{e}$ is the L_2 norm of $\mathbf{e}$.
[3] Gauss–Markov theorem.

1. One-Way ANOVA Example

The simplest example of such a model is the classic Q group one-way ANOVA model:

$$Y_{qj} = \mu + \alpha_q + \epsilon_{qj}, \tag{8}$$

where Y_{qj} is the jth observation in group $q = 1, \ldots, Q$. This model clearly does not uniquely specify the parameters. For any given μ and α_q, the parameters $\mu' = \mu + d$ and $\alpha'_q = \alpha_q - d$ give an equivalent model for any constant d. Similarly, for any set of least squares estimates $\hat{\mu}, \hat{\alpha}_q$. Here there is one degree of freedom in the model and the design matrix has rank Q, one less than the number of columns (the number of parameters). If the data vector $\mathbf{Y}$ has observations arranged by group, then for three groups ($Q = 3$), the design matrix and parameter vectors are

$$X = \begin{bmatrix} 1 & 1 & 0 & 0 \\ \vdots & \vdots & \vdots & \vdots \\ 1 & 1 & 0 & 0 \\ 1 & 0 & 1 & 0 \\ \vdots & \vdots & \vdots & \vdots \\ 1 & 0 & 1 & 0 \\ 1 & 0 & 0 & 1 \\ \vdots & \vdots & \vdots & \vdots \\ 1 & 0 & 0 & 1 \end{bmatrix} \quad \boldsymbol{\beta} = \begin{bmatrix} \mu \\ \alpha_1 \\ \alpha_2 \\ \alpha_3 \end{bmatrix}.$$

Clearly this matrix is rank deficient: the first column is the sum of the others.

2. Parameter Estimates

A set of least squares estimates may be found by imposing constraints on the estimates, or by using a pseudoinverse technique (which essentially implies a constraint). In either case it is important to remember that the actual estimates obtained depend on the particular constraint or pseudoinverse method chosen. This has implications for inference (see Section II.F); it is meaningful to consider only functions of the parameters that are independent of the particular constraint chosen.

3. Parameters for One-Way ANOVA Example

Consider the one-way ANOVA example. One possible constraint is $\hat{\mu} = 0$, effected by eliminating the first column of the design matrix, giving a design matrix of full rank. Then the least squares estimates are $\hat{\mu} = 0$, $\hat{\alpha}_q = \overline{Y}_{q\bullet}$, the mean of the group q observations.[4] Another constraint is a "sum-to-zero" constraint on the fitted group effects: $\sum_{q=1}^{Q} \hat{\alpha}_q = 0$.

This constraint implies that any one group's fitted effect is minus the sum of the others, so the constraint can be effected by expressing the effect for (say) the last group in terms of the others and eliminating it from the design. For three groups this gives $\hat{\alpha}_3 = -\hat{\alpha}_1 - \hat{\alpha}_2$, resulting in design matrix

---

[4] The standard statistical "bar and bullet" notation denotes that the mean has been taken over the values of the subscripts replaced by bullets.

X and parameter vector $\boldsymbol{\beta}$ as

$$
X = \begin{bmatrix} 1 & 1 & 0 \\ \vdots & \vdots & \vdots \\ 1 & 1 & 0 \\ 1 & 0 & 1 \\ \vdots & \vdots & \vdots \\ 1 & 0 & 1 \\ 1 & -1 & -1 \\ \vdots & \vdots & \vdots \\ 1 & -1 & -1 \end{bmatrix} \qquad \boldsymbol{\beta} = \begin{bmatrix} \mu \\ \alpha_1 \\ \alpha_2 \end{bmatrix}.
$$

In this case $\hat{\mu} = \Sigma_{j=1}^{Q}(\overline{Y}_{q\bullet})/Q$, the mean of the group means (equal to the overall mean $\overline{Y}_{\bullet\bullet}$ if all groups have equal size). The group effects are estimated by $\hat{\alpha}_q = \overline{Y}_{q\bullet} - \hat{\mu}$, the mean of the group q observations after the overall mean has been subtracted.

Alternatively, a pseudoinverse method can be used, using $\mathrm{pinv}(X^{\top}X)$ in place of $(X^{\top}X)^{-1}$ in Eq. (7). A set of least squares estimates are then given by $\hat{\boldsymbol{\beta}} = \mathrm{pinv}(X^{\top}X)X^{\top}\mathbf{Y} = \mathrm{pinv}(X)\mathbf{Y}$. The pseudoinverse function implemented in MATLAB gives the Moore–Penrose pseudoinverse.[5] This results in the least squares parameter estimates with the minimum sum of squares (minimum L_2 norm $\|\hat{\boldsymbol{\beta}}\|_2$). For the one-way ANOVA model, this can be shown to give parameter estimates $\hat{\mu} = \Sigma_{j=1}^{Q}(\overline{Y}_{q\bullet})/(1 + Q)$ and $\hat{\alpha}_q = \overline{Y}_{q\bullet} - \hat{\mu}$, a rather strange constraint!

By cunning construction of the design matrix, the Moore–Penrose pseudoinverse can be utilised to impose particular constraints. For example, reparameterising the one-way ANOVA model (Eq. (8)) by expressing the group effects relative to their mean results in the imposition of sum-to-zero constraints. The model is then

$$
Y_{qj} = \mu + (\alpha_q - \overline{\alpha}_q) + \epsilon_{qj}, \tag{9}
$$

with design matrix (for three groups)

$$
X = \begin{bmatrix} 1 & 1 - 1/3 & -1/3 & -1/3 \\ \vdots & \vdots & \vdots & \vdots \\ 1 & 1 - 1/3 & -1/3 & -1/3 \\ 1 & -1/3 & 1 - 1/3 & -1/3 \\ \vdots & \vdots & \vdots & \vdots \\ 1 & -1/3 & 1 - 1/3 & -1/3 \\ 1 & -1/3 & -1/3 & 1 - 1/3 \\ \vdots & \vdots & \vdots & \vdots \\ 1 & -1/3 & -1/3 & 1 - 1/3 \end{bmatrix} \qquad \boldsymbol{\beta} = \begin{bmatrix} \mu \\ \alpha_1 \\ \alpha_2 \\ \alpha_3 \end{bmatrix}.
$$

---

[5] If X is of full rank, then $\mathrm{pinv}(X^{\top}X)$ is an inefficient way of computing $(X^{\top}X)^{-1}$.

The least squares estimates using the Moore–Penrose pseudoinverse are then those of the sum-to-zero constraints considered above. The point to note here is that the design matrix still has a column for each effect, and has the same structure as the design matrix for the "plain" model. Thus, this implicit constraining is useful if one wishes to impose a particular constraint, but maintain the form of the design matrix. Implicit sum-to-zero constraints are used in SPM for subject effects, to give sensible adjusted values.

E. Geometrical Perspective

The vector of observed values $\mathbf{Y}$ defines a single point in $\mathscr{R}^J$, J-dimensional Euclidean space. $X\tilde{\boldsymbol{\beta}}$ is a linear combination of the columns of the design matrix X. The columns of X are J vectors, so $X\tilde{\boldsymbol{\beta}}$ for given $\tilde{\boldsymbol{\beta}}$ defines a point in $\mathscr{R}^J$. This point lies in the subspace of $\mathscr{R}^J$ spanned by the columns of the design matrix, the X space. The dimension of this subspace is rank (X). (Recall that the space spanned by the columns of X is the set of points $X\tilde{\boldsymbol{\beta}}$ for all $\tilde{\boldsymbol{\beta}} \in \mathscr{R}^L$.) The residual sum of squares for parameter estimates $\tilde{\boldsymbol{\beta}}$ is the distance from $X\hat{\mathbf{Y}}$ to $\mathbf{Y}$. Thus, the least squares estimates correspond to the point in the space spanned by the columns of X that is nearest to the data $\mathbf{Y}$. The perpendicular from $\mathbf{Y}$ to the X space meets the X space at $\hat{\mathbf{Y}} = X\hat{\boldsymbol{\beta}}$. It is now clear why there are no unique least squares estimates if X is rank-deficient; for then any point in the X space can be obtained as infinitely many linear combinations of the columns of X.

If X is of full rank, then define the *hat* matrix as $H = X(X^\top X)^{-1}X^\top$. Then $\hat{\mathbf{Y}} = H\mathbf{Y}$, and geometrically H is a projection onto the X space. Similarly, the residual forming matrix is $R = (I - H)$ for I the identity matrix. Thus $R\mathbf{Y} = \mathbf{e}$, and R is a projection onto the space orthogonal to the X plane.

As a concrete example, consider a simple linear regression with three observations. The observed datum $\mathbf{Y} = (Y_1, Y_2, Y_3)^\top$ defines a point in three-dimensional Euclidean space ($\mathscr{R}^3$). The model (Eq. (2)) leads to a design

matrix $X = \begin{bmatrix} 1 & x_1 \\ 1 & x_2 \\ 1 & x_3 \end{bmatrix}$. Provided that the x_js are not all the same, the columns

of X span a two-dimensional subspace of $\mathscr{R}^3$, a plane (Fig. 1).

F. Inference

1. Residual Sum of Squares

The residual variance σ^2 is estimated by the residual mean square, the residual sum of squares divided by the appropriate degrees of freedom:

$$\hat{\sigma}^2 = \frac{\mathbf{e}^\top \mathbf{e}}{J - p} \sim \sigma^2 \frac{\chi^2_{J-p}}{J - p}, \text{ where } p = \text{rank}(X).$$

2. Linear Combinations of the Parameter Estimates

It is not too difficult to show that the parameter estimates are normally distributed: for X of full rank $\hat{\boldsymbol{\beta}} \sim \mathscr{N}(\boldsymbol{\beta}, \sigma^2(X^\top X)^{-1})$. From this result it follows that for $\mathbf{c}$ a column vector of L weights

$$\mathbf{c}^\top \hat{\boldsymbol{\beta}} \sim \mathscr{N}(\mathbf{c}^\top \boldsymbol{\beta}, \sigma^2 \mathbf{c}^\top (X^\top X)^{-1}\mathbf{c}). \tag{10}$$

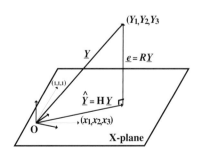

FIGURE 1 Geometrical perspective on three-point linear regression.

Furthermore, $\hat{\boldsymbol{\beta}}$ and $\hat{\sigma}^2$ are independent (Fisher's Law). Thus, prespecified hypotheses concerning linear compounds of the model parameters $\mathbf{c}^\top \boldsymbol{\beta}$ can be assessed using

$$\frac{\mathbf{c}^\top \hat{\boldsymbol{\beta}} - \mathbf{c}^\top \boldsymbol{\beta}}{\sqrt{\hat{\sigma}^2 \mathbf{c}^\top (X^\top X)^{-1} \mathbf{c}}} \sim t_{J-p} \tag{11}$$

That is, the hypothesis $\mathcal{H}: \mathbf{c}^\top \boldsymbol{\beta} = d$ can be assessed by comparing

$$T = (\mathbf{c}^\top \hat{\boldsymbol{\beta}} - d)/(\sqrt{\hat{\sigma}^2 \mathbf{c}^\top (X^\top X)^{-1} \mathbf{c}})$$

with a Student's t distribution with $J - p$ degrees of freedom.

3. Estimable Functions, Contrasts

Recall (Section II.D) that if the model is overdetermined (*i.e.*, X is rank deficient), then there are infinitely many parameter sets describing the same model. Constraints or the use of a pseudoinverse technique pull out only one set of parameters from infinitely many. Therefore, when examining linear compounds $\mathbf{c}^\top \boldsymbol{\beta}$ of the parameters it is imperative to consider only compounds that are invariant over the space of possible parameters. Such linear compounds are called contrasts.

In detail [6], a linear function $\mathbf{c}^\top \boldsymbol{\beta}$ of the parameters is estimable if there is a linear unbiased estimate $\mathbf{c}'^\top \mathbf{Y}$ for some constant vector of weights $\mathbf{c}'$. That is $\mathbf{c}^\top \boldsymbol{\beta} = \mathsf{E}[\mathbf{c}'^\top \mathbf{Y}]$, so for an estimable function the natural estimate $\mathbf{c}^\top \hat{\boldsymbol{\beta}}$ is unique whatever solution $\hat{\boldsymbol{\beta}}$ of the normal equations is chosen (Gauss–Markov theorem). Further, $\mathbf{c}^\top \boldsymbol{\beta} = \mathsf{E}[\mathbf{c}'^\top \mathbf{Y}] = \mathbf{c}'^\top X \boldsymbol{\beta} \Rightarrow \mathbf{c} = \mathbf{c}'^\top X$, so $\mathbf{c}$ is a linear combination of the rows of X.

A *contrast* is an estimable function with the additional property $\mathbf{c}^\top \hat{\boldsymbol{\beta}} = \mathbf{c}'^\top \hat{\mathbf{Y}} = \mathbf{c}'^\top \mathbf{Y}$. Now $\mathbf{c}'^\top \hat{\mathbf{Y}} = \mathbf{c}'^\top \mathbf{Y} \Leftrightarrow \mathbf{c}'^\top H\mathbf{Y} = \mathbf{c}'^\top \mathbf{Y} \Leftrightarrow \mathbf{c}' = H\mathbf{c}'$ (since H is symmetric), so $\mathbf{c}'$ is in the X space. Thus a contrast is an estimable function whose $\mathbf{c}'$ vector is a linear combination of the columns of X. Thus for a contrast it can be shown that $\mathbf{c}^\top \hat{\boldsymbol{\beta}} \sim \mathcal{N}(\mathbf{c}^\top \boldsymbol{\beta}, \sigma^2 \mathbf{c}'^\top \mathbf{c}')$. Using a pseudo-inverse technique, $H = X\text{pinv}(X^\top X)X^\top$, so $\mathbf{c}' = H\mathbf{c}' \Rightarrow \mathbf{c}'^\top \mathbf{c}' = \mathbf{c}'^\top X\text{pinv}(X^\top X)X^\top \mathbf{c}' = \mathbf{c}^\top \text{pinv}(X^\top X)\mathbf{c}$ since $\mathbf{c} = \mathbf{c}'^\top X$ for an estimable function.

The above shows that the distributional results given above for unique designs (Eqs. (10) and (11)) apply for contrasts of the parameters of nonunique designs, where $(X^\top X)^{-1}$ is replaced by a pseudoinverse.

It remains to characterise which linear compounds of the parameters are contrasts. For most designs, contrasts have weights that sum to zero over the levels of each factor. For the one-way ANOVA with parameter vector $\boldsymbol{\beta} = (\mu, \alpha_1, \ldots, \alpha_Q)^\top$, the linear compound $\mathbf{c}^\top \boldsymbol{\beta}$ with weights vector $\mathbf{c} = (c_0, c_1, \ldots, c_Q)$ is a contrast if $c_0 = 0$ and $\sum_{q=1}^Q c_q = 0$. Given that the indeterminacy in condition effects in this model is up to the level of an additive constant, the form of the contrast is intuitively correct. Contrasts of this form include no contribution from a constant added to all the condition effects. Other models and the form of appropriate contrasts are discussed in the next section (Section III).

4. Extra Sum of Squares Principle

The extra sum of squares principle provides a method of assessing general linear hypotheses and comparing models in a hierarchy. See Draper and Smith [4] for derivations and details.

Suppose we have a model with parameter vector $\boldsymbol{\beta}$ that can be partitioned into two, $\boldsymbol{\beta} = [\boldsymbol{\beta}_1^\top : \boldsymbol{\beta}_2^\top]$, and suppose we wish to test $\mathcal{H}: \boldsymbol{\beta}_1 = \mathbf{0}$. The corresponding partitioning of the design matrix X is $X = [X_1 : X_2]$, and the full model is

$$\mathbf{Y} = [X_1 \vdots X_2] \begin{bmatrix} \boldsymbol{\beta}_1 \\ \vdots \\ \boldsymbol{\beta}_2 \end{bmatrix} + \boldsymbol{\epsilon},$$

which when $\mathscr{H}$ is true reduces to the reduced model: $\mathbf{Y} = X_2\boldsymbol{\beta}_2 + \boldsymbol{\epsilon}$. Denote the residual sum of squares for the full and reduced models by $S(\boldsymbol{\beta})$ and $S(\boldsymbol{\beta}_2)$, respectively. The extra sum of squares due to $\boldsymbol{\beta}_1$ after $\boldsymbol{\beta}_2$ is then defined as $S(\boldsymbol{\beta}_1|\boldsymbol{\beta}_2) = S(\boldsymbol{\beta}_2) - S(\boldsymbol{\beta})$. Under $\mathscr{H}$, $S(\boldsymbol{\beta}_1|\boldsymbol{\beta}_2) \sim \sigma^2\chi_p^2$ independently of $S(\boldsymbol{\beta})$, where the degrees of freedom are $p = \text{rank}(X) - \text{rank}(X_2)$. (If $\mathscr{H}$ is not true, then $S(\boldsymbol{\beta}_1|\boldsymbol{\beta}_2)$ has a noncentral χ^2 distribution, still independent of $S(\boldsymbol{\beta})$.) Therefore, the following F statistic expresses evidence against $\mathscr{H}$:

$$F = \frac{(S(\boldsymbol{\beta}_2) - S(\boldsymbol{\beta}))/(p - p_2)}{S(\boldsymbol{\beta})/(J - p)} \sim F_{p-p_2, J-p}, \tag{12}$$

where $p = \text{rank}(X)$ and $p_2 = \text{rank}(X_2)$. Significance can then be assessed by comparing this with the appropriate F distribution.

G. Adjusted Values

Sometimes, designs may be partitioned into effects of interest ($\boldsymbol{\beta}_1$) and confounding effects ($\boldsymbol{\beta}_2$). It is then possible to adjust the observed data for the confounding effects, giving adjusted values $\tilde{\mathbf{Y}} = \mathbf{Y} - X_2\hat{\boldsymbol{\beta}}_2$.

III. MODELS FOR PET

With the details of the general linear model covered, we turn our attention to some actual models used in functional brain mapping and discuss the practicalities of their application. The terminology of SPM is introduced. As the approach is massively univariate, we must consider a model for each and every voxel. Bear in mind that in the massively univariate approach of SPM, the same model form is used at every voxel simultaneously, with different parameters for each voxel. This fact leads to the notion of image regression and a multivariate perspective on the massively univariate approach, which is covered in Section V. Model selection issues are raised in Section III.G.

We shall concentrate on PET, with its mature family of standard statistical experimental designs. fMRI requires extensions to the general linear model theory (presented below, in Section IV) and special design considerations (discussed in Chapter 18).

Although most PET functional mapping experiments are across subjects, many of the key concepts are readily demonstrated within the framework of a single subject experiment. Hence, for simplicity of exposition, the initial emphasis is on single subject experiments.

A. Global Changes

Global cerebral blood flow (gCBF) varies, both between subjects and over time in a single individual. If qualitative "count" measurements of relative activity (rA) are being used as an indicator of rCBF, then changes in the global activity gA reflect changes in the administered dose and head fraction as well as changes in gCBF. Therefore, changes in regional cerebral blood flow (or rA) measurements across experimental conditions (measured at different times and (possibly) pooled over subjects) are confounded by global changes.

In the remainder of this chapter, we shall refer to regional cerebral blood flow, regarding rA as an indicator of rCBF unless the discussion calls for a distinction.

Consider a simple single subject activation experiment, where a single subject is scanned repeatedly under both baseline (control) and activation (experimental) conditions. Inspection of rCBF alone at a single voxel may not indicate an experimentally induced effect, whereas consideration of gCBF for the respective scans may clearly differentiate between the two conditions (Fig. 2).

1. Measurement of gCBF

The global cerebral blood flow is adequately measured as the mean rCBF over all intracerebral voxels. If Y_j^k is the rCBF at voxel $k = 1, \ldots, K$ of scan j, then denote the gCBF by $g_j = \overline{Y}_j^\bullet = (\sum_{k=1}^K Y_j^k)/K$.

2. Proportional Scaling

Conceptually the simplest way to account for global changes is to adjust the data by scaling all scans to have the same gCBF, usually chosen to be 50 ml/min/dl. This gives adjusted rCBF at voxel k of $Y_j^k = Y_j^k/(g_j/50)$. The adjusted data are then used as raw data for analysis.

On a graph of rCBF against gCBF, the adjusted values are the point where the line joining the observed rCBF to the origin intercepts gCBF = 50 (Fig. 3a).

A single subject activation study would then be assessed using a two-sample t statistic on the adjusted rCBF at each voxel. Let Y_{qj}^k denote the adjusted rCBF at voxel k of scan $j = 1, \ldots, M$ under condition $q = 0, 1$. The model is then (from Eq. (4)): $Y_{qj}^{\prime k} = \alpha_q^k + \epsilon_{qj}^k$, where $\epsilon_{qj}^k \overset{iid}{\sim} \mathcal{N}(0, \sigma_k^2)$. Multiplying through by $g_j/50$ we arrive at

$$Y_{qj}^k = \frac{g_j}{50} \times \alpha_q^k + \epsilon_{qj}^{\prime k}. \tag{13}$$

This is a proportional regression (Fig. 3b). Activation corresponds to a change in slope. However, this is a weighted regression, since the residual variance is weighted by the global flow: $\epsilon_{qj}^{\prime k} \overset{iid}{\sim} \mathcal{N}(0, (g_j/50)^2 \times \sigma_k^2)$. Proportional scaling is not as simple as it first appears!

3. Modeling (ANCOVA)

A more rigorous approach is to explicitly model the effect of global changes. We [7] proposed that for normal ranges of cerebral blood flow the relationship between regional and global flow would be well approximated by a straight line. For repeat scans of an individual under exactly the same conditions, the model is a simple regression at each voxel,

$$Y_j^k = \mu^k + \zeta^k(g_j - \bar{g}_\bullet) + \epsilon_j^k, \tag{14}$$

where we assume normality of the errors, $\epsilon_q^k \overset{iid}{\sim} \mathcal{N}(0, \sigma_k^2)$. The error variance σ_k^2 is allowed to vary between voxels. There is substantial evidence against an assumption of constant variance (homoscedasticity) at all points of the brain. This fact is perhaps to be expected, considering the different constituents and activities of grey and white matter, which is unfortunate, as the small sample sizes leave few degrees of freedom for variance estimation. If homoscedasticity could be assumed, variance estimates could legitimately be pooled

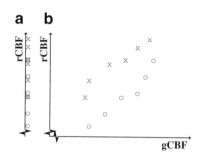

FIGURE 2 Single subject activation experiment, illustrative plots of rCBF at a single voxel: (a) dot-plots of rCBF, (b) plot of rCBF vs gCBF. Both plots indexed by condition: $\bigcirc$, baseline; $\times$, active.

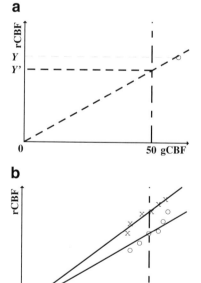

FIGURE 3 (a) Adjustment by proportional scaling. (b) Simple single subject activation as a t test on adjusted rCBF. Weighted proportional regression.

across all voxels. This would give an estimate with degrees of freedom sufficiently high that the variability of the estimate is negligible. *t* Statistics based on such a variance estimate are approximately normally distributed, the approximation failing only in the extreme tail of the distribution. This approach has been developed by Worsley *et al.* [8].

If the (mean corrected) global values are considered as confounding covariates, adjusted values at voxel k could be constructed as $Y_j'^k = Y_j^k - \hat{\zeta}^k(g_j - \bar{g}_\bullet)$. However, the modeling approach is to include gCBF explicitly as a covariate, not to use adjusted values as raw data.

Consider the simple single subject activation experiment, and suppose an activation experimental condition induces a constant increase of rCBF over the baseline condition regardless of gCBF. Then, the activation condition can be added to the model as a simple additive effect, giving an ANCOVA model (Fig. 4),[6]

$$Y_{qj}^k = \alpha_q^k + \zeta^k(g_{qj} - \bar{g}_\bullet) + \epsilon_{qj}^k, \tag{15}$$

where $\epsilon_{qj}^k \overset{iid}{\sim} \mathcal{N}(0, \sigma_k^2)$. Activation corresponds to a change in intercept.

4. Scaling verses Modeling

Clearly a choice must be made: scaling or ANCOVA. Many authors have debated this issue, yet still no consensus exists.

Due to the weighting of the variance in the proportional regression model, the "extra sum-of-squares" F test is inappropriate for comparing a proportional regression with a more general linear regression for repeat scans on a single individual under identical conditions (*i.e.*, comparing the model of Eq. (13) for one condition with that of Eq. (14)).

For normal subjects under normal conditions the range of gCBF exhibited is small and located far from zero. Therefore, for quantitative rCBF data on normal subjects under normal conditions, a simple regression model affords better modeling of the true relationship between regional and global flows than a proportional regression.

If qualitative "count" measurements are being used as indicators of rCBF, then gA can vary considerably even if the actual gCBF is fairly stable. Possible reasons for this are differences in introduced dose, scanner sensitivity, subject head fraction, or similar. Clearly, for constant gCBF the relationship between regional and global activity is proportional. More importantly, the greater the introduced dose, the greater the variance in the regional activity (since this is Poisson in nature), again suggesting the appropriateness of the proportional model. In this case proportional scaling also stabilises the variance. The variance stabilising properties of the proportional scaling approach is the only substantial reason for not using ANCOVA type modeling approaches.

For a single subject activation study, provided that the introduced dose is constant, the ANCOVA model is preferred over proportional scaling and two sample *t* test even for "count" data. There is little evidence against the "parallel lines" assumption of an additive activation effect. For multisubject experiments on the same scanner using the same protocol and dosage, current experience is that the ANCOVA style approach is adequate. Recent authors have found little empirical difference between parallel analyses using proportional scaling and ANCOVA on the same data.

---

[6] ANCOVA is the standard way to account for an (independent) confounding covariate in a two sample problem.

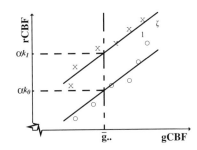

Figure 4 Single subject activation experiment, illustrative plot of ANCOVA model (Eq. (15)) for rCBF *vs* gCBF.

Special considerations apply if there are condition dependent changes in gCBF.

5. Global Differences

Implicit in allowing for changes in gCBF (either by proportional scaling or ANCOVA) when assessing condition specific changes in rCBF is the assumption that gCBF is independent of condition. Clearly, since gCBF is calculated as the mean intracerebral rCBF, an increase of rCBF in a particular brain region must cause an increase of gCBF unless there is a corresponding decrease of rCBF elsewhere in the brain. Similar problems can arise when comparing a group of subjects with a group of patients with brain atrophy, or when comparing pre- and postoperative rCBF.

If gCBF is increased by a large activation that is not associated with a corresponding deactivation, then comparison at a common gCBF will make nonactivated regions (whose rCBF remained constant) appear falsely deactivated, and the magnitude of the activation will be similarly decreased. (Figure 5a illustrates the scenario for a simple single subject activation experiment using ANCOVA.) In such circumstances a better measure of background change should be sought, for instance by examining the flow in brain regions known to be unaffected by the stimulus.

If gCBF actually varies considerably between conditions, as in pharmacological activation studies, then testing for a condition effect after allowing for global changes involves extrapolating the relationship between regional and global flow outside the range of the data. This extrapolation might not be valid, as illustrated in Fig. 5b.

B. Adjusted Data

Adjusted rCBF data are useful for illustrative plots of the nature of an effect, confounding effects having been removed. Therefore SPM partitions the model parameters (at each voxel) into effects of interest (β_1^k) and effects of no interest (β_2^k), with corresponding partitioning of the design matrix. Adjusted data are then computed as $\mathbf{Y}^k - X_2\hat{\beta}_2^k$. Since the gCBF is entered mean corrected (a centered covariate), the adjustment is to the mean gCBF of $\bar{g}_{\bullet}$. For qualitative count data, the entire dataset is usually scaled such that the mean global activity is 50, the nominal gCBF value, thus putting the adjusted data in the correct physiological scale.

C. Models

In the following sections, possible models for PET functional mapping experiments are presented. In describing the models used for various experiments, ANCOVA style models shall be used, with gCBF included as a confounding covariate. The corresponding ANOVA models for data adjusted by proportional scaling can be obtained by omitting the global terms. Voxel level models are presented in the usual statistical notation, alongside the SPM description and example design matrix "images." The form of contrasts for each design are indicated, and some practicalities of the SPM interface are discussed.

a

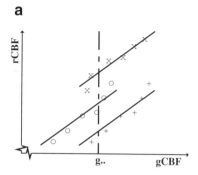

b

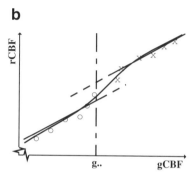

FIGURE 5 Single subject activation experiment, illustrative (ANCOVA) plots of rCBF *vs* gCBF at a single voxel showing potential problems with global changes: (a) Large activation inducing increase in gCBF. ○, Rest; ×, active condition values if this is a truly activated voxel (in which case the activation is underestimated); +, active condition values were this voxel not activated (in which case an apparent deactivation is seen). (b) Large change in gCBF between conditions. The apparent activation relies on linear extrapolation of the baseline and active condition regressions (assumed to have the same slope) beyond the range of the data. The actual relationship between regional and global for no activation may be given by the curve, in which case there is no activation effect.

D. Single Subject Models

1. Single Subject Activation Design

The simplest experimental paradigm is the simple single subject activation experiment. The ANCOVA model for this design was discussed in the previous section on global normalisation. This model extends to more than two conditions in the obvious way. Suppose there are Q conditions, with M_q scans under condition Q. Let Y_{qj}^k denote the rCBF at voxel k in scan $j = 1$, ..., M_q under condition $q = 1, ..., Q$. The model is

$$Y_{qj}^k = \alpha_q^k + \zeta^k(g_{qj} - \bar{g}_{\bullet\bullet}) + \epsilon_{jq}^k. \tag{16}$$

There are $Q + 1$ parameters, the Q condition effects (of interest), and the global regression effect (of no interest), giving parameters $\boldsymbol{\beta}^k = (\alpha_1^k, ...,$ $\alpha_Q^k, \zeta^k)^\top$. In this model, replications of the same condition are modeled with a single effect. This leaves $N - Q - 1$ residual degrees of freedom, for $N = \Sigma\, M_q$ the total number of scans.

Allowable contrasts are linear compounds $\mathbf{c}^\top \boldsymbol{\beta}^k$ for which the weights sum to zero over the condition effects; *i.e.*, $\Sigma_{q=1}^Q c_q = 0$. For example, to test $\mathcal{H}^k : \alpha_1^k = (\alpha_2^k + \alpha_3^k)/2$ against the one sided alternative $\overline{\mathcal{H}}^k : \alpha_1^k >$ $(\alpha_2^k + \alpha_3^k)/2$, appropriate contrast weights would be $\mathbf{c} = (1, -\frac{1}{2}, -\frac{1}{2}, 0, ..., 0)^\top$. The global regression parameter is uniquely determined, and its value could be assessed using contrast weights $\mathbf{c} = (0, ..., 0, 1)^\top$. However, the global confound is of no interest. SPM partitions the design into effects of interest and (confounding) effects of no interest and only prompts for contrast weights for the effects of interest (in this case requesting a Q vector). Further, SPM ensures that the weights given specify a contrast by subtracting their mean.

2. Design Matrix "Images"

Throughout SPM, linear models are represented by grayscale "images" of the design matrix used. Together with the list of scans, this image specifies the model at a glance. (Clearly the ordering of the scans is important, since each row of the design matrix corresponds to a particular scan. Reordering the rows gives the same model provided the scans are similarly reordered.)

A design matrix image for a single subject activation study with four scans under each of three conditions is shown in Fig. 6. The first three columns contain indicator variables (with values zero and one) indicating the condition. The last column contains the respective (mean corrected) gCBF values. The scans corresponding to this design matrix have been ordered such that all the scans for each condition appear together. Obviously the actual experiment would be carried out with a suitably randomised condition presentation order.

In the greyscale design matrix images, -1 is black, 0 mid-gray, and $+1$ white. Columns containing covariates are scaled by subtracting the mean (zero for centered covariates) and dividing the resulting values by their absolute maximum, giving values in $[0,1]$. (Design matrix blocks containing factor by covariate interactions (Section III.D.6) are scaled such that the covariate values lie in $[0,1]$, thus preserving the "padding" zeros' representation as mid-grey.)

3. Single Subject Parametric Design

Consider the single subject parametric experiment where a single covariate of interest, or "score," is measured. For instance, the covariate may be a physiological variable, a task difficulty rating, or a performance score. It is

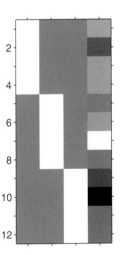

FIGURE 6 Example design matrix "image" for a three-way ANCOVA design for a single subject activation experiment of four scans in each of three conditions.

desired to find regions where the rCBF values are highly correlated with the covariate, taking into account the effect of global changes. Figure 7a depicts the situation. If Y_j^k is the rCBF at voxel k of scan $j = 1, \ldots, J$ and s_j is the independent covariate, then a simple ANCOVA style model is a multiple regression with two covariates:

$$Y_j^k = \mu^k + \varrho^k(s_j - \bar{s}_\bullet) + \zeta^k(g_j - \bar{g}_\bullet) + \epsilon_j^k. \tag{17}$$

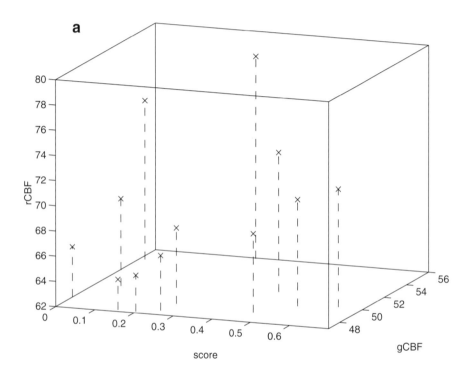

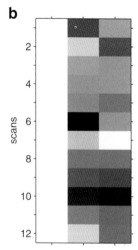

FIGURE 7 Single subject parametric experiment (Section III.D.3): (a) Plot of rCBF *vs* score and gCBF. (b) Design matrix "image" for Eq. (17), illustrated for a 12-scan experiment.

Here, ϱ is the slope of the regression plane in the direction of increasing score. In SPM this is a "single subject: covariates only" design. The design is uniquely specified, so any linear combination of the three parameters is a contrast. SPM designates ϱ as the only effect of interest, so only a single contrast weight is requested. The only sensible options are $+1$ (for rCBF increasing with score) and -1 (for rCBF decreasing as the score increases). There are three model parameters, leaving $J - 3$ residual degrees of freedom. The design matrix (Fig. 7b) has three columns, a column of 1s corresponding to μ^k and two columns containing the (mean corrected) score and global covariates.

This simple model assumes a linear relationship between rCBF and the covariate (and other explanatory variables). More general relationships may be modeled by including other functions of the covariate. These functions of the covariate are essentially new explanatory variables, which if linearly combined still fit in the framework of the general linear model. For instance, if an exponential relationship is expected, $\ln(s_j)$ would be used in place of s_j. Fitting powers of covariates as additional explanatory variables leads to polynomial regression. In this chapter, we shall restrict our attention to simple linear relationships.

4. Simple Single Subject Activation Revisited

As discussed in the general linear modeling section (Section II), it is often possible to reparameterise the same model in many ways. As an example, consider a simple (two condition, $Q = 2$) single subject activation experiment. The model (Eq. (16)) may be rewritten with an overall mean as

$$Y_{qj}^k = \mu^k + \alpha_q^k + \zeta^k(g_{qj} - \bar{g}_{\bullet\bullet}) + \epsilon_{jq}^k. \tag{18}$$

Now the model is overdetermined, and we see why attention must be restricted to contrasts whose weights sum to zero over levels of the condition effects α_q^k. Consider a sum-to-zero constraint on the condition effects. For two conditions this implies $\alpha_1^k = -\alpha_2^k$. Substituting for α_2^k, the resulting design matrix has a column of ones for the overall mean, a column containing $+1$s and -1s indicating the condition $q = 1$ or $q = 2$, respectively, and a column containing the (centered) gCBF. The corresponding parameter vector is $\boldsymbol{\beta}^k = (\mu^k, \alpha_1^k, \zeta^k)^\top$. An example design matrix image is shown in Fig. 8. Clearly this is the same design matrix as that for a parametric design with score covariate indicating the condition as active or baseline with $+1$ or -1, respectively.[7] The hypothesis of no activation at voxel k, $\mathcal{H}^k: \alpha_1^k = 0$ can be tested against the one-sided alternatives $\overline{\mathcal{H}}^k: \alpha_1^k > 0$ (activation) and $\overline{\mathcal{H}}^k: \alpha_1^k < 0$ with contrast weights $(0, 1, 0)$ and $(0, -1, 0)$, respectively. This example illustrates how the SPM interface may be used to enter "hand-built" blocks of design matrix as noncentered covariates.

5. Single Subject: Conditions and Covariates

Frequently there are other confounding covariates in addition to gCBF that can be added into the model. In SPM these appear in the design matrix as an additional covariate column adjacent to the global flow column. Care must be taken to enter the covariates in the same order that the scans were specified. As a simple example, a linear time component could be modeled simply by entering the scan number as covariate.

---

[7] In SPM94 this was how simple single subject activation studies were routinely entered.

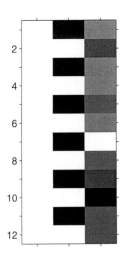

FIGURE 8 Example design matrix "image" for single subject simple activation experiment with 6 scans in each of two conditions, formulated as a parametric design (Eq. (18), Section III.D.4). The 12 scans are ordered alternating between baseline and activation conditions.

6. Factor by Covariate Interactions

A more interesting experimental scenario is when a parametric design is repeated under multiple conditions in the same subject(s). A specific example would be a PET language experiment in which, during each of 12 scans, lists of words are presented. Two types of word list (the two conditions) are presented at each of six rates (the parametric component). This is a "factor by covariate" design. Interest may lie in locating regions where there is a difference in rCBF between conditions (accounting for changes in presentation rate), the *main* effect of condition; locating regions where rCBF increases with rate (accounting for condition), the main effect of rate; and possibly assessing evidence for condition specific responses in rCBF to changes in rate, an interaction effect.[8] Let Y_{qrj}^k denote the rCBF at voxel k for the jth measurement under rate $r = 1, \ldots, R$ and condition $q = 1, \ldots, Q$, with s_r the rate covariate (some function of the rates). A suitable model is

$$Y_{qrj}^k = \alpha_q^k + \varrho_q^k(s_{qr} - \bar{s}_{\bullet\bullet}) + \zeta^k(g_{qrj} - \bar{g}_{\bullet\bullet\bullet}) + \epsilon_{qrj}^k. \tag{19}$$

Note the q subscript on the voxel covariate effect parameter ϱ_q^k. Ignoring for a moment the global flow, the model describes two simple regressions with common error variance (Fig. 9a). The SPM interface describes such factor by covariate interactions as "factor specific covariate fits." The interaction between condition and covariate effects is manifest as different regression slopes for each condition. There are Q condition effects, Q covariate parameters, one for each condition, and one global regression parameter, giving five degrees of freedom for the two-condition example. A design matrix image for the two-condition example is shown in Fig. 9b. The factor by covariate interaction takes up the third and fourth columns, corresponding to the parameters ϱ_1^k

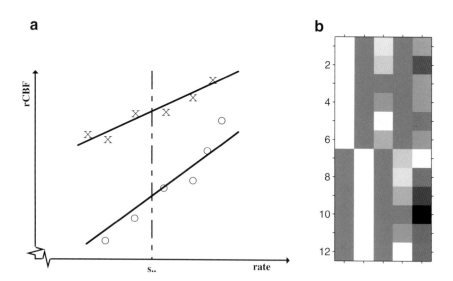

a

b

FIGURE 9 Single subject experiment with conditions, covariate, and condition by covariate interaction (Section III.D.6): (a) Illustrative plot of rCBF *vs* score. (b) Design matrix "image" for Eq. (19). Both illustrated for the two-condition 12-scan experiment described in the text. The scans have been reordered by condition.

[8] Two experimental factors *interact* if the level of one affects the expression of the other.

and ϱ_2^k, the covariate being split between the columns according to condition; the remaining cells are filled with zeros.

As with the activation study model, contrasts have weights which sum to zero over the condition effects. In the present example there are $2Q$ effects of interest, the Q condition effects, and the Q covariate parameters, so SPM prompts for contrast weight vectors of length $2Q$, the first Q weights corresponding to the condition effects. For the two-condition word presentation example, contrast weights $[0\ 0\ 1\ 0]$ assess the hypothesis that there is no covariate effect in condition one, with large values indicating evidence of a positive covariate effect. Weights $[0\ 0\ \frac{1}{2}\ \frac{1}{2}]$ address the hypothesis that there is no average covariate effect across conditions, against the one-sided alternative that the average covariate effect is positive. Weights $[0\ 0\ -1\ +1]$ address the hypothesis that there is no condition by covariate interaction, that is, that the regression slopes are the same, against the alternative that the condition two regression is steeper.

Conceptually, weights $[-1\ +1\ 0\ 0]$ and $[+1\ -1\ 0\ 0]$ assess the hypothesis of no condition effect against appropriate one-sided alternatives. However, the comparison of main effects is confounded in the presence of an interaction: In the above model, both gCBF and the rate covariate were centered, so the condition effects α_q^k are the heights of the respective regression lines at the mean gCBF and mean rate covariate. Clearly if there is an interaction, then any differences in the condition effects (the separation of the two regression lines) depends on where you look at them. Were the rate covariate not centered, the comparison would be at mean gCBF and zero rate, possibly yielding a different result.

Thus main effects of condition in such a design must be interpreted with caution. If there is little evidence for a condition dependent covariate effect then there is no problem. Otherwise, the relationship between rCBF and other design factors should be examined to assess whether the perceived condition effect is sensitive to the level of the covariate.

E. Multisubject Designs

Frequently, experimentally induced changes of rCBF are subtle, such that analyses must be pooled across subjects to find statistically significant evidence of an experimentally induced effect. Further, (for appropriate models) the use of samples of subjects allows inference to be extended to the population from which they were sampled.

The simple single subject designs presented above must be extended to account for the effect of individual subjects. The simplest type of subject effect is an additive effect, a block effect in the parlance of experimental design. That is, all subjects respond in the same way, save for an overall shift in rCBF (at each voxel). We extend our notation by adding subscript i for subjects, so Y_{iqj}^k is the rCBF at voxel k of scan j under condition q on subject $i = 1, \ldots, N$.

1. Multisubject Activation (Replications)

For instance, the single subject activation model (Eq. (16)) is extended by adding subject effects γ_i^k, giving

$$Y_{iqj}^k = \alpha_q^k + \gamma_i^k + \zeta^k(g_{iqj} - \bar{g}_{\bullet\bullet\bullet}) + \epsilon_{iqj}^k. \tag{20}$$

A schematic plot of rCBF *vs* gCBF for this model is shown in Fig. 10a. In SPM terminology, this is a "multisubject: replication of conditions" design. The parameter vector at voxel k is $\boldsymbol{\beta}^k = (\alpha_1^k, \ldots, \alpha_Q^k, \gamma_1^k, \ldots, \gamma_N^k, \zeta^k)^\top$. The design matrix (Fig. 10b) has Q columns corresponding to the subject effects, each containing a (1) for scans for that subject. (Similarly a multisubject parametric design could be derived from the single subject case (Section III.D.3) by including appropriate additive subject effects.)

In this case it is clear that the model is overdetermined. Adding a constant to each of the condition effects and subtracting it from each of the subject effects gives the same model. Bearing this in mind, it is clear that contrasts must have weights that sum to zero over both the subject effects and the condition effects. Subject effects are designated as confounding and not of interest, so SPM prompts only for contrast weights for the Q condition effects.

2. Condition by Replication Interactions

The above model assumes that (accounting for global and subject effects) replications of the same condition give the same (expected) response. There are many reasons why this assumption may be inappropriate, such as time effects or learning effects. Time effects can be modeled by including appropriate functions of the scan number as confounding covariates. With multisubject designs we have sufficient degrees of freedom available to enable the consideration of replication by condition interactions. Such interactions imply that the (expected) response to each condition is different between replications (having accounted for other effects in the model). Usually in statistical models, interaction terms are added to a model containing main effects. However, such a model is so overdetermined that the main effects may be omitted, leaving just the interaction terms. The model is

$$Y_{iqj}^k = \alpha\vartheta_{(qj)}^k + \gamma_i^k + \zeta^k(g_{iqj} - \bar{g}_{\bullet\bullet\bullet}) + \epsilon_{iqj}^k, \tag{21}$$

where $\alpha\vartheta_{(qj)}^k$ is the interaction effect for replication j of condition q, the condition-by-replication effect. As with the previous model, this model is overdetermined (by one degree of freedom), and contrasts must have weights which sum to zero over the condition-by-replication effects. There are as many of these condition-by-replication terms as there are scans per subject. (An identical model is arrived at by considering each replication of each experimental condition as a separate condition.) If the scans are reordered such that the jth scan corresponds to the same replication of the same condition in each subject, then the condition-by-replication corresponds to the scan number. With this feature in mind it is usually simplest to reorder scans when using such a model. An example design matrix for five subjects scanned 12 times is shown in Fig. 11, where the scans have been reordered. In SPM this is termed a multisubject: conditions only design.

This is the "classic" SPM ANCOVA we described in 1990 [7] and implemented in the original SPM software. It offers great latitude for specification of contrasts. Appropriate contrasts can be used to assess main effects, specific forms of interaction, and even parametric effects. For instance, consider the verbal fluency data set described by Friston *et al.* [9]. Five subjects were scanned 12 times, 6 times under each of two conditions, word shadowing (condition A) and intrinsic word generation (condition B). The scans were reordered to ABABABABABAB for all subjects. (The actual condition presentation order was randomly allocated for each subject in blocks of two scans. That is, successive pairs of scans were chosen as AB or BA on the toss of a

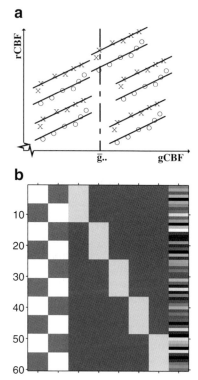

FIGURE 10 Multisubject activation experiment, replication of conditions (Section III.E.1), model Eq. (20). Illustrations for a five subject study, with six replications of each of two conditions per subject: (a) Illustrative plot of rCBF *vs* gCBF. (b) Design matrix "image": The first two columns correspond to the condition effects, the next five to the subject effects, the last to the gCBF regression parameter. The design matrix corresponds to scans ordered by subject and by condition within subjects.

coin.) Then a contrast with weights (for the condition-by-replication effects) of $(-1, 1, -1, 1, -1, 1, -1, 1, -1, 1, -1, 1)$ assesses the hypothesis of no main effect of word generation (against the one-sided alternative of activation). A contrast with weights of $(5\frac{1}{2}, 4\frac{1}{2}, 3\frac{1}{2}, 2\frac{1}{2}, 1\frac{1}{2}, \frac{1}{2}, -\frac{1}{2}, -1\frac{1}{2}, -2\frac{1}{2}, -3\frac{1}{2}, -4\frac{1}{2}, -5\frac{1}{2})$ is sensitive to linear decreases in rCBF over time, independent of condition, and accounting for subject effects and changes in gCBF. A contrast with weights of $(+1, -1, +1, -1, +1, -1, -1, +1, -1, +1, -1, +1)$ assesses the interaction of time and condition, subtracting the activation in the first half of the experiment from that in the latter half.

3. Interactions with Subject

It is also possible to consider interactions with the subject effect. While it is usually reasonable to use ANCOVA style models to account for global flow, with regression parameter constant across conditions, the multisubject models considered thus far assume that this regression parameter is constant across subjects. It is quite possible that rCBF at the same location for different subjects will respond differentially to changes in gCBF—a subject by gCBF covariate interaction. The gCBF regression parameter can be allowed to vary by subject. Extending the multisubject activation (replication) model (Eq. (20)) in this way gives

$$Y_{iqj}^k = \alpha_q^k + \gamma_i^k + \zeta_i^k(g_{iqj} - \bar{g}_{\bullet\bullet\bullet}) + \epsilon_{iqj}^k. \tag{22}$$

A schematic plot of rCBF vs gCBF for this model and an example design matrix image are shown in Fig. 12. In the terminology of the SPM interface, this is an "ANCOVA by subject." The additional parameters are of no interest, and contrasts are as before.

Similarly, the SPM interface allows subject by covariate interactions, termed "subject specific fits." Currently, SPM does not allow subject by condition interactions. If the parameters of interest are allowed to interact with subject effects, then account must be taken of variation between subjects. Essentially, the subject effects are *random effects*, since subjects are sampled from some population about which we wish to infer. In all the models considered thus far, the relevant variation is within subjects, and the variation of the subject effects can be ignored. A rigorous discussion of such *mixed effects* models is beyond the scope of this chapter. For details, see any intermediate level statistical treatment of the design of experiments.

F. Multistudy Designs

The last class of SPM models we consider are the "multistudy" models. In these models, subjects are grouped into two or more studies. The multistudy designs fit seperate condition effects for each study. In statistical terms this is a split plot design. As an example consider two multisubject activation studies, the first with five subjects scanned 12 times under two conditions (as described above in Section III.E.1), the second with three subjects scanned 6 times under three conditions. An example design matrix image for a model containing study specific condition effects, subject effects and study specific global regression (termed "ANCOVA by study" in SPM) is shown in Fig. 13. The first two columns of the design matrix correspond to the condition effects for the first study, the next two to the condition effects for the second study, the next eight to the subject effects, and the last to the gCBF regression

a

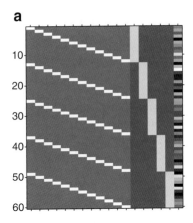

FIGURE 11 Multisubject activation experiment, "classic" SPM design, where each replication of each experimental condition is considered as a seperate condition (Eq. (21)). Illustration for five subjects, each having 12 scans, the scans having been ordered by subject, and by condition and replication within subject. Design matrix "image": The first 12 columns correspond to the "condition" effects, the next 5 to the subject effects, the last to the gCBF regression parameter.

parameter. (The corresponding scans are assumed to be ordered by study, by subject within study, and by condition within subject.)

Such multistudy designs are overdetermined by numerous degrees. An additional consideration for split-plot designs is the variation between subjects in each study. SPM assesses only variation within individuals and therefore cannot be used to assess main effects of study; that is, differences between condition across study cannot be assessed. The only exception to this is the degenerate case when there is only one scan per subject, in which case the model reduces to that of a single subject experiment. Valid contrasts for multistudy designs in SPM are contrasts whose weights, when considered for each of the studies individually, would define a contrast for the study. Thus, contrasts must have weights which sum to zero over the condition effects within each study.

There remain three types of useful comparison available. The first is a comparison of condition effects within a single study, carried out in the context of a multistudy design; the contrast appropriate for the study of interest is entered and padded with zeros for the other study's condition effects, *e.g.*, $(1, -1, 0, 0, 0)$ for the first study in our example. The second is an average effect across studies; contrasts for a particular effect in each of the studies are concatenated, the combined contrast assessing a mean effect across studies. For example, if the second study in our example has the same conditions as the first, plus an additional condition, then such a contrast would be $(-1, 1, -1, 1, 0)$. Last, differences of contrasts across studies can be assessed, such as differences in activation. The contrasts for the appropriate main effect in each study are concatenated, with some study's contrasts negated. In our example, $(-1, 1, 1, -1, 0)$ would be appropriate for locating regions where the first study activated more than the second, or where the second deactivated more than the first.

Assumption of model fit in this case includes the assumption that the error terms have equal variance (at each voxel) across studies. For very different study populations, or studies from different scanners or protocols (possibly showing large differences in the measured gA between studies), this assumption may be tenable only after scaling the values from all studies to have the same global activity.

G. Model Selection

In fitting a general linear model to a data set and then assessing questions in terms of hypotheses on the parameters of the model, it is implicitly assumed that the model fits. That is, that errors are independent and normally distributed with zero mean.

1. Problems of Assessing Model Adequacy

The usual tools for assessing the adequacy of model fit are predominantly graphical methods for a univariate linear model, for instance plots of residuals against fitted values to illustrate unmodelled structure or non-homogeneous residual variance, or plots of residuals against expected order statistics from a standard normal distribution (normal scores) to assess the validity of the normality assumption (sometimes called Q–Q plots). It is impractical to apply these methods routinely given that they would have to be employed for each voxel separately. Although various diagnostic statistics can be used to summarise the information in such plots (for instance the Shapiro–Wilks test

a

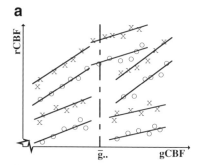

b

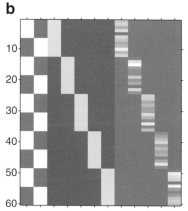

FIGURE 12 Multisubject activation experiment, replication of conditions, ANCOVA by subject (Model Eq. (22)). Illustrations for a five subject study, with six replications of each of two conditions per subject: (a) Illustrative plot of rCBF *vs* gCBF. (b) Design matrix "image": The first two columns correspond to the condition effects, the next five to the subject effects, the last five the gCBF regression parameters for each subject. The design matrix corresponds to scans ordered by subject and by condition within subjects.

for normality, using the correlation of residuals and normal scores), the small number of observations (in PET) means that such tests have extremely low power, particularly considering the multiple comparisons problem of testing at each voxel simultaneously.

2. Ill Fitting Models

If the model does not fit, for whatever reason, then the model assumptions do not hold and subsequent inferences may not be valid. Consider an appropriate model, one that fits. If a reduced model is fitted (with some effects omitted), then the omitted effects contribute to the residual error, introducing structure into the residuals in defiance of their assumed independence. Usually, this results in increases of residual variance. However, the model has fewer parameters than the appropriate one, so the residual degrees of freedom are greater, implying increased confidence in the variance estimate. So, the variance (usually) goes up according to the omitted effects, but so do the degrees of freedom. Increasing variance and increasing degrees of freedom affect significance in opposite directions (for the same effect size), so in general all that can be concluded is that ensuing tests are invalid. However, the effect of increasing degrees of freedom is more pronounced for small degrees of freedom. For low degrees of freedom the omission of terms may lead to more lenient tests despite an increase in residual variance.

If additional parameters are added to a model that is already adequate, then the (redundant) extra parameters reduce the degrees of freedom available for the estimation of residual variance. The reduced residual degrees of freedom result in reduced confidence in the variance estimates, manifesting as larger P values for the same effect.

Further, it is quite possible that different models will be appropriate for data at different voxels. Thus, the pertinent approach is to choose a model for all voxels that includes all the effects relevant for voxels individually.

3. Model Selection

For a limited set of explanatory variables (factors and covariates), the set of possible models for each voxel can be arranged into a hierarchy. Pairs of models at successive levels of the hierarchy differ by the inclusion/omission of a single term (factor, covariate, interaction effect, etc.). Related models in such a hierarchy can be compared using an extra sum-of-squares F test (Section II.F.4). Using this procedure various schemes for model selection can be developed. See Draper and Smith [4] for details. The simplest are *forward selection* and *backward selection*. In the latter, the saturated model at the top of the hierarchy is chosen as a starting point. This model contains all plausible effects. This full model is then compared in turn with each of those in the next lower level of the model hierarchy (models derived from the current model by the omission of a single term), giving an F statistic for the successive null hypotheses that the omitted effects are redundant in the model. If any of these comparisons is nonsignificant, then the terms corresponding to the lowest significance are dropped from the model. This continues until no nonsignificant terms are found, or until a minimal model is reached. The forward selection method is analogous.

In applying this (univariate) procedure to the problem of finding a simultaneous model for all voxels in a functional mapping experiment, there remains the problem of multiple comparisons. For each pair of models an F statistic is obtained for each voxel, giving an F statistic image that must be

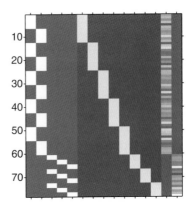

FIGURE 13 Design matrix "image" for the example multistudy activation experiment described in Section III.F.

assessed. In this application interest lies in assessing whether there is any evidence for any voxel that the larger model is required. It is not necessary to locate the particular voxels involved. Therefore, an omnibus test procedure with only weak control over experiment-wise Type I error is required, such as the "sum-of-squares" or "excedance proportion" tests described by Worsley *et al.* [10]. A backwards selection procedure using the latter test was proposed by Holmes [11]. Alternatively, the dimensionality of the data may be reduced by taking the first few principle components and multivariate models selected on the reduced data using multivariate techniques.

4. Practical Model Selection

Currently, no formal model comparison is available in the SPM package. Therefore, a more pragmatic approach must be taken. An alternate heuristic perspective on a forwards selection procedure is this. Adding effects to a model improves the modeling of the data, removing components of the error at the expense of residual degrees of freedom. The best model provides an optimal trade-off between modeling and "spending" degrees of freedom. A pragmatic approach from an investigator's point of view is to start with a basic model, and successively add terms in a sensible order, while assessing the significance of a contrast of interest at each step. The "optimal" model will be the one that gives the most significant results. Clearly this approach is less than ideal, both statistically and practically. In particular, different models might indicate significant effects in different regions.

The most important consideration in statistical experimental design is the actual design of the experiment. This may seem circular, but frequently experiments are designed with little thought for what statistical analyses will be carried out.

A related but distinct topic is randomisation. In conducting designed experiments we wish to be able to attribute any observed effects to experimentally manipulated conditions. Usually this attribution can be guaranteed only if conditions are randomly allocated to a presentation order for each subject in a sensible manner (equivalently, experimental conditions are allocated to scan slots randomly). Further this randomisation should be appropriately balanced, both across and within subjects. With such random allocation of conditions, any unexpected effects are randomly scattered between the conditions and therefore only contribute to error.

H. SPM Specifics

1. Partitioning of the Design, Contrast Specification

In general, for PET, SPM orders effects as (i) mean μ (if required), (ii) condition effects, (iii) other effects of interest (entered as covariates of interest), (iv) confounding subject (block) effects, and (v) other confounding effects (entered as covariates of no interest), including gCBF if an ANCOVA style global normalisation is chosen. Effects in categories (ii) and (iii) are classed as of interest, and contrast weights are requested only for these parameters, weights for other parameters being taken as zero. For the designs implemented in SPM, the contrast weights corresponding to the condition effects must sum to zero. The package therefore ensures these weights specify a contrast by removing their mean. The exact design matrix and contrasts used are printed by the package for inspection, and "bar charts" of contrasts are appended to design matrix images when presented with statistic images.

2. Adjusted Values

For the computation of adjusted values, any overall mean parameter (i) is left in the adjusted values, so the confounding effects ($\boldsymbol{\beta}_2^k$) removed from the data to form the adjusted data are those in categories (iv) and (v).

For multisubject models the overdetermination of the models presents a problem. The adjusted values are not uniquely determined, since the degree of latitude in the model corresponds to the addition/subtraction of a constant between the subject effects, designated as confounding, and the condition effects, designated of interest (or the overall mean if the design is parametric with no conditions). To give sensible adjusted values the subject effects are constrained to sum to zero. Rather than explicitly constrain the design matrix, leading to design matrix images that are potentially confusing, the subject effects are expressed relative to their mean (Section II.D.3), and the Moore–Penrose pseudoinverse is used to apply the constraint implicitly. This implicit constraint is exhibited in design matrix images, the subject block having a darker background and grey patches where the indicator 1s should be.

3. Alternative Hypotheses

Since the methods of assessing t statistic images (described in Chapter 5) examine only large t values, the alternative hypotheses in SPM are one sided. A two-sided test can be obtained by specifying contrasts for increases and decreases (one is the negative of the other) and assessing both the resulting t statistic images at half the significance level, easily carried out by doubling any P values obtained.

I. *F* Statistic for Any Effects of Interest

An F statistic using the extra sum of squares principle for the omnibus hypothesis that there are no effects of interest ($\mathcal{H}^k : \boldsymbol{\beta}_1^k = \mathbf{0}$) is computed for each voxel. The resulting F statistic image shows regions where there is evidence of some effect of interest. In SPM, this F statistic is thresholded (corresponding to a voxel level tail probability of 0.05 under $\mathcal{H}^k$) to identify voxels for which adjusted data, model parameters and statistics are saved for subsequent inspection. This is purely a data reduction device.

IV. FUNCTIONAL MRI

The analysis of functional magnetic resonance time series (fMRI) presents additional statistical problems. In this section some extensions to the basic general linear model theory for the analysis of fMRI time series are presented. A detailed discussion of design issues for fMRI is presented in Chapter 18, so only the simplest analysis will be considered here.

Again, a linear model is used to model the time series $\mathbf{Y}^k = (Y_1^k, \ldots, Y_j^k, \ldots, Y_J^k)$ of J observations at voxel k:

$$\mathbf{Y}^k = X\boldsymbol{\beta}^k + \boldsymbol{\epsilon}^k. \tag{23}$$

(In this section we shall drop the voxel superscript k and consider the model at a single voxel.) If the model fits the data well, then it is reasonable to assume that the errors are normally distributed with zero mean. However, the errors are slightly correlated, precluding use of the standard theory of Section II.

Since an fMRI signal for a point response has the form of the haemodynamic response function, the signal is optimally recovered if the fMRI time series is smoothed by convolution with the haemodynamic response function (matched filter theorem). This theorem suggests temporally smoothing the time series. Thus, the time series data at each voxel $\mathbf{Y}$ are convolved with a Gaussian kernel of $\tau = \sqrt{8}$ sec, leading to

$$KY = KX\boldsymbol{\beta} + K\boldsymbol{\epsilon}. \tag{24}$$

Here the convolution is expressed by the Toeplitz matrix K with the discretised Gaussian smoothing kernel on the leading diagonal, $K_{ij} \propto \exp(-(i-j)^2/2\tau^2)$. The components of the error vector are assumed independent $\epsilon_j \stackrel{iid}{\approx} \mathcal{N}(0, \sigma^2)$, such that the autocovariance of the smoothed errors is completely specified by K and σ. Although the raw errors are slightly correlated, this autocorrelation is swamped by the smoothing making the assumption tenable.

There is a large literature on the topic of serial correlation in regression, for example Watson [12] and Seber [13]. We brought the approach to functional imaging and review it here [14, 10]. Assuming X is of full-rank, the least squares estimates of $\boldsymbol{\beta}$ are:

$$\hat{\boldsymbol{\beta}} = (X^{*\top}X^*)^{-1}X^{*\top}KY, \tag{25}$$

where $X^* = KX$. Although not fully optimal, $\hat{\boldsymbol{\beta}}$ is unbiased, with variance

$$\mathrm{var}[\hat{\boldsymbol{\beta}}] = \sigma^2(X^{*\top}X^*)^{-1}X^{*\top}VX^*(X^{*\top}X^*)^{-1} \tag{26}$$

for $V = KK^\top$. This equation implies the following test statistic for a linear compound $\mathbf{c}^\top\hat{\boldsymbol{\beta}}$ of the parameters at voxel k,

$$T = \mathbf{c}^\top\hat{\boldsymbol{\beta}}/(\mathbf{c}^\top\hat{\sigma}^2(X^{*\top}X^*)^{-1}X^{*\top}VX^*(X^{*\top}X^*)^{-1}\mathbf{c})^{1/2}, \tag{27}$$

with σ^2 estimated in the usual way by dividing the residual sum of squares by its expectation,

$$\hat{\sigma}^2 = \mathbf{e}^\top\mathbf{e}/\mathrm{trace}(RV), \tag{28}$$

where $\mathbf{e} = RKX$ is the vector of residuals and R the residual forming matrix. Here $\mathsf{E}[\hat{\sigma}^2] = \sigma^2$, and $\mathrm{var}[\hat{\sigma}^2] = 2\sigma^4(\mathrm{trace}(RV\,RV))/(\mathrm{trace}(RV)^2)$, so the effective degrees of freedom are then

$$\nu = \frac{2\mathsf{E}[\hat{\sigma}^2]^2}{\mathrm{var}[\hat{\sigma}^2]} = \frac{\mathrm{trace}(RV)^2}{\mathrm{trace}(RV\,RV)}. \tag{29}$$

By analogy with the χ^2 approximation for quadratic forms [15], the null distribution of T may be approximated by a t distribution with ν degrees of freedom.

In this time series setting, the columns of a design matrix can be thought of as discretised reference waveforms. For a single subject activation experiment of alternating epochs of baseline and activation conditions, a minimal design would have only two degrees of freedom, a mean for each condition, with conditions associated with scans reflecting the haemodynamic lag. One possible design matrix X for this scenario has a column of 1s and a column containing a boxcar waveform of 0s (for rest epoch scans) and 1s (for active epoch scans) lagged 8 sec.[9] There is also evidence of global effects in fMRI,

---

[9] Clearly a lagged boxcar is a crude approximation of the haemodynamic response to neuronal activation. However, its simplicity and success have ensured its use. More refined approaches are discussed in Chapter 18.

so it would be pertinent to add the global measurement as a confounding covariate, leading to the design matrix (after convolution) shown in Fig. 14. The null hypothesis of no activation corresponds to zero amplitude of the boxcar waveform. The amplitude of the boxcar reference waveform is the only parameter of interest, so SPM prompts for contrast weight vectors of length one. Appropriate contrast weights are then $[+1]$ and $[-1]$ for alternative hypotheses of activation and deactivation, respectively.

V. A MULTIVARIATE PERSPECTIVE

The massively univariate approach outlined above involves fitting univariate linear models to the data at each voxel. Crucially, the same model form is used at each voxel; only the parameters are different. The model at voxel k is of the form

$$\mathbf{Y}^k = X\boldsymbol{\beta}^k + \boldsymbol{\epsilon}.$$

The values of the explanatory variables relate to each scan, the same explanatory variables are used for each voxel. Thus, the design matrix is the same for every voxel. Therefore, the models for all intracerebral voxels $k = 1, \ldots, K$ can be expressed in a single matrix equation as

$$Y = X\beta + \epsilon,$$

where $Y = (\mathbf{Y}^1 \vdots \ldots \vdots \mathbf{Y}^k \vdots \ldots \vdots \mathbf{Y}^K)$ is the data matrix, arranged with scans in rows, one column per voxel. $\beta = (\boldsymbol{\beta}^1 \vdots \ldots \vdots \boldsymbol{\beta}^k \vdots \ldots \vdots \boldsymbol{\beta}^K)$ is the matrix of parameters, each column containing the parameters for a single voxel. Similarly the error matrix ϵ has ϵ^k as its kth column. This equation therefore constitutes an image regression.

The least squares estimates for all the voxels may be simultaneously obtained as $\hat{\beta} = (X^\top X)^{-1} X^\top Y$.

This is the form of a multivariate regression. In multivariate regression it is usually assumed that the vectors ϵ_j of errors associated with the jth observation (the jth row of the error matrix ϵ) have a k-variate multivariate normal distribution with zero mean and variance–covariance matrix Σ [16]. The massively univariate approach of SPM assumes only that the marginal distributions are normal: $\epsilon_j^k \overset{iid}{\sim} \mathcal{N}(0, \sigma_k^2)$. Therefore we differentiate image regression from multivariate regression.

However, the random field approaches to assessing the significance of statistic images implicitly assume that the statistic images are discrete random fields. This in turn implies that the images of residual errors are Gaussian random fields, which in turn implies that the error vectors are multivariate normal.

Standard multivariate analyses of (raw) neuroimaging data are not possible. This is due to the fact that the number of variates (voxels) observed is much greater than the number of observations (scans). This fact results in a singular estimate of Σ, precluding most multivariate procedures that utilise the determinant of the variance–covariance estimate. However, multivariate analyses are possible if the dimensionality of the data set is reduced, a topic pursued in Chapter 7.

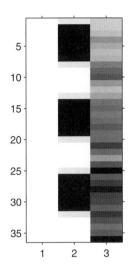

FIGURE 14 Example "image" of a smoothed fMRI design matrix KX, for 36 scans consisting of six epochs of 6 scans each with conditions alternating between epochs, starting with baseline. The time series was cut from the middle of a longer experiment, so the epoch immediately prior to the first was under the active condition.

VI. CONCLUDING REMARKS

The fixed effects general linear model provides a single framework for many statistical tests and models, giving great flexibility for experimental design and analysis. The SPM software package uses "image regression" to compute statistic images for prespecified hypotheses regarding contrasts of the parameters of a general linear model fitted at each voxel. This facility presents a useful tool for functional neuroimage analysis.

References

1. M. J. R. Healy. "Matrices for Statistics." Oxford Univ. Press, Oxford, 1986.
2. R. F. Mould. "Introductory Medical Statistics," 2nd ed. Institute of Physics Publishing, London, 1989.
3. C. Chatfield. "Statistics for Technology." Chapman & Hall, London, 1983.
4. N. R. Draper and H. Smith. "Applied Regression Analysis," 2nd ed. Wiley, New York, 1981.
5. B. J. Winer, D. R. Brown, and K. M. Michels. "Statistical Principles in Experimental Design," 3rd ed. McGraw Hill, New York, 1991.
6. H. Scheffé. "The Analysis of Variance." Wiley, New York, 1959.
7. K. J. Friston, C. D. Frith, P. F. Liddle, R. J. Dolan, A. A. Lammertsma, and R. S. J. Frackowiak. The relationship between global and local changes in PET scans. *J. Cereb. Blood Flow Metab.* **10**, 458–466 (1990).
8. K. J. Worsley, A. C. Evans, S. Marrett, and P. Neelin. A three-dimensional statistical analysis for CBF activation studies in human brain. *J. Cereb. Blood Flow Metab.* **12**, 900–918 (1992).
9. K. J. Friston, A. P. Holmes, K. J. Worsley, J. P. Poline, C. D. Frith, and R. S. J. Frackowiak. Statistical parametric maps in functional imaging: A general linear approach. *Hum. Brain Mapping* **2**, 189–210 (1995).
10. K. J. Worsley and K. J. Friston. Analysis of fMRI time-series revisited—Again. *Neuroimage* **2**, 173–181 (1995).
11. A. P. Holmes. "Statistical Issues in Functional Neuroimaging." Ph.D. thesis, Univ. of Glasgow, 1994.
12. G. S. Watson. Serial correlation in regression analysis: I. *Biometrika* **42**, 327–341 (1955).
13. G. A. F. Seber. "Linear Regression Analysis." Wiley, New York, 1977.
14. K. J. Friston, A. P. Holmes, J-B. Poline, P. J. Grasby, S. C. R. Williams, R. S. J. Frackowiak, and R. Turner. Analysis of fMRI time series revisited. *Neuroimage* **2**, 45–53 (1995).
15. F. E. Satterthwaite. An approximate distribution of estimates of variance components. *Biometrics* **2**, 110–114 (1946).
16. C. Chatfield and A. J. Collins. "An Introduction to Multivariate Analysis." Chapman & Hall, London, 1980.

CHAPTER FIVE

MAKING STATISTICAL INFERENCES

I. INTRODUCTION

Statistical methods used to analyse functional neuroimaging data are essential for a proper interpretation of the results of experiments that ultimately aim at a better understanding of the neuroanatomy of human brain function. The analysis of functional imaging experiments often involves the formation of a statistical parametric map (SPM). The conceptual idea of SPMs was first introduced by Friston *et al.* [6]. In such maps, the value at each position or voxel is a statistic that expresses evidence against a null hypothesis of no experimentally induced activation at that voxel.

The construction of an SPM can be decomposed into three main steps:

- Spatial transformations. In the most general case, functional imaging experiments require the acquisition of data from several subjects or several groups of subjects. Sophisticated techniques have been designed to normalise the anatomy of different brains into a standard stereotactic space [2,5]. Spatial smoothing is also usually performed to allow for interindividual gyral variation and to improve the signal to noise ratio. Note that smoothing does not always improve the signal to noise ratio and the relationship between smoothing and sensitivity is discussed further in this chapter.
- Construction of an SPM. This is a key step because it requires the (generally nonunique) modeling of effects of interest or of no interest for the experimental protocol analysed. The general linear model (GLM) offers the flexibility needed. This step is fully described in [14], the output of which is a three-dimensional (3D) statistic image or "map" formed of thousands of correlated Student t statistics.
- Statistical inference from the SPM. This step is the focus of this chapter.

Images contain a great number of voxels so that the SPMs are not directly interpretable. An essential step is to find a way to correct for the multiple comparison problem. A difficulty with this correction lies in the nonindependence of voxel intensities due to both the initial resolution of images and to postprocessing, especially smoothing. The nonindependence of voxels cannot be treated by "Bonferroni" procedures that treat voxels as if they were independent because they are much too stringent and would wipe out statistically reliable activation signals from the results.

Since the first attempts to analyse a voxel based activation map, a number of statistical techniques have been developed for the analysis of SPMs. Essential to the development of these techniques is Gaussian random field theory, which deals with the behaviour of stochastic processes defined over a space of any dimensions (D). Usually, D is 3 (analysis of a volume) but can be greater (*e.g.*, search over time, with potential application of fMRI, or search over scale space, multifiltering strategy). In this chapter we review for the general reader some important tests that (based on results from this field of mathematics) can be used for the assessment of significant activations in SPMs. These techniques have become increasingly important because they are general, require very little computation and provide an extensive characterisation of the different kinds of response expected in activation studies.

This chapter is organized in (almost) chronological order and we will show that this order also corresponds to the different kinds of risk of error associated with the different statistical tests described. These tests can be looked upon as a hierarchy of procedures with decreasing localising power but potentially increasing sensitivity.

We briefly review some important extensions to these statistical tests and introduce alternative nonparametric approaches which do not use random fields theory and are free from any assumptions [13]. Finally we discuss relevant issues related to image smoothness.

II. TESTING FOR THE INTENSITY OF AN ACTIVATION IN SPMs

A. Theory

Friston *et al.* [7] proposed a procedure to address the multiple comparison problem in 1991. Using very basic results on random processes found in [4], they derived a test for bidimensional (2D) processes that efficiently controlled for nonindependence in the data.

Building on this result, Worsley *et al.* [24] used a mathematically more conventional procedure to extend the test in three or more dimensions.

We describe briefly how this result was achieved, emphasising assumptions about the volume or image to be analysed, and then critically assess validity of these correction procedures whilst proposing practical guidelines. Although results are available for different random fields [25], we will concentrate on the use of the results established for Gaussian random fields. t Maps, usually generated by testing contrasts, are therefore transformed to Gaussianized t maps using a voxel by voxel t-to-Z probability transformation such that $\Phi(Z) = \Psi(t)$, where $\Phi(\cdot)$ is the standard normal cumulative density function (CDF) and $\Psi(\cdot)$ the Student t distribution with appropriate degrees of freedom.

To test for the significance of an activation intensity in an SPM, it is necessary to assess the probability that the maximum value in the map (Z_{max}) is greater than a given threshold t under the null hypothesis (when no activation is present). To approximate this probability Worsley *et al.* used the expected Euler characteristic $E[\chi_t]$ of a binarized map thresholded at t. The Euler characteristic is a geometric measure that, loosely speaking, counts the number of connected components minus the number of "holes" in a volume of the image V. At high thresholds this characteristic simply counts the number of regions above t. Moreover, for such high thresholds, suprathreshold clusters are independent and the number of clusters C_t above t follows approximately a Poisson distribution ([1], pp. 161) with mean $\mathsf{E}[\chi_t]$; i.e.,

$$\Pr(C = x) = 1/x!(\mathsf{E}[\chi_t])^x e^{-\mathsf{E}[\chi_t]} = \Upsilon(x, \mathsf{E}[\chi_t]). \tag{1}$$

For high t, we have

$$\Pr(Z_{\max} \geq t) \approx \Pr(\chi_t \geq 1) \approx 1 - e^{-\mathsf{E}[\chi_t]} \approx \mathsf{E}[\chi_t], \tag{2}$$

where χ_t is defined over a compact convex subset V of $\mathscr{R}^D$ whose boundary has zero Lebesgue measure (λ). The expected Euler characteristic is

$$\mathsf{E}[\chi_t] = \lambda(V)|\Lambda|^{1/2}(2\pi)^{-(D+1)/2}He_D(t)e^{-t^2/2}, \tag{3}$$

where $\lambda(V)$ is the volume or image being analysed. (V and Λ are measured with the same units. We make the simplification $V = \lambda(V)$ in the rest of the chapter.) $He_D(t)$ is the Hermite polynomial of degree D in t ($He_0(t) = 1$; $He_1(t) = t$; $He_2(t) = t^2 - 1$). Notice that the "threshold" t here is not set by the user; the value of t is simply the local maximum or indeed any value that is tested, as opposed to the threshold used for spatial extent tests (see Section III).

Λ is the variance-covariance matrix of the partial derivative of the process in the D directions of space and is crucial for the assessment of $\mathsf{E}[\chi_t]$ and therefore to the calculation of P values. In three dimensions (x, y, z), we have

$$\Lambda = \begin{pmatrix} \mathrm{var}\left(\dfrac{\partial X}{\partial x}\right) & \mathrm{cov}\left(\dfrac{\partial X}{\partial x}, \dfrac{\partial X}{\partial y}\right) & \mathrm{cov}\left(\dfrac{\partial X}{\partial x}, \dfrac{\partial X}{\partial z}\right) \\[2ex] \mathrm{cov}\left(\dfrac{\partial X}{\partial x}, \dfrac{\partial X}{\partial y}\right) & \mathrm{var}\left(\dfrac{\partial X}{\partial y}\right) & \mathrm{cov}\left(\dfrac{\partial X}{\partial y}, \dfrac{\partial X}{\partial z}\right) \\[2ex] \mathrm{cov}\left(\dfrac{\partial X}{\partial x}, \dfrac{\partial X}{\partial z}\right) & \mathrm{cov}\left(\dfrac{\partial X}{\partial y}, \dfrac{\partial X}{\partial z}\right) & \mathrm{var}\left(\dfrac{\partial X}{\partial z}\right) \end{pmatrix}. \tag{4}$$

For an image (or volume) generated by white noise smoothed by a Gaussian point spread function (PSF) with dispersion Σ (leading to a Gaussian autocovariance function with dispersion 2Σ), we have $\Lambda = (\Sigma^{-1}/2)$. In most cases, the PSF can be assumed to be aligned with the coordinate axes of the volume analysed, giving null off-diagonal elements for Λ and Σ. In this case the full width at half maximum (FWHM) of the PSF relates to $|\Lambda|$ with

$$|\Lambda|^{-1/2} = (4\ln(2))^{-D/2} \prod_{i=1}^{D} \mathrm{FWHM}_i,$$

leading to the definition of resolution elements (RESELS),

$$V|\Lambda|^{1/2} = \mathrm{RESELS}(4\log_e 2)^{D/2},$$

where RESELS are equal to the volume of the search region divided by the product of the FWHMs of the PSF in each dimension [26]. Note that even when the actual form of the PSF is unknown (and possibly not Gaussian), smoothness values are often described in terms of FWHM. The smoothness parameter is usually defined as $|\Lambda|^{-1}$ such that it relates simply to the FWHM

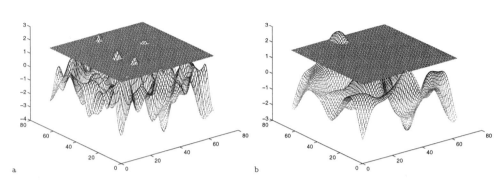

FWHM = 5.9; SD(derivative) = 0.28; u = 2   FWHM = 11.8; SD(derivative) = 0.14; u = 2

FIGURE 1   2D illustration of the relationship between the variance (or standard deviation) of the derivative of the SPM and the width of the kernel. (a) Little smoothing and (b) large smoothing. FWHM is in pixels (identical in x and y).

of a Gaussian kernel and is assessed using the partial derivatives of the SPM, a valid procedure as long as the PSF of the SPM is aligned with the coordinate axes (see Fig. 1 for an illustration). Note that this estimation is itself subject to noise (see Section VII).

A formula very similar to (3) was established by V. P. Nosko [15], formally proved by A. M. Hasofer [11] and reported in [1, pp. 133]. It gives an asymptotic result for the expected number $M_t(V)$ of maxima above a level t in V as

$$\mathsf{E}[M_t(V)] = V|\Lambda|^{1/2}(2\pi)^{-(D+1)/2}t^{D-1}e^{-t^2/2}[1 + O(1/t)]. \qquad (5)$$

Clearly, for high t, Eqs. (3) and (5) give similar results. In the current implementation of SPM software (that we will denote as SPM96 to avoid confusion with the statistical maps themselves) Eq. (5) is used as it gives slightly more conservative results.

B. Assumptions

For Eqs. (2) and (3) to hold, several assumptions have to be made: a discrete SPM approximates a continuous, zero-mean, unit variance, homogeneous, smoothed Gaussian random field (GRF); the threshold t is high; and the volume V is large compared to the resolution of the map.

1. The zero-mean and unit variance conditions hold under the null hypothesis, provided the statistical model used is correct.

2. The homogeneity condition implies that both the statistical and the spatial characteristics of the volume are constant with position. This might be of concern with 3D acquisition but is still a very reasonable first approximation. However, effects of nonstationarity of the PSF due to both instrumental or physiological factors still need to be assessed.

3. Strictly speaking, a random field is Gaussian if the joint distribution of any subset of points has a multivariate Gaussian distribution. This implies that at the univariate level each point or position should have a Gaussian distribution. In SPM96, this is ensured by the voxel by voxel t-to-Z transformation. At the multivariate level the condition is satisfied when the degrees of freedom (df) of the t statistic are large enough (*e.g.*, $df \geq 30$). In general, it is difficult to address the validity of this assumption for lower degrees of

freedom and results provided by Worsley [25] for *t* fields should be used when working with low *df*. However, spatial or temporal smoothing, usually applied to increase signal to noise ratio, minimises the risk of breaching the multivariate Gaussian assumption. Worsley [24] showed that with $df \leq 3$ singularities will almost certainly occur in any continuous random *t* field.

4. How high should *t* be? Although Eqs. (3) and (5) hold only for high *t*, these results are used in such a way that for small *t*, the probability computed by Eq. (2) is high and therefore not generally of interest.

5. A discrete lattice should approximate a continuous smoothed random field well and allow for a good estimation of the smoothness of an SPM. The estimation can be obtained when sampling is high compared to the resolution of an SPM. For Gaussian PSFs, we find that a good smoothness estimation is obtained when the FWHM in any direction is at least 2 or 3 times greater than the voxel size. In PET, the resolution of the original image volumes usually ensures that this is the case even when postprocessing smoothing is fairly low (≈ 6 mm FWHM). For fMRI, where the resolution of the data is high, when the method is applied to raw data the assessment of this smoothness fails. However, because we are dealing with an underlying biological signal that is smooth we can get around the problem simply by undersampling the fMRI maps or applying a small amount of spatial filtering to ensure validity of the assumption.

6. Results presented by Worsley and Friston [26, 7] are accurate for search volumes *V* that are large compared to the resolution of the SPM (practically at least three or four times the FWHM of the SPM). Results accurate for any volume have been developed by Worsley *et al.* [23]. When analysing the brain volume, current estimations based on the equations described above are accurate enough.

C. Discussion

The significance test we have presented provides strong control over type I errors at the *voxel level*. Strong control over type I errors is obtained if the probability of falsely rejecting any hypothesis is less than the given level α, regardless of the truth of other hypotheses. See [12] for rigorous definitions. Note that rejecting the null hypothesis at any voxel also rejects the so-called "omnibus hypothesis" (is there any signal in the entire volume?). As noted above, this test has been extended to other types of random field by Worsley *et al.* [25], *e.g.*, χ^2, *F*, and *t* fields. *F* fields have potentially important applications for model selection at the voxel level. An example of such an application is the "nonlinear" regression that tests for the best model that describes the relationship between the measured brain response (regional perfusion) and a noncategorical parameter (*e.g.*, rate of presentation, see [3]).

III. TESTING FOR THE SIGNIFICANCE OF THE SPATIAL EXTENT OF AN ACTIVATION

A. Theory

The previously described procedure tests for the significance of a simple increase in intensity of an activation in an SPM. Early work using Monte Carlo simulations [18] suggested that using information about the spatial properties of potential brain signals, and testing for the significance of the spatial extent of activated regions above a given threshold, could greatly improve the sensitivity of functional imaging experiments. We present here a theoretical test that again uses results from Gaussian random field theory [10].

The first step is to start with asymptotic results for the distribution (and expectation) of an area n_u of regions defined by thresholding an SPM at u. These results derived by Nosko [15–17] are also reported in [1, pp. 158]. They show that at high threshold u the conditional distribution of n_u is such that

$$\lim_{u \to \infty} P(|\Lambda|^{1/2}(2\pi)^{-1}u^2 n_u^{2/D} > v | n_u > 0) = \exp(-v).$$

However, this approximate distribution significantly overestimates the area n_u. To correct for this overestimation, Friston *et al.* [10] used the fact that the expected area $E[n_u]$ can also be derived from results previously described in Section II:

$$E[n_u] = V\Phi(-u)/E[M_u(V)].$$

Where $E[M_u(V)]$ is the number of expected regions above u given by Eq. (5) and $V\Phi(-u)$ the number of expected voxels above u. The corrected distribution for n_u then becomes

$$\Pr(n_u > v) = \exp(-\beta v^{2/D}), \tag{6}$$

with

$$\beta = \left(\frac{\Gamma(D/2 - 1)E[M_u(V)]}{V\Phi(-u)} \right)^{2/D}$$

and $\Phi(\cdot)$ the standard normal CDF.

This formula establishes the distribution of an area n_u given the occurrence of a region above u. The parameter we are primarily interested in is the maximum value of n_u, $n_{u\max}$, in V. The probability of having a maximum value of n_u greater than v is simply one minus the probability that all the $M_u(V)$ suprathreshold regions in V have areas less than v, times the probability of having $M_u(V)$ regions. Using Eqs. (1) and (6) we obtain

$$\Pr(n_{u\max} > v) = \sum_{i=1}^{\infty} \Pr(M_u(V) = i)\,(1 - \Pr(n_u < v)^i)$$

$$= 1 - \exp(- E[M_u(V)]\,\Pr(n_u \geq v)) \tag{7}$$

$$= 1 - \exp(- E[M_u(V)]\,\exp(-\beta v^{2/D})),$$

with β as defined above. For a full development of these equations see [10].

B. Discussion

1. Improved Sensitivity

Generally, as expected, the test provides an improved sensitivity compared to intensity testing alone, although this is not necessarily the case. A power analysis [10] shows that, if the underlying signal to be detected is wider than the resolution of the SPM, power increases with a low threshold (assuming a Gaussian shaped underlying signal). However, if signal width is smaller than the noise PSF, power increases with high values of u and an optimal sensitivity is found for the intensity test. As all kinds of signal are potentially present in an SPM, it seems that the optimal procedure is to use either a series of thresholds or combined criteria. The next section deals specifically with this question.

2. The Loss of Voxelwise Control over the Risk of Error

It is essential to note that the new extent test does not provide control of the risk of error at the voxel level and therefore individual voxels cannot be declared as "significantly activated" within a region. The localising power of the extent test has moved from the voxel level to the region (cluster) level. The localising power depends on u since high thresholds provide better localisation and greater insurance that nonactivated parts of the brain are not grouped with activated regions by the thresholding process. Although nothing can be said at the voxel level, the interpretation of results will clearly be different depending on threshold (the higher the threshold, the greater is the chance that most of the voxels in the cluster are part of an underlying signal). Indeed, an essential parameter is the expected number of voxels in noise $E[n_u]$ that should be compared to the observed number of voxels forming a suprathreshold region. This comparison will help quantify the regional specificity of the test. Another good indicator is the probability of occurrence based on the voxel by voxel test as computed in Section II for voxels with an intensity u.

3. How High Should t Be to Ensure the Validity of Analysis?

It is difficult to generalise since the magnitude of t that guarantees validity depends on the smoothness ($|\Lambda|^{-1}$). However, in most PET studies, t values between 2.5 and 3 can be used safely as demonstrated by simulations. In fMRI experiments that generally have higher spatial resolution, safe values should be higher (≥ 3).

4. Effect of Smoothing on Detection

Interestingly, smoothing has an opposite effect on the sensitivity of the extent test compared to the voxel intensity test described in Section II. This is because as smoothing increases, the probability that $Z_{\max}$ crosses the level t by chance decreases. Clearly, when smoothing increases the probability that a large region occurs above u by chance increases as well. This is illustrated in Fig. 12 which plots, for fixed values of t or area n, the probability of occurrence by chance (noise only case) as a function of smoothness. It is usually the case that greater smoothing improves the detection of significant activation at the voxel level while relatively small degrees of low pass filtering tend to improve the sensitivity of spatial extent detection. This last observation is only generally true and results depend on the shape of the activated area: for instance, filters that are too large will wipe out peaky signals.

Although no assumption has been made about the shape of the spatial autocovariance function of an SPM, because of the nature of this extent test, it is likely to be more sensitive to the nonstationarity of the PSF than the intensity test. In terms of implementation, a connectivity scheme has to be chosen for $D \geq 2$. We recommend an 18-connectivity scheme for $D = 3$ and a 4-connectivity scheme for $D = 2$.

IV. TESTING FOR BOTH PEAK HEIGHT AND SPATIAL EXTENT

A. Rationale

The sections above show that sensitivity to Gaussian signals depends on the choice of intensity thresholds, u, wide signals being best detected with low thresholds, sharp signals with high thresholds. Not only is it generally impossible to predict which test would be best for a particular analysis, but, because of the complexity of the underlying anatomy of the brain, several kinds of signal (wide or sharp) might occur simultaneously. It is also not valid to use both tests without correcting for the implicit multiple comparison involved. If the two tests were independent, a simple "Bonferroni" correction would be appropriate. However, the maximum intensity and spatial extent of a region above u are not independent and such corrections would lead to an overconservative test. In the next section we develop a test based on both spatial extent and peak intensity of regions above u.

B. Method

In this section we describe a combined test based on two parameters (peak height and spatial extent).

First, we derive an approximation for the probability that a given cluster will have a spatial extent S greater than s_0, and maximum intensity or peak height H greater than h_0 [21], using results from Gaussian random field theory. The derivation of this result is based on modeling the shape of a region above u (near a local maximum) as an inverted paraboloid. The first terms of the Taylor expansion of the processes' second derivative are then used to obtain an approximate distribution for the conditional distribution of n_u, knowing the height h_u above u. We use this approximation and the known marginal distribution of h_u (h_u has an approximate exponential distribution with mean $1/u$ [1, Chap. 6] to get an approximate conjoint distribution,

$$\mathrm{P}(n_u \ge s_0, h_u \ge h_0) \approx \int_{h=h_0}^{\infty} \Psi_\nu\{\nu ac|\Lambda|^{-1/2}u^{-D/2}h^{D/2}/s_0\}\, ue^{-uh}\, dh, \qquad (8)$$

where Ψ_ν is one minus the χ^2 cumulative distribution function with degrees of freedom $\nu = 4u^2/D$, given by

$$\Psi_\nu(x) = \int_x^{\infty} \frac{t^{\nu/2-1}e^{-t/2}}{2^{\nu/2}\Gamma(\nu/2)}\, dt.$$

Figure 2 shows the match between the theoretical approximation and the conjoint distribution derived with simulations of white noise convolved with a Gaussian PSF.

Second, a way of combining the spatial extent and the maximum intensity is chosen in order to select events (an occurrence of a cluster) that will be rejected at a given risk of error under the null hypothesis of pure noise. We note that there are an almost infinite number of possibilities for this step: in a two-parameter testing procedure a statistical threshold becomes a curve in a plane.

For our proposed combined test, the risk of error is simply defined as the minimum of the risk for spatial extent n_u and the risk for maximum peak

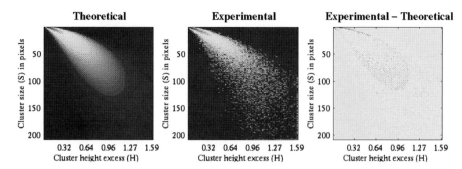

FIGURE 2 (Left) Theoretical (predicted) bivariate distribution of spatial extent and peak height for regions occurring above an image threshold of $t = 3$ in a $64 \times 64 \times 32$ volume ($128 \times 128 \times 64$ mm³) with resolution 17.5 mm in x and y, and 12.5 mm in z. Data intensity is presented on a log scale to increase the visibility of the tail of the distribution. (Middle) Observed bivariate distribution of spatial extent and peak height under the same conditions as above. (Right) Difference between the two.

height H. This gives a rejection area defined by

$$\min\{\Pr(n_u \geq s_0), P(H \geq h_0)\} = \text{constant},$$

which leads to the probability of rejection of a given cluster:

$$\Pr_{\text{joint}} = \Pr(n_u \geq s_0) + \Pr(H \geq h_0) - \Pr(n_u \geq s_0, H \geq h_0). \tag{9}$$

We then use $\Pr_{\text{joint}}$, the probability that the spatial extent and peak height probability of a single cluster falls in the rejection area to compute the probability that at least one cluster is rejected in the volume V. If k clusters occur in the volume V, the probability that at least one of them will be rejected is simply

$$\Pr(\text{rejection}|C = k) = (1 - (1 - \Pr_{\text{joint}})^k).$$

Summing over k, weighted by the probability that $C = k$, we get

$$\Pr(\text{rejection}) = \sum_{k=0}^{\infty} (1 - (1 - \Pr_{\text{joint}})^k) \mathsf{E}[M_t(V)]^k e^{-\mathsf{E}[M_t(V)]}/k!$$
$$= 1 - e^{-\mathsf{E}[M_t(V)]\Pr_{\text{joint}}}. \tag{10}$$

Simulations in pure noise for various values of u and various resolutions show that the conjoint test protects against type I risk of error α (except if the threshold is very low ($u = 2$) and the α-risk greater than 0.15). Figure 3 shows the expected *versus* observed risk of error in 3D for various thresholds.

The sensitivity of the combined test was assessed for three simulated signals: a sharp signal, an extended signal, and a signal with approximately the same probability of being detected by either the intensity test (in Section II) or the spatial extent test (Section III). Results (presented in Fig. 4) show that the conjoint test should generally increase the overall sensitivity of analyses, as well as increase their validity by correcting for the implicit multitesting procedure.

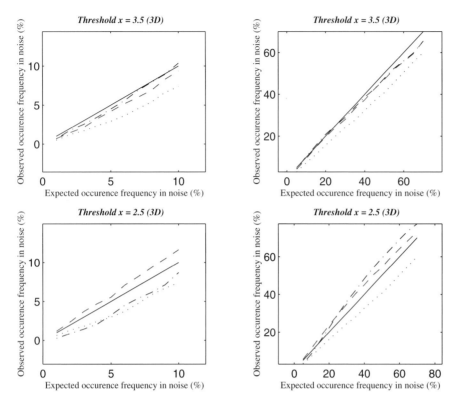

FIGURE 3 Expected *versus* observed risk of error with two thresholds u in 3D volumes ($64 \times 64 \times 32$ voxels or $128 \times 128 \times 64$ mm^3) at a fixed resolution (FWHM$_{xy}$ = 14.1 mm and FWHM$_z$ = 11.8 mm). (Top) High intensity threshold (t = 3.5). (Bottom) Low threshold (t = 2.5). (Left) Risk of error between 1 and 10%. (Right) Risk of error varying between 10 and 70%. The dashed line shows the results from the spatial extent test, the dotted line from the peak height test, and the dot and dashed line from the combined test. The solid line corresponds to the $y = x$ line. Results were assessed using 3×10^3 simulations.

C. Discussion

As for the spatial extent test, the risk of error is determined at the region level. In fact, the two tests are conceptually very similar but the conjoint test is more general. Note that it is always possible to know whether a suprathreshold region is unlikely to occur because of its size or its height, giving further information on the type of regional activation observed.

Also, note that to derive Eq. (9), slightly stronger hypotheses were required. It is assumed that the PSF, resulting from both the image reconstruction apparatus and postprocessing filtering, can be modeled by a Gaussian function. The robustness of the conjoint test with regard to this assumption remains to be evaluated.

The conjoint test may prove to be an interesting alternative to multifiltering strategies [19, 27] (these methods are not presented in this short review). These strategies have ultimately a similar goal, which is to detect signals of various sizes in one statistically valid procedure. The conjoint (or bivariate) test, however, has the advantage of requiring fewer computations and should

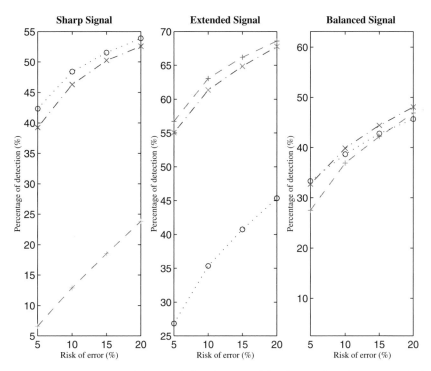

Figure 4 Percentage of detected signal *versus* risk of error for three types of signal in 3×10^3 3D volumes ($64 \times 64 \times 32$ voxels or $128 \times 128 \times 64$ mm^3). (Left) Sharp peak. (Middle) Extended signal. (Right) "Balanced" signal. The dashed line shows the results from the spatial extent test, the dotted line from the peak height test and the dot and dashed line from the combined test. Volume resolution was FWHM$_{xy}$ = 14.1 mm FWHM$_z$ = 11.8 mm and threshold $t = 3$.

preserve better the spatial resolution of large signals, an important feature for the analysis of fMRI data.

V. TESTING FOR THE SIGNIFICANCE OF A SET OF REGIONS

This section extends the previous tests and describes a new level of inference that is, in general, more sensitive but has less localising power. The test is based on the number of suprathreshold regions of size greater than k_u compared to the expected number of such regions. Control of the risk of error at the region level cannot be obtained, and control over the risk of error now has to be considered at the set-level.

We first review the operational equations and then report power analyses [8].

A. Theory

Let C_{nu} be the number of regions defined with a threshold u and area greater than n occurring in V. To test for this number we compute the probability of having C_{nu} regions *or more* of size n_u *or more* in V. This is also one minus the probability of obtaining less than C_{nu} regions with size greater than n_u,

$$\Pr(C_{nu} \geq c) = \sum_{i=0}^{c-1} \sum_{j=i}^{\infty} \Pr(C_{\odot u} = j) \binom{j}{i} \Pr(n_u \geq n)^i \Pr(n_u < n)^{j-1}$$

$$= 1 - \sum_{i=0}^{c-1} Y \left(\mathsf{E}[\chi_u] \Pr(n_u \geq n) \right), \tag{11}$$

where $\Pr(C_{\odot u} = j)$ is the probability of getting j regions above u of any size ($_\odot$ denotes any value here) in V, given Eq. (1), which also defines $Y(\odot)$. The second equality above can be seen directly by noting that the number of clusters of size n_u or more is a restriction of the process defined by the number of clusters (with any size) and therefore also follows a Poisson law. The mean of this process is simply the mean of the original process times the probability $\Pr(n_u \geq n)$.

The equation is very general and reduces to the intensity test (Section II) and to the spatial extent test (Section III) with appropriate parameters. If $n = 0$ and $c = 1$ then (11) reduces to the probability found in Section II (probability of having at least one cluster of unspecified size). If $c = 1$ and n_u is left unspecified, then the test reduces to the spatial extent test.

B. Power Analysis

We use a simulated "activation signal" that can be modeled mathematically and is physiologically plausible. Brain signals are modeled by a Gaussian random process (and therefore distributed), of a certain width f (expressed as a proportion of the smoothness of noise) and height (variance σ^2). Using this model, we can compute the probability of the alternative hypothesis depending on the parameters σ. The smoothness under the alternative hypothesis is [10]

$$u^* = u \left(1 + \sigma^2\right)^{-1/2}$$

$$|\Lambda^*|^{-1/2} = |\Lambda|^{-1/2} \left[\frac{(1 + \sigma^2)}{(1 + \sigma^2/(1 + f^2))} \right]^{1/2}.$$

For a given risk of error, α, given by $\Pr_{|\Lambda|}(C_{nu} \geq x)$, the sensitivity of the test is simply the probability $\Pr_{|\Lambda^*|}(C_{nu^*} \geq x)$. Using this model, we simply vary the parameters $u, |\Lambda|$, and n to assess the power of the different tests. Traditionally, sensitivity is plotted against the risk α. These plots are called receiving operator curves (ROC). Figure 5 shows the result of this power analysis.

In Figs. 6 and 7 we illustrate the use of such tests in a PET dataset (a verbal fluency experiment). In this case $u = 3.2$, and the spatial extent threshold was the expected value given the smoothness and the volume analyzed (eight voxels). The most sensitive test was that at the set level of inference, but note that among eight clusters in the SPM, one or two are expected to occur by chance (expected number: 1.4). For the second region listed in Fig. 7 the conjoint test was much more significant than the test on intensity (because of the cluster size) and performed approximately as well for the other clusters.

C. Discussion

Clearly, results obtained with the set level of inference should be interpreted with caution when reporting the anatomical localisation of regions forming

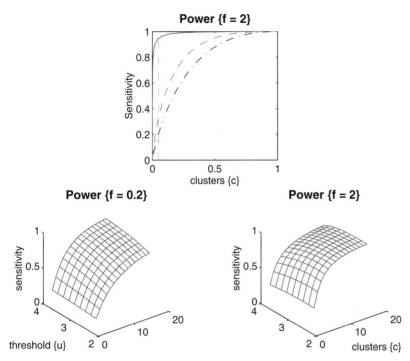

FIGURE 5 (Top) ROC curve for set-level inference with $u = 2.8$ and $n = 16$ voxels. $\mathrm{Pr}_{|\Lambda|}(C_{nu} \geq x)$ where $|\Lambda|$ corresponds to a FWHM of 3 voxels and the volume $V = 64^3$. Signal amplitude $\sigma = 0.3$ and width $f = 2$. The dashed and broken lines correspond to the equivalent cluster and voxel-level ROC curves, respectively. (Bottom) Three-dimensional plot of power ($\alpha = 0.05$) as a function of cluster number c and threshold u, for the same smoothness, volume V, and σ. (Left) $f = 0.2$ and right $f = 2$.

the significant set. However, if the number of observed regions (above u and of size greater than n_u) is much greater than the predicted number (*e.g.*, 0.5 regions expected, 5 observed) then it makes sense to report all the clusters if only descriptively. Conversely, if 5 clusters are observed but 2.5 are expected by chance, it is difficult to elaborate on the regional specificity of the results, and the set-level of inference gives information that is only slightly more precise than an omnibus test, thus providing very little regional information.

The set level of inference can be extended using a conjoint probability for both peak height and spatial extent. Simply, $\mathrm{Pr}(n_u \geq n)$ is changed for $\mathrm{Pr}_{\mathrm{joint}} = \sigma_{\mathrm{joint}}$ in Eq. (11). This manoeuver will not add another parameter (peak height); the set will simply be formed by clusters that have a probability less than a chosen value of α_{joint} (for instance $\alpha_{\mathrm{joint}} = 0.4$, either because of the height or the extent above u).

VI. NONPARAMETRIC APPROACHES: STATISTICAL *NON*PARAMETRIC MAPPING (SnPM)

A. Rationale and Method

Recently, nonparametric multiple comparisons procedures have been introduced for the assessment of functional mapping experiments, based on ran-

SPM{Z}

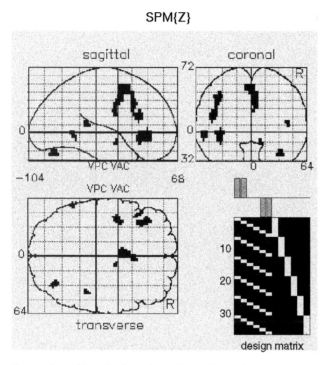

FIGURE 6 "Glass brain" view of an SPM of a verbal fluency experiment showing activation in the medial frontal cortex. The design matrix of the experiment is shown in the bottom right corner (see [14] for full details on the design matrices). Figure 7 presents the statistical results associated with this SPM.

set-level {c}	cluster-level {k,Z}	voxel-level {Z}	location {mm}
0.000 (8)	0.028 (27, 4.78)	0.018 (4.78)	-46 24 20
	0.006 (126, 4.68)	0.027 (4.68)	-2 8 48
		0.173 (4.20)	4 16 32
		0.889 (3.46)	4 14 44
	0.031 (76, 4.61)	0.037 (4.61)	-36 24 -8
		0.154 (4.24)	-36 32 0
	0.129 (26, 4.33)	0.108 (4.33)	32 -74 -24

Height threshold {u} = 3.20, p = 0.001	Volume {S} = 53132 voxels or 625 Resels
Extent threshold {k} = 8 voxels	Degrees of freedom due to error = 25
Expected voxels per cluster, E{n} = 8.2	Smoothness = 9.8 11.2 12.5 mm {FWHM}
Expected number of clusters, E{m} = 1.4	= 4.1 4.8 5.3 {voxels}

FIGURE 7 This table presents an example of the SPM96 statistical results with the set, cluster, and voxel level of inference (n_u is denoted k in this table). Note the relative sensitivity of these three tests and the loss of regional specificity.

domisation or permutation test theory [13]. By considering appropriate permutations of the labeling of scans (labeling as "rest" and "active," or by some associated covariate such as scan score) and computing statistic images for each labeling, a permutation distribution for the entire statistic image can be obtained. From this null distribution of the statistic image, given the data and appropriate null hypothesis, the permutation distribution of any statistic summarising the statistic image can be found. Summarising each statistic image by its maximum statistic gives the permutation distribution for Z_{max}, the $100(1 - \alpha)$th percentile of which is the appropriate critical threshold for a single threshold test at level α. Summarising each statistic image by the size of the largest cluster of voxels with values above a prespecified threshold gives the permutation distribution of S_{max}, and appropriate critical suprathreshold cluster sizes. Strong control over experimentwise type I error is maintained (at the appropriate level) in both cases.

In addition to the usual attractions of nonparametric methods, namely minimal assumptions, guaranteed validity and exactness, flexibility and intuitiveness, the approach is especially attractive for small data sets such as those from single subject PET studies. Statistic images with low degrees of freedom exhibit high (spatial) frequency noise therefore the statistic image is rough. The properties of such statistic images are not well approximated by continuous random fields with the same distributions. Continuous fields have features smaller than the voxel dimensions, leading to critical thresholds for single threshold tests that are conservative for lattice representations of the continuous field. An extreme example is a three-dimensional strictly stationary continuous random t field with 3 degrees of freedom, which almost certainly has a singularity [24].

The noise in low degree of freedom statistic images results from variability of the residual variance estimate. In PET it is reasonable to assume that the residual variability is approximately constant over small localities, suggesting that variance estimates could be locally pooled. A weighted local pooling of variance estimates is a smoothing of the estimated variance image (since the degrees of freedom are the same at every voxel). An example of a smoothed variance image for a PET dataset is shown in Fig. 8a, where weights from an isotropic three-dimensional Gaussian kernel of FWHM 12

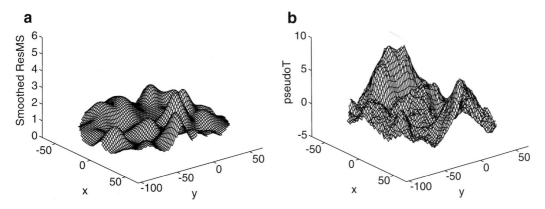

Figure 8 Statistic images for PET data set: (a) Mesh plot (intercommisural plane) of estimated variance image smoothed with an isotropic Gaussian kernel of FWHM 12 mm, truncated at the edge of the intracerebral volume. (b) Mesh plot of "pseudo" t statistic computed with smoothed variance estimate.

mm were used (the kernel was truncated at the edges of the intracerebral volume). Clearly variance estimates at proximate voxels are not independent. A theoretical distribution for such smoothed variance images has proved elusive, thus precluding further parametric analysis. The "pseudo" t statistic image formed with such a variance image is shown in figure 8b, and is much smoother than the original variance map (not shown). Figure 9 illustrates the results obtained with a pseudo t-statistic.

B. Results and Discussion

The ability to consider statistic images constructed with smoothed variance estimates appears to make the nonparametric approach considerably more powerful than the parametric approaches discussed. Nonparametric results for a PET data set are shown in Fig. 9a. One thousand permutations (including the actual allocation) of the 12! possible permutations of scan scores were considered, and the (approximate) permutation distribution of the maximum pseudo t statistic computed. The resulting single threshold test identifies many more significant voxels than the parametric single threshold test using the expected Euler characteristic on the "Gaussianised" t statistic (Fig. 9b).

Using raw t statistic images, the nonparametric approach on the whole agrees largely with parametric approaches, which is a comforting observation. Disadvantages of the nonparametric approach are a greater need for computer resources and a possible limitation when dealing with too small a number of relabelings.

Alternatively, the variance estimate can be improved by including more scans in the SPM96 analysis, taken from other subjects, while tests of the appropriate statistical contrast include only the actual subjects "of interest." This procedure assumes that physiological and instrumental noise variances are similar across pooled subjects (and that experimental effects have been removed using multilinear regression [14]). This assumption would not usually apply for patient studies. An example of such an analysis with normal subjects is given in [20].

VII. DISCUSSION AND CONCLUSION

A. Which Test Should Be Used and When

As the nature of a signal is unknown, it is impossible to predict which would be the best procedure to use for a given data set. Although, strictly speaking, it might not be valid to use several tests concurrently, the complex relationship between them and their nested aspect, should ensure that the risk of error is not exessively increased by the multitesting procedure. In future, Monte Carlo simulation will assess the extent of departure from the α risk of false positives chosen by the experimenter. We summarise the tests described above (Fig. 10) by a schematic unidimensional graph. Figure 11 gives an overview of the characteristics of the tests. For completeness we have added "omnibus" tests in this figure that give a probability value for the general overall pattern of the SPM although they are not described in this chapter (see Worsley *et al.* and Friston *et al.* [28, 9]).

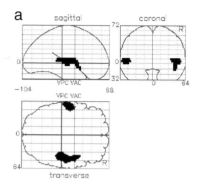

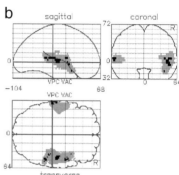

FIGURE 9 (a) "Glass brain" views of the significant voxels at $\alpha = 0.05$ from a nonparametric single threshold test using "pseudo" t statistic images. (b) Orthogonal "glass brain" views of the significant voxels at $\alpha = 0.05$ for the same PET dataset using the parametric approach. The smoothness of the "Gaussianized" t statistic image was estimated at $16.4 \times 17.5 \times 13.5$ mm, equivalent to 273 RESELS, for 66,689 intracerebral voxels. Voxels above the critical threshold $u_{\alpha=0.05}$ are shown black. Suprathreshold clusters of voxels were identified using a primary threshold of $\Phi^{-1}(1-0.001)$, identifying two significantly large clusters of voxels, shown translucent grey.

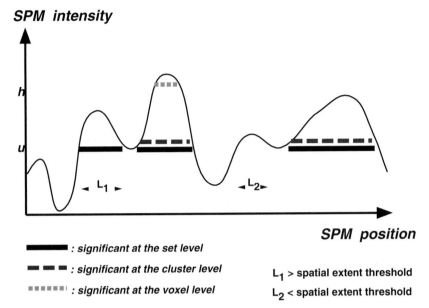

FIGURE 10 Symbolic representation of the intensity test, the cluster size (or conjoint) test, and the test over a set of regions.

B. Sensitivity and Specificity

In statistical analyses the risk of error is usually chosen to be 5%. We emphasize that this is an *arbitrary* threshold that may be too stringent on some occasion.

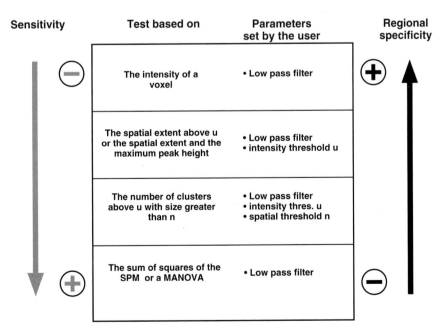

FIGURE 11 Overview of the characteristics of the hierarchy of test proposed for statistical inference in SPM. Note that the sensitivity is only *generally* increasing and in some cases more regionally specific tests will also be more sensitive.

In any case, a failure to reject the null hypothesis is never proof that the alternative hypothesis is untrue. In other words, we can never be sure that a region is not activated. We therefore recommend a discussion of results that do not reach the 5% level but are improbable under the hypothesis of noise only (risk of error of 5 to 20% for instance).

C. How Do We Choose the Parameters?

The more parameters used by the tests, the more difficult it is to choose optimal values for them *a priori*. Currently, three parameters must be chosen: the FWHM of the Gaussian kernel used for smoothing (affecting directly $|\Lambda|$), the threshold u (for the cluster level of inference), and the area n used in the set level of inference. An obvious way of proceeding is to acquire experience by analysing standard data sets and then fixing the parameters to some appropriate values.

However, this procedure would require that the volume analysed (V) and the smoothness parameter remain identical from one study to another. As this is not generally the case, we suggest setting u and n using statistical thresholds. For instance, u can be set such that, given V *and* $|\Lambda|^{-1/2}$, we have $\Pr(Z_{max} \geq u) = \xi$, where ξ will depend on the regional specificity required for the experiment (*e.g.*, for high regional specificity, $\xi = 0.75$). In an analogous way, n can be set using the expected area above u ($\mathsf{E}[n_u]$) as a reference: $n_u = \zeta\mathsf{E}[n_u]$ where $\zeta \leq 1$ for a moderate regional specificity. Future versions of SPM96 software will provide default values based on a desired regional specificity. Note that repeatedly trying different parameters will invalidate the confidence level to an unknown degree and should therefore be avoided. Note also that no correction is made for the number of contrasts performed; the risk of error is set per contrast.

D. Smoothness Variability

It is essential to note that in general the value of $|\Lambda|$ and the variance of an SPM are the only values that need to be estimated when assessing the significance of activation in SPMs (there is no error of measure on the volume V). An error on the assessment of Λ directly influences the estimation of the significance of results. Using the frequency (spectral) representation of the process (*i.e.*, the SPM, denoted X) we were able to derive the variance of the estimate of the smoothness. The principle of this computation is the following. We first assume that the PSF of the SPM is known and use this to compute the variance covariance matrix of the vector $\mathbf{U}$,

$$\mathbf{U} = (U_1, U_2, \ldots, U_{D+1}) = \left(\widehat{\mathrm{var}}(X(\mathbf{x})), \widehat{\mathrm{var}}\left(\frac{\partial X}{\partial x_1}\right), \widehat{\mathrm{var}}\left(\frac{\partial X}{\partial x_2}\right), \ldots\right),$$

where $\mathbf{x} = (x_1, x_2, \ldots, x_D)$ are the D dimensions of the space and $\hat{}$ signifies that the variance is only estimated from the data (as the sum of squares divided by the number of data points). The smoothness estimation is a simple function of the vector $\mathbf{U}$, say $f(\mathbf{U})$ and once the variance covariance matrix of its component have been found we use the Taylor expansion to obtain an estimate of the variance of $f(\mathbf{U})$ (where $f(\mathbf{U}) = (\widehat{\mathrm{var}}(X(\mathbf{x})))^D|\Lambda|^{-1}$ in

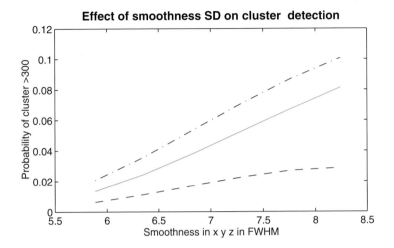

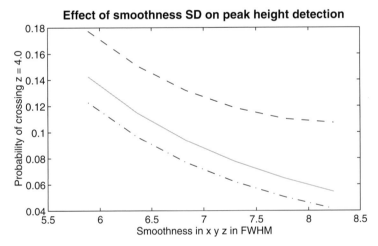

FIGURE 12 (Top) Variation of cluster size probability for a 3D process (or SPM) with the smoothness defined as the FWHM of a Gaussian kernel (defined in *pixels*) and the variation of the smoothness estimate (dashed line, $+2$ standard deviation, σ_Λ; dotted and dashed line, $-2\sigma_\Lambda$). Threshold for the cluster definition was 2.8, size of the SPM: 510^4 pixels. (Bottom) Variation of the Z value probability for 2D data for $Z = 4$ with the smoothness value and with the variation σ_Λ of its estimate (dashed line, $+2\sigma_\Lambda$; dotted and dashed line, $-2\sigma_\Lambda$).

D dimensions):

$$\text{var}(f(\mathbf{U})) = \sum_{i,j\in(1,\ldots,D+1)} \frac{\partial f(\mathbf{U})}{\partial U_i}\frac{\partial f)\mathbf{U})}{\partial U_j}\widehat{\text{cov}}(U_i, U_j).$$

For instance, using this approximation, we found that the standard deviation of the smoothness estimation σ_Λ was around 25% of the smoothness value (using common values for PET experiments). Figure 12 shows the effect of this uncertainty on the P values obtained with the intensity or the cluster size tests.[1]

---

[1] Note that the variance of the process (the SPM) is often known but is assessed in a more general case and therefore the estimation of $\widehat{\text{var}}(X(\mathbf{x}))$ can be "included" in the smoothness estimation. In other words, the smoothness estimation has generally to include the map variance estimation.

E. Smoothness Estimation on the Residuals

In SPM95 smoothness is assessed on Gaussianised t maps (G-tm) that are not generally free of physiological signal. This technique has two major drawbacks. First, the estimation is not stable (the variance of the estimate being far from negligible [22]) and second, the signal in the Gt-m will bias any estimation. A rigorous method that overcomes these drawbacks based on previously derived theoretical results [26] is presented here and implemented in SPM96. To free the smoothness estimation from signal introduced by an experimental design we propose using the residual processes that are left after removing the effects modeled in the design matrix. We make the assumption that the smoothness of these fields will approximate the smoothness of the component processes of the t field under the null hypothesis. The residual fields are defined by

$$R_i(\mathbf{x}) = Y_i(\mathbf{x}) - \hat{Y}_i(\mathbf{x}) = Y_i(\mathbf{x}) - D\hat{\beta}(\mathbf{x}),$$

where $\mathbf{x}$ is a location in space, i indexes the ith observation, D (denoted X in [14]) is the design matrix of the experiment, the $\hat{\beta}$ are the estimated effects, Y_i are the original values (scans), and $\hat{Y}_i$ the fitted values. The R_i are free from all linear effects explicitly modeled in the analysis. We first demonstrate (using simulated stationary Gaussian smoothed processes) that smoothnesses of residual fields R_i and of original fields Y_i are equivalent and that this holds whatever the degrees of freedom (df) in R_i. The smoothness of 36 R_i using noise only random fields (8.2, 8.2, 5.9 FWHM in (x, y, z)) was assessed for a series of design matrices of decreasing rank, giving 7, 15, and 25 df. We then used results derived by Worsley *et al.* to relate the smoothness $|\Lambda|$ of the original component fields (estimated with R_i) to the smoothness $|\Lambda^\dagger|$ of the Gaussianised t fields with $|\Lambda^\dagger| = \lambda_{n'}\Lambda\sigma^2$ with σ^2 the variance of the original processes and $\lambda_{n'}$ a correction factor defined in [26] that depends on the number of independent residual fields n'.

Table 1 presents the theoretical (Theo) smoothness values for the Gaussianised t fields (*i.e.*, true values corrected by $\lambda_{n'}$), the values estimated using 36 R_i (Res) and the values estimated using t maps (Gt-m) (with random orthogonal contrasts). It is seen that the values assessed on t maps and on the residual maps are good estimates. However, we also demonstrate that the smoothness estimate can be biased under an alternative hypothesis, by assessing its value using the Gt-m of a data set in which half of the images contain a cubic signal (size $17 \times 17 \times 9$ voxels, and magnitude set to 0.3

TABLE 1

Theoretical *vs* Estimated (on Residuals and Gt-m) Smoothness

	$df = 7$			$df = 15$			$df = 25$		
	Theo.	Res.	Gt-m.	Theo.	Res.	Gt-m.	Theo.	Res.	Gt-m.
x	7.5	7.6 (0.1)	7.9 (0.2)	7.9	8.0 (0.1)	7.8 (0.2)	8.1	8.1 (0.1)	8.3 (0.2)
y	7.5	7.7 (0.1)	7.7 (0.1)	7.9	8.0 (0.1)	8.2 (0.2)	8.1	8.2 (0.1)	8.1 (0.2)
z	5.4	5.6 (0.1)	5.3 (0.1)	5.7	5.8 (0.1)	5.6 (0.2)	5.8	5.8 (0.1)	5.8 (0.2)

Note. Values in pixels FWHM. Res., (SDM) 36 processes, and Gt-m, (SD) over random contrasts.

noise SD). The contrast used to create the t fields (25 df) tested for the main activation effect. These simulations show that the discrepancy between the theoretical value and the Gt-m estimate is important: Theo, (8.1, 8.1, 5.8); Gt-m, (10.1, 10.4, 7.1) FWHM in (x, y, z). Assessing the smoothness of the residuals fields provides a much better estimate: (8.1, 8.0, 5.8). Recent work has further refined this method and smoothness in SPMs is now assessed using normalized residuals.

F. A priori Hypothesis

It should be noted that with a prior hypothesis about the localisation of signal, *i.e.*, if a precise position (x, y, z) is tested, it is possible to use noncorrected P values. If the precise localisation is not known, but a larger circumscribed region is interrogated for the occurrence of an activation, the p value should be corrected for that volume (for instance using the results derived by Worsley for small regions [23]). More often than not several hypotheses about the localisation are possible and therefore a correction (Bonferroni) should be made for the number of regions to be interrogated to ensure the validity of the statistical procedures.

G. Testing for Commonalities

Often, the question of experimental interest relates to the commonalities between two SPMs. A simple way of dealing with this problem is to look for voxels that have a low probability of occurrence in both SPMs. If the components of the design matrix (see Chapter 4 for description of the design matrix) used to produce the SPMs are orthogonal then the resulting P values in the conjoint map are the product of the P values in the original SPMs.

References

1. R. Adler, "The Geometry of Random Fields." Wiley, New York, 1981.
2. John Ashburner and Karl J. Friston. "Spatial Transformation of Images," Chap. 2, pp. 1–12. Functional Imaging Laboratory, London, 1996. (http://www.fil.ion.ucl.ac.uk/spm)
3. Christian Buechel and Karl J. Friston. "Effective Connectivity in Neuroimaging," Chap. 6, pp. 1–15. Functional Imaging Laboratory, London, 1996. (http://www.fil.ion.ucl.ac.uk/spm)
4. D. R. Cox and H. D. Miller. "The Theory of Stochastic Processes." Chapman and Hall, London, 1990.
5. K. J. Friston, J. Ashburner, C. D. Frith, J.-B. Poline, J. D. Heather, and R. S. J. Frackowiak. Spatial registration and normalization of images. *Hum. Brain Mapping* **2**, 165–89 (1996). (http://www.fil.ion.ucl.ac.uk/spm)
6. K. J. Friston, C. D. Frith, P. F. Liddle, R. J. Dolan, A. A. Lammertsma, and R. S. J. Frackowiak. The relationship between global and local changes in PET scans. *J. Cereb. Blood Flow Metab.* **10**, 458–466 (1990).
7. K. J. Friston, C. D. Frith, P. F. Liddle, and R. S. J. Frackowiak. Comparing functional (PET) images: The assessment of significant change. *J. Cereb. Blood Flow Metab.* **10**, 690–699 (1991).
8. K. J. Friston, J.-B. Poline, A. P. Holmes, C. J. Price, and C. D. Frith. Detecting activations in PET and fMRI: Levels of inference and power. *NeuroImage* **4**, 223–235 (1996).
9. K. J. Friston, J.-B. Poline, S. Strother, A. P. Holmes, C. D. Frith, and R. S. J.

Frackowiak. A multivariate analysis of PET activation studies. *Hum. Brain Mapping*, in press (1996).

10. K. J. Friston, K. J. Worsley, R. S. J. Frackowiak, J. C. Mazziotta, and A. C. Evans. Assessing the significance of focal activations using their spatial extent. *Hum. Brain Mapping* **1**, 214–220 (1994).

11. A. M. Hasofer. The mean number of maxima above high levels in gaussian random fields. *J. Appl. Prob.* **13**, 377–379 (1976).

12. Y. Hochberg and A. C. Tamhane. "Multiple Comparisons Procedures." Wiley, New York, 1987.

13. A. P. Holmes, R. C. Blair, J. D. G. Watson, and I. Ford. Non-parametric analysis of statistic images from functional mapping experiments. *J. Cereb. Blood Flow Metab.* **16**, 7–22 (1996).

14. A. P. Holmes, J.-B. Poline, and K. J. Friston. "Statistical Models and Experimental Design," Chap. 3, pp. 1–20. Functional Imaging Laboratory, London, 1996. (http://www.fil.ion.ucl.ac.uk/spm)

15. V. P. Nosko. The characteristics of excursions of Gaussian homogeneous random fields above a high level. *In* "Proceedings, USSR–Japan Symposium on Probability, Harbarovsk, 1969, pp. 216–222. Novosibirsk, 1969.

16. V. P. Nosko. "On Shines of Gaussian Random Fields." Technical report, Vestnik Moscow. Univ. Ser. I. Mat. Meth., 1970. [in Russian]

17. V. P. Nosko. Local structure of gaussian random fields in the vicinity of high level shines. *Sov. Math. Dok* **10**, 1481–1484 (1976).

18. J.-B. Poline and B. M. Mazoyer. Analysis of individual positron emission tomography activation maps by detection of high signal-to-noise ratio pixel clusters. *J. Cereb. Blood Flow Metab.* **13**, 425–437 (1993).

19. J.-B. Poline and B. M. Mazoyer. Enhanced detection in brain activation maps using a multi filtering approach. *J. Cereb. Blood Flow Metab.* **14**, 639–641 (1994).

20. J.-B. Poline, R. Vandenberghe, A. P. Holmes, K. J. Friston, and R. S. J. Frackowiak. Reproducibility of PET activation studies: Lessons from a multi-centre european experiment. *NeuroImage* **4**, 34–54 (1996).

21. J.-B. Poline, R. Vandenberghe, A. P. Holmes, and K. J. Friston, Combining spatial extent and peak intensity to test for activations in functional imaging. Submitted for publication.

22. J.-B. Poline, K. J. Worsley, A. P. Holmes, R. S. J. Frackowiak, and K. J. Friston. Estimating smoothness in statistical parametric maps: Variability of p-values. *J. Comput. Assist. Tomogr.* **19**(5), 788–796 (1995).

23. K. J. Worsley, S. Marrett, P. Neelin, K. J. Friston, and A. Evans. "A Unified Statistical Approach for Determining Significant Signals in Images of Cerebral Activation," Academic Press, San Diego, 1995.

24. K. J. Worsley. Instability of localisation of cerebral blood flow activation foci with parametric maps. *J. Cereb. Blood Flow Metab* **13**(6), 1041–1042 (1993). [In reply to S. F. Taylor, S. M. Minoshima, and R. A. Koeppe]

25. K. J. Worsley. Local maxima and the expected euler characteristic of excursion sets of χ^2, f, and t fields. *Adv,. Appl. Prob.* **26**, 13–42 (1994).

26. K. J. Worsley, A. C. Evans, S. Marrett, and P. Neelin. A three-dimensional statistical analysis for CBF activation studies in human brain. *J. Cereb. Blood Flow Metab.* **12**, 900–918 (1992).

27. K. J. Worsley, S. Marrett, P. Neelin, and A. C. Evans. A three-dimensional statistical analysis for CBF activation studies in human brain. *J. Cereb. Blood Flow Metab.* **12**, 900–918 (1992).

28. K. J. Worsley, J.-B. Poline, R. S. J. Frackowiak, and K. J. Friston, A test for distributed, non focal brain activation. *NeuroImage* **2**, 183–194 (1995).

CHAPTER SIX

CHARACTERISING DISTRIBUTED FUNCTIONAL SYSTEMS

I. INTRODUCTION

This chapter is concerned with the characterisation of imaging data from a multivariate perspective. This means that the observations at each voxel are considered conjointly with explicit reference to the interactions among brain regions. The concept of functional connectivity is introduced and provides the basis for understanding what eigenimages represent and how they can be interpreted. Having considered the nature of eigenimages and variations on their applications we then turn to a related approach that, unlike eigenimage analysis, is predicated on a statistical model. This approach is called multivariate analysis of variance (MANCOVA) and uses canonical variates analysis to create canonical images. In contradistinction to previous chapters this and the next chapter are less concerned with functional segregation but more with functional integration. The integrated and distributed nature of neurophysiological responses to sensorimotor or cognitive challenge makes a multivariate perspective particularly appropriate and provides a complementary characterisation of activation studies.

II. FUNCTIONAL INTEGRATION AND CONNECTIVITY

A landmark meeting that took place on the morning of August 4th, 1881, highlighted the difficulties of attributing function to a cortical area, given the dependence of cerebral activity on underlying connections [1]. Goltz, although accepting the results of electrical stimulation in dog and monkey cortex, considered the excitation method inconclusive in that the movements elicited might have originated in related pathways, or current could have spread to distant centres. Despite advances over the past century, the question remains: Are the physiological changes elicited by sensorimotor or cognitive challenges explained by functional segregation or by integrated and distributed changes mediated by neuronal connections? The question itself calls for a framework within which to address these issues. *Functional and effective connectivity* are concepts critical to this framework.

A. Origins and Definitions

In the analysis of neuroimaging time series functional connectivity is defined as the "*temporal correlations between spatially remote neurophysiological events*" [2]. This definition provides a simple characterization of functional interactions. The alternative is effective connectivity (*i.e.*, "*the influence one neuronal system exerts over another*") [3]. These concepts originated in the analysis of separable spike trains obtained from multiunit electrode recordings [4,5]. Functional connectivity is simply a statement about the observed correlations; it does not comment on how these correlations are mediated. For example, at the level of multiunit microelectrode recordings, correlations can result from stimulus-locked transients evoked by a common afferent input, or reflect stimulus-induced oscillations, phasic coupling of neural assemblies mediated by synaptic connections [6]. Effective connectivity is closer to the notion of a connection and can be defined as the influence one neural system exerts over another at either a synaptic (*cf.* synaptic efficacy) or a cortical level. Although functional and effective connectivity can be invoked at a conceptual level in both neuroimaging and electrophysiology they differ fundamentally at a practical level. This is because the time scales and nature of neurophysiological measurements are very different (seconds *vs* milliseconds and haemodynamics *vs* spike trains). In electrophysiology it is often necessary to remove the confounding effects of stimulus-locked transients (that introduce correlations not causally mediated by direct neural interactions) in order to reveal an underlying connectivity. The confounding effect of stimulus-evoked transients is less problematic in neuroimaging because promulgation of dynamics from primary sensory areas onward is mediated by neuronal connections (usually reciprocal and interconnecting). However, it should be remembered that functional connectivity is not necessarily due to effective connectivity (*e.g.*, common neuromodulatory input from ascending aminergic neurotransmitter systems or thalamo-cortical afferents) and, where it is, effective influences may be indirect (*e.g.*, polysynaptic relays through multiple areas).

III. EIGENIMAGES, MULTIDIMENSIONAL SCALING, AND OTHER DEVICES

In what follows we introduce a number of techniques (eigenimage analysis, multidimensional scaling, partial least squares, and generalised eigenimage analysis) using functional connectivity as a reference. Emphasis is placed on the relationships between these techniques. For example, eigenimage analysis is equivalent to principal component analysis and the variant of multidimensional scaling considered here is equivalent to principal coordinates analysis. Principal components and coordinates analyses are predicated on exactly the same eigenvector solution and from a mathematical perspective are essentially the same thing.

A. Measuring a Pattern of Correlated Activity

Here we introduce a simple way of measuring the amount a pattern of activity (representing a connected brain system) contributes to the functional connectivity or variance–covariance observed in imaging data. Functional connectivity is defined in terms of correlations or covariances (correlations are normalised covariances). The point to point functional connectivity between one voxel and another is not usually of great interest. The important aspect of a covariance structure is the pattern of correlated activity subtended by (an enormous number of) pairwise covariances. In measuring such patterns it is useful to introduce the concept of a *norm*. Vector and matrix norms serve the same purpose as absolute values for scalar quantities. In other words, they furnish a measure of distance. One frequently used norm is the 2-norm, which is the length of a vector. The vector 2-norm can be used to measure the degree to which a particular pattern of brain activity contributes to a covariance structure. If a pattern is described by a column vector ($\mathbf{p}$), with an element for each voxel, then the contribution of that pattern to the covariance structure can be measured by the 2-norm of $\mathbf{M}$. $\mathbf{p} = |\mathbf{M} \cdot \mathbf{p}|_2 \cdot \mathbf{M}$ is a (mean corrected) matrix of data with one row for each successive scan and one column for each voxel ($^\mathrm{T}$ denotes transposition):

$$|\mathbf{M} \cdot \mathbf{p}|_2^2 = \mathbf{p}^\mathrm{T} \cdot \mathbf{M}^\mathrm{T} \cdot \mathbf{M} \cdot \mathbf{P}. \tag{1}$$

Put simply, the 2-norm is a number that reflects the amount of variance–covariance or functional connectivity that can be accounted for by a particular distributed pattern. If time-dependent changes occur predominantly in regions described by the pattern ($\mathbf{p}$) then the correlation between the pattern of activity and $\mathbf{p}$ *over space* will vary substantially *over time*. The 2-norm measures this temporal variance in the spatial correlation. The pattern $\mathbf{p}$ can be used to define the functional connectivity of interest. For example, if one were interested in the functional connectivity between left dorsolateral prefrontal cortex (DLPFC) and left superior temporal region one could test for this interaction using the 2-norm in Eq. (1) where $\mathbf{p}$ had large values in the frontal and temporal regions. This approach has been used to demonstrate abnormal prefronto-temporal integration in schizophrenia [7], an example we shall return to below.

It should be noted that the 2-norm measures only the pattern of interest. There may be many other important patterns of functional connectivity. This fact begs the question "what are the most prevalent patterns of coherent activity?" To answer this question one turns to eigenimages or spatial modes.

B. Eigenimages and Spatial Modes

In this section the concept of eigenimages or spatial modes is introduced in terms of patterns of activity ($\mathbf{p}$) defined in the previous section. We show that spatial modes are simply those patterns that account for the most variance–covariance (*i.e.*, have the largest 2-norm).

Eigenimages or spatial modes are most commonly obtained using singular value decomposition (SVD). SVD is an operation that decomposes an original time series ($\mathbf{M}$) into two sets of orthogonal vectors (patterns in space and patterns in time) $\mathbf{V}$ and $\mathbf{U}$, where

$$[\mathbf{U} \quad \mathbf{S} \quad \mathbf{V}] = \mathrm{SVD}\{\mathbf{M}\}$$

such that

$$\mathbf{M} \qquad = \mathbf{U} \cdot \mathbf{S} \cdot \mathbf{V}^\mathrm{T}. \tag{2}$$

U and **V** are unitary orthogonal matrices (the sum of squares of each column is unity and all the columns are uncorrelated) and **S** is a diagonal matrix (only the leading diagonal has nonzero values) of decreasing singular values. The singular value of each eigenimage is simply its 2-norm. Because SVD maximises the largest singular value, the first eigenimage is the pattern that accounts for the greatest amount of the variance–covariance structure. In summary, SVD and equivalent devices are powerful ways of decomposing an imaging time series into a series of orthogonal patterns that embody, in a stepdown fashion, the greatest amounts of functional connectivity. Each eigenvector (column of **V**) defines a distributed brain system that can be displayed as an image. The distributed systems that ensue are called eigenimages or spatial modes and have been used to characterise the spatiotemporal dynamics of neurophysiological time series from several modalities, including multiunit electrode recordings [8], EEG [9], MEG [10], PET [2], and functional MRI [11].

Many readers will notice that the eigenimages associated with the functional connectivity or covariance matrix are simply principal components of the time series. In the EEG literature one sometimes comes across the Karhunen–Loeve expansion which is employed to identify spatial modes. If this expansion is in terms of eigenvectors of covariances (and it usually is), then the analysis is formally identical to the one presented above.

One might ask what the column vectors of **U** in Eq. (2) correspond to. These vectors are the time-dependent profiles associated with each eigenimage. They reflect the extent to which an eigenimage is expressed in each experimental condition or over time. These vectors play an important role in the functional attribution of distributed systems defined by eigenimages. This point and others will be illustrated in the next section.

C. Mapping Function into Anatomical Space—Eigenimage Analysis

To illustrate the approach, we will use a standard word generation study. The data were obtained from five subjects scanned 12 times whilst performing one of two verbal tasks in alternation. One task involved repeating a letter presented aurally at one per 2 secs (word shadowing). The other was a paced verbal fluency task, where subjects responded with a word that began with the letter presented (intrinsic word generation). To facilitate intersubject pooling, the data were realigned and spatially normalised and smoothed with an isotropic Gaussian kernel (FWHM of 16 mm). The data were then subject to an ANCOVA (with 12 conditions, subject effects and global activity as a confound). Voxels were selected using the omnibus F ratio to identify those significant at $P < 0.05$ (uncorrected). The adjusted time series from each of these voxels formed a mean corrected data matrix **M** with 12 rows (one for each condition) and one column for each voxel.

The images data matrix **M** was subject to SVD as described in the previous section. The distribution of eigenvalues (Fig. 1, bottom left) suggests that only two eigenimages are required to account for most of the observed variance–covariance structure. The first mode accounted for 64% and the second for 16% of the variance. The first eigenimage (the first column of **V**) is shown in Fig. 1 (top) along with the corresponding vector in time (the first column of **U**, bottom right). The first eigenimage has positive loadings in the anterior cingulate, the left DLPFC, Broca's area, the thalamic nuclei, and the cerebellum. Negative loadings were seen bitemporally and in the posterior

eigenimage 1 {–ve}

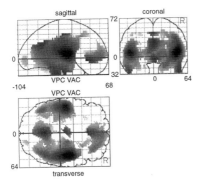

eigenimage 1 {+ve}

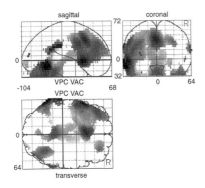

Eigenimage analysis:

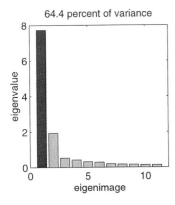

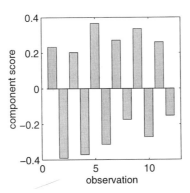

FIGURE 1 Eigenimage analysis the PET activation study of word generation. (Top) Positive and negative components of the first eigenimage (*i.e.*, first column of **V**). The maximum intensity projection display format is standard and provides three views of the brain in the stereotactic space of Talairach and Tournoux [20] (from the back, from the right, and from the top). (Bottom left) Eigenvalues (singular values squared) of the functional connectivity matrix reflecting the relative amounts of variance accounted for by the 11 eigenimages associated with these data. Only two eigenvalues are greater than unity and to all intents and purposes the changes characterising this time series can be considered two-dimensional. (Bottom right) The temporal eigenvector reflecting the expression of this eigenimage over the 12 conditions (*i.e.*, the first column of **U**).

cingulate. According to **U** this eigenimage is prevalent in the verbal fluency tasks with negative scores in word shadowing. The second spatial mode (not shown) had its highest positive loadings in the anterior cingulate and bitemporal regions (notably Wernicke's area on the left). This mode appears to correspond to a highly nonlinear, monotonic time effect with greatest prominence in earlier conditions.

The post hoc functional attribution of these eigenimages is usually based on their time-dependent profiles (**U**). The first mode may represent an intentional system critical for the intrinsic generation of words in the sense that the key cognitive difference between verbal fluency and word shadowing is the intrinsic generation as opposed to extrinsic specification of word representations and implicit mnemonic processing. The second system, which includes the anterior cingulate, seems to be involved in habituation, possibly of attentional or perceptual set.

There is nothing "biologically" important about the particular spatial modes obtained in this fashion, in the sense that one could "rotate" the eigenvectors such that they were still orthogonal and yet gave different eigenimages. The uniqueness of the particular solution given by SVD is that the first eigenimage accounts for the largest amount of variance–covariance and the second for the greatest amount that remains and so on. The reason that the eigenimages in the example above lend themselves to such a simple interpretation is that the variance introduced by experimental design (intentional) was substantially greater than that due to time (attentional) and both these sources were greater than any other effect. Other factors that ensure a parsimonious characterization of a time series with small numbers of well defined modes include (i) smoothness in the data and (ii) using only voxels that show a nontrivial amount of change during the scanning session.

D. Mapping Anatomy into Functional Space—Multidimensional Scaling

In the previous section the functional connectivity matrix was used to define associated eigenimages or spatial modes. In this section functional connectivity is used in a different way, namely, to constrain the proximity of two cortical areas in some functional space. The objective here is to transform anatomical space so that the distance between cortical areas is directly related to their functional connectivity. This transformation defines a new space whose topography is purely functional in nature. This space is constructed using multidimensional scaling or principal coordinates analysis [12].

Multidimensional scaling (MDS) is a descriptive method for representing the structure of a system. Based on pairwise measures of similarity or confusability [13,14]. The resulting multidimensional spatial configuration of a system's elements embody, in their proximity relationships, comparative similarities. The technique was developed primarily for the analysis of perceptual spaces. The proposal that stimuli be modeled by points in space, so that perceived similarity is represented by spatial distances, goes back to the days of Isaac Newton [15]. The implementation of this idea, however, is relatively new [14].

Imagine K measures from n voxels plotted as n points in a K-dimensional space (K-space). If they have been normalized to zero mean and unit sum of squares, these points will fall on a K-1 dimensional sphere. The closer any two points are to each other, the greater their correlation or functional connectivity (in fact the correlation is a cosine of the angle subtended at the origin).

The distribution of these points embodies the functional topography. A view of this distribution that reveals the greatest structure is simply obtained by rotating the points to maximise their apparent dispersion (variance). In other words one looks at the subspace with the largest "volume" spanned by the principal axes of the n points in K-space. These principal axes are given by the eigenvectors of $\mathbf{M} \cdot \mathbf{M}^T$, *i.e.*, the column vectors of $\mathbf{U}$, from Eq. (2):

$$\mathbf{M} \cdot \mathbf{M}^T = \mathbf{U} \cdot \mathbf{S}^2 \cdot \mathbf{U}^T.$$

Let $\mathbf{Q}$ be the matrix of desired coordinates derived by simply projecting the original data ($\mathbf{M}^T$) onto axes defined by $\mathbf{U}$:

$$\mathbf{Q} = \mathbf{M}^T \cdot \mathbf{U} \tag{3}$$

Voxels that have a correlation of unity will occupy the same point in MDS space. Voxels that have independent dynamics (correlation = 0) will be $\sqrt{2}$ apart. Voxels that are negatively but totally correlated (correlation = -1) will be maximally separated (by a distance of 2). Profound negative correlations denote a functional association that is modeled in MDS functional space as diametrically opposed locations on the hypersphere. In other words, two regions with profound negative correlations will form two "poles" in functional space.

Following normalisation to unit sum of squares over each column $\mathbf{M}$ (the adjusted data matrix from the word generation study above) the data are subjected to singular value decomposition according to Eq. (2) and the coordinates $\mathbf{Q}$ of the voxels in MDS functional space are computed as in Eq. (3). Recall that only two eigenvalues exceed unity (Fig. 1, left), suggesting a functional space that is essentially two dimensional. The locations of voxels in this two-dimensional subspace are shown in Fig. 2 (lower row) by rendering voxels from different regions in different colours. The anatomical regions corresponding to the different colours are shown in the top row. Anatomical regions were selected to include those parts of the brain that showed the greatest variance during the 12 conditions. Anterior regions (Fig. 2, right) include the mediodorsal thalamus (blue), the dorsolateral prefrontal cortex (DLPFC), Broca's area (red), and the anterior cingulate (green). Posterior regions (Fig. 2, left) include the superior temporal regions (red), the posterior superior temporal regions (blue), and the posterior cingulate (green). The corresponding functional spaces (Fig. 2, lower rows) reveal a number of things about the functional topography elicited by this set of activation tasks. First, each anatomical region maps into a relatively localised portion of functional space. This preservation of local contiguity reflects the high correlations within anatomical regions due, in part, to smoothness of the original data and to high degrees of intraregional functional connectivity. Second, the anterior regions are almost in juxtaposition, as are posterior regions; however, the confluence of anterior and posterior regions forms two diametrically opposing poles (or one axis). This configuration suggests an anterior–posterior axis with prefronto-temporal and cingulo-cingulate components. One might have predicted this configuration by noting that the anterior regions had high positive loadings on the first eigenimage (see Fig. 1), while the posterior regions had high negative loadings. Third, within the anterior and posterior sets of regions certain generic features are evident. The most striking is the particular ordering of functional interactions. For example, the functional connectivity between posterior cingulate (green) and superior temporal regions (red) is high and similarly for the superior temporal (red) and posterior temporal regions (blue),

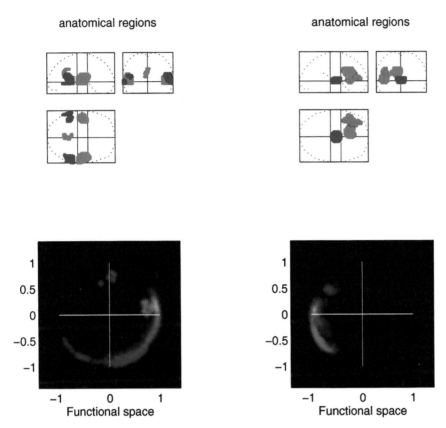

FIGURE 2 Classical or metric scaling analysis of the functional topography of intrinsic word generation in normal subjects. (Top) Anatomical regions categorised according to their colour. The designation was by reference to the atlas of Talairach and Tournoux [20]. (Bottom) Regions plotted in a functional space following the scaling transformation. In this space the proximity relationships reflect the functional connectivity between regions. The colour of each voxel corresponds to the anatomical region to which it belongs. The brightness reflects the local density of points corresponding to voxels in anatomical space. This density was estimated by binning the number of voxels in 0.02 "boxes" and smoothing with a Gaussian kernel of full width at half maximum of 3 boxes. Each colour was scaled to its maximum brightness.

yet the posterior cingulate and posterior temporal regions show very little functional connectivity (they are $\sqrt{2}$ apart or equivalently subtend 90° at the origin).

These results are consistent with known anatomical connections. For example DLPFC–anterior cingulate connections, DLPFC–temporal connections, bitemporal commissural connections, and mediodorsal thalamic–DLPFC projections have all been demonstrated in nonhuman primates [16]. The mediodorsal thalamic region and DLPFC are so correlated that one is embedded within the other (purple area). This is pleasing given the known thalamo-cortical projections to DLPFC.

E. Functional Connectivity between Systems—Partial Least Squares

Hitherto we have been dealing with functional connectivity between two voxels. The same notion can be extended to functional connectivity between two systems by noting that there is no fundamental difference between the dynamics of one voxel and the dynamics of a distributed system or pattern. The functional connectivity between two systems is simply the correlation or covariance between their time-dependent activity. The time-dependent activity of a system or pattern $\mathbf{p}$ is given by

$$\mathbf{m}_p = \mathbf{M} \cdot \mathbf{p};$$

therefore

$$\rho_{pq} = \mathbf{m}_q^T \cdot \mathbf{m}_p = \mathbf{q}^T \cdot \mathbf{M}^T \cdot \mathbf{M} \cdot \mathbf{p}, \tag{4}$$

where ρ_{pq} is the functional connectivity between the systems described by vectors $\mathbf{p}$ and $\mathbf{q}$. Consider next functional connectivity between two systems in separate parts of the brain, for example the right and left hemispheres. Here the data matrices ($\mathbf{M}_p$ and $\mathbf{M}_q$) derive from different sets of voxels and Eq. (4) becomes

$$\rho_{pq} = \mathbf{m}_q^T \cdot \mathbf{m}_p = \mathbf{q}^T \cdot \mathbf{M}_q^T \cdot \mathbf{M}_p \cdot \mathbf{p}. \tag{5}$$

If one wanted to identify the intrahemispheric systems that showed the greatest interhemispheric functional connectivity (*i.e.*, covariance) one would need to identify the set of vectors $\mathbf{p}$ and $\mathbf{q}$ that maximise ρ_{pq} in Eq. (5). SVD finds yet another powerful application in doing just this, where

$$[\mathbf{U} \quad \mathbf{S} \quad \mathbf{V}] \quad = \mathrm{SVD}\{\mathbf{M}_q^T \cdot \mathbf{M}_p\},$$

such that

$$\mathbf{M}_q^T \cdot \mathbf{M}_p \quad = \mathbf{U} \cdot \mathbf{S} \cdot \mathbf{V}^T$$

and

$$\mathbf{U}^T \cdot \mathbf{M}_q^T \cdot \mathbf{M}_p \cdot \mathbf{V} = \mathbf{S}. \tag{6}$$

The first columns of $\mathbf{U}$ and $\mathbf{V}$ represent the singular images that correspond to the two systems with the greatest amount of functional connectivity (the singular values in the diagonal matrix $\mathbf{S}$). In other words, SVD of the (generally asymmetric) covariance matrix, based on time series from two anatomically separate parts of the brain, yields a series of paired vectors (paired columns of $\mathbf{U}$ and $\mathbf{V}$) that, in a stepdown fashion, define pairs of brain systems that show the greatest functional connectivity. See Friston [7] for further details. This particular application of SVD is also know as partial least squares and has been proposed for analysis of designed activation experiments where the two data matrices comprise (i) an imaging time series and (ii) a set of behavioural or task parameters [17]. In this application the paired singular vectors correspond to (i) a singular image and (ii) a set of weights that give the linear combination of task parameters that show the maximal covariance with the corresponding singular image.

F. Differences in Functional Connectivity—Generalised Eigenimages

In this section we introduce an extension of eigenimage analysis using the solution to the generalised eigenvalue problem. This problem involves finding the eigenvector solution that involves two functional connectivity or covariance matrices and can be used to find the eigenimage that is maximally expressed in one time series relative to another. In other words, it can find a pattern of distributed activity that is most prevalent in one data set and least expressed in another. The example used to illustrate this idea is fronto-temporal functional disconnection in schizophrenia.

The notion that schizophrenia represents a disintegration or fraction-ation of the psyche is as old as its name, introduced by Bleuler [18] to convey a *"splitting"* of mental faculties. Many of Bleuler's primary processes, such as *"loosening of associations"* emphasize a fragmentation and loss of coherent integration. In what follows we assume that this mentalistic *"splitting"* has a physiological basis, and furthermore that both the mentalistic and physiologi-cal disintegration have precise and specific characteristics that can be under-stood in terms of functional connectivity.

The idea is that although localised pathophysiology in cortical areas may be a sufficient explanation for some signs of schizophrenia it does not suffice as a rich or compelling explanation for the symptoms of schizophrenia. The conjecture is that symptoms such as hallucinations and delusions are better understood in terms of abnormal interactions or impaired integration between different cortical areas. This dysfunctional integration, expressed at a physio-logical level as abnormal functional connectivity, is measurable with functional neuroimaging and observable at a cognitive level as a failure to integrate perception and action that manifests as clinical symptoms. The distinction between a regionally specific pathology and a pathology of interaction can be seen in terms of a first order effect (*e.g.*, hypofrontality) and a second order effect that exists only in the relationship between activity in the prefrontal cortex and some other (*e.g.*, temporal) region. In a similar way psychological abnormalities can be regarded as first order (*e.g.*, a poverty of intrinsically cued behaviour in psychomotor poverty) or second order (*e.g.*, a failure to integrate intrinsically cued behaviour and perception in reality distortion).

1. The Generalised Eigenvalue Solution

Suppose that we want to find a pattern embodying the greatest amount of functional connectivity in normal subjects that, relatively speaking, was not evident in schizophrenia (*e.g.*, fronto-temporal covariance). To achieve this result we identify an eigenimage that reflects the most functional connectivity in normal subjects relative to a schizophrenic group (**d**). This eigenimage is obtained by using a generalised eigenvector solution,

$$\mathbf{C}_1^{-1} \cdot \mathbf{C}_2 \cdot \mathbf{d}_1 = \mathbf{d} \cdot \lambda$$

or

$$\mathbf{C}_2 \cdot \mathbf{d}_1 \qquad = \mathbf{C}_1 \mathbf{d} \cdot \lambda,$$

where $\mathbf{C}_1$ and $\mathbf{C}_2$ are the two functional connectivity matrices. The generalised eigenimage (**d**) is essentially a single pattern that maximizes the ratio of the 2-norm measure [Eq. (1)] when applied to $\mathbf{C}_1$ and $\mathbf{C}_2$. Generally speaking these matrices could represent data from two [groups of] subjects or from the same subject[s] scanned under different conditions. In the present example we use connectivity matrices from normal subjects and people with schizophrenia showing pronounced psychomotor poverty.

The data were acquired from two groups of six subjects. Each subject was scanned six times during the performance of three word generation tasks (A B C C B A). Task A was a verbal fluency task, requiring subjects to respond with a word that began with a heard letter. Task B was a semantic categorisation task in which subjects responded "man made" or "natural," depending on a heard noun. Task C was a word shadowing task in which subjects simply repeated what was heard. In the current context the detailed nature of the tasks is not very important. They were used to introduce variance and covariance in activity that could support an analysis of functional connectivity.

The groups comprised six normal subjects and six schizophrenic patients. The schizophrenic subjects produced less than 24 words on a standard (1-min) FAS verbal fluency task (generating words beginning with the letters "F", "A", and "S"). The results of a generalised eigenimage analysis are presented in Fig. 3. As expected the pattern that best captures differences between the two groups involves prefrontal and temporal cortices. Negative correlations between left DLPFC and bilateral superior temporal regions are found (Fig. 3, top). The amount to which this pattern was expressed in each individual group is shown in the bottom panel of Fig. 3 using the appropriate 2-norm $\|\mathbf{d} \cdot \mathbf{C} \cdot \mathbf{d}\|$. It is seen that this eigenimage, whilst prevalent in normal subjects, is uniformly reduced in schizophrenic subjects.

G. Summary

In the preceding sections we have seen how eigenimages can be framed in relation to functional connectivity and the relationship between eigenimage analysis, multidimensional scaling, partial least squares, and generalised eigenimage analysis. All these techniques are essentially descriptive, in that they do not allow one to make any statistical inferences about the characterisations that obtain. In the second half of this chapter we turn to multivariate techniques that do embody statistical inference and explicit hypothesis testing. We will introduce canonical images, which can be thought of as statistically informed eigenimages pertaining to a particular effect introduced by experimental design. We have seen that patterns can be identified using the generalised eigenvalue solution that are maximally expressed in one covariance structure relative to another. Consider the advantage of using this approach where the first covariance matrix reflects the effects of interest, and the second embodies covariances due to error. This application generates canonical images, and is considered in the following sections.

IV. MANCOVA AND CANONICAL IMAGE ANALYSIS

A. Introduction

In the following sections we review a general multivariate approach to the analysis of functional imaging studies. This analysis uses standard multivariate techniques to make statistical inferences about activation effects and to describe important features of these effects. Specifically we introduce MANCOVA and canonical variates analysis (CVA) to characterise activation effects and address special issues that ensue. This approach characterises the brain's response in terms of functionally connected and distributed systems in a similar fashion to eigenimage analysis. Eigenimages figure in the current analysis in the following way. A problematic issue in multivariate analysis of functional imaging data is that the number of samples (*i.e.*, scans) is usually very small in relation to the number of components (*i.e.*, voxels) of the observations. This issue is resolved by analysing the data not in terms of voxels but

positive

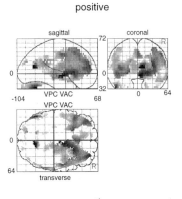

negative

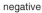
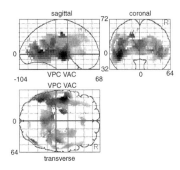

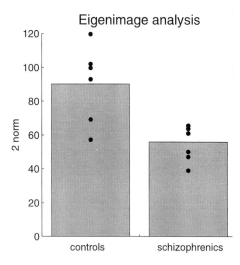

FIGURE 3 Generalized eigenimage analysis of the schizophrenic and control subjects. (Top upper and lower) Positive and negative loadings of the first eigenimage that is maximally expressed in the normal group and minimally expressed in the schizophrenic group. This analysis used ^{15}O PET activation studies of word generation with six scans per subject and six subjects per group. The activation study involved three word generation conditions (word shadowing, semantic categorisation, and verbal fluency) each of which was presented twice. The grey scale is arbitrary and each image has been normalised to the image maximum. The display format is standard and represents a maximum intensity projection. This eigenimage is relatively less expressed in the schizophrenic data. This point is made by expressing the amount of functional connectivity attributable to the eigenimage in (each subject in) both groups, using the appropriate 2-norm (bottom).

in terms of eigenimages, because the number of eigenimages is much smaller than the number of voxels. The importance of multivariate analysis that ensues can be summarised as follows: (i) Unlike eigenimage analysis it provides for statistical inferences (based on a *P* value) about the significance of the brain's response in terms of some hypothesis. (ii) The approach implicitly takes account of spatial correlations in the data without making any assumptions. (iii) The canonical variates analysis produces generalised eigenimages (canonical images) that capture the activation effects, while suppressing the effects of noise or error. (iv) The theoretical basis is well established and can be found in most introductory texts on multivariate analysis.

Although useful, in a descriptive sense, eigenimage analysis and related approaches are not generally considered as "statistical" methods that can be used to make statistical inferences; they are mathematical devices that simply identify prominent patterns of correlations or functional connectivity. It must be said, however, that large sample, asymptotic, multivariate normal theory could be used to make some inferences about the relative contributions of each eigenimage (*e.g.*, tests for nonsphericity) if a sufficient number of scans were available. In what follows we observe that MANCOVA with canonical variates analysis combines many of the attractive features of statistical parametric mapping and eigenimage analysis. Unlike statistical parametric mapping, MANCOVA is multivariate. In other words, it considers as one observation all voxels in a single scan. The importance of this multivariate approach is that effects due to activations, confounding effects and error effects are assessed both in terms of effects at each voxel and interactions among voxels. This feature means that one does not have to assume anything about spatial correlations (*cf.* stationariness with Gaussian field models) to assess the significance of an activation effect. Unlike statistical parametric mapping these correlations are explicitly included in an analysis. The price one pays for adopting a multivariate approach is that inferences cannot be made about regionally specific changes (*cf.* statistical parametric mapping). This is because the inference pertains to all the components (voxels) of a multivariate variable (not a particular voxel or set of voxels).

In general, multivariate analyses are implemented in two steps. First, the significance of a hypothesised effect is assessed in terms of a *P* value, and second, if justified, the exact nature of the effect is determined. The analysis here conforms to this two stage procedure. When the brain's response is assessed to be significant using MANCOVA, the nature of this response remains to be characterised. We propose that CVA is an appropriate way of doing this. The canonical images obtained with CVA are similar to eigenimages but are based on both the activation and error effects. CVA is closely related to denoising techniques in EEG and MEG time series analyses that use a generalised eigenvalue solution. Another way of looking at canonical images is to think of them as eigenimages that reflect functional connectivity due to activations when spurious correlations due to error are discounted.

B. Dimension Reduction and Eigenimages

The first step in multivariate analysis is to ensure that the dimensionality (number of components or voxels) of the data is smaller than the number of observations. Clearly for images this is not the case, because there are more voxels than scans; therefore the data have to be transformed. The dimension reduction proposed here is straightforward and uses the scan-dependent expression $\mathbf{X}$ of eigenimages as a reduced set of components for each multivariate observation (scan), where

$$[\mathbf{U} \quad \mathbf{S} \quad \mathbf{V}] = \text{SVD}\{\mathbf{M}\}$$

and

$$\mathbf{X} = \mathbf{U} \cdot \mathbf{S}. \tag{7}$$

As above $\mathbf{M}$ is a large matrix of corrected voxel values with one column for each voxel and one row for each scan. Here "corrected" implies mean correction and removal of any confounds using linear regression. The eigenimages constitute the columns of $\mathbf{U}$, another unitary orthonormal matrix, and their expression over scans corresponds to the columns of the matrix $\mathbf{X}$. $\mathbf{X}$ has one column for each eigenimage and one row for each scan. In our work we use only the J columns of $\mathbf{X}$ and $\mathbf{U}$ associated with eigenvalues greater than unity (after normalising each eigenvalue by the average eigenvalue).

C. The General Linear Model Revisited

Recall the general linear model from previous chapters,

$$\mathbf{X} = \mathbf{G}\beta + \mathbf{e}, \tag{8}$$

where the errors $\mathbf{e}$ are assumed to be independent and identically normally distributed. The design matrix $\mathbf{G}$ has one column for every effect (factor or covariate) in the model. The design matrix can contain both covariates and indicator variables reflecting an experimental design. β is the parameter matrix with one column vector of parameters for each mode. Each column of $\mathbf{G}$ has an associated unknown parameter. Some of these parameters will be of interest; the remaining parameters will not. As before we will split $\mathbf{G}$ (and β) into two partitions $\mathbf{G} = [\mathbf{H} \ \mathbf{D}]$ and similarly $\beta = [\alpha^T \gamma^T]^T$ with estimators $\mathbf{b} = [\mathbf{a}^T \mathbf{g}^T]^T$. Here effects of interest are denoted by $\mathbf{H}$ and confounding effects of no interest by $\mathbf{D}$. Equation (8) can be expanded,

$$\mathbf{X} = \mathbf{H} \cdot \alpha + \mathbf{D}\gamma + \mathbf{e}, \tag{9}$$

where $\mathbf{H}$ represents a matrix of 0s or 1s depending on the level or presence of some interesting condition or treatment effect (*e.g.*, the presence of a particular cognitive component) or the columns of $\mathbf{H}$ might contain covariates of interest that could explain the observed variance in $\mathbf{X}$ (*e.g.*, dose of apomorphine or "time on target"). $\mathbf{D}$ corresponds to a matrix of indicator variables denoting effects that are not of any interest (*e.g.*, of being a particular subject or block effect) or covariates of no interest (*i.e.*, "nuisance variables" such as global activity or confounding time effects).

D. Statistical Inference

Significance is assessed by testing the null hypothesis that the effects of interest do not significantly reduce the error variance when compared to the remaining effects alone (or alternatively the null hypothesis that α is zero). The null hypothesis can be tested in the following way. The sum of squares and products matrix (SSPM) due to error $\mathbf{R}(\Omega)$ is obtained from the difference between actual and estimated values of $\mathbf{X}$,

$$\mathbf{R} = \mathbf{R}(\Omega) = (\mathbf{X} - \mathbf{G} \cdot \mathbf{b})^{\mathrm{T}}(\mathbf{X} - \mathbf{G} \cdot \mathbf{b}), \qquad (10)$$

where the sums of squares and products due to effects of interest is given by

$$\mathbf{T} = (\mathbf{H} \cdot \mathbf{a})^{\mathrm{T}} \cdot (\mathbf{H} \cdot \mathbf{a}). \qquad (11)$$

The error sum of squares and products under the null hypothesis $\mathbf{R}(\Omega_0)$, *i.e.*, after discounting the effects of interest ($\mathbf{H}$), are given by

$$\mathbf{R}(\Omega_0) = (\mathbf{X} - \mathbf{D} \cdot \mathbf{g})^{\mathrm{T}} \cdot (\mathbf{X} - \mathbf{D} \cdot \mathbf{g}). \qquad (12)$$

Clearly if $\mathbf{D}$ does not exist this simply reduces to the sum of squares and products of the response variable ($\mathbf{X}^{\mathrm{T}}\mathbf{X}$). The significance can now be tested with

$$\Lambda = |\mathbf{R}(\Omega)|/|\mathbf{R}(\Omega_0)|, \qquad (13)$$

where Λ is Wilk's statistic (known as Wilk's Lambda). A special case of this test is Hotelling's T^2 test and applies when $\mathbf{H}$ simply compares one condition with another [19]. Under the null hypothesis, after transformation, Λ has a χ^2 distribution with degrees of freedom $J \cdot h$. The transformation is given by

$$-(r - ((J - h + 1)/2)) \cdot \log(\Lambda) \sim \chi^2(J \cdot h),$$

where r is the degrees of freedom associated with error terms, equal to the number of scans (I) minus the number of effects modeled $= I - \mathrm{rank}(\mathbf{G})$. J is the number of eigenimages in the J-variate response variable $\mathbf{X}$ and h are the degrees of freedom associated with effects of interest $= \mathrm{rank}(\mathbf{H})$.

E. Characterising the Effect

Having established that the effects of interest are significant (*e.g.*, differences among two or more activation conditions) the final step is to characterise these effects in terms of their spatial topography. This characterisation uses canonical variates analysis or CVA. The objective is to find a linear combination (compound or contrast) of the components of $\mathbf{X}$, in this case the eigenimages, that best express the activation effects when compared to error effects. More exactly we want to find $\mathbf{c}_1$ such that the variance ratio,

$$(\mathbf{c}_1^{\mathrm{T}} \cdot \mathbf{H} \cdot \mathbf{c}_1)/(\mathbf{c}_1^{\mathrm{T}} \cdot \mathbf{R} \cdot \mathbf{c}_1),$$

is maximised [19]. Let $\mathbf{Z}_1 = \mathbf{X} \cdot \mathbf{c}_1$; where $\mathbf{Z}_1$ is the first canonical variate and $\mathbf{c}_1$ is a canonical image (defined in the space of the spatial modes) that maximises this ratio. $\mathbf{c}_2$ is the second canonical image that maximises the ratio subject to the constraints of $\mathrm{Cov}\{\mathbf{c}_1 \ \mathbf{c}_2\} = 0$ (and so on). The matrix of canonical images $\mathbf{c} = [\mathbf{c}_1 \ \mathbf{c}_2 \ \ldots \ \mathbf{c}_J]$ is given by solution of the generalised eigenvalue problem,

$$\mathbf{T} \cdot \mathbf{c} = \mathbf{R} \cdot \mathbf{c} \cdot \Theta, \qquad (14)$$

where Θ is a diagonal matrix of eigenvalues. Voxel-space canonical images $\mathbf{C}$ are obtained by rotating the canonical image in the columns of $\mathbf{c}$ back into voxel-space with the original eigenimages $\mathbf{V}$:

$$\mathbf{C} = \mathbf{V} \cdot \mathbf{c}. \qquad (15)$$

The columns of **C** now contain the voxel values of the canonical images. The kth column of **C** (the kth canonical image) has an associated canonical value equal to the kth leading diagonal element of Θ times r/h. Note that the "activation" effect is a multivariate one, with J components or canonical images. Normally only a few of these components have large canonical values and only these need be reported. There are procedures based on distributional approximations of Θ that allow inferences about the dimensionality of a response (number of canonical images). We refer the interested reader to Chatfield and Collins [19] for further details.

F. Relationship to Eigenimage Analysis

When applied to adjusted data eigenimages [2] correspond to the eigenvectors of **T**. These have an interesting relationship to the canonical images: On rearranging Eq. (14),

$$\mathbf{R}^{-1} \cdot \mathbf{T} \cdot \mathbf{c} = \mathbf{c} \cdot \Theta,$$

we note that the canonical images are eigenvectors of $\mathbf{R}^{-1} \cdot \mathbf{T}$. In other words, an eigenimage analysis of an activation study returns the eigenvectors that express the most variance due to the effects of interest—eig(**T**). A canonical image, on the other hand, expresses the greatest amount of variance due to the effects of interest relative to error—eig($\mathbf{R}^{-1} \cdot \mathbf{T}$). In this sense a CVA can be considered an eigenimage analysis that is "informed" by the estimates of error effects.

G. An Illustrative Application

In this section we consider an application of the above theory to the word generation study in normal subjects used in previous sections. We assessed the significance of condition-dependent effects by treating each of the 12 scans as a different condition. Note that we do not consider the six-word generation (or word shadowing) conditions as replications of the same condition. In other words, the first time one performs a word generation task is a different condition from the second time and so on. The (alternative) hypothesis adopted here states that there is a significant difference among the 12 conditions, but does not constrain the nature of this difference to a particular form. The most important differences will emerge from the CVA. Clearly one might hope that these differences will be due to word generation, but they might not be. This hypothesis should be compared with a more constrained hypothesis that considers the conditions as six replications of word shadowing and word generation. This latter hypothesis is more directed and explicitly compares word shadowing with word generation. This comparison could be tested in a single subject. The point is that the generality afforded by the current framework allows one to test very constrained (*i.e.*, specific) hypotheses or rather general hypotheses about some unspecified activation effect. We choose the latter case here because it places more emphasis on canonical images as descriptions of what has actually occurred during the experiment.

The design matrix partition for effects of interest **H** has 12 columns representing the 12 different conditions. We designated subject effects, time, and global activity as uninteresting confounds **D**. The corrected data were reduced to 60 eigenvectors as described above. The first 14 eigenvectors had (normalised) eigenvalues greater than unity and were used in the subsequent analysis. The resulting matrix **X**, with 60 rows (one for each scan) and 14 columns (one for each eigenimage) was subject to MANCOVA. The significance of the condition effects was assessed with Wilk's Lambda. The threshold for condition or activation effects was set at $P = 0.02$. In other words, the probability of there being no differences among the 12 conditions was 2%.

H. Canonical Variates Analysis

The first canonical image and its expression in each condition is shown in Fig. 4. The top panels show this system to include anterior cingulate and Broca's area, with more moderate expression in the left posterior inferotemporal regions (right). The positive components of this canonical image (left) implicate ventro-medial prefrontal cortex and bitemporal regions (right greater than left). One important aspect of these canonical images is their highly distributed yet structured nature, reflecting the distributed integration of many brain areas. The canonical variate expressed in terms of mean condition effects is seen in the bottom panel of Fig. 4. This variate is simply $\mathbf{a} \cdot \mathbf{c}_1$. It is pleasing to note that the first canonical variate corresponds to the difference between word shadowing and verbal fluency.

Recall that the eigenimage in Fig. 1 reflects the main pattern of correlations evoked by the mean condition effects and should be compared with the first canonical image in Fig. 4. The differences between these characterisations of activation effects are informative. The eigenimage is totally insensitive to the reliability or error attributable to differential activation from subject to subject, whereas the canonical image does reflect these variations. For example, the absence of the posterior cingulate in the canonical image and its relative prominence in the eigenimage suggests that this region is implicated in some subjects but not in others. The subjects that engage the posterior cingulate must do so to some considerable degree because the average effects (represented by the eigenimage) are quite substantial. Conversely the medial prefrontal cortical deactivations are a much more generic feature of activation effects than would have been inferred on the basis of the eigenimage analysis. These observations beg the question "which is the best characterisation of functional anatomy?" Obviously, there is no simple answer but the question speaks to an important point. A canonical image characterises a response relative to error, by partitioning the observed variance (in the J larger spatial modes) into effects of interest and a residual variation about these effects (error). This partitioning is determined by experimental design, a hypothesis, and the inferences that are sought. An eigenimage does not embody any concept of error and is not constrained by any hypothesis.

I. Summary

These sections have described a multivariate approach to the analysis of functional imaging studies. This analysis uses standard multivariate techniques to make statistical inferences about activation effects and to describe the important features of these effects. More specifically, the proposed analysis uses MANCOVA with Wilk's Lambda to test for specific effects of interest (*e.g.*, differences among activation conditions) and CVA to characterise these distributed responses. The generality of this approach is assured by the generality of the linear model used. The design and inferences sought are embodied in the design matrix and can, in principle, accommodate most parametric

canonical image 1 {+ve}

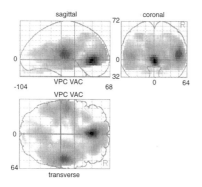

canonical image 1 {−ve}

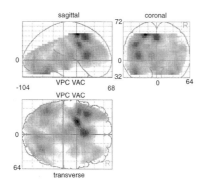

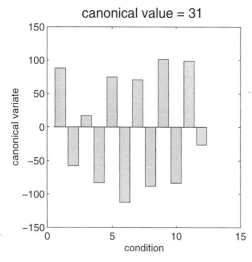

FIGURE 4 (Top) The first canonical image displayed as maximum intensity projections of the positive and negative components. The display format is standard and provides three views of the brain from the front, the back, and the right-hand side. The grey scale is arbitrary and the space conforms to that described in the atlas of Talairach and Tournoux [20]. (Bottom) The expression of the first canonical image (*i.e.*, the canonical variate) averaged over conditions. The odd conditions correspond to word shadowing and the even conditions correspond to word generation. This canonical variate is clearly sensitive to the differences evoked by these two tasks.

statistical analyses. This multivariate approach differs fundamentally from statistical parametric mapping, because the concept of a separate voxel or region of interest ceases to have meaning. One scan represents one observation (not 10^5 voxels). In this sense the statistical inference is about the whole image volume not any component of it. This feature precludes statistical inferences about regional effects made without reference to changes elsewhere in the brain. This fundamental difference ensures that SPM and multivariate approaches are likely to be regarded as distinct and complementary approaches to functional imaging data.

There are many potential applications of the analysis presented above. One particularly interesting application concerns the ability to test various models in a comprehensive and direct fashion. Hitherto there has been no "omnibus" test for a particular neurophysiological response or model of this response that did not rely on some assumptions about the multivariate structure of the data (*e.g.*, Gaussian fields). Wilk's statistic could provide this test. For example, the controversy over an appropriate model for removing confounding effects of global activity on regional effects has been dogged by the lack of any compelling comparative assessment of different models. Wilk's statistic could, in principle, be used to resolve this issue by explicitly testing hierarchies of models (a succession of extra effects modeled in the design matrix).

An attractive neuroscience application of the multivariate approach considered here pertains to the significance of interaction terms in a design matrix. Cognitive subtraction is based on the assumption that extra components of a task can be inserted without affecting preexisting components. In order to verify the assumptions behind cognitive subtraction one needs to demonstrate that these interactions can be ignored when modeling the brain's response. This can be effected simply and rigorously using Wilk's statistic to show that interaction terms in the design matrix are not significant (here one would treat the interaction terms as effects of interest and the remaining effects of no interest). Of course, if the interactions were significant this leads to a richer understanding of functional anatomy and provides a basis for more sophisticated experimental designs. We take up this theme again in the next chapter.

References

1. C. G. Phillips, S. Zeki, and H. B. Barlow. Localization of function in the cerebral cortex. Past, present and future. *Brain* **107**, 327–361 (1984).
2. K. J. Friston, C. D. Frith, P. F. Liddle, and R. S. J. Frackowiak. Functional connectivity: The principal component analysis of large (PET) data sets. *J. Cereb. Blood Flow Metab.* **13**, 5–14 (1993).
3. K. J. Friston, C. D. Frith, and R. S. J. Frackowiak. Time-dependent changes in effective connectivity measured with PET. *Hum. Brain Mapping* **1**, 69–80 (1993).
4. G. L. Gerstein and D. H. Perkel. Simultaneously recorded trains of action potentials: Analysis and functional interpretation. *Science* **164**, 828–830 (1969).
5. A. Aertsen and H. Preissl. Dynamics of activity and connectivity in physiological neuronal networks. *In* "Non Linear Dynamics and Neuronal Networks" (H. G. Schuster Publishers Inc., Ed.), pp. 281–302. H, G. Schuster, New York, 1991.
6. G. L. Gerstein, P. Bedenbaugh, and A. M. H. J. Aertsen. Neuronal assemblies IEEE. *Trans. Biomed. Eng.* **36**, 4–14 (1989).
7. K. J. Friston, S. Herold, P. Fletcher, D. Silbersweig, C. Cahill, R. J. Dolan, P. F.

Liddle, R. S. J. Frackowiak, and C. D. Frith. Abnormal fronto-temporal interactions in schizophrenia. *In* "Biology of Schizophrenia and Affective Disease" (S. J. Watson, Ed.), ARNMD Series, Vol. 73, 1994.

8. G. Mayer-Kress, C. Barczys, and W. Freeman. Attractor reconstruction from event-related multi-electrode EEG data. *In* "Mathematical Approaches to Brain Functioning Diagnostics" (I. Dvorak and A. V. Holden, Ed.). Manchester Univ. Press, New York, 1991.

9. R. Friedrich, A. Fuchs, and H. Haken. Modelling of spatio-temporal EEG patterns. *In* "Mathematical Approaches to Brain Functioning Diagnostics" (I. Dvorak and A. V. Holden, Ed.). Manchester Univ. Press, New York, 1991.

10. A. Fuchs, J. A. S. Kelso, and H. Haken. Phase transitions in the human brain: Spatial mode dynamics. *Int. J. Bifurcation Chaos* **2,** 917–939 (1992).

11. K. J. Friston, P. Jezzard, R. S. J. Frackowiak, and R. Turner. Characterizing focal and distributed physiological changes with MRI and PET. *In* "Functional MRI of the Brain." Society of Magnetic Resonance in Medicine, Berkeley CA. pp. 207–216. 1993.

12. J. C. Gower. Some distance properties of latent root and vector methods used in multivariate analysis. *Biometrika* **53,** 325–328 (1966).

13. W. S. Torgerson. "Theory and Methods of Scaling." Wiley, New York, 1958.

14. R. N. Shepard. Multidimensional scaling, tree-fitting and clustering. *Science* **210,** 390–398 (1980).

15. I. Newton. "Opticks," Book 1, part 2, prop. 6. Smith and Walford, London, 1704.

16. P. S. Goldman-Rakic. Topography of cognition: Parallel distributed networks in primate association cortex. *Ann. Rev. Neurosci.* **11,** 137–156 (1988).

17. A. R. McIntosh, F. L. Bookstein, J. V. Haxby, and C. L. Grady. Spatial pattern analysis of functional brain images using partial least squares. *NeuroImage* **3,** 143–157 (1996).

18. E. Bleuler. Dementia Praecox or the group of schizophrenias. *In* "The Clinical Roots of the Schizophrenia Concept" (J. Cutting and M. Shepherd, Eds.). Cambridge Univ. Press, UK, 1913. [Translated into English 1987]

19. C. Chatfield and A. J. Collins. "Introduction to Multivariate Analysis," pp. 189–210. Chapman and Hall, London, 1980.

20. P. Talairach and J. Tournoux. "A Stereotactic Coplanar Atlas of the Human Brain." Thieme, Stuttgart, 1988.

CHAPTER SEVEN

CHARACTERISING FUNCTIONAL INTEGRATION

I. INTRODUCTION

In the past decade functional neuroimaging has been extremely successful in establishing functional segregation as a principle of organisation in the human brain. Functional segregation is usually inferred by the presence of activation foci in change or statistical parametric maps. The nature of the functional specialisation is then attributed to the sensori-motor or cognitive process that has been manipulated experimentally. Newer approaches have addressed the integration of functionally specialised areas by characterising neurophysiological activations in terms of distributed changes [1–6]. These approaches have introduced a number of concepts into neuroimaging (*e.g.*, functional and effective connectivity, eigenimages, spatial modes, information theory, multidimensional scaling) and their application to issues in imaging neuroscience (*e.g.*, functional systems, cortical integration, associative plasticity, and nonlinear cortical interactions). The study of effective connectivity will also gain importance for relating cognitive theories (*e.g.*, attention) to brain operations. For example, categorical comparisons of functional brain imaging data suggest modulation of extrastriate cortical areas by attentional processes [7]. It would be very compelling to demonstrate modulation of the responsiveness of such areas in terms of attention-dependent changes in the interactions or effective connectivity among visual areas.

The aim of this chapter is to review some key applications of effective connectivity in terms of functional imaging. In neuroimaging, functional connectivity is defined as the temporal correlations between remote neurophysiological events, whereas effective connectivity is defined as the influence one neural system exerts over another. Functional connectivity is simply a statement about the observed correlations; it does not provide any direct insight into how these correlations are mediated. For example, at the level of multiunit microelectrode recordings, correlations can result from stimulus-locked transients, evoked by a common afferent input, or reflect stimulus-induced oscillations–phasic coupling of neural assemblies, mediated by synaptic connections [8]. To clarify this distinction let us consider a simple example. The reticular formation in the brainstem is highly interconnected with different cortical structures. Increased activity in this brainstem structure will therefore lead to highly correlated brain activity in the cortical terminal fields of its projections, despite the fact that they are not directly connected. Eigenimage analysis of the cortical functional imaging data without similar data from the brain stem would reveal a functional network of cortical areas. Although these results can be misleading, they would be correct in the context of how functional connectivity is defined. This example shows the teleological weakness of functional connectivity and speaks to the importance of directly modeling causal interactions by using effective connectivity.

We will introduce the notion of effective connectivity and consider some of the validation issues that ensue. Some of the more powerful applications of effective connectivity are concerned with changes in connectivity (*e.g.*, time-dependent changes during procedural learning). Such an application is illustrated by characterising nonlinear interactions between striate (V1) and extrastriate (V2) cortices using fMRI data from a single-subject photic stimulation study. A modulatory interaction between V2 and V1 serves as an example of activity-dependent change in effective connectivity.

One method used to estimate effective connectivity is the application of structural equation modeling to functional brain imaging data. This technique combines an anatomical (constraining) model and the interregional covariances of measured activity. The ensuing functional model represents the influence of regions on each other through the putative anatomical connections. These influences can be either direct or indirect. Changes in effective connectivity after surgical disruption of subcortical structures in the human motor system of Parkinson's disease patients serve as an example to illustrate this technique. This chapter will conclude with a critique of proposed models of effective connectivity.

II. ORIGINS AND DEFINITIONS

The concept of effective connectivity originated in the analysis of separable spike trains obtained from multiunit electrode recordings [8–11].

Effective connectivity is closer to the intuitive notion of a connection than functional connectivity and can be defined as the influence one neural system exerts over another [3], at either a synaptic (*cf.* synaptic efficacy) or a cortical level. In electrophysiology there is a close relationship between effective connectivity and synaptic efficacy: *"It is useful to describe the effective connectivity with a connectivity matrix of effective synaptic weights. Matrix elements $[C_{ij}]$ would represent the effective influence by neuron j on neuron i"* [8]. It has also been proposed that *"the [electrophysiological] notion of effective connectivity should be understood as the experiment and time-dependent, simplest possible circuit diagram that would replicate the observed timing relationships between the recorded neurons"* [11].

Although functional and effective connectivity can be invoked at a conceptual level in both neuroimaging and electrophysiology they differ fundamentally at a practical level. This is because the time scales and nature of the neurophysiological measurements are very different (seconds *vs* milliseconds and haemodynamics *vs* spike trains). In electrophysiology it is often necessary to remove the confounding effects of stimulus-locked transients (that introduce correlations not causally mediated by direct neural interactions) in order to reveal the underlying connectivity. The confounding effect of stimulus-evoked transients is less problematic in neuroimaging because the promulgation of dynamics from primary sensory areas onwards is mediated by neuronal connections (usually reciprocal and interconnecting). However, it should be kept in mind that functional connectivity is not necessarily due to effective connectivity as described above using the example of the reticular formation.

III. THE BASIC LINEAR MODEL

Functional connectivity is an operational definition. Effective connectivity is not; it depends on two models: a mathematical model, describing how areas are connected, and a neuroanatomical model, describing which areas are connected. We shall consider linear and nonlinear models. Perhaps the simplest model of effective connectivity expresses the haemodynamic change at one voxel as a weighted sum of changes elsewhere. The weights or coefficients can then be identified with effective connectivity: For example, let the activity of voxel i be m_i, then

$$m_i = \Sigma C_{ij} \cdot m_j + e_i$$

or in matrix notation

$$\mathbf{m_i} = \mathbf{M} \cdot \mathbf{C_i} + \mathbf{e}, \qquad (1)$$

where $\mathbf{C_i}$ is a column vector of effective connection estimates from all locations to the one in question (i). $\mathbf{e}$ is an error term. If one selects a point (i) in the brain and asks, what is the effective connection strength between the location chosen and all other locations, then one wants to know the values of $\mathbf{C_i}$. The least squares solution for $\mathbf{C_i}$ is [12]

$$\mathbf{C_i} = (\mathbf{M}^T \cdot \mathbf{M})^{-1} \cdot \mathbf{M}^T \cdot \mathbf{m_i}. \qquad (2)$$

This solution can be regarded as a linear regression, such that the effective connectivity reflects the amount of rCBF variability at i attributable to rCBF changes at location j. Implicit in this interpretation is a mediation of the influence by neuronal connections with an effective strength equal to C_{ij}. There are many issues that deserve comment when estimating effective connectivity in this way. First, the fact that there are only a few observations (*e.g.*, 12 in a PET study is not uncommon) but many thousand voxels in each image means that the equations are very underdetermined. This problem is dealt with by finding a solution with the minimum 2-norm [13]. This in turn is equivalent to solving equations in a space defined by the eigenimages (see Chapter 6). Mathematically,

$$\mathbf{m_i} = \mathbf{M} \cdot \mathbf{v} \cdot \mathbf{a_i} + \mathbf{e} \qquad (3)$$

is solved for $\mathbf{a_i}$, where $\mathbf{C_i} = \mathbf{v} \cdot \mathbf{a_i}$. As in Chapter 6 $\mathbf{v} = [\mathbf{v}^1 \ldots \mathbf{v}^r]$ is a matrix of r eigenimages and $\mathbf{M} \cdot \mathbf{v} = \mathbf{u} \cdot \mathbf{s}$. Only the r (or less) eigenvectors with nonzero (or large) eigenvalues are used, giving

$$\mathbf{C_i} = \mathbf{v} \cdot \mathbf{s}^{-2} \cdot \mathbf{v}^T \mathbf{M}^T \cdot \mathbf{m_i} = \mathbf{v} \cdot \text{pinv}(\mathbf{M} \cdot \mathbf{v}) \cdot \mathbf{m_i}, \qquad (4)$$

where pinv(.) denotes the pseudoinverse. Provisional experience suggests that the linear model [Eq. (1)] can be well behaved. One explanation is that the dimensionality (the number of things that are going on) of the physiological changes can be small. In fact, the distribution of eigenvalues associated with the PET study of Chapter 6 suggested a dimensionality of two. In other words, the brain responds to simple and well organised experiments in a simple and well organised way. In the PET example, despite measurements in thousands of voxels there were substantial changes in only two eigenimages.

Generally, however, neurophysiology is nonlinear and the adequacy of linear models must be questioned (or at least qualified). Consequently, we focus on a nonlinear model of effective connectivity that is an extension of the linear framework presented in this section. This model was designed to answer a specific but important question about modulatory interactions in visual cortex.

IV. NONLINEAR EFFECTIVE CONNECTIVITY BETWEEN V1 AND V2

A. Modulatory Interactions in Visual Cortex

Reversible cooling experiments in monkey visual cortex during visual stimulation have demonstrated that neuronal activity in V2 depends on forward inputs from V1. Conversely, neuronal activity in V1 is modulated by feedback or reentrant connections from V2 to V1 [14–16]. Evidence for these functional asymmetries is found in the work of Schiller and colleagues [14,15]. Retinotopically, corresponding regions of V1 and V2 are reciprocally connected in the monkey. V1 provides a crucial input to V2, in the sense that visual activation of V2 cells depends on input from V1. This dependency has been demonstrated by reversibly cooling (deactivating) V1 while recording from V2 during visual stimulation [14,16]. In contrast, cooling V2 has a more modulatory effect on V1 unit activity. *"Most cells became less responsive to visual stimulation, while a few became more active during cooling"* [15]. The cells in V1 that were most affected by V2 deactivation were in the infragranular layers, suggesting that V2 may use this pathway to modulate the output from V1. Similar conclusions about the return pathway between V5 and V2 were drawn by Girard and Bullier [16]. Because, in the absence of V1 input, these reentrant connections do not constitute an efficient drive to V2 cells, their role is most likely *"to modulate the information relayed through area 17"* (V1) [16].

B. A Nonlinear Model of Effective Connectivity

To examine the interactions between human V1 and V2 using fMRI, we used a nonlinear model of effective connectivity, extended to include a modulatory interaction [cf. Eq. (1)]:

$$m_i = \Sigma(C_{ij}^O \cdot m_j + C_{ij}^M \cdot m_j m_i). \tag{5}$$

This model has two terms that allow for the activity in area i to be influenced by activity in area j. The first represents an effect that depends only on afferent input from area j. This is the activity in j scaled by C_{ij}^O. The coefficient C_{ij}^O is referred to as an obligatory connection strength, in the sense that a change in area j results in an obligatory response in area i. Conversely, the second term reflects a modulatory influence of area j on area i. The coefficient determining the size of this effect (C_{ij}^M) is referred to as a modulatory connection strength, because the overall effect depends on both the afferent input ($C_{ij}^M \cdot m_j$) and intrinsic activity (m_i).

This equation, or model, can be interpreted from two points of view: (i) by analogy with the nonlinear behaviour that characterizes voltage-dependent channels in electrophysiology or, (ii) in terms of classical (pharmacological) neuromodulation where postsynaptic responsiveness is modulated without a direct effect on postsynaptic membrane potential. The voltage-dependent analogy is obtained by considering m_i as the postsynaptic potential and m_j as a depolarising current. According to Eq. (5) a high C_{ij}^M reflects a greater sensitivity to changes of input at higher levels of intrinsic activity. In electrophysiological terms this translates as a change of postsynaptic depolarisation, in response to a fixed depolarising current, that increases with depolarisation. This characteristic is typical of voltage-dependent interactions [17]. The intrinsic activity-dependent effect, determined by the value of C_{ij}^M, provides an intuitive sense of how to estimate C_{ij}^M. The estimation involves measuring the difference in sensitivity between states with high and low intrinsic activity at the location of interest.

Let us imagine we were able to "fix" the activity in V1 at a low level and measure the connectivity between V2 and V1 assuming a simple linear relationship [Eq. (1)]. A value for the sensitivity of V1 to V2 changes could be obtained, say C1. Now, if the procedure were repeated with V1 activity fixed at a high level, a second (linear) estimate would be obtained (C2). In the presence of a substantial modulatory interaction between V2 and V1 the second estimate will be higher than the first. This is because the activity intrinsic to V1 is higher and V1 should be more sensitive to inputs from V2. In short C2 − C1 provides an estimate of the modulatory influence of V2 on V1. The activity of V1 can be fixed *post hoc* by simply selecting a subset of data in which V1 activity is confined to some small range.

An estimate of effective connection strengths of both an obligatory and a modulatory nature can be obtained for the connections between all voxels and a reference location in the following way: for any reference location (i) assume that a subset of the time series can be selected so that m_i is limited to some small range about its mean ($\langle m_i \rangle$). For this subset Eq. (5) can be approximated by Eq. (1) (omitting error terms for clarity),

$$
\begin{aligned}
m_i &\approx \Sigma\, C_{ij}^O \cdot m_j + \langle m_i \rangle \Sigma\, C_{ij}^M \cdot m_j \\
&\approx \mathbf{m_j} \cdot (\mathbf{C^O} + \langle \mathbf{m_i} \rangle \mathbf{C^M}) \\
&\approx \mathbf{m_j} \cdot \mathbf{C},
\end{aligned}
\tag{6}
$$

where $\mathbf{C} = \mathbf{C^O} + \langle \mathbf{m_i} \rangle \cdot \mathbf{C^M}$. Now assume that two such subsets are selected, one with a high mean ($\langle \mathbf{m_i} \rangle_2$) and one with a low mean ($\langle \mathbf{m_i} \rangle_2$), giving two solutions for $\mathbf{C}$ ($\mathbf{C_2}$ and $\mathbf{C_1}$), then

$$
\mathbf{C^M} \approx (\mathbf{C_2} - \mathbf{C_1})/(\langle \mathbf{m_i} \rangle_2 - \langle \mathbf{m_i} \rangle_1)
\tag{7}
$$

(a similar expression for $\mathbf{C^O}$ can be derived) [18]. Again the estimate of ($\mathbf{C_2} - \mathbf{C_1}$) is computed in the space defined by the spatial modes in the same way as in Eq. (4),

$$
(\mathbf{C_2} - \mathbf{C_1}) = \mathbf{v} \cdot (\mathrm{pinv}(\mathbf{M_2} \cdot \mathbf{v}) \cdot \mathbf{m_{2i}} - \mathrm{pinv}(\mathbf{M_1} \cdot \mathbf{v}) \cdot \mathbf{m_{1i}}),
\tag{8}
$$

where the subscripts 1 and 2 denote subsets of the time series selected on the basis of intrinsic activity (m_i) being low or high. This general approach to characterising nonlinear systems with a piece-wise series of locally linear models has proved to be a fruitful strategy in many instances [19]. See [20] for a conceptually related approach to multichannel EEG recordings.

The hypothesis that asymmetrical nonlinear V1–V2 interactions would characterize cortical activity in human visual cortex can be formulated in terms of C_{ij}^{M}: We predicted that anatomically (i) the modulatory component of effective connections to V1 would be regionally specific and include V2 and that functionally (ii) the forward modulatory influences from V1 to V2 would be smaller than the reciprocal influences.

The data used in this analysis were a time series of 64 gradient-echo EPI coronal slices (5 mm thick, with 64×64 voxels, $2.5 \times 2.5 \times 5$ mm) through the calcarine sulcus and extrastriate areas. Images were obtained every 3 sec from a normal male subject using a 4.0T whole body system, fitted with a small (27 cm diameter) z-gradient coil (TE, 25 msec; acquisition time, 41 msec). Photic stimulation (at 16 Hz) was provided by goggles fitted with 16 light emitting diodes. The stimulation was off for the first 10 scans (30 sec), on for the second 10, off for the third, and so on. Images were reconstructed without phase correction. The data were interpolated to 128×128 voxels. Each interpolated voxel thus represented $1.25 \times 1.25 \times 5$ mm of cerebral tissue. The first 4 scans were removed to eliminate magnetic saturation effects and the remainder were realigned. The result of this preprocessing was a mean corrected data matrix **M** with 60 rows (one for each scan) and 2160 columns (one for each voxel).

C. Regional Specificity of Modulatory Connections to V1

A reference voxel was chosen in V1, according to the atlas of Talairach and Tournoux [21], and the effective connection strengths $C_{V1,j}^{M}$ were estimated according to Eq. (7), allowing a map of $C_{V1,j}^{M}$ (and $C_{V1,j}^{O}$) to be constructed. This map provides a direct test of the hypothesis concerning the topography and regional specificity of modulatory influences on V1. The lower row in Fig. 1 shows maps of $C_{V1,j}^{O}$ and $C_{V1,j}^{M}$ (for a reference voxel in V1 on the right) and reflect the degree to which the area exerts an obligatory (left) or modulatory (right) effect on V1 activity. These maps have been thresholded at $Z = 1.64$ after normalization to a standard deviation of unity. This corresponds to an uncorrected threshold of $P = 0.05$.

The obligatory connections to the reference voxel derive mainly from V1 itself, both ipsilaterally and contralaterally, with a small contribution from contiguous portions of V2. The effective connectivity from contralateral V1 should not be overinterpreted given that (i) the source of many afferents to V1 (the lateral geniculate nuclei) were not included in the field of view and that (ii) this finding can be more parsimoniously explained by "common input." As predicted, and with remarkable regional specificity, the modulatory connections were most marked from ipsilateral V2, dorsal and ventral to the calcarine fissure (Brodmann's area 18 according to the atlas of Talairach and Tournoux [Talairach, 1988, No. 102]) (note that "common input" cannot explain interactions between V1 and V2 because the geniculate inputs are restricted to V1).

D. Functional Asymmetry in V2–V1 and V1–V2 Modulatory Connections

To address the functional asymmetry hypothesis the modulatory connection strengths between two extended regions (two 5×5 voxel squares) in ipsilateral V1 and V2 were examined. The estimates of effective connection strengths

anatomy

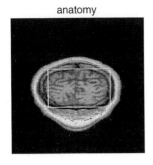

physiological variance

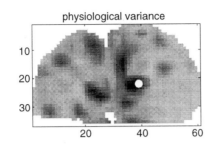

source of obligatory effects

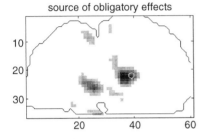

source of modulatory effects

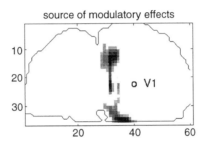

FIGURE 1 Maps of the estimates of obligatory and modulatory connection strengths to V1. (Top left) Anatomical features of the coronal data used. This image is a high resolution anatomical MRI scan of the subject that corresponds to the fMRI slices. The box defines the position of a (36×60 voxel) subpartition of the fMRI time series selected for analysis. (Top right) The location of the reference voxel is designated as V1 (white dot). This location is shown on a statistical parametric map of physiological variance (calculated for each voxel from the time series of 60 scans). The image has been scaled to its maximum. (Lower right and lower left) Maps of $C_{V1,j}^{O}$ and $C_{V1,j}^{M}$. The images have been scaled to unit variance and thresholded at $P = 0.05$ (assuming, under the null hypothesis of no effective connectivity, that the estimates have a Gaussian distribution). The reference voxel in V1 is depicted by a circle. The key thing to note is that V1 is subject to modulatory influences from ipsilateral and extensive regions of V2.

were based on haemodynamic changes in all areas and a subset of connections between the two regions were selected to compare the distributions of forward and backward modulatory influences. Figure 2 shows the location of the two regions (this time on the right) and the frequency distribution of the estimates for connections from the V1 box to the V2 box (broken line) and the corresponding estimates for connections from V2 to V1 (solid line). There is a remarkable dissociation, with backward modulatory effects (V2 to V1) being much greater than forward effects (V1 to V2). This can be considered a confirmation of the functional asymmetry hypothesis.

V. STRUCTURAL EQUATION MODELING

Structural equation modeling or path analysis is a technique developed in economics, psychology and the social sciences. The basic idea is different from the usual statistical approach of modeling individual observations. In multiple regression, or ANOVA, the regression coefficients or the error variance derive

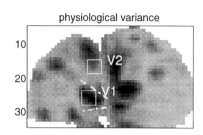

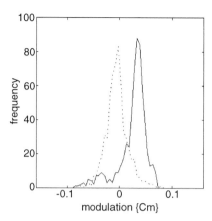

FIGURE 2   Graphical presentation of a direct test of the hypothesis concerning the asymmetry between forward and backward V1–V2 interactions. (Left) A map of physiological variance showing the positions of two boxes defining regions in V1 and V2. The broken lines correspond (roughly) to the position of the V1/V2 border according to the atlas of Talairach and Tournoux [21]. The value of C_{ij}^M were computed for all voxels in either box and Euclidean normalized to unity over the image. The frequency distribution of C_{ij}^M connecting the two regions is presented on the right. The backward connections (V2 to V1, solid line) are clearly higher than the corresponding forward connections (V1 to V2, broken line).

from the minimisation of the sum of squared differences of the predicted and observed dependent variables. Structural equation modeling approaches data from a different perspective. Instead of considering variables individually the emphasis lies on the variance–covariance structure. Thus models are solved in structural equation modeling by minimising the difference between an observed variance–covariance structure and one implied by a structural or path model. In the past few years structural equation modeling has been applied to functional brain imaging. McIntosh and Gonzales-Lima [1] demonstrated the dissociation between ventral and dorsal visual pathways for object and spatial vision using structural equation modeling of PET data in the human. In this chapter we will focus on the theoretical background of structural equation modeling and demonstrate an adaptation of this technique to functional brain imaging with a PET study by Grafton [22]. This study examined the effect of pallidotomy on the effective connectivity of the motor system in Parkinson patients.

In terms of neural systems a measure of covariance represents the degree to which activities of two or more regions are related (*i.e.*, functional connectivity). The study of variance–covariance structures in neuroscience has a major advantage compared to applications of this technique in other fields; the interconnection of the dependent variables (regional activity of brain areas) is anatomically determined and the activation of each region can be directly measured with functional brain imaging. This is a major difference to "classical" structural equation modeling in the behavourial sciences where models are highly hypothetical and contain latent variables which represent a concept (*e.g.*, intelligence) that cannot be measured directly. Latent variables also speak to the link between structural equation modeling and factor analysis, a somewhat controversial technique [23]. Eschewing latent variables in the adaptation of structural equation modeling to functional imaging needs avoids this controversy and makes path analysis a reasonably straightforward tool [1].

A. Models

As mentioned above structural equation modeling minimises the difference between the observed S and implied covariance matrix Σ. The variance–covariance structure **S** of the observed variables is given by

$$S = (1/(N-1)) \cdot \mathbf{y}^{\mathrm{T}} \cdot \mathbf{y}, \tag{9}$$

where **y** is a N by p matrix of deviation (from the mean) scores of P observed variables with N observations and $\mathbf{y}^{\mathrm{T}}$ is **y** transpose. The matrix **S** is square and symmetric with the sample variances down its main diagonal and the covariances off the diagonal.

Consider a model in which variables **x** are "caused" by a set of independent variables **z** (Fig. 3). This could also be construed as a set of variables **x** with residual influences **z** (outside the model). In addition the variables **x** may cause each other.

Algebraically, the model for **x** is

$$\mathbf{x} = \mathbf{x} \cdot \mathbf{B} + \mathbf{z} \cdot \mathbf{I}, \tag{10}$$

where **B** is a matrix of unidirectional path coefficients and **I** is the identity matrix. Here **x** appears on both sides of the equation. The equation reduces to

$$\mathbf{x} = \mathrm{inv}(\mathbf{I} - \mathbf{B}) \cdot \mathbf{z}. \tag{11}$$

Looking at the variance–covariance structure and omitting the denominator $(1/(N-1))$ we have

$$\mathbf{x}^{\mathrm{T}} \cdot \mathbf{x} = (\mathrm{inv}(\mathbf{I} - \mathbf{B}) \cdot \mathbf{z})^{\mathrm{T}} \cdot (\mathrm{inv}(\mathbf{I} - \mathbf{B}) \cdot \mathbf{z}) = \mathrm{inv}(\mathbf{I} - \mathbf{B})^{\mathrm{T}} \cdot \mathbf{C} \cdot (\mathrm{inv}(I - B)), \tag{12}$$

where

$$\mathbf{C} = \mathbf{z}^{\mathrm{T}} \cdot \mathbf{z}.$$

B is not symmetric because structural equation modeling allows asymmetric connections. **C** is a diagonal matrix and contains the residual variances. If interaction between residual influences were incorporated in the model, their covariances would appear (symmetrically) off the leading diagonal in **C** (not shown in Fig. 3). This follows from the fact that **C** is equal to $\mathbf{z}^{\mathrm{T}} \cdot \mathbf{z}$, which is the variance–covariance structure of **z**. The denominator $(1/N - 1)$ is omitted for clarity. The solution of Eq. (12), $\mathbf{x}^{\mathrm{T}} \cdot \mathbf{x}$ is the implied variance–covariance structure Σ. Parameters in **C** and **B**, that are to be estimated, are called free parameters.

B. Estimation

The free parameters are estimated by minimising a function of S and Σ. To date, the most widely used objective function for structural equation modeling is the maximum likelihood (ML) function:

$$F_{\mathrm{ML}} = \log|\Sigma| + \mathrm{tr}(S \cdot \mathrm{inv}(\Sigma)) - \log|S| - p, \tag{13}$$

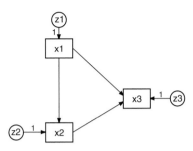

FIGURE 3 Simple path model to demonstrate the mathematical background of structural equation modeling. x are observed variables, the (unidirectional) path coefficients between variables **x** constitute matrix **B**. The 1 at each path between **z** and the corresponding variable **x** denotes the fact that **z** are residual variances, that are not explained by the model. The path coefficients for the connections from **z** to **x** are therefore, one, which is simply the identity matrix (Eq. 10).

where tr(.) is the trace of the matrix and p is the number of free parameters. Starting values can be provided for the free parameters or estimated by a least squares approach [24]. The simplest method of determining the parameters is the method of "steepest decent." The major problem of steepest descent is that the second derivative of the function being minimised is not taken into account. This is important because the curvature of the function—which determines its behaviour near the minimum—depends on these derivatives. The Newton–Raphson method, or other methods that overcome this disadvantage are therefore used in most structural equation modeling implementations. The use of different starting values can help to find the global maximum during minimisation.

An important issue in structural equation modeling is the determination of the underlying anatomical model. Different objective methods can be combined. Categorical comparisons between different conditions, eigenimages highlighting structures of functional connectivity in conjunction with nonhuman electrophysiological and anatomical studies have been used [22,24]. A model is always a simplification of reality therefore absolutely correct models either do not exist or would be too complicated to understand. In the context of effective connectivity one has to find a compromise between complexity, anatomical accuracy, and interpretability. There are also mathematical constraints on the model. If the number of free parameters (unknowns) exceeds the number of observed covariances the system is underdetermined and no single solution exists.

C. Statistical Inference

Statistical inference in structural equation modeling can address two points. The goodness of overall fit of the model, *i.e.*, how significantly different is the implied from the observed variance–covariance structure, and the difference between different models (*e.g.*, object *versus* spatial vision [1]). In the context of multivariate, normally distributed variables, the minimum of the maximum likelihood fit function times the number of observations minus one, follows a χ^2 distribution with $(q/2) \cdot (q + 1) - p$ degrees of freedom [25]. p is the number of free parameters and q is the number of observed variables. The null hypothesis is that the model is not able to reproduce an observed variance–covariance structure. If the χ^2 goodness of fit is statistically insignificant, the model is able to reproduce the observed variance–covariance structure. In traditional structural equation modeling applications the goodness of fit revealed by the χ^2 value is used to prove that a hypothesised model is tenable, given the data. Goodness of fit estimation by the minimum of the maximum likelihood objective function is one target of major criticism of structural equation modeling. In contrast to "classical" path analysis, the validation of models used in the context of functional brain imaging relies on neuroanatomy. Therefore, goodness of fit estimation plays only a minor role. However, the goodness of fit measure might be useful in comparing different models with each other. This so-called "stacked model" approach can be used to compare different models (*e.g.*, data from different groups or conditions) in the context of structural equation modeling. A so called "null-model" is constructed in which the estimates of all free parameters are constrained to be the same for both groups. The alternative model allows the free parameters to differ between groups. The significance of the differences between models is expressed by the difference of the χ^2 goodness of fit indicator.

How are path coefficients interpreted? The path coefficients calculated by the minimisation procedure outlined above depend upon the units in which the variables are measured. Although all variables in functional imaging procedures are measured in the same units, the direct comparison of path coefficients between two different groups might be misleading due to different scaling (*e.g.*, global blood flow in PET). In this case a standardised path coefficient is calculated. This is equal to the path coefficient times the ratio of the standard deviations of the two connected variables (the standard deviation of the caused variable constituting the denominator). The standardised coefficient shows the mean response in units of standard deviation of the dependent variable for a standard deviation change in an explanatory variable, whilst other variables in the model are held constant [25].

A major limitation of current applications of structural equation modeling is the restriction to linear models. This limitation can be overcome by introducing additional variables containing a nonlinear function (*e.g.*, $f(x) = x^2$) of the original variables [26]. Interactions of variables can be incorporated in a similar fashion, wherein a new variable, containing the product of the two interacting variables, is introduced as an additional influence.

VI. AN EXAMPLE: PATH ANALYSIS OF THE HUMAN MOTOR SYSTEM

The motor system is one of the best understood systems in the human. This is due to two factors: (i) An understanding of the system is largely based on anatomical and electrophysiological results from primate research. (ii) A wide variety of movement disorders in the human places this system at the centre of active clinical research. Parkinson's disease is characterised by the triad of bradykinesia, rigidity, and tremor. In the normal state subcortical excitatory and inhibitory influences on thalamocortical projections are in balance. In hypokinetic movement disorders like Parkinson's disease, there is an imbalance of excitatory and inhibitory influences culminating in excess inhibition of the same movement related thalamocortical neurons. It is known that a lesion of the posteroventral globus pallidus (GPi) can improve tremor, rigidity, and hypokinesia in Parkinson's disease [27]. Grafton *et al.* [22] studied patients with Parkinson's disease before and after pallidotomy with a $H_2^{15}O$ PET activation study, using a simple grasping paradigm. The functional model of the human motor system was based on the Alexander and DeLong model [28] (Fig. 4). As mentioned above, structural equation modeling decomposes covariances instead of correlations. If one specifies correlations, as in this example, the standard deviations are required to estimate the path coefficients. The results of our estimation differ from those published in Grafton *et al.* [29]. This is due to the fact that LISREL, the software package used by Grafton *et al.* uses correlations as covariances. The problem is that the original sampling theory designed to analyse covariance structures is built around the multivariate sampling distribution of elements of a covariance matrix. This sampling distribution is not the same as the multivariate distribution of the elements of a correlation matrix. To see this, simply regard the diagonal, which contains fixed ones in a correlation matrix, but contains random variables in a covariance matrix. This difference also affects the fixed residual variances of the SMA and MOTOR variable (0.25 in Grafton *et al.* [29]). We fixed the observed variance of those variables at the observed variance divided by four

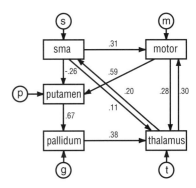

FIGURE 4 Structural equation model of the human cortical–subcortical motor network according to Alexander and DeLong [28]. Values for a visually guided grasping task before pallidotomy are shown. The values of the estimated path coefficients are standardised. The standardised coefficient shows the mean response in standard deviation units of the dependent variable for a one standard deviation change in an explanatory variable, holding constant the other variables in the model [25]. Note that although some path coefficients are constrained to be equal (*i.e.*, SMA to thalamus and SMA to MOTOR) the standardised coefficient can differ. The data shown are part of Grafton *et al.* [22].

(Figs. 3 and 4). Our estimation is calculated by the program AMOS (version 3.51), that uses standard deviations to build an internal covariance matrix.

To obtain stable results the number of regions and free parameters had to be less than the number of observations ($n = 10$). Therefore, additional constraints were applied. The residual variances affecting motor cortex were fixed, based on the assumption that external influences on these cortical regions could be treated as constant across subjects and time. In addition, recursive pathways between cortical structures and the thalamus were constrained to be equal.

The results of the parameter estimation using AMOS (SmallWaters Corporation, Chicago, IL) before pallidotomy are shown in Fig. 4. The overall pattern of regional interactions shows dramatic changes after pallidotomy (Fig. 5). Using the stacked model approach, both models were significantly different. A decrease in the projection from the thalamus to SMA/cingulate motor areas is evident (*e.g.*, thalamus—SMA: 0.20 before and -0.04 after pallidotomy). These changes affect preferentially the mesial motor areas and only indirectly involve the primary motor cortex. This result is in accord with previous studies of Parkinson's disease [30]. Consistent with the effect of pallidotomy, output from the globus pallidus to the thalamus decreased (0.38 before *vs* -0.14 after surgery). These results show that functional imaging techniques, like PET, are sensitive enough to identify disruption of neural connections. Furthermore, an integrational data analysis can be helpful in examining a neuronal network as a whole and can show changes that are not always apparent when images are compared categorically.

VII. ISSUES OF VALIDITY

A major criticism of path analysis is the validity of the model. The issue of construct validity applies to most models of effective connectivity. The difficulty in proving that a model is correct does not pertain only to effective connectivity. Every discussion of functional imaging experiments trying to explain results of categorical comparisons on the basis of connected networks faces this problem. This debate can also be seen from a different angle. A simple subtraction paradigm in functional imaging most often reveals more than one site of activation. It is necessary to have a hypothesis about interconnections between these regions (functional/anatomical model) to explain the integration of the observed (spatially remote) activations. Structural equation modeling and other techniques of estimating effective connectivity can be seen as a "reverse" approach, where an anatomical model is specified and can then be tested under different experimental conditions. The technique has been successfully applied (for instance) comparing object to spatial vision as shown in a study by McIntosh and Gonzales-Lima [24]. Structural equation modeling of PET data is limited by the fact that only a few observations are available. In the future, path analysis (and the concept of effective connectivity in general) will benefit from the acquisition of long time-series data sets using fMRI.

The measurements used in all examples of this chapter were hemodynamic in nature. This limits an interpretation at the level of neuronal interactions. However, the analogy between the form of nonlinear interaction between V1 and V2 activity and voltage-dependent connections is a strong one. It is possible that the modulatory impact of V2 on V1 is mediated by predominantly voltage-dependent connections. The presence of horizontal

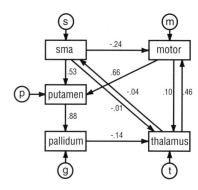

FIGURE 5 Estimation of path coefficients of the human motor system during a visually guided grasping task. The results for patients suffering from Parkinson's disease *after* pallidotomy are shown. Pallidotomy is associated with an attenuation in the projection from the globus pallidus to the thalamus and a marked change in the thalamo-cortical connections to the SMA motor areas. The data shown are part of Grafton *et al.* [22].

voltage-dependent connections within V1 has been established in cat striate cortex [31]. We know of no direct electrophysiological evidence to suggest that extrinsic backward V2 to V1 connections are voltage-dependent; however, our results are consistent with this suggestion. An alternative explanation for modulatory effects, that does not necessarily involve voltage-dependent connections, can again be found in the work of Aertsen and Preissl [11]. Recall that they concluded effective connectivity varies strongly with, or is modulated by, pool activity. The mechanism relates to the efficacy of subthreshold EPSPs in establishing dynamic interactions as a function of postsynaptic depolarisation, which in turn depends on the tonic background of activity. This formulation clearly relates to the idea that sensitivity to afferent input increases with intrinsic activity. The original presentation of these results and a fuller discussion can be found in Friston et al. [18].

It is also important to clarify the terms "excitatory" and "inhibitory" effects in the context of effective connectivity. The conclusion that a positive path coefficient from region A to B reflects a predominantly excitatory pathway between A and B is wrong. As mentioned before, all measurements are haemodynamic in nature and one has to keep in mind that both excitation and inhibition can lead to an increase of regional cerebral blood flow.

This chapter has reviewed some basic concepts of effective connectivity in relation to neuroimaging data. Methods currently used to assess effective connectivity have been demonstrated. The first example showed that nonlinear interactions can be characterised using simple extensions of linear models. In the second example, structural equation modeling was introduced as a device that allows one to combine observed changes in cortical activity and anatomical models. Both examples concentrated on changes of effective connectivity and allowed a comprehensive description of the interacting areas of a network on a functional level. Although less than mature this approach to analysis of neuroimaging data and of regional interactions is an exciting endeavour that deserves to attract more attention.

References

1. A. R. McIntosh, C. L. Grady, L. G. Ungerleider, J. V. Haxby, S. I. Rapoport, and B. Horwitz. Network analysis of cortical visual pathways mapped with PET. *J. Neurosci.* **14,** 655–666 (1994).
2. K. J. Friston, C. D. Frith, P. F. Liddle, and R. S. J. Frackowiak. Functional connectivity: The principal component analysis of large (PET) data sets. *J. Cereb. Blood Flow Metab.* **13,** 5–14 (1993).
3. K. J. Friston, C. D. Frith, and R. S. J. Frackowiak. Time-dependent changes in effective connectivity measured with PET. *Hum. Brain Mapping* **1,** 69–80 (1993).
4. A. R. McIntosh and F. Gonzalez-Lima. Structural modelling of functional neural pathways mapped with 2-deoxyglucose: Effects of acoustic startle habituation on the auditory system. *Brain Res.* **547,** 295–302 (1991).
5. B. Horwitz, C. Grady, J. Haxby, *et al.* Object and spatial visual processing: Intercorrelations of regional cerebral blood flow among posterior brain regions. *J. Cereb. Blood Flow Metab.* **11,** S380 (1991).
6. B. Horwitz, A. R. McIntosh, J. V. Haxby, *et al.* Altered brain functional interactions during visual processing in Alzheimer type dementia. *NeuroReport* **6,** 2287–2292 (1995).
7. M. Corbetta, F. M. Miezin, S. Dobmeyer, G. L. Shulman, and P. S. E. Petersen. Selective and divided attention during visual discrimination of shape, colour, and speed: Functional anatomy by positron emission tomography. *J. Neurosci.* **13,** 1202–1226 (1991).

8. G. L. Gerstein, P. Bedenbaugh, and A. Aertsen. Neuronal assemblies. *IEEE Trans. Biomed. Eng.* **36,** 4–14 (1989).

9. G. L. Gerstein and D. H. Perkel. Simultaneously recorded trains of action potentials: Analysis and functional interpretation. *Science* **164,** 828–830 (1969).

10. P. M. Gochin, E. K. Miller, C. G. Gross, and G. L. Gerstein. Functional interactions among neurons in inferior temporal cortex of the awake macaque. *Exp. Brain Res.* **84,** 505–516 (1991).

11. A. Aertsen and H. Preissl. "Dynamics of Activity and Connectivity in Physiological Neuronal Networks." VCH, New York, 1991.

12. K. G. Binmore. "Mathematical Analysis." Cambridge Univ. Press, Cambridge, 1982.

13. G. H. Golub and C. F. Van Loan. "Matrix Computations," 2nd ed. pp. 241–248. Johns Hopkins Univ. Press, Baltimore and London, 1991.

14. P. H. Schiller and J. G. Malpeli. The effect of striate cortex cooling on area 18 cells in the monkey. *Brain Res.* **126,** 366–369 (1977).

15. J. H. Sandell and P. J. Schiller. Effect of cooling area 18 on striate cortex cells in the squirrel monkey. *J. Neurophysiol.* **48,** 38–48 (1982).

16. P. Girard and J. Bullier. Visual activity in area V2 during reversible inactivation of area 17 in the macaque monkey. *J. Neurophysiol.* **62,** 1287–1301 (1988).

17. L. B. Haberly. "Olfactory Cortex." Oxford Univ. Press, Oxford, 1991.

18. K. J. Friston, L. G. Ungerleider, P. Jezzard, and R. Turner. Characterizing modulatory interactions between V1 and V2 in human cortex with fMRI. *Hum. Brain Mapping* **2,** 211–224 (1995).

19. A. A. Tsonis. "Chaos: From Theory to Applications," Plenum, New York and London, 1992.

20. M. Palus, I. Dvorak, and I. David. Remarks on spatial and temporal dynamics of EEG. *In* "Mathematical Approaches to Brain Imaging Diagnostics" (I. Dvorak and A.V. Holden, Eds.), Vol. pp. 369–385, Manchester Univ. Press, Manchester and New York, 1991.

21. P. Talairach and J. Tournoux. "A Stereotactic Coplanar Atlas of the Human Brain." Thieme, Stuttgart, 1988.

22. S. T. Grafton, J. Sutton, W. Couldwell, M. Lew, and C. Waters. Network analysis of motor system connectivity in Parkinson's disease: Modulation of thalamocortical interactions after pallidotomy. *Hum. Brain Mapping* **2,** 45–55 (1994).

23. C. Chatfield and A. J. Collins. "Introduction to Multivariate Analysis." Chapman and Hall, London, 1995.

24. A. R. McIntosh and F. Gonzalez-Lima. Structural equation modelling and its application to network analysis in functional brain imaging. *Hum. Brain Mapping* **2,** 2–22 (1994).

25. K. A. Bollen. "Structural Equations with Latent Variables." Wiley, New York, 1989.

26. D. A. Kenny and C. M. Judd. Estimating nonlinear and interactive effects of latent variables. *Psychol. Bull.* **96,** 201–210 (1984).

27. L. V. Laitinen, A. T. Bergenheim, and M. I. Hariz. Leksell's posteroventral pallidotomy in the treatment of Parkinson's disease. *J. Neurosurg.* **76,** 53–61 (1992).

28. G. E. Alexander, M. D. Crutcher, and M. R. DeLong. Basal ganglia thalamocortical circuits: Parallel substrates for motor, oculomotor, "prefrontal" and "limbic" functions. *Prog. Brain Res.* **85,** 119–146 (1990).

29. S. T. Grafton, J. Sutton, W. Couldwell, M. Lew, and C. Waters. Network analysis of motor system connectivity in Parkinson's disease: Modulation of thalamocortical interactions after pallidotomy. *Hum. Brain Mapping* **2,** 45–55 (1994).

30. I. H. Jenkins, W. Fernandez, E. D. Playford, A. J. Lees, R. S. J. Frackowiak, R. E. Passingham, and D. J. Brooks. Impaired activation of the supplementary motor area in Parkinson's disease is reversed when akinesia is treated with apomorphine. *Ann. Neurol.* **32,** 749–757 (1992).

31. J. A. Hirsch and C. D. Gilbert. Synaptic physiology of horizontal connections in the cat's visual cortex. *J. Neurosci.* **11,** 1800–1809 (1991).

CHAPTER EIGHT

A Taxonomy of Study Design

I. INTRODUCTION

This chapter is concerned with the way in which methods presented in previous chapters are implemented in terms of experimental design, and the sort of questions they are used to address. In this chapter we review different sorts of experimental design and examine some of the assumptions about the relationship between cognitive function and neurobiology. We start with a simple taxonomy of experimental design that includes (i) categorical, (ii) parametric, and (iii) factorial designs. Each of these designs is discussed from a conceptual viewpoint and illustrated using an exemplar activation study. The remaining sections of the chapter focus on parametric and factorial designs by considering specific examples of their use. For parametric designs we have chosen nonlinear regression and show how curvilinear relationships between task parameters and evoked haemodynamic responses can be characterised. The example of factorial designs is chosen to address problems with cognitive subtraction and the validity of pure insertion.

II. A TAXONOMY OF EXPERIMENTAL DESIGN

A. Categorical Designs

The tenet of the categorical approach is that the difference between two tasks can be formulated as a separable cognitive or sensorimotor component and that the regionally specific differences in brain activity identify a corresponding functionally specialised area. Early applications of subtraction range from the functional anatomy of word processing [1] to functional specialisation in extrastriate cortex [2]. The latter studies involved presenting visual stimuli with and without some specific sensory attribute (*e.g.*, colour, motion, *etc.*). The areas highlighted by subtraction were identified with homologous areas in monkeys that showed selective electrophysiological responses to equivalent visual stimuli. Cognitive subtraction is conceptually simple and is a very effective device for mapping functional anatomy. When used in the context of serial subtraction, however, it depends on the assumption that cognitive states differ in components that can be purely inserted or removed with no interaction between them, both at the level of a function and at the level of its neural implementation. The possible fallibility of this assumption (see below) has prompted the exploration of other experimental designs.

B. Parametric Designs

The premise with parametric designs is that regional physiology will vary monotonically and systematically with the amount of cognitive or sensorimotor processing. Examples of this approach include the experiments of Grafton *et al.* [3], who demonstrated significant correlations between regional cerebral blood flow (rCBF) and the performance of a visually guided motor tracking task (using a pursuit rotor device) in the primary motor area, supplementary motor area, and pulvinar thalamus. The authors associated this distributed network with early procedural learning. On the sensory side we [4] have demonstrated a remarkable linear relationship between rCBF in periauditory regions and frequency of aural word presentation. Significantly, this correlation was not observed in Wernicke's area where rCBF appeared to correlate not with the discriminative attributes of the stimulus, but with the presence or absence of semantics. This nonlinear relationship between stimulus presentation frequency and evoked response speaks to the importance of modelling nonlinear associations explicitly in an analysis. This theme will be taken up again below.

Time-dependent changes in physiology are clearly central to studies of learning and memory. Many animal models of procedural learning depend on habituation and adaptation, at either a behaviourial or an electrophysiological level. In the context of functional imaging, physiological adaptation to a challenge is simply the change in rCBF activation with time. This is an interaction of the effect with time.

C. Factorial Designs

At its simplest an interaction is basically a change in a change. Interactions are associated with factorial designs where two factors are combined in the same experiment. The effect of one factor on the effect of another is assessed by an interaction term (two factors interact if the level of one factor affects the effect of another). Factorial designs have a wide range of applications. The first PET experiment of this sort was perhaps the simplest imaginable and examined the interaction between motor activation (sequential finger opposition paced by a metronome) and time (rest–performance pairs repeated three times) [5]. Significant adaptation was seen in the cerebellar cortex (ipsilateral to the hand moved) and cerebellar nuclei. These results are consistent with the electrophysiological studies of Gilbert and Thach [6], who demonstrated a reduction in simple and complex spike activity of Purkinje cells in the cerebellum during motor learning in monkeys. Psychopharmacological activation studies are examples of a factorial design [7]. In these studies subjects perform a series of baseline-activation task pairs before and after the administration of a centrally acting drug. The interaction term reflects a modulatory drug effect on the task-dependent physiological response. Such studies are providing an exciting insight into the relationship between cognition and neurotransmitter function in man [8]. A further example of factorial designs includes experiments designed to examine the interaction between cognitive processes, for example dual task interference paradigms. An early example of this approach involved an analysis of encoding of episodic verbal material (using paired associates). Memory and control tasks were performed under two conditions, an easy and a difficult manual distractor task. Encoding is generally confounded with priming. However, due to the differential impact of the distractor task on encoding and priming, we were able to make inferences about encoding *per se* using the interaction effects [9].

The examples cited above all involve the use of factorial designs where each factor has a number of discrete or categorical levels. These designs have facilitated studies of adaptation, neuromodulation, and interference at a cognitive level. It is, of course, possible to combine parametric and factorial designs, wherein a task or stimulus parameter is varied under two or more conditions. For example, the frequency of stimuli can be manipulated under different forms of attentional set [10]. Interaction effects in this context can be thought of as a change in the slope of a regression of haemodynamic response on the task parameter under different conditions. This sort of design has clear applications for examining changes of sensitivity of a particular area to stimulation under different conditions. We will return to factorial designs and their relationship to "cognitive interactions" below.

All the examples cited above use statistical parametric maps (SPMs) in conjunction with the general linear model. The following section provides an illustration of the basic differences between categorical, parametric, and factorial approaches to the same data.

III. AN ILLUSTRATIVE EXAMPLE USING PET DATA

A. The Data

The data were obtained from five subjects scanned 12 times whilst performing one of two verbal tasks in alternation. One task involved repeating a letter presented aurally at one per 2 sec (word shadowing). The other was a paced verbal fluency task, in which the subjects responded with a word that began with a presented letter (intrinsic word generation). To facilitate intersubject pooling, data were realigned, spatially normalised and smoothed with an isotropic Gaussian kernel (FWHM of 16 mm). In this case there are five subjects and 12 conditions. We removed the confounding effect of global activity by designating global activities as covariates of no interest. This example is equivalent to a one-way ANCOVA with a blocked design [11]. There are thus 12 condition-specific effects, five subject effects, and a covariate effect. By specifying appropriate contrasts we tested for different effects of a categorical, parametric, or factorial nature.

B. Categorical or Subtractive Approach

In this example we address the effects of activations due to intrinsic word generation or, equivalently, deactivations due to word repetition (extrinsic word generation). Following the philosophy of cognitive subtraction this comparison is effected by subtracting the word shadowing from the verbal fluency conditions to assess activations associated with cognitive components in word

generation that are not present in word shadowing (*e.g.*, the intrinsic generation of word representations and the "working memory" for words already
produced). Having estimated the 12 condition-specific (and all other) effects
using the general linear model the effect of verbal fluency *vs* word shadowing
was assessed using a contrast that was 1 in all the verbal fluency conditions,
-1 in the word generation conditions, and 0 elsewhere $[1 -1 1 -1 \ldots -1$
$0\,0\,0\,0\ldots]$. The results of this analysis are presented in Fig. 1 which shows the
design matrix, the contrast and the resulting SPM$\{Z\}$. The results demonstrate
significant activations of the left anterior cingulate, left dorsolateral prefrontal
cortex, operculum and related insula, thalamus, and extrastriate areas
(among others).

C. A Parametric Approach

In this example we tested for monotonic, nonlinear (exponential) time effects
using the contrast depicted in Fig. 2. The results of this analysis identify
bilateral foci in the temporal regions and prefrontal cortices that show monotonic decreases of activity. These decreases are task-independent. This example is trivial in its conception but is used here to introduce the notion of a
parametric approach to the data. Parametric approaches test for systematic
relationships between neurophysiology and sensorimotor, psychophysical,
pharmacological, or cognitive parameters. These systematic relationships are
not constrained to be linear or additive and may show very nonlinear behaviour, reflecting complex interactions at a physiological or cognitive level.

D. A Factorial Approach

This example looks at regionally specific interactions, in this instance between
an activation effect due to intrinsic word generation and time. The contrast
used is depicted in Fig. 3 and shows a typical mirror symmetry. This contrast
highlights those regions that deactivate early in the experiment and activate
towards the end. In other words, those areas that show a time-dependent
augmentation of their activation. The areas implicated include left frontal
operculum, insula, thalamus, and left temporal cortex. Note that these regional
results suggest a true physiological "adaptation" in the sense that it is the
physiological response (to a task component) that shows a time-dependent
change (contrast this with the task-independent changes of the previous section). In this example we have described a time-dependent reorganisation of
physiological responses to the same task. It is tempting to call this plasticity;
however, the term plasticity means many things to many people and hence it
should be used carefully [12].

E. Summary

Experimental design has been briefly reviewed using a taxonomy of activation
studies that distinguishes between categorical (subtractive), parametric (dimensional), and factorial (interaction) designs. Subtraction designs are well
established in functional mapping but are predicated on possibly untenable
assumptions about the relationship between brain dynamics and the functional
processes that ensue. For example, even if, from a functionalist perspective,
a cogntive component can be added without interaction among preexisting
components the brain's implementation of these processes will almost certainly

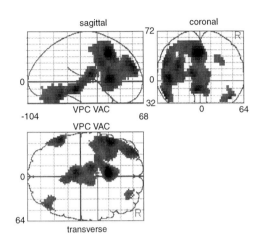

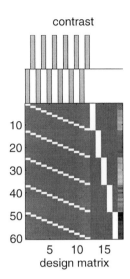

A categorical analysis

set–level {c}	cluster–level {k,Z}	voxel–level {Z}	uncorrected	location {mm}
0.000 (5)	0.000 (2980, 6.35)	0.000 (6.35)	0.000	−4 16 44
		0.000 (5.80)	0.000	−46 18 4
		0.000 (5.44)	0.000	−34 52 20
	0.000 (1007, 5.67)	0.000 (5.67)	0.000	−6 −34 −12
		0.000 (5.44)	0.000	−14 −12 12
		0.003 (4.86)	0.000	2 −40 −12
	0.001 (330, 5.50)	0.000 (5.50)	0.000	−52 −58 −20
		0.012 (4.55)	0.000	−50 −72 −16
		0.084 (4.02)	0.000	−44 −72 −28
	0.003 (135, 4.98)	0.002 (4.98)	0.000	44 −74 −24
		0.010 (4.59)	0.000	34 −70 −24
		0.172 (3.79)	0.000	50 −64 −20
	0.032 (56, 4.34)	0.026 (4.34)	0.000	30 46 28

Height threshold {u} = 3.20, p = 0.001   Volume {S} = 55027 voxels or 149.6 Resels

Extent threshold {k} = 35 voxels   Degrees of freedom due to error = 43

Expected voxels per cluster, E{n} = 35.3   Smoothness = 15.7 19.6 19.1 mm {FWHM}

Expected number of clusters, E{m} = 0.3   = 6.7 8.3 8.1 {voxels}

FIGURE 1   A subtraction analysis. (Top right) Design matrix: This is an image representation of the design matrix. "Contrast" is the contrast or vector defining the linear compound of parameters tested. The contrast is displayed over the column of the design matrix that corresponds to the effect[s] in question. The design matrix here includes condition, subject (block), and one confounding covariate (global activity) effects. The contrast can be seen to test for differences between the verbal fluency (even) and word shadowing (odd) conditions. (Top left) SPM{Z}: This is a maximum intensity projection of the SPM{t} following transformation to the Z score. (Bottom) Tabular data of "significant" regions are presented (in terms of set, cluster, and voxel level inferences).

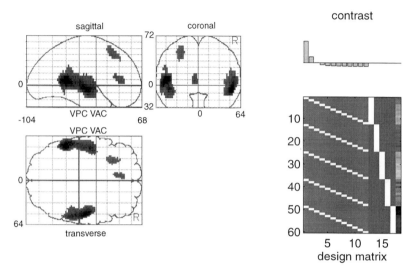

A parametric analysis

set–level {c}	cluster–level {k,Z}	voxel–level {Z}	uncorrected	location {mm}
0.000 (4)	0.000 (851, 5.50)	0.000 (5.50)	0.000	−48 −48 8
		0.000 (5.25)	0.000	−54 −40 4
		0.005 (4.74)	0.000	−44 −10 −4
	0.001 (653, 5.35)	0.000 (5.35)	0.000	50 −18 −4
		0.006 (4.72)	0.000	52 −32 4
		0.027 (4.33)	0.000	52 −40 0
	0.110 (66, 3.96)	0.101 (3.96)	0.000	−6 34 8
		0.260 (3.65)	0.000	−8 26 12
	0.092 (105, 3.88)	0.133 (3.88)	0.000	−26 22 44
		0.422 (3.45)	0.000	−28 34 40

Height threshold {u} = 3.20, p = 0.001	Volume {S} = 55027 voxels or 149.6 Resels
Extent threshold {k} = 35 voxels	Degrees of freedom due to error = 43
Expected voxels per cluster, E{n} = 35.3	Smoothness = 15.7 19.6 19.1 mm {FWHM}
Expected number of clusters, E{m} = 0.3	= 6.7 8.3 8.1 {voxels}

FIGURE 2 A parametric analysis. The format of this figure is the same as for Fig. 1 and shows the results of testing for a nonlinear (exponential) decreasing monotonic time effect using a contrast of the condition effect estimates.

show profound interactions. This conclusion follows from the observation that neural dynamics are nonlinear. Parametric approaches avoid many of the shortcomings of "cognitive subtraction" by testing for systematic relationships between neurophysiology and sensorimotor, psychophysical, pharmacological or cognitive parameters. These systematic relationships are not constrained to be linear or additive and may show very nonlinear behaviour. The fundamental difference between subtractive and parametric approaches lies in treating a cognitive process, not as a categorical invariant, but as a dimension or attribute that can be expressed to a greater or lesser extent. It is anticipated that

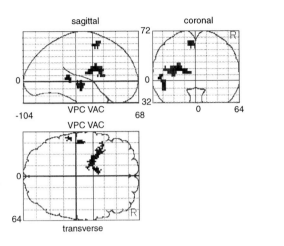

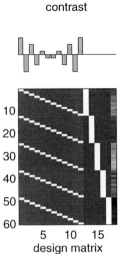

A factorial analysis

set–level {c}	cluster–level {k,Z}	voxel–level {Z}	uncorrected	location {mm}
0.633 (4)	0.414 (125, 3.49)	0.380 (3.49)	0.000	−24 −2 16
		0.785 (3.05)	0.001	−30 6 16
		0.932 (2.81)	0.003	−14 −8 12
	0.844 (31, 2.98)	0.837 (2.98)	0.001	−8 0 52
		0.982 (2.60)	0.005	−8 10 56
	0.895 (15, 2.89)	0.893 (2.89)	0.002	−54 −38 4
	0.917 (30, 2.85)	0.915 (2.85)	0.002	−48 −18 −4

Height threshold {u} = 2.40, p = 0.008   Volume {S} = 55027 voxels or 149.6 Resels

Extent threshold {k} = 8 voxels   Degrees of freedom due to error = 43

Expected voxels per cluster, E{n} = 79.7   Smoothness = 15.7 19.6 19.1 mm {FWHM}

Expected number of clusters, E{m} = 4.4   = 6.7 8.3 8.1 {voxels}

Figure 3 A factorial analysis. The format of this figure is the same as for Fig. 2 and shows the results of testing for an interaction between activations due to verbal fluency and time. The contrast used detects regions whose response to verbal fluency increases with time. The results of this analysis can be reported only descriptively because the *P* values do not survive a correction for the volume analyzed.

parametric designs of this type will find an increasing role in psychological and psychophysical activation experiments. Finally, factorial experiments provide a rich way of assessing the affect of one manipulation on the effects of another. The designs can be used to examine a variety of effects; we have mentioned adaptation, neuromodulation, and dual task interference as three compelling examples. The assessment of differences in activations between two or more groups represents a further question about regionally specific interactions.

The limiting case of this example is where one group contains only one subject. This may be one way to proceed with single subject analyses, in that the interesting thing about an individual's activation profile is how it relates to some normal profile or a profile obtained from the same subject in different situations or at a different time. These differences in activations are interactions.

IV. NONLINEAR PARAMETRIC APPROACHES

Parametric study designs can reveal information about the relationship between a study parameter (*e.g.*, word presentation rate) and regional perfusion. The brain's responses in relation to study parameters may be nonlinear; therefore, linear regressions, as often used in the analysis of parametric studies, may not characterise them properly. We describe here a method that fits nonlinear functions of stimulus or task parameters to rCBF responses, using second order polynomials. This technique is implemented in the context of the general linear model and SPM. We consider the usefulness of statistical inferences, based on SPM{F}, about differences between nonlinear responses as an example of a factorial approach to parametric designs. We will illustrate these points with a PET activation study using an auditory paradigm of increasing word presentation rate.

A. Theoretical Background

Digital signal processing utilises many different techniques to characterise discrete signals by a combination of a number of basis functions. Well known examples are the Fourier expansion and the polynomial expansion. We adapt this technique to characterise activations in terms of a set of basis functions of a given parameter (*e.g.*, study parameter or response) and show how such responses can be approximated by a small number of such basis functions. In what follows we use a second order polynomial expansion of the task parameters. Recall the basic equation of the general linear model:

$$\mathbf{X} = \mathbf{G}\boldsymbol{\beta} + \mathbf{e}. \tag{1}$$

$\mathbf{G}$ is the design matrix, which has one row for every scan and one column for every modeled (*i.e.*, "designed") effect, $\boldsymbol{\beta}$ is the parameter matrix which has one row for each column of $\mathbf{G}$ and one column for every voxel in the volume, and $\mathbf{e}$ is the matrix of error terms. In this case the polynomial basis functions are the explanatory variables used to model the rCBF responses $\mathbf{X}$ and comprise the first two columns of $\mathbf{G}$. The first two rows of $\mathbf{b}$ (the least squares estimates of $\boldsymbol{\beta}$) are the coefficients of the second order polynomial that best model the relationship between rCBF and the variable in question. To test the overall significance of the polynomial regression we test the null hypothesis in the usual way using the F statistic (see Chapter 4). The ensuing SPM{F} can be interpreted as an image of the significance of the variance explained by the effects of interest (*i.e.*, the polynomials in $\mathbf{G}$) relative to error.

The probability of getting one or more voxels with a certain F value in a given SPM{F} is the same as the probability that the largest F value of the

SPM{F} is greater than this F value. At high thresholds this probability equals the expected number of maxima. Therefore, the problem of calculating a corrected P value can be reduced to finding the expected number of maxima at or above this threshold. Worsley *et al.* [13] derived an equation for the probability that the largest F value of the SPM{F} is greater than a threshold f given the smoothness of the underlying Gaussian component processes,

$$P(F_{\max} \geq f) \rightarrow \frac{\lambda(C) \det(\Lambda)^{1/2}\Gamma(\frac{1}{2}(m + n - N))(m - 1)!}{(2\pi)^{1/2N}2^{1/2(N-2)}\Gamma(\frac{1}{2}m)\Gamma(\frac{1}{2}n)(m - N)!}\left(\frac{nf}{m}\right)^{-1/2(m-N)},$$

where n and m are the degrees of freedom of the F statistic, N is the dimension, $\lambda(C)$ is the Lebesgue measure of C (the number of voxels in the volume), and Λ is the variance–covariance matrix of the first derivative of the underlying Gaussian component processes. $P(F_{\max} > F)$ corresponds to the corrected P value.

This general approach to parametric studies can also be extended to compare the nonlinear responses of different groups. To test for differences, the polynomials appear twice in the design matrix. First the functions are replicated in both groups; in the second partition the polynomials are inverted for the second group. This partition models differential responses and, effectively, represents the interactions. These nonlinear interactions can be designated as the effects of interest and the resulting SPM{F} depicts the significance of the differential response.

B. An Example

A patient, who had recovered from severe aphasia after an infarction largely confined to the left temporal lobe and involving the whole of the superior temporal gyrus, was scanned 12 times while listening to words presented at different rates. To illustrate a comparison of regressions between different subjects, a normal subject was studied using the same paradigm. The SPM{F} reflecting the significance of a nonlinear relationship between word presentation rate and evoked response in the patient is shown in Fig. 4 (top). As an example of one of the many forms of such a nonlinear relationship, the adjusted and fitted responses from a voxel (at −34, 40, and 24 mm) are shown in the bottom left panel. This region shows a highly nonlinear (inverted U) rCBF response in relation to word presentation rate.

Figure 5 demonstrates statistical inferences about nonlinear differences in rCBF responses between the two subjects. The first two columns of the design matrix are the effects of interest (*i.e.*, differences). Confounding effects are the commonalities (columns 3 and 4), subject or block effects (columns 5 and 6), and global activity (column 7). There are two maxima apparent in the SPM{F}. To demonstrate a nonlinear interaction we have chosen a voxel in the left hippocampus (−18, −26, and −12 mm). Note the deactivation in relation to increasing word presentation rate in the normal subject compared to the patient who shows an activation.

C. Summary

Nonlinear fitting techniques allow detection of activations in brain regions that might not be so evident using simple (*i.e.*, linear) regression. The general

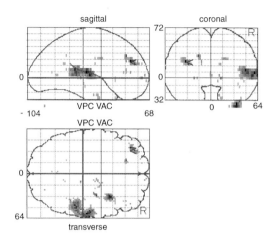

SPM{F}: p < 0.002 {uncorrected}

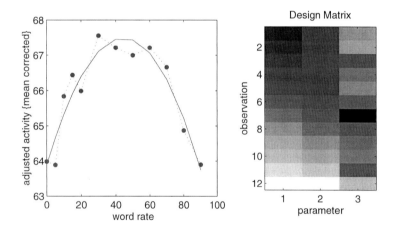

FIGURE 4   SPM{F} for polynomial regression in the patient who had recovered from an ischemic infarction in the territory of the left middle cerebral artery. Voxels over a threshold of $F = 15$ are shown. The regression is for a voxel in a left frontal region ($x = -34$, $y = 40$, and $z = 24$ mm); $F = 20$, df 2, 8, $P < 0.001$ (uncorrected).

approach using polynomial expansions avoids predefined fit functions and can model a family of nonlinear rCBF responses, without specifying the exact form of the relationship. Different brain areas can show differential responses to a study parameter that can then be used to characterise each area involved in a task. Although we have restricted our model to a second order polynomial regression, other basis functions could be used. The use of cosine basis functions has some advantages in modelling ceiling or floor effects; however, the interpretation of polynomial coefficients (*i.e.*, a decomposition into linear and nonlinear effects) is more intuitive than interpreting the coefficients of cosine basis functions. This fact may be important in experimental analysis where the introduction of nonlinearity (the second order term) considerably improves a fit. In general, questions pertaining to the number and type of basis functions are questions of model selection.

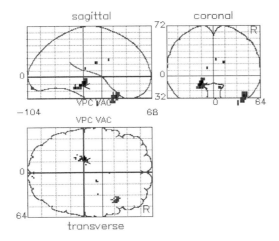

SPM{F}: p < 0.001 {uncorrected}

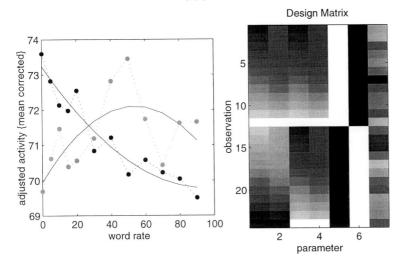

FIGURE 5 SPM{F}, regression plot, and design matrix for the differences of rCBF responses in the patient (grey dots) and a control (dark dots) subject. Voxels over a threshold of $F = 10$ are shown. Regression for differential rCBF responses at a voxel x; -18 mm; y; -26 mm; and z; -12 mm are shown; $F = 17$, $df\, 2, 17$, $P < 0.0005$ (uncorrected).

V. SUBTRACTION, FACTORIAL DESIGNS, AND PURE INSERTION

A. Introduction

This section represents a critique of cognitive subtraction as a conceptual framework for the design of brain activation experiments and allows us to demonstrate the potential usefulness of factorial designs. Subtraction designs are well established and powerful devices in mapping cognitive neuroanatomy [1] but are predicated on possibly untenable assumptions about the relationship between brain dynamics and the functional processes that ensue (and where these assumptions may be tenable they are seldom demonstrated to be so). Concerns with cognitive subtraction can be formulated in terms of the relationship between cognitive processes and their neuronal implementation.

We suggest that nonlinear systems like the brain do not behave in a fashion this is consistent with pure insertion. We illustrate our point with a simple example—the functional anatomy of phonological retrieval during object naming.

B. Cognitive Subtraction, Pure Insertion, and Additive Factors

Cognitive subtraction involves the successive elaboration of a task by adding separable cognitive components and measuring the resulting increases of neuronal activity elicited by these tasks. The physiological activations that obtain on serial subtraction of such measurements are then identified with the added cognitive components. The approach predicated on pure insertion assumes that each cognitive component evokes an "extra" physiological activation that is the same irrespective of the cognitive or physiological context. Pure insertion is an idea that underlies the original Donders subtractive method and has proven itself in many situations, for example in the psychophysics of reaction time measurements during the detection of visual targets embedded in a background of distractors. The linear (additive) relationship between reaction time and the number of distractors has been used to infer a "serial search" of the visual field [14]. Compelling examples of pure insertion usually involve an empirical demonstration of this additive relationship between a perceptual or cognitive process and a phenomenal brain measure (*e.g.*, reaction time). However, pure insertion in the context of brain activation experiments is an *a priori* assumption that has not been validated in any physiological sense. We present here an evaluation, in physiological terms, of cognitive subtraction by focusing on pure insertion. This evaluation follows Sternberg's proposal [15] to use additivity and interaction within factorial designs (the additive factor method) to address the issue.

Pure insertion is implicit in serial subtraction. The idea is that as a new cognitive component (A) is added to a task, the implementation of preexisting components (*e.g.*, B) remains unaffected. If this were not the case the difference between tasks that did, and did not, include component B would depend on the presence of component A. In other words, pure insertion requires that one cognitive component does not affect the effect of another. In factorial designs pure insertion is another way of saying that the interaction terms are negligible. The fact that interactions can be measured, using functional imaging [5], means that the validity of pure insertion can now be addressed empirically. In this section we use a simple factorial design to demonstrate that the physiological brain does not conform to pure insertion.

C. The Nonlinear Brain and Interactions

Even if, from a functionalist perspective, a cognitive component can be added without interacting with preexisting components, the brain's implementation of these processes will almost certainly show profound interactions. This conclusion follows from the observation that neural dynamics are nonlinear [16]. Nearly all theoretical and computational neurobiology is based on this observation. The point is that although a cognitive science model describing functions may include serial and additive elements, the implementation of those functions does not. Consequently, the structure of the cognitive components (functional model) and the brain's physiological implementation are not isomorphic and the mapping of one onto the other is problematic. Put boldly, cognitive science may be an internally consistent discipline, but it has no necessary or defined relation to measurements of brain function. Cognitive subtraction makes some strong assumptions about this relationship which are difficult to reconcile with basic neurobiology.

One of the innumerable examples of nonlinear brain dynamics that confound cognitive subtraction is modulation; from classical neuromodulation to large-scale modulatory interactions between different cortical areas. A particularly relevant example is the modulatory role of attention on perceptual processing, for example the responsiveness of V5 to motion in the visual field [17]. It is likely that responsiveness is enhanced by selectively attending to motion [18]. V5 activation therefore represents an interaction between visual motion and selective attention. Consider now an experiment in which visual motion is presented with and without selective attention for motion. The resulting difference in physiological activation of V5 would, in terms of cognitive subtraction, be attributed to selective attention for motion. This would be a fallacious conclusion because the differential responses of V5 represent an interaction between visual analysis of a particular attribute and selective attention to that attribute. In neuronal terms this interaction might be described in terms of a modulation of V5 responsiveness to motion in the visual field, mediated by afferents from some higher order area. The fallacy would be revealed by repeating the experiment in the absence of visual motion. In this instance "selective attention for motion" should not activate V5 because there are no motion-dependent responses to modulate. This second experiment would demonstrate an interaction between "selective attention for motion" and "visual motion" using a factorial experimental design. The V5 example highlights the close relationship between functional interactions (between different cognitive or sensorimotor components) and statistical interactions that can be inferred using factorial designs. It should be said that we do not consider "attention" a cognitive component (although the "control" of attention can be) but our point is clearly illustrated by this example. Furthermore, a motion stimulus may not be necessary to demonstrate a modulatory effect of attention. For example, "imagined" motion could interact with selective attention in an analogous way. This sort of experiment would speak to an intimate relationship between imagery and attention.

Similar conclusions have been reached in neuropsychology. A patient with acquired dyslexia without dysgraphia was found to have a deficit in accessing phonology from semantics and a mild deficit in attending selectively to components of compound visual stimuli. These deficits interacted to severely disrupt her ability to name the components of visual arrays, despite the fact that she could name each component when presented it in isolation (a symptom of attentional dyslexia). This example *"highlights the importance of interactions between deficits as being a major contributory factor to some neuropsychological syndromes"* [19]. In summary, pure insertion discounts both functional and physiological interactions and therefore represents a very restrictive precondition for cognitive subtraction.

D. Cognitive Subtraction *versus* Factorial Designs

We suggest that a more powerful approach to cognitive neuroanatomy is to consider interactions explicitly, both in terms of a cognitive model and in terms of experimental design and analysis. This suggestion acknowledges that the conjunction or integration of two or more cognitive processes may require an active physical implementation. For example, naming an object involves object recognition, phonological retrieval, and the integration of the two, where that integration calls upon separable brain processes. Put more simply, phonological retrieval influences object recognition, and *vice versa,* and these effects are physiologically measurable. This perspective requires a factorial design in which the interaction term represents nonadditive (*i.e.,* nonlinear) physiological concomitants of naming a recognised object that is independent of the activations produced by recognising or naming alone. This is the example we use to illustrate our ideas below.

E. An Empirical Example

The example chosen uses the same data to address the question, "is the inferotemporal region implicated in phonological retrieval during object naming?" from a subtraction perspective and from a factorial perspective. Considerable evidence from neuroanatomy and unit-electrode recordings suggests that neurons in the inferotemporal cortex of animals respond selectively to specific objects in the visual field or have the appropriate responses to do so [20–22]. On the basis of this and other evidence it might be hypothesised that inferotemporal regions are functionally specialised for object recognition in man. Furthermore, lesion studies in man have shown that the ability to name objects is impaired when the inferotemporal regions are damaged. For example, De Renzi *et al.* [23] studied the neuropsychological correlates of inferior temporal ischaemic damage. As well as alexia, subjects were impaired in naming objects and photographs. This evidence suggests that the integrity of the inferotemporal cortex may be necessary for phonological retrieval (among other things) in object naming.

Consider the problem of designing an experiment to identify brain areas selectively activated by phonological retrieval during object naming. The cognitive processes involved in such a task include visual analysis, object recognition, phonological retrieval, and speech. Suppose that we are not concerned with the sensorimotor aspects of the task but wish to test a hypothesis that the inferotemporal regions are involved in both object recognition and phonological retrieval. In this case we need a series of tasks that, on successive subtraction, isolate these two cognitive components (*i.e.,* three tasks). The tasks used were:

A. Saying "yes" when presented with a coloured shape (**visual analysis and speech**);
B. Saying "yes" when presented with a coloured object (**visual analysis, speech, and object recognition**);
C. Naming a visually presented coloured object (**visual analysis, speech, object recognition, and phonological retrieval**).

Subtraction of task A from task B should identify brain regions associated with object recognition and subtraction of task B from task C should identify regions implicated in phonological retrieval. The hypothesis is that both subtractions should activate the left inferotemporal regions (among other regions). The data were obtained from six subjects scanned 12 times (every 8 min) whilst performing one of four different tasks (the three tasks, A, B, C, and a further task, D, to be described below). The subjects were instructed to respond with either "yes" (tasks A and B) or a name (tasks C and D). In the analysis we are concerned only with differential responses in the left inferotemporal region. Therefore, we make no correction for multiple nonindependent comparisons in other brain regions.

Significantly activated voxels ($P < 0.05$ uncorrected) in the subtraction of task A from task B included, as predicted, a small focus in the left inferotemporal region. No significant activations were detected in the second subtraction, comparing tasks B and C. From our current perspective the key thing to note is that the inferotemporal regions showed no further activation due to phonological retrieval. Figure 6 shows the activity of a voxel in the inferotemporal region (-48, -24, -32 mm, BA 20—according to the atlas of Talairach and Tournoux [24]) during the three tasks (A, B, and C). On the basis of these results one might conclude that the inferotemporal regions are specialised for (implicit) object recognition and that this cognitive component is sufficient to explain the activations even in the context of naming the objects. In other words, there is no evidence for differential responses in the inferotemporal regions due to phonological retrieval. These results show that phonological retrieval does not, in itself, activate the infero-temporal region. The conclusion is that the inferotemporal regions cannot be implicated in phonological retrieval (as far as can be measured with functional imaging).

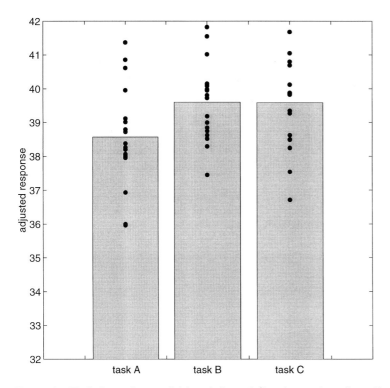

FIGURE 6 Task-dependent activities. Adjusted (for the confounding effects of global activity and the subject or block effect) rCBF equivalents for the three tasks (A, B, and C). The bars represent mean activity and the dots are the individual data points from each scan. Note that there is activation in passing from task A to B but not in going from task B to C. These data were taken from a voxel in the left inferotemporal regions (-48, -18, -24 mm according to the atlas of Talairach and Tournoux).

F. A Critical Reevaluation Using a Factorial Approach

The forgoing conclusion is wrong because it assumes pure insertion and hence has to lead to the inference that activation due to object recognition is the same, irrespective of whether phonological retrieval is present or not. In order to say that phonological retrieval does not activate the infero-temporal region (as found in the second subtraction) one has to assume that the activation due to object recognition is the same as in the first subtraction (*i.e.*, object recognition in the absence of phonological retrieval). To validate this assumption we need to measure activations due to object recognition in the presence of phonological retrieval. This can be effected by comparing tasks that involve phonological retrieval with and without object recognition. This comparison required a fourth condition:

> D. Name the colour of a presented shape (**visual analysis, speech, and phonological retrieval**).

Subtraction of task A and task B gives the activations due to object recognition in the absence of phonological retrieval and subtraction of task D from task C gives recognition-dependent activation in the context of phonological retrieval. Pure insertion requires these activations to be the same and this is not the case. Figure 7 (top) shows that activation in the context of phonological retrieval is far greater than under conditions without phonological retrieval. In other words, phonological retrieval can be thought of as modulating the recognition-dependant responses of the inferotemporal region and in this sense the inferotemporal regions clearly contribute to phonological retrieval.

There is an alternative and equivalent perspective on this interaction that considers the inferotemporal activations induced by phonological retrieval with and without object recognition. Figure 7 (bottom) shows that, in the absence of object recognition, phonological retrieval deactivates the inferotemporal regions, whereas in the context of object recognition, this effect is nullified if not reversed. These data come from a voxel in BA 20 (-48, -18, -24 mm). In summary, inferotemporal responses do discriminate between situations where phonological retrieval is present or not and can be directly implicated in this cognitive process. These differential responses are expressed at the level of interactions and are revealed only with a factorial experimental design.

Using the same statistical model as in the previous analysis we tested for the main effect of object recognition, the main effect of phonological retrieval, and the interaction between them, by using the appropriate contrasts. The SPM reflecting the interaction effects is shown in Fig. 8 where significant voxels are rendered onto a magnetic resonance imaging scan (white areas are significant at $P < 0.05$ uncorrected). This interaction effect depicts augmented activation due to a conjunction of phonological retrieval and object recognition and allows us to confirm that the inferotemporal region is implicated in phonological retrieval during object naming.

V. CONCLUSION

We have presented a deliberately emphatic critique of cognitive subtraction and in particular the notion of pure insertion upon which serial subtraction relies. The main contention is that pure insertion may, or may not, be a valid

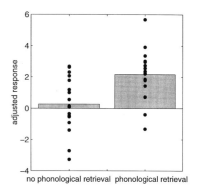

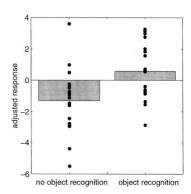

FIGURE 7 Modulation of task-dependent activations. (Top) The activations due to object recognition with (right) and without (left) phonological retrieval. For this graph the differences were obtained by subtracting the adjusted activities in the first second and third occurrence of the two tasks in each subject. (Bottom) The same but comparing the activation due to phonological retrieval with (right) and without (left) object recognition. As in the previous figure the bars represent mean activity and the dots are the individual data points from each scan.

sagittal

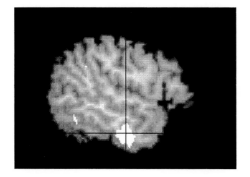

coronal

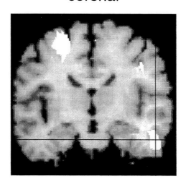

transverse {left = right}

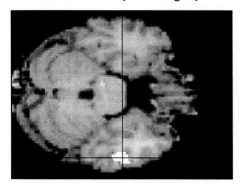

FIGURE 8 Factorial SPM. White areas correspond to voxels that showed a significant interaction [*i.e.*, (C–D)–(B–A)] at $P < 0.05$ (uncorrected) rendered onto a MRI scan in standard space [24].

cognitive science level description, but it is almost certainly not valid in relation to the brain's implementation of cognitive functions. This conclusion follows from the fact that the brain is a highly nonlinear system and, phenomenologically, does not conform to additive or linear principles. Pure insertion disallows any interactions and yet these interactions are evident, even in the simplest experiments. To illustrate this point we have used a factorial experiment designed to elucidate the functional anatomy of object recognition and phonological retrieval. We show that pure insertion can be an inappropriate and misleading assumption. In so doing we are able to demonstrate that inferotemporal activations, due to object recognition, are profoundly modulated by phonological retrieval of the object's name. This interaction clearly implicates the inferotemporal regions in phonological retrieval during object naming, despite the absence of a main effect of phonological retrieval in the same region. By avoiding cognitive subtraction and using a factorial design of this sort we were able to reconcile our functional imaging results with lesion deficit studies [23].

It is interesting to speculate that cognitive processes may express themselves only at the level of interactions. For example, the *semantics* (memory or knowledge of meaning) of a word may be realised only by the interaction, or integration, between a particular phonology (word) and an associated percept, intention, affect or action (*e.g.*, for nouns, the interaction between phonology, and object recognition). If this is the case, there would be no "semantic centre" *per se*, but semantics would be subtended by interactions between a set of cortical regions subserving subordinate components (*e.g.*, phonological retrieval and object recognition). In this regard it is noteworthy that in semantic dementia, which is associated with progressive loss of semantic knowledge, the atrophy seen on magnetic resonance images is often maximal in the infero-lateral temporal cortex [25]. Although very conjectural, this perspective is consistent with conclusions based on lesion data [26].

In conclusion we suggest that the effect of a cognitive component (that is independent of all other components) is best captured by the main effect of that component and that the integration of various components (*i.e.*, the expression of one cognitive process is the context of another) is embedded in interaction terms. Brain regions can be functionally specialised for integration in the sense that they can demonstrate significant interactions in terms of their physiological responses. If we are right then brain activations are only part of the story in mapping cognitive anatomy. Regionally specific interactions may hold the key for a more complete and richer characterisation.

References

1. S. E. Petersen, P. T. Fox, M. I. Posner, M. Mintun, and M. E. Raichle. Positron emission tomographic studies of the processing of single words. *J. Cogn. Neurosci.* **1,** 153–170 (1989).

2. C. J. Lueck, S. Zeki, K. J. Friston, N. O. Deiber, P. Cope, V. J. Cunningham, A. A. Lammertsma, C. Kennard, and R. S. J. Frackowiak. The colour centre in the cerebral cortex of man. *Nature* **340,** 386–389 (1989).

3. S. Grafton, J. Mazziotta, S. Presty, K. J. Friston, R. S. J. Frackowiak, and M. Phelps. Functional anatomy of human procedural learning determined with regional cerebral blood flow and PET. *J. Neurosci.* **12,** 2542–2548 (1992).

4. C. J. Price, R. J. S. Wise, S. Ramsay, K. J. Friston, D. Howard, K. Patterson, and R. S. J. Frackowiak. Regional response differences within the human auditory cortex when listening to words. *Neurosci. Lett.* **146,** 179–182 (1992).

5. K. J. Friston, C. Frith, R. E. Passingham, P. Liddle, and R. S. J. Frackowiak. Motor practice and neurophysiological adaptation in the cerebellum: A positron tomography study. *Proc. R. Soc. London B* **248,** 223–228 (1992a).

6. P. F. C. Gilbert and W. T. Thach. Purkinje cell activity during motor learning. *Brain Res.* **128,** 309–328 (1977).

7. K. J. Friston, P. Grasby, C. Bench, C. Frith, P. Cowen, P. Little, R. S. J. Frackowiak, and R. Dolan. Measuring the neuromodulatory effects of drugs in man with positron tomography. *Neurosci. Lett.* **141,** 106–110 (1992b).

8. P. Grasby, K. J. Friston, C. Bench, P. Cowen, C. Frith, P. Liddle, R. S. J. Frackowiak, and R. Dolan. Effect of the 5-HT1$_A$ partial agonist buspirone on regional cerebral blood flow in man. *Psychopharmacology* **108,** 380–386 (1992).

9. P. C. Fletcher, C. D. Frith, P. M. Grasby, T. Shallice, R. S. J. Frackowiak, and R. J. Dolan. Brain systems for encoding and retrieval of auditory–verbal memory. *Brain* **118,** 401–416 (1995).

10. C. D. Frith, and K. J. Friston. The role of the thalamus in "top down" modulation of attention to sound. *NeuroImage* **4,** 210–215 (1996).

11. K. F. Friston, C. D. Frith, P. F. Liddle, R. J. Dolan, A. A. Lammertsma, and R. S. J. Frackowiak. The relationship between global and local changes in PET scans *J. Cereb. Blood Flow Metab.* **10,** 458–466 (1990).

12. R. S. J. Frackowiak. Plasticity in the human brain: Insights from functional imaging. *The Neuroscientist* **2,** 353–362 (1996).

13. K. J. Worsley. Local Maxima and the expected Euler characteristic of excursion sets of c^2, F and t fields. *Adv. Appl. Prob.* **26,** 13–42 (1994).

14. A. Treisman and J. Souther. Search asymmetry: A diagnostic for preattentive processing of separable features. *J. Exp. Psychol. Gen.* **114,** 285–310 (1985).

15. S. Sternberg. The discovery of processing stages: Extension of Donders method. *Acta Psychol.* **30,** 276–315 (1969).

16. A. Aertsen and H. Preissl. Dynamics of activity and connectivity in physiological neuronal Networks. *In* "Non Linear Dynamics and Neuronal Networks" (H. G. Schuster, VCH Publishers, Eds.), pp. 281–302. H. G. Schuster, VCH Publishers, New York, NY, 1991.

17. S. Zeki, J. D. G. Watson, C. J. Lueck, K. J. Friston, C. Kennard, and R. S. J. Frackowiak. A direct demonstration of functional specialisation in human visual cortex. *J. Neurosci.* **11,** 641–649 (1991).

18. M. Corbetta, F. M. Miezin, S. Dobmeyer, G. L. Shulman, and S. E. Petersen. Selective and divided attention during visual discrimination of shape, color and speed. Functional anatomy by positron emission tomography. *J. Neurosci.* **11**(8), 2383–2402 (1991).

19. C. J. Price and G. W. Humphreys. Attentional dyslexia: The effect of co-occurring deficits. *Cogn. Neuropsychology* **10,** 569–592 (1993).

20. L. G. Ungerleider and M. Mishkin. Two cortical visual systems. *In* "Analysis of Visual Behaviour" (D. J. Ingle, M. A. Goodale, and R. J. W. Mansfield, Eds.), pp. 549–586. MIT Press, Cambridge, MA, 1982.

21. R. Desimone, T. D. Albright, C. G. Gross, and C. Bruce. Stimulus selective properties of inferior temporal neurons in the macaque. *J Neurosci.* **4,** 2051–2062 (1984).

22. D. I. Perret, A. J. Mistlin, D. D. Potter, P. A. J. Smith, A. S. Head, A. J. Chitty, R. Broenimann, A. D. Milner, and M. A. Jeeves. Functional organization of visual neurones processing face identity. *In* "Aspects of Face Processing" (H. Ellis, M. A. Jeeves, F. Newcombe, and A. W. Young, Eds.), pp. 187–198. Martinus Nijhoff, Dordrecht, 1986.

23. E. De Renzi, A. Zambolin, and G. Crisi. The pattern of neuropsychological impairment associated with left posterior cerebral artery territory infarcts. *Brain* **110,** 1088–1116 (1987).

24. J. Talairach and P. Tournoux. A Co-planar stereotaxic atlas of a human brain. Thieme, Stuttgart, 1988.

25. J. R. Hodges, K. Patterson, S. Oxbury, and E. Funnell. Semantic dementia: progressive fluent aphasia with temporal lobe atrophy. *Brain* **115,** 1783–1806 (1992).

26. J. M. Nielsen. "Agnosia, Apraxia, Aphasia: Their Value in Cerebral Localization," 2nd ed. Paul B. Hoebner, New York, 1946.

PART TWO

FUNCTIONAL ANATOMY

CHAPTER NINE

DYNAMISM OF A PET IMAGE: STUDIES OF VISUAL FUNCTION

I. INTRODUCTION

We take the title from Giacomo Balla's "Dynamism of a Dog." Balla wanted to import the dynamic element into painting, "to displace from A to B what before had been immobile," as Umberto Boccioni tells us (see Zeki and Lamb [1]). He therefore created several paintings of the same kind, "Dynamism of a Dog" being but one example (Fig. 1). These represented motion statically, leaving it to the imagination of the beholder to perceive the dynamic element. Images derived from positron emission tomography (PET) are similarly static. However, can the beholder use his imagination to perceive a dynamic element in them? And once perceived, can that dynamic element be harnessed to generate new and interesting ideas about the brain, leading to new experiments?

We think it would be fair to say that anyone looking at functional images of the visual cortex would find it hard not to see a strong dynamic element in the relationship between V1 and the specialised visual areas of the brain. Something is known about the anatomy underlying that dynamic element, but little is known of the detailed physiological mechanisms involved. This is not surprising. The question of a dynamic relationship between V1 and the specialised areas has hardly been posed and therefore the element itself has not been recognised. This chapter therefore is an attempt to highlight the dynamism of the static functional images and describe an experiment or two on how the dynamic interpretation that we gave to our static functional images helped us to extract more information from the visual cortex. We hope that no one will be too censorious if we rely mainly on work done in our laboratory. This is not to belittle the achievements of others but only to have the protection of writing about what we know best.

II. THE VISUAL PATHWAYS AND FUNCTIONAL SPECIALISATION IN HUMAN VISUAL CORTEX

It has long been known that the major visual input to the brain is through the primary visual cortex, area V1. Studies in the macaque monkey have

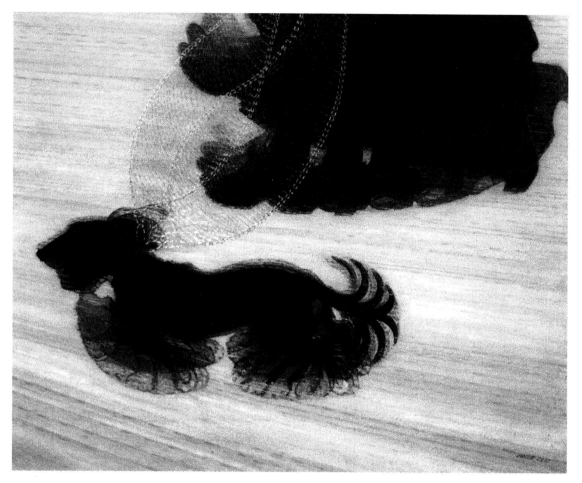

FIGURE 1 *"Dynamism of a Dog"* by Giacomo Balla (Albright-Knox Art Gallery, Buffalo).

shown that V1 has multiple, parallel outputs to the visual areas surrounding it [2], areas that are specialised to process different kinds of visual signals [3–7]. Neurobiologists may disagree about the total number of visual areas in the cortex; they may even disagree about what in fact constitutes an appropriate definition of a visual area (see, for example, Zeki [3]). However, all would nevertheless agree that the so-called visual "association" cortex is made up of many different visual areas. Equally, they may disagree about which of the many visual areas surrounding V1 receive parallel outputs from it and hence about the number of parallel outputs leaving V1, but all would agree that parallelism is a fundamental strategy used by the visual cortex. Since the early 1970s, the number of visual areas has increased sharply. As a consequence, neurophysiologists may disagree about the extent to which the visual areas of the prestriate cortex are specialised to undertake different functions, but all would agree that there is some degree of specialisation. Most may not want to go as far as us, when we say that these findings will almost certainly entail a major revision of ill-defined concepts such as agnosia, whether of the apperceptive or associative variety, and that it will require a major reappraisal, too, of the direct and explicit contribution that each area is capable of making to conscious visual perception [8] as well as of controversial concepts such as blindsight. Most may not even agree with us that our present picture of the visual cortex also entails a revision of the old concept of a neat separation between seeing and understanding, that there are large areas of vision in which these two faculties overlap [8]. However, most would also agree, we hope, that our present concept of the cortical involvement in vision is vastly different from that prevalent even in the early 1970s and that there is a genuine interest in reexamining the doctrines of vision inherited from the past and derived from the then known anatomy and physiology of the primate visual cortex.

III. PARALLELISM AND DYNAMIC FUNCTIONAL IMAGES

It is within the context of parallelism and functional specialisation that one gets the first hint of dynamism in a PET image, at least for colour and motion [9]. If V1 is a segregator of visual signals in the human brain, just as it is in the monkey, parcelling out different signals to different visual areas for further processing, as the parallel outputs from V1 and direct recordings from it show [2,10], then it follows that V1 must be in a dynamic rather than a fixed relationship with the different visual areas, sending signals to them on a "need to know" basis. Hence, if the signals are related to static objects and to colour, then one would expect a greater activation of those subdivisions of V1 that are concerned with colour and little activation of those subdivisions concerned with motion; one would equally expect that the output from V1 would be selective rather than general, and related to areas that are destined, through their specialisation, to receive the relevant signals; in the example given above, V1 would not need to send any signals to V5, from which it follows that V1 should be active whether one stimulates with, say, colour or motion, but that it should channel colour and motion signals to different visual areas. This is largely, but not exactly, what is observed. Thus the use of motion and colour stimulation activates different areas within the prestriate cortex, thereby giving direct and unequivocal support to the notion of a functional specialisation in human visual cortex and of a parallel output from V1 to the specialised areas [9]. However, this picture shows that the relationship between V1 and individual visual areas may be more variable than the static functional image or the static anatomical results at first suggest.

Dynamic Relationship between V1 and V5 Derived from PET Images

Given the known anatomy linking V1 to V5, the cortical area specialised for visual motion, one might suspect that every activation of V5 would entail a parallel activation of V1. However, our studies, as well as those of others, of the visual motion system have shown that this is not always the case. In our first PET study to identify V5 [9], the activity in V1 did not reach significance, while that in V5 did (Fig. 2). This result was similar to results obtained by others (for example, Tootell et al. [11]). We are always tempted to seek the easy solution, and hence we supposed, like others, that both the moving and the stationary stimuli that we used activated V1 about equally and that the activities therefore cancelled out in the comparison images. However, in our subsequent and more detailed study of V5 [12], we found that area V1 was

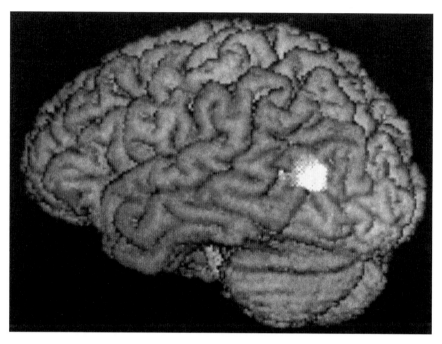

FIGURE 2   Area V5 on the surface of the human cortex is shown here in white.

active and indeed more so than V5. The solution to this apparent discrepancy is not easy, since our stimuli were the same in the two studies; it may lie in the state of the brain, in the sensitivity of scanning, or in the method of analysis. Although we cannot pinpoint a reason for this difference, the result nevertheless highlights the fact that not every activation of V5 entails as vigorous a parallel activation of V1, which in turn implies that the relationship between V1 and V5 may be a variable one.

IV. THE ANATOMY OF THE CONNECTIONS BETWEEN V1 AND V5

The relationship between V1 and V5 in the monkey is fairly complex, anatomically at least. It involves (a) the visual input from segregated cells, mainly in layer 4B but also in upper layer 6, of V1 to V5 [13,7]; (b) the return projection from V5 back to V1, which is more diffusely distributed within the territory of layer 4B and does not respect the territory of cells within 4B projecting to V5 [7]; and (c) a direct visual input that by-passes V1 and uses the superior colliculus and the pulvinar to terminate directly in V5 [14,15]. This does not exhaust all the possible anatomical interactions between V1 and V5. For example, there are reciprocal connections between V2 (itself receiving signals from layer 4B) and V5 [16]. It would be hard to imagine that these pathways are not involved also in motion perception and easy to believe that they may not all be activated at the same time, that their activation may be motion-task dependent. Thus the static anatomical picture derived from experimental anatomy and from functional imaging studies suggests the possibility of a dynamic relationship between V1 and V5. One way of confirming this is to supplement the functional data with other studies.

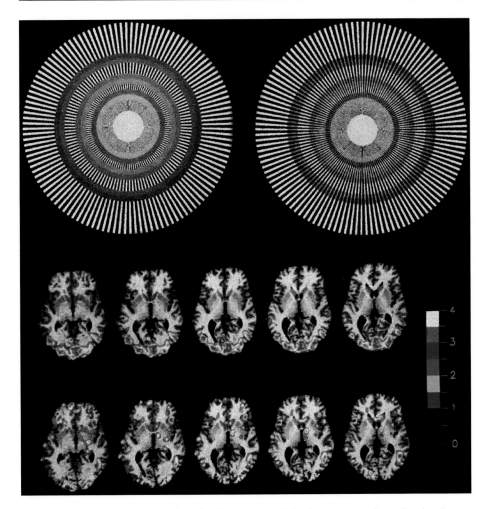

FIGURE 3   When most people view the figure on the left, they see an enigmatic, circular motion in the grey rings. This illusion can be destroyed by making the spokes intersect the rings. This can provide a stimulus for a PET scan. When subjects placed in the scanner are shown the two images, and the activity patterns are contrasted, increased activity is detected in an area (arrowed) very close to the area V5 which is detected using moving dots. From Zeki *et al.* [8].

Other anatomical studies also suggest that the relationship between V1 and V5 may be more variable than we suppose. For example, when the change in cerebral activity of subjects who see motion in the rings of Leviant's *Enigma* figure is measured, the largest increase is found in and around area V5, with no detectable increase in V1 or in V2 [8] (Fig. 3). When the same subjects view coherent motion, activity is found in both V1 and V5. This does not prove that V1 is inactive during the perception of phenomenal motion, since it may have been equally active when subjects were looking at the Leviant figure as well as its control, and that the activity in V1 thus cancelled out in the final images. However, it does show that the balance of activity between V1 and V5 is not the same as in the condition when the same subjects see objective motion. Nor is such an interpretation of the static pictures limited to the motion system. Interesting in this regard is our study of the brain activity related to the perception of the "illusory" Kanizsa triangle [17]. Here we found, just like Hirsch *et al.* [18], that the activity was almost entirely restricted to V2 (and possibly V3), without a parallel activation of V1 and without any activation in the frontal lobe, which is what one might expect if the interpretation of the Kanizsa picture as a triangle were dependent upon some higher order cognitive hypothesis, as has been suggested [19]. This is not the place to discuss the possible reasons for the restriction of the activation to V2 [17]; instead we emphasise yet again that the balance of activity between V1 and areas of the prestriate cortex with which it connects can be variable and stimulus dependent.

A. How Dependent Are Visual Areas on V1?

A variable relationship implies a certain degree of autonomy, for if the relationship were fixed then every activation of one area would entail an activation of the other. By contrast, if the relationship is variable, it becomes plausible to suppose that the variability is an expression of the fact that, for some activities at least, one area can be wholly or partially independent of the other while other activities may require a greater or lesser cooperation between the two (or more) areas. The results given above thus draw attention to the possibility that the visual areas may be capable of acting more autonomously than we generally suppose, or at least to be able to act to some degree without pre- or postprocessing by V1. This is not such an outrageous idea, for the results of Rodman *et al.* [20] and Girard *et al.* [21] have shown that the characteristic of V5, directional selectivity, is maintained after removal or inactivation of V1. The maintenance of the characteristic of V5 in these conditions is almost certainly due to the normal functioning of the pathway that reaches V5 from the pulvinar without passing through V1, although Bullier *et al.* [22] have concluded that the information transmitted through the latter pathway "*may not reach consciousness.*"

Perhaps the most convincing of our functional imaging studies in this regard comes from the study of GY [23], a patient who had been rendered hemianopic through damage to his occipital lobe sustained at the age of 8, and one who had been studied in detail by others [24,25] and had been shown to suffer from blindsight, a condition in which subjects blinded by lesions in V1 are reported to be able to discriminate visual stimuli with high accuracy without having any conscious awareness of having seen anything at all. Here, we thought, was an opportunity to show that, under such conditions, there would be no activity within V5. This would constitute one small step, though not a conclusive one, towards establishing not only the preeminent role of the cortex in conscious vision and in the acquisition of knowledge but also the importance of preprocessing by V1 and hence of the dependence of the visual areas on V1, at least for conscious vision, as asserted in the blindsight literature [26,27], for it has been our contention that the primary role of vision is the acquisition of knowledge and that knowledge can be acquired only in the conscious state, and with cortical involvement [28]. Here then was the opportunity to show that, with no cortical involvement, only a blindsight type of discrimination, but not conscious vision, is possible.

However, our high expectations were soon dashed. It turned out that, under the conditions in which we tested him, GY was perfectly conscious of what he was seeing, crude though that was, and could discriminate consciously and report verbally with the highest accuracy the direction of motion of high contrast stimuli, provided they were moving at high speeds [23], thus rendering questionable the assertion in the blindsight literature that V1 is necessary for conscious perception [26] and that *"Patients with lesions up to and including primary visual cortex can show ... no conscious vision"* [27]. Under these conditions, V5 and the two areas that are coactivated with it in the normal subject [12,29] were also active in GY, without, of course, a parallel activation of V1. In other words, the entire experiment was turned on its head. Not only was GY conscious of motion in his blind field but his V5 was active. When we asked GY to describe what he had seen, he replied that it was "a shadow," similar to what a normal person would see if he closed his eyes, looked out of the window and moved his hands in front, the use of the word "shadow" being reminiscent of Riddoch's description of what his subjects had seen as being *"vague and shadowy"* [30]. He was asked the same question 2 years later and said that it was more of a "feeling" (see below); when the possible discrepancy between the two descriptions was pointed out, he replied that, in the earlier statement, he had used language that he thought might be best understood. Our contention [23] that GY can have a conscious dimension to his visual motion has recently been confirmed in the studies of Weiskrantz *et al.* [31] and leads us to postulate that V1 is not necessary for conscious visual experience, at least of fast visual motion. Whether it is necessary for other kinds of visual experience is not a subject that we have studied.

B. The Perils of Ignoring Published Evidence

This was surprising and unexpected, but it should not have been. Instead of being surprised, we should have recalled what Riddoch had said in his 1917 paper, where he had given the first and most detailed description of patients rendered hemianopic by lesions in V1, who could nevertheless see motion [30]. They were, he wrote, *"... immediately conscious of 'something' moving when the object was oscillated"* [in their scotomatous fields] and *"... the consciousness of 'something moving' kept up a continual desire to turn the head."* However, this conscious experience was for visual motion only because his patients, who had *"great difficulty in describing the nature of the movement that they see: it is so vague and shadowy,"* were nevertheless *"... quite sure that neither shape nor colour can be attributed to [the movement]."* Riddoch tried to account for his phenomenon by supposing that tissue within V1 had been spared, an obviously unsatisfactory explanation [32]. Such an implausible explanation is presumably one reason why Holmes [33] found it so easy to dismiss his work and why most others do not refer to it. However, Holmes himself, in the same paper, had described a patient (Case 11) in whom *"there was a considerable return of vision in the periphery ... but he was generally conscious only of the movement"* [our emphasis], although Holmes seems to have ignored this patient in challenging Riddoch's conclusion. We had read and quoted both papers [32] and could not therefore plead ignorance which is, in any case, no defence in law. Perhaps we concentrated too much on Riddoch's explanation; perhaps we were more impressed by the syndrome of blindsight and thus ignored the repetitive use of the word conscious in Riddoch's paper; perhaps we had accepted too readily the implied reasoning of the blindsight literature, made explicit here and there [26,27], that conscious vision is not possible without V1, even though the results of blindsight studies show that, with motion at least, subjects may have a feeling of having experienced something [34,35], which leaves one wondering whether blindsight for motion is not a variant of the Riddoch phenomenon. However that may be, one can, at the very least, try to account for the syndrome that Riddoch described in terms of modern knowledge of the input to V5. Given that a crude but conscious vision for motion is possible without V1, can we attribute this to a direct activation of V5, without parallel activation of V1? The supposition was worth studying because it has important implications.

C. Dynamic Parallelism in the Visual Input to V1 and V5

The first hint that there is an input to V5 that is functionally more or less independent from that to V1 came from studies in which V5 and V1 were selectively inactivated using transcranial magnetic stimulation (TMS) [36]. We found, first, that inactivation of V5 was a more potent way of inducing a reversible akinetopsia (motion imperception) than inactivation of V1, itself a somewhat surprising finding suggesting a certain independence for V5. More interesting still was the time course of the effective inactivation: it was not the same for the two areas. To obtain an akinetopsia with inactivation of V1, the inactivating magnetic pulse had to be delivered at 60–70 msec after the appearance of the visual stimulus. By contrast, V5 inactivation produced akinetopsia only if the inactivating pulse was delivered at −20 to +10 msec before, during, or after the appearance of the moving stimulus. This suggested at once that V5 must receive visual signals before V1 and that it must receive them at the shortest known latencies, not exceeding 30–40 msec.

These conclusions were worth confirming by direct measurement, especially since they ran counter to all the evidence from the electroencephalographic (EEG) literature which had suggested instead that prestriate cortex is activated sequentially, after V1, and with latencies of about 110 msec [37]. It was nevertheless worth remeasuring with the EEG method, since our theoretical calculations, made from such evidence as was available in the literature, showed that it was possible for signals to reach visual cortex with latencies of 28 msec [36]. However, there was another striking finding that had not been exploited by the EEG studies. In reviewing our own studies and the published evidence on patients, we became aware that speed must be the critical variable in determining whether signals reach V5 or V1 first. At one end is patient LM, rendered akinetopsic following bilateral damage to her V5. Our studies [38], as well as earlier ones [39,40] had shown that, in spite of her akinetopsia, patient LM is nevertheless able to discriminate consciously slow motion, inferior in angular extent to $10°$ sec^{-1}. This suggested that V5 is critical for the discrimination of fast motion, a suggestion confirmed at once by our observation that patient GY could discriminate only fast motion [23]. By contrast, the inability of the latter to discriminate consciously anything but fast motion suggested that V1 must be in some way critical for slow motion. In this simple observation lay the key to understanding the failure of the EEG literature to reveal a fast activation of the prestriate cortex: all the EEG studies had employed slow motion only and could therefore not detect the fast component. We decided to remeasure the latency of arrival of motion-related visual signals in human visual cortex, using fast and slow motion as our stimuli. We found that fast-moving signals ($>15°$ sec^{-1}) activate prestriate cortex first while slow-moving signals ($< 5°$ sec^{-1}) activate V1 first [37] (Fig. 4). There is, in other words, a parallel input from the retina to the two areas and, whereas the two pathways may in fact terminate in V5, one does so without passing through V1, while the other uses the V1 route. The evidence led us to the concept of dynamic parallelism, by which we mean that while

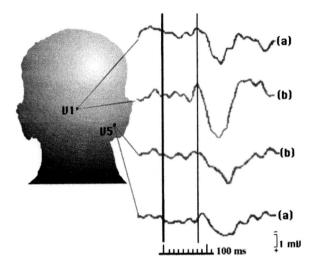

FIGURE 4   The evoked electroencephalographic (EEG) activity from electrodes placed over area V5 and V1 in the human: (a) The activity elicited by a slow moving stimulus and (b) the activity elicited by a fast moving stimulus. The vertical line allows the timing of the first negative peak to be compared between electrodes and conditions. In the fast motion condition the peak in V5 precedes the peak in V1, while in the slow motion condition the peak in V5 follows the peak in V1. Modified from ffytche *et al.* [37].

both areas can be healthy and functional in a normal brain, which area gets activated first depends upon the nature of the stimulus [37]. We need to add that three of the subjects who took part in this study were also subjects in our previous functional imaging study [12] and hence we had a good idea of where to place our EEG electrodes to record optimally from V5. Our conclusion that the recordings were from V5 is, nevertheless, still not direct, since there is no sure way of resolving the problem of spatial location with any certainty using the EEG method.

D. Does This Mean That Motion Is Perceived First?

This early arrival of signals in V5 was unexpected and implied that motion, or at least fast motion, must be perceived first. Such a conclusion was in any case consistent with the published evidence which showed that the fastest conducting fibres belong to the M system which, unlike the P system, is concerned with motion but indifferent to colour [5]. However, does this mean that motion is perceived before colour? In considering this question, we are more interested in whether motion and colour are perceived at identical times rather than which is perceived first. This may appear to be a digression from our main theme but is in fact an important point in the argument because a demonstration that the perceptual systems are independent, just like the processing systems, adds to the argument that the specialised visual areas and systems are more autonomous than we had supposed.

Temporal integration times, which essentially measure exposure times required for detection at threshold, have been measured by many different authors, using different stimuli. One can deduce almost anything one wants from them, for the simple reason that such integration times differ for different wavelengths, with different experimental designs and different tasks. Although no one has ever done so, one could—if pushed—conclude that temporal integration times for colour are shorter than for motion, but one could also conclude the reverse. Such games would be silly to play and it is healthy that no one has actually played them or predicted that motion is perceived faster than colour—or vice versa—from temporal integration times, or that at least they have kept very quiet about it if they have done so. By contrast, it has been claimed from a review of the psychophysical evidence that the motion system is faster than the colour system [5]. The evidence here seems more convincing, but also turns out to be incorrect. This is probably due to the fact that neither the psychophysical reaction nor the temporal integration times are the same thing as perceptual times; they can only give a hint—no more—about perceptual times. However, actual perceptual times are not measurable. We thought that one way around this impasse was to devise a method for measuring relative perceptual times for motion and colour, partly because we were dazzled by the rapid delivery of signals to V5 and wanted to learn whether this gives motion a substantial lead time over colour in perceptual terms.

The study, described in detail elsewhere [41], shows, unexpectedly to us, that colour is perceived before orientation and orientation before motion, giving a lead time of colour over motion of about 80 msec. The *accelerando* that the brain imposes on the motion system, by providing it with faster conducting fibres, is evidently not sufficient to overcome its in-built *ritardando* relative to the colour system. There are four conclusions to be derived from this experiment: first, that colour is not perceived at the same time as motion and that the two perceptual systems are therefore different, as are the processing systems; second, that there is no synchroniser in the brain, capable of setting the results of the operations of the two processing–perceptual systems to "time zero" and thus providing the exact temporal registration that we thought was the hallmark of our visual experience; third, that the brain therefore missynchronises and misbinds or, rather more accurately, it binds the results of its processing–perceptual systems, not what happens in real time in the world outside; fourth, and probably not last, that the delivery times of visual signals and the cortical processing leading to perception are two very different things. An early delivery does not necessarily result in faster perception, quite the contrary in the case of motion. Of these, it is the first conclusion that is the most interesting in this context because it is consistent with the notion of autonomy and variable, dynamic relationships between visual areas, the main theme of this chapter. It is this separateness, however trivial, that gives the motion system based on V5 its small degree of autonomy and it is that small degree of autonomy that imposes a dynamic relationship between it on the one hand, and V1/V2 on the other. It is presumably also this autonomy that results in a conscious correlate to activity in it.

V. THE CONSCIOUS EXPERIENCE OF VISION WITHOUT V1

Given the separateness of the motion perceptual system, it becomes interesting to ask whether it can manifest its autonomy more convincingly. What kind of evoked signal, for example, would one detect from the brain of GY following stimulation with fast motion, which he can discriminate and has a conscious awareness of, and with slow motion, which he cannot discriminate and has no awareness of? In fact, our EEG studies [42] showed that the activity evoked

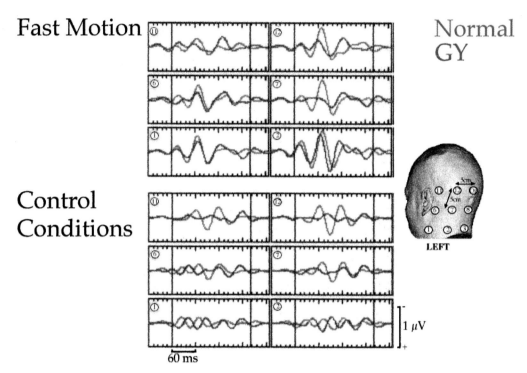

Fast Motion

Normal GY

Control Conditions

LEFT

60 ms

1 μV

FIGURE 5 The evoked EEG activity elicited by fast motion and control stimuli at six electrodes placed over the occipital cortex in patient GY (green) and two control subjects (red). In the fast motion condition, the activity recorded over the ventral occipital cortex (electrodes 1, 2 and 6) in the control subjects matches the activity elicited in GY. In the control condition the activity elicited in the control subjects is located at different electrodes (11 and 12) and is absent in GY. Modified from ffytche *et al.* [42].

in GY's brain, and more specifically from electrodes placed optimally to record from his V5, were almost entirely normal and comparable to that of normal subjects when we used the fast motion that he could consciously discriminate (Fig. 5). By contrast, we could not evoke any activity in his brain when we used stimuli which he, unlike normals, was neither capable of discriminating nor had any conscious awareness of.

A. Conscious Vision without Pre- or Postprocessing by V1

Taken together with our functional imaging experiments, as well as with our TMS and EEG studies described above, the conclusion was obvious: the motion system can and does manifest its autonomy, in that activity in V5, without pre- or postprocessing by V1 is sufficient to lead to conscious vision. This conclusion is consistent with all the evidence given above: consistent with the independent arrival of signals in V5; consistent with the survival of the characteristic of V5, directional selectivity, after deafferentation from V1; consistent with the fact that the direct motion signals that V5 receives are related to fast motion, which is the only motion that a patient such as GY can see; consistent with the earlier results of Riddoch and of Holmes; and consistent too with the studies on patient MM, who has a double hemianopia with minor central sparing following a bilateral calcarine lesion [43]. However, it is not consistent with a central dogma of blindsight theory, that conscious vision is not possible without V1 [26,27].

Caution is required, however, as one of our eminent colleagues keeps reminding us. As in normals, V3 and parietal cortex were coactivated with V5 in GY. Hence to ascribe the conscious vision to V5 alone is at present unjustified. What is more certain is that activity in a small number of visual areas, including V5, can lead to conscious vision without pre- or postprocessing by V1. These areas, in other words, are more autonomous of V1 (and of V2) than we had presumed. We hope no one misreads us to be saying that V1 is not necessary for visual perception in general or visual motion perception in particular, that, if necessary, it can be eliminated with impunity, or that the quality of motion vision in the absence of V1 is as good as in its presence. None of these statements is true. On the contrary, the quality of motion vision in the absence of V1 is poor, an observation implicit in the use of the term "residual" [24]. We are merely drawing attention to the fact that the relationship between V1 and the prestriate areas may not be quite so rigid and that the latter areas may be able to contribute more to conscious vision than we have been willing to suppose. The fast-motion vision of GY, crude though it is, is conscious and can give a crude knowledge; it satisfies the definition of vision as a knowledge seeking mechanism that we have given above.

Nor is GY the only example. Another example is patient MM, unaccountably ignored even by those who have discussed such matters at length in prestigious journals, in spite of a perfectly valid and quite remarkable description of him in respectable journals [43,44]. This patient has been examined with our French colleagues in Marseilles and we can confirm his remarkable ability to discriminate motion, but another kind of motion, optical flow, both correctly and consciously in spite of a near total blindness resulting from a bilateral lesion involving the calcarine sulcus in both hemispheres. This finding raises the question that we have discussed elsewhere [45] of another, possibly semi-independent, processing-perceptual system more specialised for optical flow. In fact, our imaging experiments [46,47] show that optical flow stimuli do not activate V5 but a more ventral zone extending to the fusiform gyrus and possibly constituting part of the V5 complex in humans.

B. Is Consciousness Also Modular?

We have emphasised above that V5 can act autonomously of V1, since it is still active in the absence of V1 and can still mediate conscious perception of visual motion, perhaps on its own and perhaps in concert with the other areas that are active. It is results like this that have led us to propose that the individual areas of the prestriate cortex can each contribute explicitly to conscious visual perception, without the need for pre- or postprocessing by V1 or indeed other visual areas [28], which is not the same thing as saying that, in the intact brain, these areas always act autonomously. However, if V5 can act in a more or less autonomous fashion and if activity in it has a conscious correlate related to motion, can other visual areas not do the same? The evidence presented above, that optical flow stimuli activate an area of the brain that is close to, but distinct from, V5, supplemented with the evidence derived from patient MM who has a conscious experience of optical flow in his blind field, but not of other kinds of motion, suggests that stimulation of the cerebral area active with optic flow stimuli may also have conscious experience as a correlate, but a different kind of conscious experience from that resulting from stimulation of V5. That in turn raises the fascinating question of whether consciousness itself is not also modular, a topic that we are currently investigating [45].

C. Conscious and Unconscious Components in the Motion Vision of GY?

This still leaves open the question of whether GYs vision has an unconscious component, a component that allows him to discriminate visual stimuli correctly, and to a high degree of accuracy, though without conscious awareness. A capacity to discriminate without conscious awareness would not modify any of the conclusions reached above—that conscious vision is possible without pre- or postprocessing by V1—but would suggest that knowledge can be acquired in the unconscious state, a bizarre situation not in accord with our definition. There is of course nothing holy about our definition, and it may be wrong or at least partially wrong; more likely, it would have to be extended, if the phenomenon of blindsight were incontrovertibly demonstrated, which it well might. The issue itself is, however, of more than passing interest which is why we are currently studying this phenomenon in GY in greater detail. Since the publication of our 1993 paper showing that GY has a conscious dimension to his motion vision [23], Weiskrantz and his colleagues have not only confirmed this but have also shown convincingly that GY is capable of discriminating to a very high degree of accuracy, without conscious awareness, if the visual stimuli are appropriately scaled. It will be especially interesting to learn whether there are particular stimulus conditions for demonstrating blindsight which would suggest that blindsight must be distinguished sharply from the Riddoch phenomenon, or whether, with the same stimulation conditions, conscious awareness itself waxes and wanes, resulting in blindsight in some test sessions and in conscious awareness of the same stimuli in others. The former would suggest that a highly specialised visual pathway, distinct from that capable of mediating a conscious correlate, is used. The latter would suggest that blindsight and conscious residual vision for motion are two aspects of the Riddoch phenomenon and would raise the interesting question of whether the brain switches from one neural system to another during the waxing and waning of consciousness, a rich if difficult question for imaging studies. Blindsight theorists usually make no reference to the Riddoch phenomenon at all, which implies that they treat the blindsight phenomenon as quite distinct from the Riddoch phenomenon. This may well turn out to be so, but it could equally well turn out not to be so. We believe, however, that there is a need to extend these observations to subjects beyond GY, as we have done in our study of conscious visual motion in blind subjects by studying patient MM. And while there is now a large number of cortically blind and scotomatous subjects who have been shown to have a conscious experience of visual motion in their blind fields [23,24,30,31,33], there is only a limited number of subjects, GY apart, in whom blindsight for motion has been demonstrated. An interesting case is that of subject DB [34]. His verbal commentary to his discrimination of a moving vertical line was *"I did not see the line ... but I could feel the movement, and I was absolutely sure of it."* That certainty implies a conscious dimension and when a subject like DB reports *"having a 'feeling' of something moving"* but asserts firmly that he does not *'see' anything"* [35], one is hard put to understand why the former (feeling) is not also a conscious experience. The problem becomes especially acute given the variation in GYs description, alluded to above, of what he experienced with visual motion—seeing shadows in one instance and having feelings in another—a variation that demands a more careful definition of what state correlates with a conscious one and the extension of the search to more subjects.

VI. THE INTERACTION BETWEEN V1 AND V5 DURING THE PERCEPTION OF FORM FROM MOTION

What started as a relatively simple enquiry into GY, with results that we thought would be predictable, ended up by immersing us into worlds that we had thought not to visit, of perceptual times, of latency of signal arrival in V5, of the relationship between evoked potentials and blood flow during conscious visual experience. The conclusion that we have drawn from these studies was unexpected. However, it is perhaps wise to also emphasise the other side of the coin, namely a strong interaction between V1 and V5 in other conditions, since it is a variable relationship that we are discussing.

The poverty of vision without V1 may be due in part to the necessity for preprocessing by V1, but it may also be due in part to postprocessing in V1. V1 not only sends a powerful projection to V5 but receives a powerful projection back from it [7] (Fig. 6). One characteristic of the latter is that, unlike the former, it is not patchy but diffuse and does not respect the territory of the cells in layer 4B projecting to V5 but also invades the territory of cells in layer 4B that project to V3 and to V2. Such a diffuse return projection is also the hallmark of the backprojection from V5 to V2 [16] (Fig. 7). It would be astonishing if such a powerful return projection were not put to some use. We have speculated elsewhere that it is one way of informing several subdivisions of V1 of the results of the operations undertaken by V5 [48]. We have also suggested that such a feed-back connection may be the kind of neural machinery needed to generate one attribute of vision from another [48]. As an example, we chose structure from motion and have used it for a functional imaging

FIGURE 6 A reconstruction of layer 4B of area V1 made by stacking straightened contours on top of each other. In this case an axonal tracer (horseradish peroxidase) had been injected into area V5. The triangles represent cells in V1 that took up the stain and thus project to V5. The stipple represents labeled terminals in V1 that come from cells in V5 that took up the stain. The scale bar is 5 mm. From Shipp and Zeki [7].

activation study (Zeki, Watson, Friston, and Frackowiak, unpublished results 1995). The rationale for this study is as follows. The oriented lines to which the cells of V3 respond so well [49,50] can be generated from differences in luminance between the oriented lines and the background (condition A); they can also be generated if a texture moves in two different directions, say to the left in the zone defined by the oriented lines and to the right in the zone defined by the background (condition B) (Fig. 8). In our functional imaging study we made the supposition that, in condition A, the orientation selective cells of V1 are stimulated first, followed by the orientation selective cells of area V3, through the direct anatomical link connecting the two areas [14,51]; in condition B the directionally selective cells of layer 4B are stimulated first, followed by an activation of area V5, which is then followed by an activation of V1 through the return connections from V5 to V1, followed finally by an activation of the same orientation selective cells of area V3. On the other hand, if one were to stimulate with uniform motion of the same textured stimulus alone (condition C), one should stimulate V1 and V5 alone. Put more briefly, area V1 will be activated once in conditions A and C and twice in condition B. Hence if one were to use human subjects to view these three conditions, one should expect that the highest activity will be in V1, in condition B. Our results, using six subjects, showed that there was a highly significant increase in blood flow (and therefore activity) within areas V1 and V2 when subjects had been viewing the form from motion stimulus compared to the weighted mean activity when they were viewing the motion stimulus alone and the form stimulus alone (Fig. 8). Although we choose to interpret this result to mean that motion is being extracted from the stimulus first, in V5, and the results of the operation thus performed in V5 are then relayed back to V1 to activate the V3 projecting cells there, we acknowledge that there may be other interpretations to this, in particular that the form from motion stimulus is a more potent one for the cells of V1 than either the form alone or the motion alone. However, whatever the exact interpretation, the results of this experiment, when compared to the results of our earlier experiment [9,12], in which subjects viewed the movement of small squares in different directions, and the results of experiments in which subjects viewed Leviant's "*Enigma*," [8] all show that area V5 is in dynamic relationship with area V1 and that the strength of that relationship may be variable, depending upon the stimulus, though they give us no hint about the intimate physiological mechanisms that control that dynamic relationship.

Figure 7   A reconstruction of layers 3 and 6 of area V2 made by stacking straightened contours on top of each other. In this case an axonal tracer (horseradish peroxidase) had been injected into area V5. The large dots represent cells in V2 that took up the stain and thus project to V5. The stipple represents labeled terminals in V2 that come from cells in V5 that took up the stain. The scale bar is 2 mm. From Shipp and Zeki [16].

Form from motion vs. form, motion

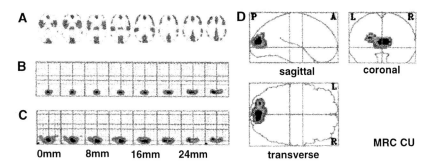

FIGURE 8 (Top) The stimuli used in this study consist of three parts. First there is a pattern of vertical lines made from black and white stripes: this is the "form" stimulus. These vertical stripes can also be defined by moving textures, the texture moving to the left in a white bar, to the right in a black bar: this is the "form-from-motion" or "FFM" stimulus. The final stimulus is a control consisting of texture moving in one direction only. (Bottom) The pattern of activation produced when the motion only and form only activation is subtracted from the FFM activation. The main activation occurs within areas V1 and V2 (Zeki *et al.* unpublished results, 1995).

VII. CONCLUSION

The series of experiments reported here started with observations of the static PET images derived from our early experiments. Just as Balla's "Dog" was one of the precursors of an art that was to lead, especially in the hands of Jean Tinguely and Alexander Calder, to kinetic art and the incorporation of actual motion into the creations of artists, so the study of static PET images has led us to an experimental journey in search of dynamism in cortical connections and its implications. From this has emerged a picture of the relationship between visual areas that is far more dynamic than we had dared to imagine. In this relationship, it is perhaps futile to think of which area, V1 or V5, is activated first, for they can both be the first to be activated, depending upon the speed of motion of the stimulus. Moreover, once V5, say, is activated first, it will have the anatomical machinery to activate V1 immediately through the return connections from V5 to V1 and perhaps be activated simultaneously by the forward input from V1 to V5, hence setting up a repetitive, ongoing dynamic relationship where the beginning and the end cease to matter because, ultimately, there is no beginning or end,

> Or say that the end precedes the beginning
> And the end and the beginning were always there,
> Before the beginning and after the end,
> And all is always now.
>
> [*T.S. Eliot, Burnt Norton*]

References

1. S. Zeki and M. Lamb. The neurology of kinetic art. *Brain* **117,** 607–636 (1994).
2. S. Zeki. The functional organization of projections from striate to prestriate visual cortex in the rhesus monkey. *Cold Spring Harbour Symp. Quant. Biol.* **40,** 591–600 (1975).
3. S. Zeki. Functional specialization in the visual cortex of the monkey. *Nature* **274,** 423–428 (1978).
4. S. Zeki. The cortical projections of foveal striate cortex in the rhesus monkey. *J. Physiol.* (*London*) **277,** 227–244 (1978).
5. M. S. Livingstone and D. H. Hubel. Psychophysical evidence for separate channels for the perception of form, color, movement, and depth. *J. Neurosci.* **7,** 3416–3468 (1987).
6. E. A. DeYoe and D. C. Van Essen. Concurrent processing streams in monkey visual-cortex. *Trends Neurosci.* **11,** 219–226 (1988).
7. S. Shipp and S. Zeki. The organization of connections between areas V5 and V1 in macaque monkey visual cortex. *Eur. J. Neurosci.* **1,** 309–332 (1989).
8. S. Zeki, J. D. G. Watson, and R. S. J. Frackowiak. Going beyond the information given—the relation of illusory visual-motion to brain activity. *Proc. R. Soc. London B* **252,** 215–222 (1993).
9. S. Zeki, J. D. G. Watson, C. J. Lueck, K. J. Friston, C. Kennard, and R. S. J. Frackowiak. A direct demonstration of functional specialization in human visual-cortex. *J. Neurosci.* **11,** 641–649 (1991).
10. M. S. Livingstone and D. H. Hubel. Specificity of intrinsic connections in primate primary visual cortex. *J. Neurosci.* **4,** 2830–2835 (1984).
11. B. H. Tootell, J. B. Reppas, K. K. Kenneth, R. Malach, R. T. Born, and T. J. Brady. Functional analysis of human MT and related visual cortical areas using magnetic resonance imaging. *J. Neurosci.* **15,** 3215–3230 (1995).
12. J. D. G. Watson, R. Myers, R. S. J. Frackowiak, J. V. Hajnal, R. P. Woods, J. C. Mazziotta, S. Shipp, and S. Zeki. Area-V5 of the human brain—Evidence from a combined study using positron emission tomography and magnetic-resonance-imaging. *Cereb. Cortex* **3,** 79–94 (1993).
13. J. S. Lund, R. D. Lund, A. E. Hendrickson, A. M. Bunt, and A. F. Fuchs. The origin of efferent pathways from the primary visual cortex, (area 17), of the

macaque monkey as shown by retrograde transport of horseradish peroxidase. *J. Comp. Neurol.* **164,** 287–304 (1975).

14. B. G. Cragg. The topography of the afferent projections in circumstriate visual cortex studied by the Nauta method. *Vision Res.* **9,** 733–747 (1969).

15. G. P. Standage and L. A. Benevento. The organization of connections between the pulvinar and visual area MT in the macaque monkey. *Brain Res.* **262,** 288–294 (1983).

16. S. Shipp and S. Zeki. The organization of connections between areas V5 and V2 in macaque monkey visual cortex. *Eur. J. Neurosci.* **1,** 333–354 (1989).

17. D. H. ffytche and S. Zeki. Brain activity related to the perception of illusory contours. *Neuroimage* **3,** 104–108 (1996).

18. J. Hirsch, R. L. Delapaz, N. R. Relkin, J. Victor, K. Kim, T. Li, P. Borden, N. Rubin, and R. Shapley. Illusory contours activate specific regions in human visual-cortex—evidence from functional magnetic-resonance-imaging. *Proc. Nat. Acad. Sci. USA* **92,** 6469–6473 (1995).

19. R. Gregory. Cognitive contours. *Nature* **23,** 51–52 (1972).

20. H. R. Rodman, C. G. Gross, and T. D. Albright. Afferent basis of visual response properties in area MT of the macaque. I. Effects of striate cortex removal. *J. Neurosci.* **9,** 1033–1050 (1989).

21. P. Girard, P. A. Salin, and J. Bullier. Response selectivity of neurons in area MT of the macaque monkey during reversible inactivation of area V1. *J. Neurophysiol.* **67,** 1437–1446 (1992).

22. J. Bullier, P. Girard, and P. A. Salin. The role of area 17 in the transfer of information to extrastriate visual cortex. *In* "Cerebral Cortex Volume 10: Primary Visual Cortex in Primates" (A. Peters and K. S. Rockland, Eds.), pp. 301–330. Plenum, New York, 1994.

23. J. L. Barbur, J. D. G. Watson, R. S. J. Frackowiak, and S. Zeki. Conscious visual-perception without V1. *Brain* **116,** 1293–1302 (1993).

24. I. M. Blythe, C. Kennard, and K. H. Ruddock. Residual vision in patients with retrogeniculate lesions of the visual pathways. *Brain* **110,** 887–905 (1987).

25. L. Weiskrantz. Side glances at blindsight: recent approaches to implicit discrimination in human cortical blindness. *Proc. R. Soc. London B* **239** (1989).

26. A. Cowey and P. Stoerig. The neurobiology of blindsight. *Trends Neurosci.* **14,** 140–145 (1991).

27. P. Steorig. Varieties of vision: From blind responses to conscious recognition. *Trends Neurosci.* **19,** 401–406 (1996).

28. S. Zeki. "A Vision of the Brain." Blackwell, Oxford, 1993.

29. P. Dupont, G. A. Orban, B. De Bruyn, A. Verbruggen, and L. Mortelmans. Many areas in the human brain respond to visual motion. *J. Neurophysiol.* **72,** 1420–1424 (1994).

30. G. Riddoch. Dissociations of visual perception due to occipital injuries, with especial reference to appreciation of movement. *Brain* **40,** 15–57 (1917).

31. L. Weiskrantz, J. L. Barbur, and A. Sahraie. Parameters affecting conscious *versus* unconscious visual-discrimination with damage to the visual-cortex (V1). *Proc. Natl. Acad. Sci. USA* **92,** 6122–6126 (1995).

32. S. Zeki. Cerebral akinetopsia (visual-motion blindness)—A review. *Brain* **114,** 811–824 (1991).

33. G. Holmes. Disturbances of vision by cerebral lesions. *Br. J. Ophthalmol.* **2,** 353–384 (1918).

34. L. Weiskrantz. "Blindsight." Clarendon Press, Oxford, 1986.

35. L. Y. Weiskrantz. The Ferrier lecture: Outlooks for blindsight: Explicit methodologies for implicit processes. *Proc. R. Soc. London. B* **239,** 247–278 (1990).

36. G. Beckers and S. Zeki. The consequences of inactivating areas V1 and V5 on visual-motion perception. *Brain* **118,** 49–60 (1995).

37. D. H. ffytche, C. N. Guy, and S. Zeki. The parallel visual-motion inputs into areas V1 and V5 of human cerebral-cortex. *Brain* **118,** 1375–1394 (1995).

38. S. Shipp, B. M. de Jong, J. Zihl, R. S. J. Frackowiak, and S. Zeki. The brain activity related to residual motion vision in a patient with bilateral lesions of V5. *Brain* **117,** 1023–1038 (1994).

39. R. H. Hess, C. L. Baker, and J. Zihl. The motion-blind patient—low-level spatial and temporal filters. *J. Neurosci.* **9,** 1628–1640 (1989).

40. C. L. Baker, R. Hess, and J. Zihl. The motion-blind human patient—peripheral filters. *J. Physiol.* (*London*) **396,** 63 (1988).

41. K. Moutoussis and S. Zeki. A direct demonstration of perceptual asynchrony in vision. *Proc. R. Soc. London B.* **264,** 393–399 (1997).

42. D. H. ffytche, C. N. Guy, and S. Zeki. Motion specific responses from a blind hemifield. *Brain* **119,** 1971–1982 (1996).

43. M. Ceccaldi, D. Mestre, M. Brouchon, M. Balzamo, and M. Poncet. Autonomie déambulatoire et perception visuelle du mouvement dans un cas de cécité corticale quasi totale. *Rev. Neurol.* (*Paris*) **148,** 343–349 (1992).

44. D. R. Mestre, M. Brouchon, M. Ceccaldi, and M. Poncet. Perception of optical-flow in cortical blindness–A case-report. *Neuropsychologia* **30,** 783–795 (1992).

45. S. Zeki. "Parallel processing, asynchronous perception and a distributed system of consciousness in vision." Submitted for publication.

46. R. J. Howard, M. Brammer, I. Wright, P. W. Woodruff, E. T. Bullmore, and S. Zeki. A direct demonstration of functional specialization within motion-related visual and auditory-cortex of the human brain. *Curr. Biol.* **6,** 1015–1019 (1996).

47. B. M. de Jong, S. Shipp, B. Skidmore, R. S. J. Frackowiak, and S. Zeki. The cerebral activity related to the visual perception of forward motion in depth. *Brain* **117,** 1039–1054 (1994).

48. S. Zeki and S. Shipp. Modular connections between areas V2 and V4 of macaque monkey visual cortex. *Eur. J. Neurosci.* **1,** 494–506 (1989).

49. S. Zeki. The third visual complex of rhesus monkey prestriate cortex, *J. Physiol.* (*London*) **277,** 245–272 (1978).

50. A. Burkhalter and D. C. Van Essen. Processing of color, form and disparity information in visual areas VP and V2 of ventral extrastriate cortex in the macaque monkey. *J. Neurosci.* **6,** 2237–2351 (1986).

51. S. Zeki. Representation of central visual fields in prestriate cortex of monkey. *Brain Res.* **14,** 271–291 (1969).

CHAPTER TEN

MAPS OF SOMATOSENSORY SYSTEMS

I. INTRODUCTION

Each of the novel functional neuroimaging techniques to become available in the past 30 years has been immediately applied to the mapping of somatosensory systems [1–4]. Somatosensory stimulation, under psychophysically controlled conditions, allows assessment of the nature of the relationship between manipulation of stimulus characteristics (*e.g.*, frequency, amplitude) and the physiological response in the brain (indexed by, for example, rCBF, rCMRglc, or $rCMRO_2$). The historical primacy of mapping studies of the somatosensory systems has had the consequence that functional imaging data derived from diverse imaging techniques, from the nontomographic xenon-133 technique to state-of-the-art PET and fMRI, are available for comparison. The literature data are therefore not homogeneous and may need to be reinterpreted in a historical perspective, depending on when and how they were collected. Mapping of the somatosensory systems poses special challenges for spatial and temporal resolution of functional neuroimaging methods. A fine grained cartography or temporal characterisation of the individual somatosensory areas is beyond the present potential of state-of-the-art PET or fMRI. However, the spatial resolution and anatomical accuracy of the most recent techniques are now sufficient to allow a description of the properties of major functional components of the somatosensory system and their interactions. Therefore, we predict that there will be further interest in studies of somatosensory systems with the more modern functional imaging techniques in future years.

In this chapter, we review current knowledge about the functional mapping of human somatosensory systems. We will be primarily concerned with cortical brain mapping as evaluation of the functional characteristics of subcortical grey nuclei (of structures such as the thalamus) is still difficult. Given the limited data about submodalities of the somatosensory systems (*e.g.*, proprioception, touch, nociception, temperature sense, *etc.*), when necessary we will refer to results of functional imaging studies of the motor system. This seems appropriate because there are several aspects of somatosensory function that contribute to motor function. Human anatomical, electrophysiological, and lesional data will be presented together with a short-review of the anatomy of monkey somatosensory areas. Subsequently the contribution of functional imaging to the understanding of the somatosensory system will be reviewed.

We shall also review information on brain mapping of the vestibular system. We will take the opportunity to discuss interactions between vestibular system signals and other somatosensory representations in the generation of a mental body representation referring also to the neuropsychological syndrome of unilateral neglect. The hierarchy between somatosensory areas will be addressed by reference to the role of different cortical areas to the conscious perception of touch.

II. HOW IS SOMATIC SENSORY INFORMATION COLLECTED AND CLASSIFIED?

Many different receptors exist in skin, joints, and muscles that collect somatosensory information. A detailed dissertation on the anatomy and physiology of such receptors and the psychophysics of somatosensory perception is beyond the scope of this chapter. However, before discussing the various somatosensory brain areas, we will give a short general overview of somatic sensory receptors and the afferent somatic sensory pathways from the periphery to the brain (for a more systematic introductory dissertation, see Refs. [5–9]).

There is no agreement about the classification of somatosensory cutaneous receptors in the periphery. Two alternative classifications exist. Melzack and Wall [10] suggest that *"skin receptors have specialised properties for the transduction of particular ranges of stimuli into (temporal) patterns of impulses rather than modality-specific information."* They also say that *"to ram receptors into one of a number of preconceived separated categories would be arbitrary and artificial."* A number of examples support this theory. In the cornea there are freely ending nerve filaments only and nevertheless touch, pain, and thermal sense (cold and warm) can be distinctively perceived [11]. In the ear, there are only freely ending and perifollicular receptors, nevertheless all four sensations are perceived. Based on these examples, Adams and Victor [12] conclude that *"the lack of organised receptors, e.g., the end-bulbs of Krause and Ruffini in the cornea and ear, makes it evident that these types of receptors are not essential for the recognition of cold and warmth, respectively, as von Frey and other early anatomists postulated."*

More recently, however, modern techniques for single peripheral nerve fiber stimulation and recording have renewed the fortunes of a theory originally associated with the name of von Frey [13], which predicates that specificity of signals transmitted to the central nervous system is a key property of somatic receptors and their afferent axons (for a review, see Turebjörk *et al.* [14]). According to this theory, distinctiveness of an (elementary) sensation is predominantly based on stimulation of specific receptors and on the fact that specific information travels along discrete neural pathways from the periphery to the central nervous system. For example, before integration, specific somatic sensory signals of touch and proprioception are kept anatomically distinct at least up to the four somatosensory areas of the primary somatosensory complex in anterior parietal cortex [5].

Turebjörk *et al.* [14], while constraining the relevance of their observations to the glabrous skin of the hand, also suggest that *"... particular patterns of nerve impulses are not necessarily determinant of the subjective quality attribute of simple tactile sensation. This conclusion does not conflict with the concept that the brain normally makes use of temporal and spatial patterns of impulses from a large number of receptors of various types to form more complex tactile percepts such as recognition of texture."*

Intermediate versions of the two theories also exist. It is generally acknowledged that *"(even though) cutaneous receptors are not specific, each responds preferentially (i.e., each has a lower threshold) to one form of stimulation in distinction to another"* [12]. Adams and Victor [12], to interpret the single peripheral nerve fibre stimulation and recording data [14] also conclude that *"more recent physiologic studies have shown that the quality of sensation depends on the type of fibre that is stimulated, even though the endings themselves are not specific."*

A. Anatomical Pathways for Different Types of Somatosensory Sensations: Touch, Proprioception, Pain, and Thermal Sense

The sense of touch is caused by mechanical stimuli of the body [5]. It is mediated by mechanoreceptors in the skin placed at different depth, with different receptive fields and different time reaction profiles to stimulation: Meissner's corpuscles and Pacini's corpuscles are rapidly adapting mechanoceptors and signal onset and offset of stimulation, while Merkel's receptors and Ruffini's corpuscles are slowly adapting receptors, that maintain information about mechanical stimulation throughout longer periods of time. Meissner's corpuscles and Merkel's receptors are placed in the superficial skin while Pacini's corpuscles and Ruffini's corpuscles are in the subcutaneous tissue (Fig. 1).

Natural stimuli generally activate different combinations of receptors and indeed there are specific sensations, such as the sensation of wetness, that arise from this compound stimulation. Tactile signals from the body travel through peripheral nerves to the dorsal root ganglia where the first order sensory neurones are located. From the dorsal root ganglia, fibres and signals are sent along the dorsal columns of the spinal cord, whose axons synapse with the cells of the dorsal nuclei (gracile and cuneate nucleii) in the medulla oblongata where second order sensory neurons of the dorsal column system are located. Ascending projections from cells of the dorsal nuclei cross and project through the medial lemniscal system to the ventral posterior nuclei of the thalamus and, finally, to the anterior parietal cortex through the internal capsule. Somatic signals from a large (anterior) part of the cranium are collected by cranial nerves V, VII, and IX and travel to specific cranial ganglia and hence to distinct nuclei in the brain stem, before reaching the ventral posteromedial thalamus (Fig. 2).

Proprioception, the perception of the position of the limbs and the sense of movement, is signaled by specific receptors and is conveyed to the cerebral cortex through the same pathway as the tactile modality. Other second order neurones for muscle spindle afferents are located in the medullary nuclei X and Z, in Clarke's column of the T1–L4 spinal cord, and in the external cuneate nucleus [6]. The peripheral receptors that mediate proprioception are located in the muscle spindles, in joints and in skin. Proprioception is essential for any kind of exploratory behaviour such as appreciating the shape of an object. Proprioception is also fundamental to the control of balance.

The feeling of pain is transmitted by three kinds of receptors called nociceptors: mechanical nociceptors are sensitive to violent, sharp mechanical

		Receptive field	
		Small, sharp borders Cutaneous	Large, obscure borders Subcutaneous
Adaptation	Fast, no static response	FA I Meissner	FA II Pacini and Golgi
	Slow, static response present	SA I Merkel	SA II Ruffini

Figure 1 Receptor types and characteristics of afferent fibers from the glabrous skin of the human hand. FA, fast adapting; SA, slowly adapting. Redrawn from Turebjörk *et al.* [14].

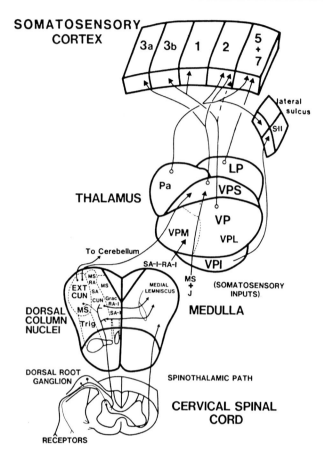

FIGURE 2 Summary illustration of the major ascending somatic sensory systems for tactile object recognition in the monkey, the dorsal-column medial lemniscal system, and the antero-lateral (spino-thalamic) system [7]. These are described in the main text. SA-I, slowly adapting receptors of type I; RA-I, rapidly adapting receptors of type I; MS, muscle-spindle receptors; CUN, nucleus cuneatus; Grac, nucleus gracilis; Trig, spinal trigeminal nucleus; VP, ventro-posterior thalamic nucleus; VPS, ventro-postero-superior thalamic nucleus; VPI, ventro-postero-inferior thalamic nucleus; VPL, ventro-postero-lateral thalamic nucleus; VPM, ventro-postero-medial thalamic nucleus; Pa, anterior pulvinar; LP, lateral-posterior complex.

stimulation; thermal nociceptors respond to thermal stimulation over 45°C or to very cold stimulation; polymodal nociceptors respond to either mechanical, thermal, or chemical stimuli, including the chemical stimulation released by damaged cells. Nociceptors are located in the skin and in the viscera and their nerves reach the dorsal ganglia either as slowly conducting myelinated fibres or as nonmyelinated fibres. Dorsal ganglia neurons enter into the spinal cord and synapse in the posterior horn where second-order neurons are located. Axons from second order neurons cross at the same level, entering into the ascending antero-lateral system. Nociceptors from viscera converge to the same neurons of the dorsal horn where afferent fibres arrive from nociceptors of the skin. This anatomical convergence explains the phenomenon of referred pain; a typical example is the pain associated with myocardial infarction that can be referred to the chest or to the left arm. From the spinal cord, pain signals are conveyed to the brain through the spino-thalamic, spino-reticular, spino-mesencephalic, and spino-cervical tracts. A small number of fibres project to the gracile and cuneate columns as well. It is still unclear how the feeling of pain is processed in the brain. Identification of human cortical areas involved in pain signal processing has been a major challenge taken up by functional imaging.

Thermal sensation is elicited by cold and warmth that stimulate specific thermal receptors. Stimulation of a cold receptor with a hot stimulus induces a sensation of cold. This is more evidence that somatic stimuli are classified correctly because specific receptors produce a labeled line code. Thermal signals travel along the same antero-lateral pain system. Both painful and thermal stimuli reach more than one thalamic nucleus, including the ventroposterolateral nucleus, the intralaminar nuclei, and the posterior nuclei.

III. SOMATOSENSORY THALAMUS

A. Specific Thalamic Nuclei

Before further processing at cortical level, all somatosensory signals are processed by specific thalamic nuclei. Current knowledge about the human somatosensory thalamus is still incomplete (but see Ohye [15]), while extensive information is available about monkey somatosensory thalamic nuclei (for a review, see Kaas [7]). A summary of the somatosensory thalamic nuclei and their distinct projections to the somatosensory areas of the monkey is given in Table 1. Illustrations for the monkey are given in Fig. 2 and for humans in Fig. 3. There is a large ventro-posterior nuclear complex (VP) with the nuclei of the posterior (PC) complex assuming more limited importance. The VP nuclear complex has been subdivided into a number of components. The ventroposteromedial (VPM) nucleus receives cutaneous inputs from the face, while the ventroposterolateral (VPL) nucleus has inputs from the rest of the body. These nuclei have a precise somatotopy. Since the work of Poggio and Mountcastle [16] it has also been recognised that inputs from receptors in deep tissues are at least partially segregated from inputs from cutaneous structures. A specific ventroposterosuperior (VPS) nucleus receives deep tissue inputs. These nuclear subdivisions project to specific subdivisions of the primary somatosensory area complex in the anterior parietal lobe, showing that signals are kept segregated to some extent from the periphery up to the primary sensory cortical areas before further integration.

In primates there is also a distinct ventroposteroinferior (VPI) nucleus whose role is not well understood. It is suspected, however, that VPI may be of functional importance as it is the major relay nucleus that projects to the second somatosensory area SII [17]. Finally there is one subdivision of the PC nuclei, the medial posterior nucleus (Pom), that has large cutaneous receptive fields and which projects to retroinsular (Ri) cortex and to granular insular (Ig) cortex, both of which are somatosensory areas (for review and illustrations, see Burton [18]).

B. Nonspecific Thalamic Nuclei Connected with Somatosensory Areas

In the monkey, associative somatosensory areas also receive projections from thalamic nuclei that do not have direct connections with second order somatic neurons. These include the (anterior) oral pulvinar (Pulo), the medial pulvinar

TABLE I

Anatomical and Physiological Properties of Somatosensory Cortices in Monkeys[a]

	Anterior parietal cortex				Posterior parietal cortex		Somatosensory cortex of the lateral sulcus		
	Area 3a	Area 3b [SI proper]	Area 1	Area 2	Area 5	Area 7b	Area SII	RetroInsular area [Ri]	Insula granular [Ig]
Localization	Post-central gyrus. Anterior depth of the CS. [7,25]	Post-central gyrus. In the depth of CS. Posterior to 3a. [7,25]	Post-central gyrus. Anterior surface of the gyrus. Posterior to 3b. [7,25]	Post-central gyrus. 2nd half of the surface of the gyrus. [7,25,48]	Cortex between PCS and IPS. [7,25,52]	Anterior half of the cortex limited by IPS, STS, and LS.	Upper [parietal] bank of LS behind the in-sula. [18,60]	Fundus of the upper and lower banks of the LS posterior to the insula. [110]	Posterior half of the insula. [84,85]
Somatotopography	Whole body fine-grained map. Tail >>> Tongue Medial >>> Lateral [7,23,25]	Whole body fine-grained map. Tail >>> Tongue Medial >>> Lateral [7,23,25]	Whole body fine-grained map. Tail >>> Tongue Medial >>> Lateral [7,23,25]	Whole body map looser than in 3b.1. Some reduplications. Tail >>> Tongue Medial >>> Lateral [7,25,48]	Both convergence and divergence within a given representa-tion (e.g. hand). Harm very large. Face smaller than in SI. [49]	Very crude body map. Limited topo-graphic organiza-tion. Hindlimb > Head-face lateral > medial [110]	Whole-body cutane-ous map. Tail >>> Head Post-Med >>> Ant-Lat [18,60]	Whole-body cutane-ous map. Tail >>>> Head Posterior >>> Anterior [110]	Very crude body map. Body >>> Face Posterior >> Anterior [85]
Receptive fields	Contralateral [7]	Contralateral [7,31]	Contralateral [7,31]	Contralateral [7]	Contralateral 58%. Bilateral 26.5%. Ipsilateral 15.5% [15,52]	Contralateral 30%. Bilateral 66%. Ipsilateral 4%. Whole body neurons. [59]	Contralateral 55%. Bilateral 39%. Ipsilateral 6% [59]	Contralateral 57%. Bilateral 41%. Ipsilateral 2% [59]	Bilateral 79%. Contralateral 23%. [85]
Cytoarchitecture	Layer IV less thick and granular than in area 3b. Giant pyramidal cells in layer V. [7,25]	Somatic koniocortex. Highly granular layers IV and III. [7,25]	Layers IV, III, and VI less densely packed with cells than area 3b. [7,25]	Layers IV and VI more dense than in area 1. [7,25]	Very similar to area 2. [49,48]	Narrow granular layer. Large layer III with large pyra-midal cells permit-ting sublamination. [110]	No hyper-granularity typical of SI. Marked blurring of lamination. [18]	Medium sized and plump layer III pyramidal cells + distinct separation of layers V and VI. [84,110]	Granular isocortical with fully demar-cated granule cell layers both in layer IV and II. [84]
Thalamic connections	VPO [7,25]	VP [7,25]	VP [7,25]	VP, VPSup, Pa [7,25,219]	VPL, VPS, Pulo, LP, Pa [18,48,219]	LP, Pulo, Pulm, MD, VL [17,87,219]	VPI, VPM [17]	Po, SG-Li, MGmc, Pulm, VPI [17,18]	VPI, Pulo, Pulm, Pom, MGmc, SG-Li [17,18,84]
Cortical efferent projections									
Feed-forward	4, 1, 5. SII [7,30,49,73]	1, 2, 5. SII 3b [7,30,49,73]	2, 3a, 5. SII 3b [7,30,49,73]	4-6, 3a, 5. SII 3b,1 [7,30,48,49,73]	6-4, 7b, Ri, Ig, SII 2 [48,73,84,220–222]	4, 6, SII, Ig 5 [46,73]	4-6, Id, Ig 3a, 3b, 1, 2, 7b, Ri [73]	SII, Ig 5 [73]	Amygdala SII, Ri [73]
Feed-back	−	−	±	+	+	6, 1, 2, 5, 7 [46]	+	+ [33]	+ [33]
Callosal connections	± with SI more con-nections for the hand than in area 3b. + with SII. [34,224,225]	± with SI. − for hand fingers. + with SII. [34,224,225]	± with SI. ± for hand fingers. + with SII. [34,224,225]	+ with SI more con-nections for the hand than in area 3b. ++ with SII. [34,224,225]	+ with SI, 4, 5, 7. + for hand fingers. [34,225]		With SI directly and through contralat-eral SII. With SII. [32–34,224,226]		
Physiological responses	Muscle spindles. Lim-ited cutaneous in-put. Neurons respon-sive during movements. [7,25,227]	Tactile cutaneous stim-uli from both RA-I and SA afferent. [7,25,229]	Tactile cutaneous stim-ulation from RA-I cutaneous recep-tors and from RA-II (Pacini) receptors. [7,23,25,164]	Stimulation of deep re-ceptors from joints and muscles. Lim-ited cutaneous input from the hand area. [7,25,164,228]	Passive and active limb movements. Specific combina-tions of positions of joints. ± response cutaneous stimuli, direction selective responses. [46,50,52,223]	Innocuous tactile 63%. Any noxious 7.5%. n.d. Any visual 19.6. n.d. 9.3%. Complex stim-ulation and atten-tion. [18,59]	Sudden high-velocity taps of hair stimula-tion. Transient stim-uli are preferred. Limited response to sustained pressure. [18,59]	Innocuous tactile 88%. Noxious 2.5%. Very robust response to mechanical stimu-lation. [18,59]	Tactile stimulation in-cluding light touch and stimulation of deep receptors. [85]
Prevalent deficit after selective lesion	n.f.	All discriminative functions but the crudest tactile dis-crimination. [42,230]	Texture discrimination rather than shape. [43]	Finger coordination and discrimination of shape and size. [42,43]	Altered guidance of arm movements on the basis of proprio-ceptive inputs. [54]	Complex body schema disorders including mild unilateral ne-glect. [46,53]	Impairment of texture and shpae discrimi-nation learning. [76]	n.f.	n.f.

a Only cortico–cortical connections within the somatosensory system are considered. Abbreviations: CS = central sulcus. Ig = granular insula. IPS = intra-parietal sulcus. LP = lateral posterior nucleus. LS = lateral sulcus. MD = Medial dorsal nucleus. MGmc = Medial geniculate nucleus, magnocellular division. Pa = Anterior Pulvinar. PCS = post-central sulcus. Po = Posterior nucleus. Pulm = Medial pulvinar nucleus. Pulo = Oral pulvinar nucleus. Ri = Retroinsular area. SG-Li = Suprageniculate Limitans nucleus. SII = Second somatosensory area. STS = superior temporal sulcus. VP = Ventroposterior nucleus. VPI = Ventroposterior inferior nucleus. VPM = Ventroposterior medial nucleus. VPO = Ventroposterior oral nucleus. VPSup = Ventroposterior superior nucleus. n.f. = not found in the literature.

[7] J. H. Kaas. Somatosensory system in "The Human Nervous System" (G. Paxinos, ed.), p. 813–844, Academic Press, San Diego (1990). [17] D. P. Friedman and E. A. Murray. Thalamic connectivity of the second somatosensory area and neighboring somatosensory fields of the lateral sulcus in the macaques. J. Comp. Neurol. 252, 348–373 (1986). [18] H. Burton. Second somatosensory cortex and related areas in "Cerebral Cortex. Sensory Motor Areas and Aspects of Cortical Connectivity" (E. G. Jones and A. Peters, eds.) vol. V, p. 31–98, Plenum Press, New York (1986). [23] J. H. Kaas. What, if anything, is SI? Organization of first somatosensory area of cortex. Physiol. Rev. 63, 206–231 (1983). [30] M. F. Shanks, R. C. A. Pearson, and T. P. S. Powell. The ipsilateral cortico–cortical connexions between the cytoarchitectonic subdivisions of the primary somatic sensory cortex in the monkey. Brain Research reviews 9, 67–88 (1985). [31] M. Sur. Receptive fields of neurons in areas 3b and 1 of somatosensory cortex in monkeys. Brain Res. 198, 465–471 (1980). [32] D. N. Pandya and L. A. Vignolo. Interhemispheric projections of the parietal lobe in the rhesus monkey. Brain Res. 15, 49–65 (1969). [33] E. A. Karol and D. N. Pandya. The distribution of the corpus callosum in the Rhesus monkey. Brain 94, 471–486 (1971). [34] H. P. Killackey, H. J. Gould, C. G. Cusick, T. P. Pons, J. H. Kaas. The relation of corpus callosum connections to architectonic fields and body surface maps in sensorimotor cortex. J. Comp. Neurol. 34, 384–419 (1983). [42] O. Hikosaka, M. Tanaka, M. Sakamoto, and Y. Iwamura. Deficits of manipulative behaviors induced by local injections of muscimol in the first somatosensory cortex of the conscious monkey. Brain Res. 325, 375–380 (1985). [43] M. Carlson. Characteristics of sensory deficits following lesions of Brodmann's areas 1 and 2 in the post-central gyrus of Macaca Mulatta. Brain Res. 204, 424–430 (1981). [46] J. Hyvärinen. Posterior parietal lobe of the primate brain. Physiol. Rev. 62, 1060–1129 (1982). [48] T. P. Pons, P. E. Garraghty, C. G. Cusick, and J. H. Kaas. The somatotopic organization of area 2 in macaque monkeys. J. Comp. Neurol. 248, 313–335 (1985). [49] R. C. A. Pearson and T. P. S. Powell. The projection of the primary somatic sensory cortex upon area 5 in the monkey. Brain Research Reviews 9, 89–97 (1985). [48] T. P. Pons and J. H. Kaas. Corticocortical connections of area 2 of somatosensory cortex in macaque monkeys. A correlative anatomical and electrophysiological study. J. Comp. Neurol. 248, 313–335 (1986). [50] F. H. Duffy and J. L. Burchfiel. Somatosensory system organizational hierarchy from single units in monkey area 5. Science 172, 273–275 (1979). [51] Y. M.Iwamura, A. Iriki, and M. Tanaka. Bilateral hand representation in postcentral somatosensory cortex. Nature 369, 554–556 (1994). [52] H. Sakata, Y. Takaoka, and A. Kawarasaki. Somatosensory properties of neurons in superior parietal cortex area 5 of the rhesus monkey. Brain Res. 64, 85–102 (1973). [53] T. L. Peele. Acute and chronic parietal lobe ablations in monkeys. J. Neurophysiol. 7, 269–286 (1944). [54] P. D. Nixon, P. Burbaud, and R. E. Passingham. Control of arm movement after bilateral lesions of area 5 in the monkey (Macaca mulatta). Exp. Brain Res. 90, 229–232 (1992). [59] C. J. Robinson and H. Burton. Somatic submodalities distribution within the second somatosensory (SII), 7b, retroinsular, postauditory and granular insular of M. fascicularis. J. Comp. Neurol. 192, 93–108 (1980). [60] C. J. Robinson and H. Burton. Somatotopographic organization in the second somatosensory area of M. fascicularis. J. Comp. Neurol. 192, 43–67 (1980). [73] D. P. Friedman, E. A. Murray, J. B. O'Neill, and M. Mishkin. Cortical connections of the lateral sulcus of macaques. Evidence for a corticolimbic pathway for touch. J. Comp. Neurol. 252, 323–347 (1986). [76] E. A. Murray and M. Mishkin. Relative contributions of area SII and area 5 to tactile discrimination. Behav. Brain. Res. 11, 67–83 (1984). [84] M. M. Mesulam and E. J. Mufson. "The Insula of Reil in Man and Monkey. Architectonics Connectivity and Function in 'Cerebral-Cortex'" (E. G. Jones and A. Peters, eds.) vol. V, p. 179–223, Plenum Press, New York (1986). [85] R. J. Schneider, D. P. Friedman, and M. Mishkin. A modality-specific somatosensory area within the insula of the rhesus monkey. Brain Res. 621, 116–120 (1993). [87] E. G. Jones and D. P. Friedman. Projection pattern of functional components of thalamic ventro-basal complex on monkey somatosensory cortex. J. Neurophysiol. 48, 521–544 (1982). [110] C. J. Robinson and H. Burton. The organization of somatosensory receptive fields in cortical areas 7b, retroinsular, postauditory, granular insular of M. fascicularis. J. Comp. Neurol. 192, 69–92 (1980). [164] J. Hyvärinen, A. Poranen, and Y. Jokinen. Influence of attentive behavior on neuronal responses to vibration in primary somatosensory cortex of the monkey. J. Neurophysiol. 43, 873–882 (1980). [219] T. P. Pons and J. H. Kaas. Connections of area 2 of somatosensory cortex with the anterior pulvinar and subdivisions of the ventroposterior complex in macaque monkeys. J. Comp. Neurol. 240, 16–36 (1985). [220] E. G. Jones, J. D. Coulter, and S. H. C. Hendry. Intracortical connectivity of architectonic fields in the somatosensory, motor and parietal cortex of monkeys. J. Comp. Neurol. 181 (1978). [221] E. G. Jones and T. P. S. Powell. An anatomical study of converging sensory pathways within the cerebral cortex of the rhesus monkey. Brain 93, 793–820 (1970). [222] D. P. Friedman, E. G. Jones, and H. Burton. Representation pattern in the second somatic sensory area of the monkey cerebral cortex. J. Comp. Neurol. 192, 21–42 (1980). [223] V. B. Mountcastle, J. C. Lynch, A. Georgopulos, H. Sakata, and C. Acuna. Posterior parietal association cortex of the monkey: command functions for operations within extrapersonal space. J. Neurophysiol. 38, 871–908 (1975). [224] H. J. Gould and J. H. Kaas. The distribution of commissural terminations in somatosensory areas I and II of the grey squirrel. J. Comp. Neurol. 196, 489–504 (1981). [225] E. G. Jones and S. H. C. Hendry. Distribution of callosal fibers around the hand representations in monkey somatic sensory cortex. Neurosci. Lett. 19, 167–172 (1980). [226] E. G. Jones and T. P. S. Powell. Connections of the somatic sensory cortex of the rhesus monkey. II. Contralateral cortical connections. Brain 92, 717–730 (1969). [227] R. J. Nelson. Responsiveness of monkey primary somatosensory cortical neurons to peripheral stimulation depends on "motor-set." Brain Res. 304, 143–148 (1984). [228] T. P. S. Powell and V. B. Mountcastle. Some aspects of the functional organization of the cortex of the postcentral gyrus of the monkey. Bull. Johns Hopkins Hosp. 105, 133–162 (1959). [229] J. Tanji and S. P. Wise. Submodality distribution in sensorimotor cortex of unanesthetized monkey. J. Neurophysiol. 45, 467–481 (1981). [230] M. Randolph and J. Semmes. Behavioral consequences of selective subtotal ablations in the postcentral gyrus of Macaca mulatta. Brain Res. 70, 55–70 (1974).

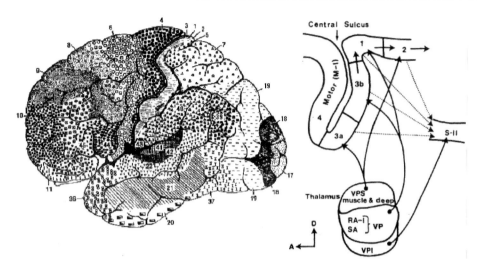

FIGURE 3 Cytoarchitectonic mapping of the lateral surface of the human cerebral hemisphere according to Brodmann [19] and thalamic afferents to areas SI and SII in humans [7]. Legends as for Fig. 2.

(Pulm) that projects to area Ri and to area 7b, and the lateral posterior nucleus (LP) which projects to somatosensory area 5. The somatosensory functional relevance of these connections is not well understood at present.

IV. SOMATOSENSORY CORTICES IN MONKEY AND HUMANS: ANATOMICAL, ELECTROPHYSIOLOGICAL AND LESIONAL STUDIES

Nine major cortical areas of the monkey brain and their human homologues with prevalent, if not exclusive, somatosensory function will be discussed; the primary somatosensory complex (areas 3a, 3b, 1, and 2), area 5, area 7b, second somatosensory area (SII), granular insula (Ig), and area Ri. The anatomical nomenclature adopted here refers to the classifications of Brodmann [19] and Vogt and Vogt [20]. A tentative summary of the properties of these areas in the monkey brain is given in Table I and therefore, in the following discussion we will focus on more general principles of organisation. A discussion of human homologues will also be presented. For human homologues Brodmann's classification will be used as this is the most widely used descriptive nomenclature in the functional imaging literature.

A. The Primary Somatosensory Complex

The anterior parietal cortex (SI-complex) has been the focus of considerable research since the beginning of the century [19–22] but only more recently has it been recognised that the four subdivisions described by Vogt and Vogt [20] were meaningful in cytoarchitectonic and in physiological terms. It is now acknowledged that the cortex buried in the posterior bank of the central sulcus (areas 3a and 3b) and on the surface of the postcentral gyrus (areas 1 and 2) represents four independent complete representations of the body [23–25]. Importantly, these different body representations are not just reduplications but are cortical representations of different somatosensory receptors; areas 3b and 1 have two mirror reversed body maps of cutaneous receptors (Fig.

4); areas 2 and 3a respond primarily to deep stimulation of joints (area 2) and muscles (area 3a).

Accordingly, in the rostro-caudal direction there are three areas of response with response differences at the borders of different architectonic fields [deep (Brodmann's area (BA) 3a) → superficial (BA 3b and 1) → deep (BA 2)]. The somatotopy of these areas corresponds to the well known arrangement [supero-mesial (tail–foot) → latero-ventral (tongue)] (Fig. 4), so that the inferior limbs are represented at the vertex, with the foot represented on the mesial wall of the postcentral gyrus, while the upper limbs and mouth are represented on the convexity, with the mouth area, tongue, and larynx at the bottom of the gyrus. Another well established organisational principle derived from studies of the somatotopy of the SI complex is that the hand and mouth areas are disproportionately larger than the trunk, a fact that reflects a greater cutaneous receptor density on the hand and in the mouth.

Detailed studies of the somatotopy of areas of the SI-complex have revealed that the fine grained organisation is far more complicated than described in the above simple scheme [26]. In area 3b there are contiguities of the body map that do not correspond to cutaneous contiguities; one such example is the contiguity of jaw, mouth, and hand–fingers that is a geographic arrangement bringing together somatosensory representations concerned with eating food.

In his provocative review article *"What, if Anything, Is SI?"* (a paraphrase of the famous article *"What, if Anything, Is a Rabbit?"* [27]) Kaas [25] has raised the question of whether any of the four areas of the monkey SI-complex could be considered a primary somatosensory cortex proper, by analogy to SI cortex of the cat and by analogy to primary visual and auditory cortices. According to Kaas [25], a candidate area for SI-proper should satisfy a number of criteria:

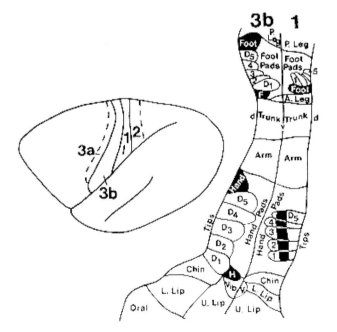

Figure 4 Architectonic fields (areas 3a, 3b, 1, 2) of primary somatosensory cortex (on the left) and representation of body surface in areas 3b and 1 for the owl monkey (on the right) [23]. The two maps are mirror-reversed, as can be seen from the location of the hand pads and finger tips.

1. architectonic distinctiveness and specific thalamic connections,
2. a systematic and complete representation of the body surface,
3. unique sensory processing at the single neurone level,
4. a unique set of connections with other structures,

and be associated with

5. specific impairment after damage and removal.

On the basis of a number of observations, Kaas' suggestion is that monkey SI-proper is area 3b. Area 3b has cytoarchitectonic features typical of other koniocortical areas such as primary auditory and visual cortices. Area 3b has laminar patterns of forward connections that mimic those of area V1 with neighbouring areas [28,29]; area 3b sends projections to areas 1, 2, 3a, and 5 in layers IV and III and there are documented backward projections to area 3b in layer 1 from areas 1 and 2 [30].

Receptive field (RF) characteristics and callosal projections also indicate that area 3b is a good candidate for SI-proper. RFs are maximally focused in area 3b, while in area 1, RFs become larger and more complex [31]. In area 2, RFs are even more complex with some reduplications. Callosal projections are unevenly distributed in area 3b with very limited connections, if any, for the hand and foot areas [32,33]. The pattern of callosal connections evolves in area 1 and reaches an even distribution in area 2, including a hand representation [34]. However, even neurons of area 2 have excitatory receptive fields restricted to the contralateral body [7].

Human cortex of the primary somatosensory complex seems fairly similar to that of the monkey [7]. Since Vogt and Vogt (1919) [20] four distinct areas are recognised whose cytoarchitectonic features and anatomical localisations are consistent with what is reported in Table 1 for the monkey brain. A schematic representation of human primary somatosensory cortex is shown in Fig. 3. An excellent microscopic illustration of human primary somatosensory complex can be found in Zilles [35].

There is neurophysiological evidence to suggest that the human cytoarchitectonic subdivisions have physiological meaning. Electrical stimulation of cutaneous afferents of the median nerve give evoked potentials in area 3b 30 msec after stimulation. A potential in area 1 is seen 5 msec after that in area 3b [36]. Gandevia *et al.* [37] stimulated muscle afferents and detected activation in a region caudal to that for cutaneous afferents, possibly in area 2. Kaukoranta *et al.* [38] have found activation of areas 3b and 3a with mixed nerve stimulation that includes both cutaneous and muscle spindle afferents.

Two methods have been used to determine somatotopy in postcentral human somatosensory cortex: direct surface recordings of evoked potentials [39,40] and observation of sensations elicited by electrical stimulation of the cortex (see Fig. 5) [41]. In the medio-lateral plane human and monkey data are substantially consistent even for some of the discontinuities found in the monkey; the head and neck are on the vertex separated from the face representation by a field for the hand and fingers. Attempts have been made recently to specify finer grained maps of the sensory representation of the human hand. Sutherling and colleagues [40] used electrocorticography with subdural electrodes in three epileptic patients and found an uneven representation of the fingers, in contrast to the classical description of Penfield and Boldrey [41]. From largest to smallest, the size of cortical representations in the three patients studied was thumb, index, middle, little, and ring fingers.

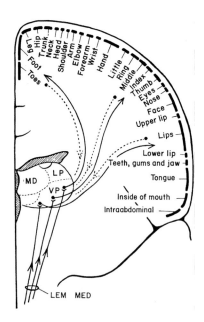

FIGURE 5 Somatotopography in human primary somatosensory cortex as revealed by electrical stimulation, according to Penfield and Jasper [57]. VP, ventro-posterior thalamic nucleus; LP, lateral-posterior complex; LEM MED, lemniscus medialis.

These findings agree better with what is seen in the monkey [23], with the exception of the thumb representation that is proportionally larger in humans. On the other hand, not much can be said about the rostro-caudal somatotopy and homologies between monkey and human. In the macaque the maps of the four architectonic fields of postcentral cortex follow a reciprocal mirror-reversed orientation (see Fig. 3) [25]. To ascertain this in humans would require invasive recordings in the depths of the central sulcus.

Damage to postcentral cortex has been studied in detail in the monkey. There is a gradient of functional impairment caused by damage from area 3b to adjoining areas. Lesions restricted to area 3b affect all kinds of tactile discrimination with sparing of very crude tactile perception [42]. On the other hand, lesions to area 1 impair texture rather than shape discrimination [43] and lesions to area 2 impair finger coordination [42] and discrimination of shape and size [43].

In humans, damage to postcentral somatosensory cortex is hardly ever restricted to one cytoarchitectonic field. Typical extensive postcentral ischemic lesions result in lasting impairment of a number of skills such as pressure sensitivity, two point discrimination, point localization, and discrimination of object shape, size, and texture [44,45]. However, primary modalities (touch, pain, temperature, and vibration sense) are relatively little affected [12]. Roland (1987) collected psychophysical curves for somatosensory detection of electrical stimuli in normal subjects and in brain damaged patients with lesion sites verified during surgery [45]. The majority of normal subjects had psychometric detection functions that were quantal such that minute increases of stimulus strength resulted in dramatic changes in the probability of detection. Patients with postcentral lesions showed an average increase of threshold to about 6 mA (normal threshold is between 0.5 and 1.0 mA), but only when the lesion involved the anterior half of the gyrus and the cortex buried in the central sulcus. The shape of the psychometric detection function was also dramatically altered, with a noisy profile and poor detection of signal. However, Roland [45] also reports that *"stimuli from 6 to 8 mA and upwards were detected by all patients"* Roland has given an anatomical interpretation to these findings. None of his patients with lesions of SI had a concurrent lesion in SII. Accordingly, he has speculated that intact neurons of SII might subserve residual tactile perception in his patients.

B. Somatosensory Areas of the Posterior Parietal Cortex

The posterior parietal region is an arbitrary subdivision of the parietal lobe that includes the cortex posterior to area 2 and excludes somatosensory cortex located in the depth of the lateral (Sylvian) fissure. In the monkey, the BAs of posterior parietal cortex are BA 5 and BA 7. These areas can be subdivided further. However, for our purposes we can consider area 5 as a single area because both area 5a and area 5b are somatosensory in function [7]. The situation may be different for area 7. Here we shall consider the anterior portion only, area 7b, the one chiefly concerned with somatosensory processing. Area 7a, which is located posteriorly to 7b, appears more concerned with visual and visuo-motor integration [7, 46].

It is not a straightforward task to establish the human homologues of these areas because different authors have called superior parietal lobules area 7 or area 5. Accordingly, homologies have to be considered within a homogeneous terminology. For example, area 7 in humans is located in superior parietal cortex and therefore is not a likely candidate for the homologue of monkey area 7. As far as the terminology of Brodmann is concerned, the human homologue of monkey BA 5 may be human BA 5 and BA 7, while BA 40 in the supramarginal gyrus is probably the human homologue of area 7b of the monkey (for a review, see Hyvärinen [46]). In addition, the inferior parietal cortex is considerably expanded in humans. In humans a cortical field located at the junction between superior temporal cortex and the supramarginal gyrus (area TPT) is related to auditory cortex [47].

Area 5 is posteriorly located to area 2 from which it cannot be easily distinguished on purely cytoarchitectonic grounds [48]. Area 5 has cutaneous and deep representations, especially of the arm, with several reduplications of somatotopic representations [49]. Only a small portion of the area receives specific thalamic connections from nuclei connected with somatosensory projections from the posterior complex [7]. Importantly, in this area there are also neurons with bilateral RFs for the hand and similar neurons have also been found in the intraparietal sulcus [50,51]. Neurons in area 5 are responsive to passive and active limb movements and specific combinations of positions of joints [52], while the response to cutaneous stimuli is marginal and the response to visual stimuli is more limited [46]. In the monkey, selective damage to area 5 causes altered guidance of arm movements on the basis of proprioceptive inputs (without visual control) and misreaching [53,54].

It is interesting that a similar syndrome has been described in a human patient by Levine *et al.* [55]. This patient, as a consequence of a right superior parietal tumour, was unable to reach a target if he could not see his moving arm. However, the same patient showed misreaching for the ipsilateral arm moving in the contralateral hemifield. This and other evidence in patients with superior parietal lobule lesions, may suggest that area 5/7 in humans has some integrative function with respect to upper limb movements based on proprioceptive information. Human area 5/7 may also have a role in visual guidance of movement. However, acquired human lesions are seldom pure and the symptoms described above are frequently confounded in more complex syndromes especially when lesions are bilateral [56]. Functional imaging may provide more information about human functional homologues of monkey area 5.

In the human literature, the mesial aspect of area 5 has been traditionally called the *supplementary sensory area*. This area was originally defined by Penfield and Jasper (1954) with intraoperative electrical stimulation studies [57]. Circumscribed lesions of this region cause acute apraxic symptoms and can leave somatosensory function substantially normal [58].

Area 7b is the anterior half of area 7 and is involved in high-order integration within the somatosensory system. Consistent with the associative nature of the region, area 7b has a crude body map with a preponderant proportion of neurons with bilateral RFs. Within the somatosensory cortices area 7 has rich intra- and interhemispheric direct connections. Thalamic connections are with nuclei that are unconnected with second order somatosensory neurons. Area 7b also has rich connections with regions outside somatosensory cortex proper, including premotor cortex and the cortex of the superior temporal sulcus [46]. Neurons in area 7b are activated predominantly by innocuous tactile stimuli and to a lesser extent by visual stimuli or noxious stimuli [59,60].

Lesions to area 7 (including area 7a) in the monkey cause complex disorders of somatosensory schemata, including signs of unilateral neglect [53], that are milder than the neglect syndrome observed in humans after parietal lesions. On the other hand, neglect is much more severe in monkeys following prefrontal lesions [61,62]. This observation has led some authors to conclude that the organisation of visuospatial perception in monkeys is substantially different from that of humans [63]. Lesions restricted to area 7b can cause impaired tactile placing and holding [64] or slight weakness and hypotonia [53] without major somatoaesthetic discriminatory deficit.

Comparison of human and monkey lesion data of the anterior half of posterior parietal cortex is not simple for the very reason that parietal cortex is also uniquely involved with language function in humans. Language functions may result in a considerable topographical redistribution of function in this cortex especially in the dominant hemisphere [12]. The crude spatial description of human lesional mapping studies is a considerable limitation to the study of monkey and human homologies with the lesion method. If we assume that the human homologue of monkey area 7b is BA 40 in the supramarginal gyrus [7,46], deficits resulting from lesions in this area can vary depending on hemisphere. Unilateral neglect, the inability to attend to lateralised stimuli in the absence of obvious sensory deficits, is much more frequent in damage to the nondominant (usually right) hemisphere (for review, see Vallar [65]). Right brain damage is also associated with a greater incidence of contra-lateral hemianaesthesia and hemiplegia that could itself be explained as the result of mild unilateral neglect [66].

Lesion data in unilateral neglect permits a distinction between the functional effects of inferior and superior parietal lesions. The same patient described above [55], who had a lesion in superior parietal cortex, did not show signs of neglect. In a series of right brain damaged patients described by Vallar and Perani [67], the maximum overlap of lesions in neglect patients was in the right inferior parietal lobule, while one of the two areas of maximum overlap in cases without neglect was in the superior parietal lobule. Firm conclusions about the exact location of lesions within the inferior parietal lobule that cause neglect are not possible given the imprecision of anatomical mapping techniques based on CT scans [65,67]. It remains to be seen whether the critical lesion that causes neglect is in the supramarginal gyrus, in the angular gyrus, or in both.

The functional impact of hemispheric asymmetry in lesions of parietal cortex is further qualified by the fact that left supramarginal gyrus or underlying white matter lesions primarily cause language disorders including conduction aphasia (for a review, see Damasio [68]) or more discrete language impairments such as deficits of verbal short-term memory [69].

C. Somatosensory Areas of the Lateral (Sylvian) Sulcus: Second Somatosensory Area (SII), Retroinsular and Postauditory Areas, and Somatosensory Insula

Area SII was first described by Adrian [70] in the cat and by Woolsey [71,72] in several other animals. In the monkey, SII localizes to the upper (parietal) bank of the lateral (Sylvian) sulcus behind the insula (Fig. 6) [18,60]. The term "second" does not necessarily imply a hierarchical position of the region with respect to the SI-complex (see below); rather the terminology serves to define an historical sequence in the identification of somatosensory areas. The cytoarchitectonic features of SII are distinctive from all fields of the SI-complex; there is no hypergranularity typical of SI and there is a marked blurring of lamination [59]. Area SII has a whole-body cutaneous map whose

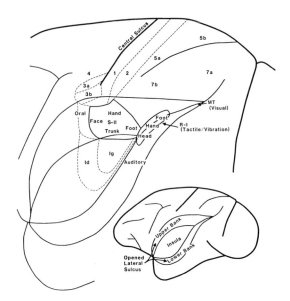

FIGURE 6 Subdivision of the somatosensory cortex in the lateral sulcus of macaque monkeys. R-I, retro-insular; Id, insula dysgranular; Ig, insula granular. From Kaas and Pons [226].

accuracy is not as crude as was initially believed [18,59]. The somatotopy of area SII is such that the face is antero-lateral and the tail (foot) in the postero-medial portion. However, SII contains many more neurons than SI that have nearly identical RFs. It is not clear whether in SII there are deformed body representations (*e.g.*, a very large hand area) as in SI [18]. Nearly 40% of the neurons have bilateral RFs, which suggests that the area may have associative functions. Area SII has rich direct connections with all somatosensory areas with the exception of area 5 [73] and receives thalamic input from a specific nucleus, the ventroposterior inferior (VPI) nucleus (Figs. 2 and 3) [17]. The functional relevance of these thalamic connections has been the subject of discussion [74]. In the monkey, neurons in SII are best activated by sudden high-velocity taps or hair stimulation [18]. In the monkey [59] and in the cat [75], transient stimuli are preferred, while most neurons show limited response to sustained pressure. Robinson and Burton [59] have observed responses to passive rotation of the joints in only three neurons, while 15% of SII neurons responded to massaging muscles or subcutaneous tissues, including joints [59].

Robinson and Burton [59] distinguish SII proper from other areas rostral to SII. Several units in these complex zones require active interaction of the animal with a sensory stimulus. A limited number of units fire in response to noxious stimuli. On the other hand, no evidence has been found of units sensitive to acoustic stimuli in SII nor in the rostral SII complex.

Lesions to area SII in monkeys have led to opposite conclusions, spanning from no evidence of deficit to evidence of specific impairment. Murray and Mishkin [76] caused complete damage to area SII in monkeys and were able to demonstrate a severe impairment of texture and shape discrimination, learning and altered size and roughness discrimination.

There is some electrophysiological evidence to suggest the location of the human homologue of monkey area SII. Penfield and co-workers [57,77] identified an area SII in awake patients by recording the sensations evoked by electrical stimulation. The stimulated sites were predominantly on the convexity near the Sylvian fissure and below the central sulcus, while access to the upper bank of the Sylvian fissure, where area SII is located in the macaque, was difficult. Lüders and co-workers [78] have recorded evoked potentials and electrically stimulated the same epileptic patient using chronically implanted electrodes. They propose that area SII is located somewhat anteriorly to the central sulcus. The early evoked potential recorded in putative human area SII was almost simultaneous with that recorded in area SI but a delay of 2.4 msec was sufficient to suggest that activity in SII could be dependent on synaptic input from SI. There is no evidence of the effect of selective damage to human area SII and indeed its localization is still a matter of debate.

Robinson and Burton [59,60] have described the somatosensory properties of the neurons of two other fields, the Ri cortex and the Pa cortex. About 80% of the neurons in these fields respond to tactile stimuli, while only a minority of the neurons (3%) respond to noxious stimuli. Robinson and Burton report that responses to touch in area Ri are as robust as, if not more robust than, those observed in area SII. Ri neurons follow faithfully a pattern of peripheral stimulation (*e.g.*, frequency of a vibratory stimulation from 64 to 256 Hz). A minority of neurons in Ri (16%) fire with acoustic stimuli. RFs in Ri neurons are very similar to those of SII. The somatotopy of Ri and Pa have not been determined precisely, though an antero-posterior gradient similar to that in SII has been proposed for Ri [59,60]. Guldin and Grusser [79] propose that Ri cortex should be divided in two components, lateral (Ri-l) and medial (Ri-m) Ri cortex. Ri-m cortex has a high proportion of neurons that are driven by vestibular stimuli. We are unaware of experiments where the effect of selective Ri or Pa damage has been examined in detail in monkeys. In humans, Brandt *et al.* [80] found that Ri cortex was the area of maximal overlap of lesions in patients with signs of vestibular dysfunction. Greenspan and Winfield [81] described a patient with altered touch and pain perception associated with a small tumor compressing the posterior insula, area Ri, and the parietal operculum.

The fact that the somatosensory insula is a brain area that is not just devoted to visceral processing is now well recognised [82–84]. Among the functions of the granular insula is the processing of somatic sensation (area Ig, the posterior half of the insula). In monkeys, the majority of somatosensory projections to the insula come from area SII [73]. Friedman and collaborators [73] and Schneider *et al.* [85] compared the role of somatosensory insula in tactile learning to the role of area TE in inferior temporal cortex for visual learning. However, area TE is purely visual [86] while early reports suggested that the insula is a multimodal area [82]. Recent evidence from Schneider *et al.* [85] has shown that a major portion of monkey area Ig is exclusively devoted to somatic processing. The somatotopy in monkey insula appears crude, with the face and head represented rostrally and the rest of the body more caudally. The large majority of insular somatosensory neurons have bilateral receptive fields. Callosal projections in the posterior portion of the insula have been shown by Karol and Pandya [33]. A specific somatosensory thalamic input exists from the ventropostero-inferior nucleus [84,87]. Optimal stimuli for activation of area Ig are tactile stimuli including light touch and stimulation of deep receptors [85]. Data about the functional effects of lesions circumscribed to area Ig in the monkey are not available.

While human data about the effect of selective lesions of individual somatosensory areas in the Sylvian sulcus and somatosensory insula are lack-

ing, there are studies that have considered the somatoaesthetic consequences
of lesions encompassing more than one area at a time. Lesions involving the
so-called ventro-lateral somatoaesthetic complex (area 40, putative area SII,
somatosensory insula) cause disorders of tactile object recognition [58]. We
[88] have proposed left hemispheric dominance for tactile matching of different
exemplars of the same meaningful object (*e.g.*, two different keys), while the
right hemisphere in this scheme is thought to be specialised for tactile matching
of nonmeaningful objects.

D. Hierarchical Organisation of Somatosensory Cortices and the Perception of Touch

Until recently, both area SI and area SII were thought to receive substantial
projections from thalamic nucleus VP. This dual projection supported the
view that tactile stimuli are processed in parallel by the two cortical regions.
This assumption remains valid for cats, rabbits, tree shrews, and galagos
in which inactivation of area SI has little effect on the responsiveness of
area SII to cutaneous stimuli [71,89–91]. However, more recently it has
been reported that in macaques the VP thalamic nucleus provides only
sparse projections to area SII [17]. In addition, monkey thalamic nucleus
VPI, that specifically projects to area SII, seems to process only vibrotactile
stimuli from pacinian receptors. These observations have led Pons and
colleagues [74,92,93] to challenge the dual projection pathway theory in
the macaque. Pons *et al.* [74] reported a study where lesions were made
to the whole hand representation in area SI of monkeys. All cytoarchitectonic
fields were damaged. Electrophysiological recordings were then performed
in the hand representation of SII which was found totally unresponsive to
cutaneous stimuli. On the other hand, there was no difficulty recording
responses to stimulation of all other body parts. Pons *et al.* [74] also
performed a control experiment in which they removed the entire SII and
made recordings from SI. No obvious alterations were found in the firing
pattern of area SI, showing that the functional dependency of SII on the
postcentral cortex is not reciprocal. The pattern of anatomical connections
from SI to SII is organised as follows: pyramidal neurons in layer III of
SI project to layer IV and lower layer III of area SII. This is the typical
arrangement of brain areas where signals are transmitted in a hierarchical
fashion, as in the visual cortices [28,29]. On the basis of their physiological
observations and of other independent anatomical findings Pons and colleagues [74,92,93] concluded that there is both a hierarchical and a serial
organisation between areas SI and SII and that, together with other
modalities, all somatosensory modalities are served by such multisynaptic
cortico-cortical sensory processing pathways. The authors suggest that this
represents *"an evolutionary shift in the organisation of somatosensory systems
from the general mammalian plan .... to a new (serial) organisation in
higher primates"* [93]. Findings similar to those of Pons *et al.* [74] in the
Rhesus monkey, have been found in marmosets [94], where selective lesions
were made to area SI. The serial pathway theory is consistent with the
original hypothesis of Mishkin [95] who postulated that SII is positioned
as an intermediary station in a serial pathway from SI to limbic areas
devoted to tactile learning.

In a further study Pons and colleagues provided additional data about
the reorganisation of SII following lesions to SI [92]. In the same monkeys

described in Pons *et al.* [74] the authors noticed that the somatotopic representations in area SII changed with time. This change involved an expansion of the representation of the foot into the area that normally contains hand representations within area SII. The effect on SII responsiveness of SI lesions involving only selected cytoarchitectonic fields can be found in Pons *et al.* [93].

A similar experiment assessed the effect of SI lesions on the responsiveness of SII in infant or juvenile macaques [96]. They found that, 1 year after a surgical lesion in the hand area of SI, substantial portions of the SII hand area became unresponsive to cutaneous stimulation of the hand in both age groups. In particular, they were unable to find responses for stimulation of the digits. However, and especially in infants, there were spared hand cutaneous receptive fields in which subsequent histochemical examination confirmed the absence of any residual input from SI. To explain their findings, Burton *et al.* [96] emphasise thalamic inputs to area SII that they believe carry somatosensory signals. They also speculate that (i) thalamic projections may change quantitatively as a function of age, (ii) thalamic cell loss due to lesions of SI may trigger remaining cells that project to SII to reinforce their connections, and (iii) SI may gate thalamic inputs to SII and this gating mechanism may be less efficient during infancy.

However, recent data indicate that the generalisation proposed by Pons *et al.* [93] about the serial arrangement of hierarchies in somatosensory cortices of primates needs to be reconsidered. Zhang *et al.* have investigated responsiveness within the hand region of SII in the marmoset monkey in association with cooling-induced, reversible inactivation of SI [97]. In contrast with the lesion study of Garraghty *et al.* [94], Zhang *et al.* have found no evidence of major changes in the responsiveness of SII after inhibition of SI [97].

We have discussed the problem of hierarchies at some length because it is relevant to the problem of whether there is a somatosensory area that has a primacy for somatosensory perception of all kinds. The neurophysiological and anatomical foundations of the serial pathway hypothesis in the adult monkey seem well documented, although the data of Zhang *et al.* suggest that this view cannot be generalised yet [97]. The logical consequence of a strict serial scheme in which signals are conveyed from the thalamus to SI, and then to SII and other somatosensory cortices, is the prediction that somatosensory (conscious) perceptions should be greatly reduced, if not abolished, following lesions to area SI. However, as discussed above, this prediction in its most extreme form has little support from studies in humans. Lesions to area SI greatly reduce discriminative skills without abolishing the capacity to perceive touch in an elementary manner (for a short review, see Kaas [7]). We do not know, however, which brain areas subserve residual perceptual skills after SI damage. These may well be beyond SII, in the insula or in the retroinsular cortex, for example, in which case there would be no inconsistency between monkey and human data. Other data that could reconcile the human and macaque literature are the behavioural observations. While area SII of monkeys cannot be activated with SI lesions, we are ignorant of even indirect behavioural observations about what, if anything, such monkeys can perceive. These questions have theoretical importance as we shall describe below a patient whose functional imaging data and perceptions suggest the possibility that parallel somatosensory inputs may reach human cerebral cortex.

V. FUNCTIONAL IMAGING STUDIES
OF SOMATOSENSORY SYSTEMS

There are few available functional imaging data that explicitly investigate the somatosensory system. A search of the literature reveals that basic elements of somatosensory function have not been explored systematically by functional imaging. We shall review in separate sections the basic somatosensory functions (light touch, vibratory sensation, kinaesthesia and proprioception) and complex somatosensory functions (*e.g.*, discrimination of texture and shape, tactile object recognition and tactile learning) [58]. A separate section will be dedicated to neurophysiological mechanisms of attention in somatosensory perception. Data pertinent to the postulated hierarchical organisation of somatosensory areas and their relationship to conscious tactile perception will be discussed at the end of the chapter together with the data of a hemianaesthesic patient originally described by Bottini *et al.* [98].

A. Elementary Somato-sensory Functions

These include vibratory sensation, the perception of light touch, kinaesthesia, proprioception, and two-point discrimination. The majority of these functions are subserved by the dorsal-column system while light touch perception is also mediated by the spino-thalamic system. The precise contribution of different human cortical areas to these sensory functions remains to be established.

1. Studies of Vibratory Sensation, Perception of Touch

Among the various stimuli used to study elementary somatosensory functions with functional imaging, vibratory stimulation has been most frequently used [2,3,99,100]. A justification for using this rather crude stimulation was that *"stimulation magnitudes are probably sufficient to activate most innocuous mechanoceptors in the skin and adjoining deeper tissues"* [99]. This argument illustrates the very reasonable preoccupation with using a stimulus that is sufficiently robust to elicit a detectable change of perfusion. In spite of its simplicity and crudeness, the paradigm of simple vibratory stimulation contrasted with a resting state has provided some interesting results [3,99]. Burton *et al.* [99] gave vibratory stimuli to each hand and foot. In all conditions, even when the stimulus was given unilaterally, activations were observed bilaterally in the SI complex, in an area identified as putative SII at the parietal operculum near the Sylvian fissure, and in the insula. The bilateral activation in SI is a slightly surprising finding as in the monkey SI complex the hand area has no callosal connections with contralateral SI (with the exception of BA 2) nor are there neurons with bilateral receptive fields [7].

Bilateral activation of human primary sensorimotor cortex has been observed several times with functional imaging for complex finger movements [4,101,102]. Colebatch *et al.* [103] have shown that activations of the ipsilateral sensorimotor cortex are significantly larger for proximal (shoulder) movements that for hand movements. The ipsilateral activations of motor and sensory cortex were interpreted as the result of activity in descending ipsilateral corticospinal fibres, but the possibility cannot be excluded that the activations observed were due to callosal projections from contralateral somatosensory cortex.

However, in the study of Burton *et al.* [99] activation of SI by vibratory stimulation was much greater in the hemisphere contralateral to the stimulated hand, suggesting that the proportion of neurons in human area SI with bilateral representations, or with callosal connections, might be relatively small or restricted to a cortical subcomponent of the SI complex (*e.g.*, BA 2). On the other hand, bilateral activation of the parietal operculum and insula is more consistent with data from monkeys that indicate that these regions have a high proportion of neurons with bilateral RFs [59,60]. Another interesting finding in Burton's data [99] is that putative SII seems to be placed in the depths of the Sylvian fissure, which is in good agreement with data from nonhuman primates and at variance with human electrophysiological recordings [57,77] and evoked-potential/electrical stimulation studies [78]. No somatotopic organisation was detectable in the Burton *et al.* [99] study in putative SII and in the insula. This result could be due to the limited spatial resolution of the PET scanner used for that study and to considerable intersubject averaging (data from up to 30 subjects were averaged).

Preliminary data on the somatotopic organisation of areas SI and SII have also been reported in a recent fMRI study [104]. The authors measured brain activity during a 3- to 5-Hz pressure stimulation delivered with a von Frey pressure aesthesiometer to the palm of the hand, the sole of the foot, and the volar forearm. In agreement with the Penfield and Rasmussen data [77], bilateral activation of putative SII was reported for all stimuli. A somatotopic representation of the hand and sole was detected in all subjects for SI. However, it was impossible to detect fine somatotopy within SII even with the relatively high spatial resolving capabilities of their fMRI scanner.

The data from St. Louis are consistent with those of Seitz and Roland [3] who delivered vibratory stimulation to the right hand. The authors measured perfusion and also oxygen extraction ratio and oxygen metabolism. They reported significant activations in contralateral SI and MI and a number of other areas that they call, respectively, area SII, retroinsular area Ri, supplementary motor area, and anterior parietal area. Homolateral activations were observed in the posterior cingulate cortex only. Marked lateralisation of the activation pattern seems somewhat in conflict with the results of Burton *et al.* [96]. Nevertheless, the sample of the study of Seitz and Roland [3] was relatively small (five observations per condition) and hence smaller homolateral activation foci seen by Burton *et al.* [99] were probably missed because of lack of statistical power.

2. The Sensory Motor Paradox

While SI activation can be easily detected following vibratory stimulation [2,3] or during sensorimotor tasks [1,103,105] greater difficulties are encountered detecting significant activations in SI by those who have used purer stimuli, such as suprathreshold electrical cutaneous stimulation [1] or suprathreshold touches delivered with a von Frey hair at 3–5 Hz frequency [106]. In these experiments Ingvar [1] and Pardo *et al.* [106] found greater activations in prefrontal cortex. This phenomenon was called the *sensory motor paradox* by Ingvar [1]. We have some data to support this observation. Two normal adult right-handed males underwent 12 perfusion measurements. The subjects received light, short tactile stimuli of the left hand during 6 of their 12 scans. Tactile stimulation was delivered with the tip of an index finger every 2 sec during scanning. Subjects explicitly confirmed, after each scan, that they had consistently perceived the tactile stimuli. Six eyes-closed resting state baseline scans were also collected. The order of experimental and control scans was counterbalanced to avoid order effects. Enough scans were collected in each condition to allow detection of significant perfusion changes because scans were collected in 3D [107,108]. To magnify common activations in the two subjects, an analysis by group was performed using SPM [109].

Comparison of touch with resting state scans revealed highly significant activations in right prefrontal cortex, ventral premotor cortex, anterior insula, and a region at the border of the retro-insular cortex and human putative SII, putamen, temporo-parietal junction, and anterior cingulate cortex (Fig. 7). Consistent with Ingvar's *sensory motor paradox* no activation was seen in the hand somatosensory cortex around the central sulcus. Indeed, significant rCBF decreases were seen bilaterally (Fig. 7) at stereotactic coordinates that are compatible with current views of the location of the hand area (right hemisphere: $x = 44$, $y = -24$, $z = 52$, Z score 3.8; left hemisphere: $x = -46$, $y = -32$, $z = 48$, Z score 4.1). Relative deactivations were more pronounced ipsilateral to a stimulated hand. It seems very unlikely that the lack of activation in SI is due to the intensity of the stimuli as other somatosensory areas such as the insula, area Ri/SII [110] and ventral premotor cortex [111], showed a very robust activation. On the other hand, physiological data in monkeys show that SI, and in particular areas 3b and 1, are activated by tactile stimuli such as light touch [7,25] and can follow the rhythm of peripheral mechanical stimulation up to 40 Hz [112]. It may be possible that human area

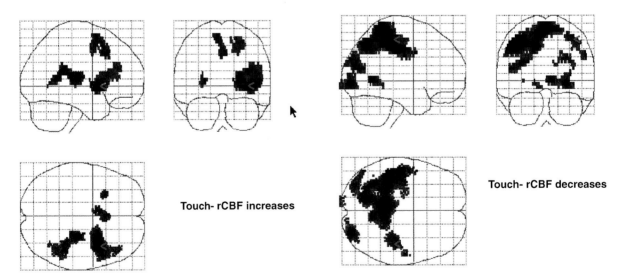

Touch- rCBF increases

Touch- rCBF decreases

FIGURE 7 The *sensory motor paradox* revisited. Patterns of activation induced by 0.5 Hz tactile stimulation of the left hand. Images are shown as integrated projections through sagittal, coronal, and transverse views of the brain. These images permit the correct location of activation patterns in three dimensions in the stereotactic space defined by Talairach and Tournoux [118]. Threshold for significance: $P < 0.001$. Activations were observed in right prefrontal cortex, ventral premotor cortex, anterior insula, at the border of the retro-insular cortex and human putative SII, putamen, temporo-parietal junction, and anterior-cingulate cortex (images on the left). Deactivations involved primarily area SI bilaterally, with more prominent deactivations in the left hemisphere (side of tactile stimulation).

SI is tuned to transient stimuli and that its temporal pattern of firing follows the temporal dynamics of stimulation faithfully. If this were the case, it is conceivable that overall neural activity during 0.5 Hz stimulation was not sufficient to cause a detectable activation because the total time without stimulation during a 60-sec scan was greater than the time of stimulation. However, this explanation does not explain deactivations observed in the SI hand area during touch scans nor the prominent activations of other somatosensory areas.

There are alternative interpretations for our paradoxical observation. One is that SI may not be crucial for detection of simple monotonic touches, as also suggested by clinical data [12]. Lesions of SI leave relatively unaffected the detection of touch, pain, temperature, and vibration. On the other hand, SI lesions alter somatosensory perception in more subtle and complex tactile discrimination tasks, such as texture appreciation.

Recent data from Ibañez *et al.* [113] and Sadato *et al.* [114] may help to interpret these results, at least in part. Ibañez *et al.* [113] studied the relationship between a linear increase of frequency of electrical stimulation to the right medial nerve at the wrist and perfusion in 10 subjects [113]. Five PET scans were performed, one at rest and the others during 0.2, 1, 2, and 4 Hz stimulation. A subgroup of six subjects had five additional scans at 8, 10, 12, 16, and 20 Hz. They found significant activations in SI only when the frequency of stimulation was 2 Hz or above. Trends towards significance were observed at lower stimulation rates. Activations reached a plateau at 4 Hz stimulation. Activation in an area that the authors identify as SII was seen at the 20-Hz stimulation rate only.

Sadato *et al.* (1996) observed a similar rate-dependent response in primary somatosensory cortex during an index-to-thumb opposition task of the right hand. No significant activation was detected at very low movement rates (0.25 and 0.50 Hz), while increasing activations were detected at slow (0.75–1 Hz), fast (2 and 2.5 Hz), and very fast rates (3 and 4 Hz) [114]. Sadato *et al.* [14] also observed activation of posterior supplementary motor area, anterior cingulate cortex, right thalamus, and right prefrontal cortex at very slow rates only.

These studies support the idea that we found no activation of SI because of the low rate of stimulation (0.5 Hz). Nevertheless, there is still no satisfactory explanation of the observed deactivation of SI and the robust activations of other somatosensory areas located along the Sylvian fissure. In summary, Ingvar's *sensory motor paradox* seems to survive the evidence of more recent studies suggesting that further experiments are needed to understand the complex relationship between activity in SI and other somatosensory areas during simple tactile stimulation.

3. Identification of Human Area SII

Activation of a human homologue of primate SII has been claimed in many studies. This claim should be treated with some caution as a complete assessment of the correspondence between a monkey area and its human homologue depends on a combination of several criteria that include macroscopic and microscopic anatomy in addition to functional information. The properties of monkey SII are summarised in Table 1 and Section IV.4. Here we recall that in the monkey SII localises to the upper (parietal) bank of the lateral (Sylvian) sulcus behind, above, and laterally to the insula, ventral to primary somatosensory cortex [59,60,73]. An illustration of the uncertainty about localization of a human homologue of SII is given by the contradictory electrophysiological findings of Penfield and Jaspers [57] and Lüders *et al.* [78]. This uncertainty was reinforced by the early functional imaging literature on somatosensory perception. As noted by Roland [115], the insular region of Fox and Appelgate [116] is called SII by Seitz and Roland [3] and the region called SII in Fox and Appelgate is called retroinsular in Seitz and Roland. Some of the inconsistencies in the functional imaging literature are probably due to the low spatial resolution of early studies when results were reported with reference to drawings from stereotactic atlases alone. Modern methods of coregistering the perfusion maps of individual subjects onto their own MRI scans and the advent of fMRI should overcome these initial problems.

An interim identification of the human homologue of SII is provided by a metaanalysis of the stereotactic coordinates of activation foci called SII by various authors. One such metaanalysis is given in Fig. 8 and Table II for the right hand or forearm. For comparison see the location of monkey area SII as illustrated in Fig. 6. We cannot include all functional mapping studies of somatosensory function as some (*e.g.*, [3,117]) do not report data according to standard stereotactic conventions. The metaanalysis suggests a mean location for SII in stereotactic space [118] in the ventral bank of the parietal operculum at the following stereotactic coordinates $x = -45$, $y = -21$,

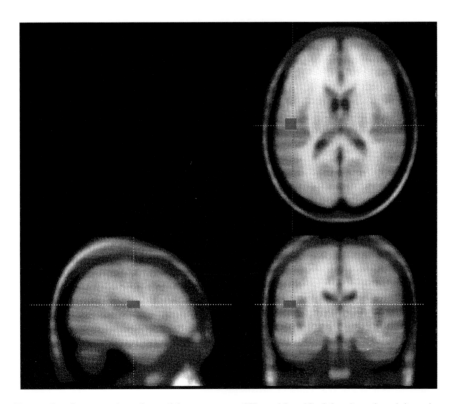

FIGURE 8 Average location of human area SII as identified by functional imaging studies reported in Table II (red region of interest). This location (the mean of stereotactic coordinates for the two hemispheres) has been superimposed on a 305-subject average MRI brain (Montreal Neurological Institute, Montreal, Canada [released with SPM96]).

Table II

Location of Putative Human Area SII for the Hand/Forearm as Revealed by Activation Studies

| Study | Task | Stereotactic coordinates | | | | | |
| | | Left | | | Right | | |
		x	y	z	x	y	z
Burton et al. (1993)[a] [99]	Vibratory stimulation of the left hand	—	—	—	44	−17	16
Burton et al. (1993)[a] [99]	Vibratory stimulation of the right hand	−42	−18	21			
Ibañez et al. (1995) [113]	20 Hz electrical stimulation of the right median nerve	−48	−22	16	—	—	—
Coghill et al. (1994) [100]	Vibratory stimuli of the forearm vs neutral (34°) thermal stimulation	−55	−26	21	42	−21	15
Coghill et al. (1994) [100]	Painful heat (48°C) stimuli of the forearm vs neutral (34°) thermal stimulation	—	—	—	36	−6	18
Stephan et al. (1994) [232]	Execution of right hand movement vs imagined movements	−38	−22	20	—	—	—
	Imagined movement of the right hand vs Motor preparation	−44	−14	24	—	—	—
	Executed movement vs Motor preparation (right hand)	−42	−22	20	50	−18	20
Bottini et al. (unpublished)	Light touch on the left hand	—	—	—	32	−36	16
Mean stereotactic coordinates		−45	−21	20	41	−20	17

[a] The coordinates reported here for the Burton et al. study (1993) are the mean coordinates of the two reported, transformed from the Talairach et al. (1967) [231] stereotactic conventions to the Talairach et al. (1988) conventions. All other stereotactic coordinates conform to Talairach et al. (1988) [188] conventions as in the original papers. Bottini et al. (unpublished) data refer to the experiment reported in Seciton V,A,2 of this chapter.

$z = 20$ for the left hemisphere and $x = 41$, $y = −20$, $z = 17$ for the right hemisphere.

In agreement with electrophysiological recordings made in monkeys [59,60], the human homologue of SII can be activated bilaterally with unilateral stimulation, although this was not an invariable finding in the functional imaging studies reviewed for Table II. Both vibratory stimulation and somatic pain seem to activate human SII.

4. Somatic Pain and Itch

Before reviewing the functional imaging literature on pain, we will summarise assumptions about the cortical contribution to pain perception of studies before functional imaging data became available. The issue of whether the cerebral cortex contributes to pain perception at all has been the focus of debate throughout the century, until functional imaging was used to study cerebral physiological responses associated with pain perception. The lesion studies of Head and Holmes [119] first suggested that pain is a diencephalic phenomenon and that the telencephalon has little to do with it. Then Penfield and Boldrey's [41] electrophysiological studies found that occasionally (11 of 800 trials) stimulation of somatosensory cortex causes pain; hence they concluded that the contribution of somatosensory cortex to pain perception is of marginal importance. On the other hand, there have never been doubts about the importance of the thalamus to pain perception, as well placed lesions to it can abolish all somatosensory perception from the contralateral hemisoma, including pain [12]. Sceptics about a cortical role for pain perception have found support in anatomical studies on monkeys. It has been shown that the thalamic nucleus VP, which projects to SI and SII, has only a small percentage of neurons that respond to painful stimuli [120], and there are few monkey SI neurons responsive to pain [121].

Other electrophysiological stimulation studies in man have proposed opposing views [39,122,123] and lesion studies have also suggested that different parts of the somatosensory cortex may play different roles in pain perception. Area SI [121,124] and the parietal operculum [81] may both contribute to the localisation and intensity discrimination of painful stimuli. Another component of pain perception, the affective response to it, may be mediated by cortical regions such as the cingulate cortex, as lesions there can greatly reduce the anxiety due to pain [125]. As a result of these observations, two separate pain systems have been proposed [120]; a medial pain system that involves the medial thalamic nuclei and their cortical projections (e.g., to the cingulate cortex) [126] and a lateral pain system that includes the ventral posterior lateral nucleus and cortical areas SI and SII [120].

In summary, at the time of the first functional imaging studies a traditional view that pain perception had little to do with the cerebral cortex seemed questionable. Nevertheless, the evidence for a dichotomous organisation of pain pathways in the brain was not definitive, nor was the assignation of specific roles in pain perception to different somatosensory areas.

Against this background, functional imaging has provided new information to attempt resolution of these issues. Unfortunately, the results of such studies have not settled any issues definitively. The two first functional imaging studies on somatic pain were published almost simultaneously. Talbot et al. [127] studied eight subjects in two conditions. In the one case subjects received a series of heat pulses at 48 to 49°C on the volar surface of the forearm. These stimuli were described by subjects as painful but tolerable. In the control condition, stimuli were clearly warm but not painful (41 to 42°C). Twelve 5-sec heat pulses were delivered in the 2 min around each 60-sec scan. Jones et al. [128] stimulated the back of the right hand at increasing temperatures: 36.3°C was experienced as warm, 41.3°C was experienced as nonpainful hot, and 46.4°C was experienced as painful hot. These mean peak temperatures were delivered in intermittent ramps so that the peak temperature was experienced for about 5 sec. An intermittent ramp of increasing heat was delivered every 15 sec over a stimulation/scan period of 3 min.

There was only one activated area common to the two studies. In a comparison between painful hot and nonpainful hot the anterior cingulate cortex (presumed BA 24) was activated. On the other hand, several areas were activated in one study but not in the other; contralateral primary somatosensory cortex and area SII in Talbot's [127] study, contralateral thalamus and lenticular nucleus in Jones' [128] study (an activation in right prefrontal cortex was just below threshold). However, thalamus and putamen were not scanned in Talbot's [127] study, as subsequently revealed by Coghill *et al.* [100].

The differences in these results were clearly of great theoretical importance as Talbot's [127] study would suggest the existence of both medial and lateral pain systems (area SI–SII and anterior cingulate cortex) in humans, whereas Jones' [128] study suggested that a medial pain system (thalamus and anterior cingulate) would be sufficient to mediate pain perception. There were differences, however, in the study design that could explain the outcomes. The temperatures of nonpainful hot and painful hot were more closely matched in Jones' study. It is therefore possible that activation of area SI–SII observed by Talbot was due to combined warmth and pain stimulation. It was unfortunate that Jones did not report results of a comparison between painful hot and warm scans because these data could have resolved that question. Nevertheless the lack of significant activations in a comparison between nonpainful hot and warm scans suggests that activations observed in the crucial comparison are not due to the perception of a temperature difference of 5°C. On the other hand, the stimulation rate in Jones' study was slower. It has been suggested [130] that the lack of S1 activation observed by Jones could be due to temporal characteristics of their stimuli, as the neurons of area S1 (in the monkey) are now believed to encode both the temporal and spatial characteristics of innocuous [46] and noxious somatic stimuli [124].

Four subsequent studies have addressed the issues left open by Talbot *et al.* [127] and Jones *et al.* [128]. Jones' results, in particular the lack of activation of SI during pain perception, was criticised [100] because (i) studies in the monkey show a small population of SI neurons that encode the intensity of noxious thermal stimulation [121], and (ii) the stimulus intensity used by Jones *et al.* only approximated the threshold for nociceptive activity in primary somatosensory cortex (of the monkey) [121]. Therefore a follow-up study was performed with the aim of replicating the SI/SII observations. This study also addressed the issue of whether brain areas activated by painful stimuli overlap with those activated by innocuous vibro-tactile stimuli in the same subjects. Nine additional subjects were studied under the following conditions: (i) neutral 34°C (control) thermal stimulation, (ii) 47–48°C painful heat stimulation, (iii) 110 Hz vibrotactile stimulation. All stimuli were given to the left hand. As previously, pain stimulation caused an activation of contralateral SI, SII, and anterior cingulate cortex. In addition the authors were able to find activation of anterior insula bilaterally, contralateral thalamus and putamen (not scanned in their previous study), and supplementary motor area. Deactivations were observed in the posterior cingulate and orbital gyri contralaterally. The pattern of activation induced by vibrotactile stimulation was very similar to that observed with painful stimulation. In particular, the stereotactic coordinates of activation in SI were virtually identical. There were also some important discrepancies. The foci of activation in SII and in the insula were somewhat more posterior, activation in SII was bilateral, and perfusion changes in SMA, anterior cingulate, and thalamus were below the threshold of significance. It would have been interesting to know the results of a direct comparison of painful and the vibratory stimulation scans. The authors concluded that *"despite the difficulty of identifying pain-related activity in human SI cortex with lesion and stimulation methods, a contra-lateral representation of pain-related activity clearly coexists with tactile representations."* Meanwhile, Kenshalo *et al.* [129] had shown that in the monkey a complete lesion of area SI disrupts the ability to discriminate the intensity of noxious heat, and the authors speculated that human area SI may be involved in the sensory-discriminative component of pain perception. However, given the equivocal stimulation and lesion results in humans, Coghill *et al.* [100] also admit that although human area SI may have a role in pain perception, *"other regions must necessarily be activated for the full experience of pain."* A confound was still present in the study design of Coghill *et al.* [100]. The difference in temperature between painful heat and warm control stimuli was even larger than in Talbot *et al.* [117] (13–14°C as opposed to 8°C). Thus, it remains possible that some of the activations seen in this experiment are due to a large temperature difference rather than to the painful nature of the stimuli *per se*.

The issue has been reexamined by Casey *et al.* [130] who noticed the temperature confound in the 1991 studies. Nine subjects were studied with warm (40°C) or painful hot stimuli (50°C) to the volar surface of the left forearm (phase 1 experiment). In nine additional subjects (phase 2 experiment) both forearms were cooled to baseline temperatures ranging from 21 to 24°C by placing saline fluid bags on each forearm and circulating cooled water through the bags between scans. The bags were removed before stimulation began. The baseline stimulus temperature was 32°C, and the experimental stimulus temperature was 40°C. No activation was detected in the phase 2 experiment when the baseline skin temperature was manipulated. On the other hand, painful hot stimuli in the phase 1 experiment elicited activations that were consistent with Coghill's findings [100], with involvement of contra-lateral cingulate cortex, S1, insula, bilateral thalamus and SII. The authors were also able to show activation of the medial dorsal midbrain in the periac-queductal grey and in the cerebellar vermis. The contention is that these results demonstrate more convincingly than others the specificity of activation patterns due to noxious heat, because in the phase 2 study no activation was detected for nonnoxious heat stimulation of similar magnitude. However, the possibility that the higher temperature stimuli used in the pain experiment were uniquely effective in activating warm receptors surrounding the site of noxious stimulation cannot be ruled out. A similar experimental control for the temperature difference confound was also incorporated in Jones' original experiment [128] with a comparison of nonpainful hot and warm scans. The amplitude of the temperature differences was smaller (5°C) in that study.

Two more recent experiments from Jones and colleagues (Derbyshire *et al.* [131,132]) have replicated their original finding of a lack of involvement of S1 in pain perception. In one study Derbyshire *et al.* [131] used Jones' stimulation technique to deliver nonpainful hot and painful-hot stimuli to a group of six healthy women and six women affected by atypical facial pain (a chronic pain syndrome with a predominant affective component). Derbyshire *et al.* [132] also reported in an abstract that they performed two additional studies on 12 subjects with two different scanners (6 subjects for each scanner). Thermal stimuli (nonpainful and painful) were delivered, using an infrared CO_2 laser, to a circular spot measuring 1 cm in diameter on the back of the subjects' right hand. During scans a constant energy was delivered for 1 msec every 2 sec corresponding to the experiences of warm, just painful, mildly painful, and mildly–moderately painful. Activation of S1 was not observed, while anterior cingulate and prefrontal cortex activation was consistently found.

To summarise, the functional imaging studies on somatic pain have certainly achieved the result of showing that the cerebral cortex contributes to the perception of pain. This involvement occurs in a distributed manner and possibly as a result, altered pain perception is seldom observed after cortical lesions, nor is it easy to alleviate chronic pain with neurosurgical manoeuvres. The distributed nature of pain-associated cortical areas may be an explanation for the difficulties with interpretation of lesion studies in humans. No agreement has been reached about the relative importance and physiological role of the various areas activated by pain, although speculations can be formulated on the basis of metaanalyses of data. Another cause of the discrepancies between results may lie in the subtraction approach used in functional imaging studies of pain. It seems possible that subtle manipulations of stimulation parameters for subtractive comparisons will be unable to isolate individual areas sufficiently to assign specific roles to them. It is also relevant that pain perception does not come on its own, as pain elicits automatic motor withdrawal responses, which are suppressed by subjects during experiments because of explicit instructions, and involuntary vegetative responses. All these factors will influence the pattern of activation of brain regions by any painful stimuli. It is possible that correlations between perfusion measurements and psychophysical variables recorded during pain may help to further address these problems. Psychopharmacological experiments, where painful stimuli and drug administration are combined may further assist our progress in understanding more mechanistic neurochemical aspects of pain related brain function.

Like pain, itch is an unpleasant somatosensory sensation. Itch elicits an instinctive reaction to scratch that is considered analogous to the reflex withdrawal during somatic pain. Brain activations associated with itch have been studied by Hsieh *et al.* [117]. They measured activations during itch induced by injections of histamine into the lateral aspect of the right upper arm. The baseline condition involved injections of saline. Following histamine injections all subjects reported a pure sensation of itch and the presence of an urge to scratch. However, subjects were instructed to remain still during scanning. Activations were observed bilaterally in anterior cingulate, ventral and dorsal premotor cortex, SMA, prefrontal cortex, and in the inferior parietal lobule of the right hemisphere, but not in SI, SII, or thalamus. The authors propose that the anterior cingulate cortex subserves a sensation of itch and believe that the lack of activation in SI, SII, and thalamus may be ascribed to an insufficient intensity of itch elicited by their stimulation. On the other hand, they believe that activation of premotor and SMA cortices may represent the intention to move or to suppress movement given the repressed urge to scratch.

5. Visceral Pain

This is a subject that has not been explored systematically, probably because studies in this area are technically difficult. Not surprisingly, until recently most visceral pain research has been invasive in nature, employing animal models. From this research, it has become established that painful stimuli are transmitted through sympathetic afferents to the dorsal root ganglia, thence principally via the spinothalamic tracts and medial pain pathway to posterior thalamus [133,134]. A significant number of vagal fibres, connecting to the nucleus of the tractus solitarius and thence to the posterior thalamus, are also involved in the afferent conduction of painful stimuli [135]. However, beyond these facts, the central connections mediating visceral pain perception and the resulting affective responses are unclear.

Rosen *et al.* [136] studied brain activity during angina pectoris, a common clinical example of visceral pain. As for other forms of visceral pain, the central nervous pathways have not been investigated in man. Twelve patients with stable angina pectoris and angiographically proven coronary artery disease were studied during anginal pain induced by intravenous infusion of dobutamine, an inotrope drug that does not cross the blood–brain barrier and has a 2.4-min half-life. All subjects experienced typical retrosternal chest pain accompanied by ischemic electrocardiographic changes during dobutamine infusion. Compared to the resting state, angina was associated with activation in the hypothalamus, periaquaductal grey, bilaterally in the thalamus, lateral prefrontal cortex, and left inferior anterocaudal cingulate cortex (BA 25). In contrast, there were bilateral deactivations in the mid-rostrocaudal cingulate cortex, fusiform gyrus, right posterior cingulate, and left parietal cortices. Several minutes after stopping dobutamine infusion, when the patients no longer experienced angina and the electrocardiographic changes had resolved, thalamic, but not cortical activation was still present. The authors proposed that the central structures activated constitute the pathways for perception of anginal pain. In addition, they speculated that the thalamus may act as a gate to afferent pain signals, with cortical activation being necessary for the sensation of pain.

There were a number of commonalities between these findings and those for somatic pain [130]—bilateral (as opposed to unilateral) thalamic activation and activation of the periaqueductal grey. However, there were also important differences that appear to be specific for visceral pain. During angina Rosen *et al.* [136] observed activations of the hypothalamus and, perhaps more importantly, activation of a totally different portion of the cingulate cortex than with somatic pain. The inferior anterocaudal cingulate cortex (BA 25) is a region that in the rat has documented connections to the nucleus of the solitary tract [137], dorsal motor nucleus of the vagus and to the sympathetic thoracic intermediolateral cell column [138]. Another difference between visceral and somatic pain was the activation of orbito-frontal cortex bilaterally. Rosen *et al.* [136] have proposed that the topographical differences in the activation of cingulate cortex between somatic and visceral pain may represent somatotopic differences in the pain pathways. Importantly, the area of the cingulate gyrus that activates during somatic pain was, if anything, deactivated during angina. This observation reinforces the specificity of the observations in both sets of studies.

Rosen's experiment was performed using pharmacological stress. Accordingly, the findings are potentially confounded with the generic effects of the drug. To control for this potential confound, the authors measured perfusion during an infusion of a dose of dobutamine that was insufficient to cause angina. Under these circumstances no activation was observed in the regions described above. Nevertheless, an objection is that the activations were due to dose-dependent specific and nonspecific pharmacological effects. A better experimental test of these assumptions has come from a subsequent study where the same paradigm was applied to patients who do not perceive pain during myocardial ischemia for unknown reasons [139]. Diabetic patients were excluded in order to minimise the risk that silent myocardial ischemia was due to peripheral nerve disease. During scans with injections of high doses of dobutamine, patients affected by silent myocardial ischemia had typical ischemic changes on ECG and also heart wall motion abnormalities revealed by echocardiography. In spite of this, none of the patients perceived pain. Under such circumstances, both thalami were activated but cortical activation was limited to a small region of the right frontal cortex. A formal comparison of the angina and silent ischemia groups revealed that activations in the angina group were significantly greater in the basal frontal cortex and the ventral cingulate cortex. On the basis of these findings Rosen *et al.* [139] suggest that, since in both angina and silent ischemia bilateral activation of the thalamus can be shown, peripheral nerve dysfunction cannot offer a complete explanation for silent ischemia. More importantly for our understanding of the basis of visceral pain perception, those cortical activations that appeared specific for ischemic cardiac pain appear necessary for the sensation of pain. In addition, this study suggests that the original findings could not be merely due to a pharmacological effect.

6. Kinesthesia and Proprioception

These are aspects of somatosensory sensation that await systematic exploration. We are aware of only one functional imaging activation study in which the effect of passive finger movements was explored. Preliminary results have been reported by Krams *et al.* [140]. The hypothesis that cortico-spinal neurons fire during passive movements was tested, an observation previously reported in monkeys [141]. Two subjects were studied during passive opposition of thumb and index finger of the right hand. During rest the investigator held the index finger and thumb of the subject's right hand without moving them. One subject was scanned during active finger–thumb opposition of the right hand as well. As expected, active finger movement produced a highly significant activation of the contralateral primary motor and sensory cortex. However, the same activation was also observed during passive finger movements. EMG recordings confirmed that voluntary motor activity occurred only during active finger–thumb movements. The authors conclude that *"activation in primary motor cortex may partly reflect synaptic activity related to afferent sensory feedback."* They also suggest that *"to interpret activation in the primary motor cortex correctly, appropriate controls for afferent sensory activation should be applied."*

B. Complex Somatosensory Functions

1. Texture and Shape Discrimination

Texture and shape discrimination are stages of somatosensory perception that combine to enable tactile object discrimination. Object recognition based on (micro)geometric features has been studied by Ginsberg and colleagues [142] in 10 subjects during rest and during a sensory-motor object discrimination task. Both regional cerebral blood flow (rCBF) and regional cerebral glucose consumption were measured. The activation task was the palpation and sorting of mah-jong tiles. Subjects were asked to discriminate by palpation among three classes of mah-jong tile; those inscribed with (1) either one or more lines, (2) one or more cycles or, (3) a Chinese character. Scanning was performed during rest and object discrimination. There were three areas in the hemisphere contralateral to the sorting hand activated in both sets of measurements; (primary) sensorimotor, superior parietal, and medial temporal cortices. With measurement of glucose consumption there were also two areas activated in the ipsilateral hemisphere; somatosensory and medial temporal cortices. Given the experimental design, however, these findings do not distinguish activations due simply to the motor aspects of the task from those related to the somatosensory perceptual aspects.

A study of brain correlates of sensory discrimination of micro- and macrogeometric attributes of objects has been reported by Roland and collaborators in brain damaged patients [45] and in normal subjects [143–145]. Microgeometry refers to small variations on an object's surface that do not alter the shape of the object itself. Roughness is one of the sensory attributes that we perceive as a result of microgeometric features of objects. Macrogeometric features of objects define their size and shape. It is currently thought that microgeometric features are appreciated through rapidly adapting Pacinian skin receptors and broad-band receptors in general. This point of view was argued by Roland and Mortensen [146] on the basis of a dynamic analysis of the palpation velocity of roughness stimuli. On the other hand, shape and length discrimination should depend on slowly adapting (narrow band) cutaneous receptors with small receptive fields. Roland [45] has suggested that lesions in the parietal operculum interfere with discrimination of roughness, whereas discrimination of length and shape is disturbed by lesions in the anterior parts of the parietal lobules. This dichotomy, together with the psychophysical dissociation between broad-band and narrow-band receptors was seen by O'Sullivan and colleagues [143] as analogous to the parvocellular/magnocellular dichotomy observed in the visual system. The authors therefore decided to explore whether it was possible to demonstrate the same dichotomy in normal subjects and to test the hypothesis that, beyond area SI, appreciation of microgeometric features would depend on different somatosensory areas than those for shape discrimination. The functional imaging experiment involved three exploratory conditions using the right hand; (1) a two-alternative forced choice discrimination task of tactile roughness of cylinders of well characterised stimulus energies, (2) a similar forced choice discrimination task for smooth cylinders of different lengths, (3) a baseline state in which subjects performed exploratory finger movements but without a stimulus to feel [143]. That particular baseline task was adopted to control for sensory feedback from joint receptors and muscle spindles. Both experimental tasks activated the anterior and posterior lips of the contralateral post-central sulcus with an extension of the activation focus backwards up to putative BA 2 and BA 5. Activation of the postcentral sulcus, over and above that in the exploratory finger motion task, was interpreted as the result of a contribution from subcomponents of area SI (BA 3b and 1) that in the monkey are more concerned with touch than with proprioceptive stimulation. However, the length discrimination task induced additional activations in the left supramarginal gyrus, in the angular gyri bilaterally, and in the left premotor cortex. These additional activations in the length discrimination task were interpreted as the result of a different sampling strategy. Hence, the areas activated by roughness discrimination were a subset of those activated by the shape discrimination task, and therefore it was not possible to demonstrate any functional separation between the central projections of broad-band and narrow-band receptors. However, the possibility cannot be excluded that a double dissociation between these projections was not found because the experimental stimuli were not pure enough to stimulate selectively one of the two classes of receptors.

To the authors' surprise, no activation was observed in any of the comparisons between scans in the parietal operculum, including human area SII, in spite of pathological evidence that roughness discrimination is impaired following lesions in that area. Nevertheless, in two subsequent papers [144,145], the same group reported finding an activation in the parietal operculum for microgeometric discrimination using exactly the same tasks as above.

2. Tactile Object Learning and Recognition

The anatomical foundations of tactile learning in monkeys have been the focus of extensive research by Mishkin and his colleagues [95]. He proposed the existence of an anatomical pathway that mediates tactile memory from SI and SII to the limbic structures of the temporal lobe, hippocampus and amygdala, through the insula [147]. This (serially) organised pathway is analogous to a visual learning pathway that accesses the limbic structures of the temporal lobe through inferior temporal cortex [86].

There is only one functional imaging experiment where tactile learning has been studied in humans. Roland *et al.* [148] described changes in regional cerebral oxidative metabolism induced by tactile learning and recognition. Normal subjects were scanned during rest, tactile learning, and tactile recognition of complicated geometrical objects. Learning and recognition were performed with the right hand. The recognition task involved frequency of exploratory movements that was twice that of tactile learning. Given the complexities of measuring oxygen metabolism, a sample population of 20 subjects was needed to cover all experimental condition pairs. Six subjects were scanned during learning and rest, six subjects were scanned during recognition and rest, eight subjects were scanned during learning and recognition. The areas activated during the experimental tasks were very similar; prefrontal and premotor cortex bilaterally, the left anterior superior parietal lobule, the supplementary motor area bilaterally, the left primary motor and somatosensory area, the anterior insula bilaterally, the lingual gyri, the hippocampus, basal ganglia, anterior parasagittal cerebellum, and the posterior lobule of the cerebellum. There were few differences. Left premotor cortex, SMA, and M1/S1 were more active during the recognition task, a finding confounded by the different rates of exploratory movement. During learning, activation in the neocerebellar cortex was greater than during recognition. On the basis of these findings, Roland and colleagues [148] suggested that the anatomical organization of tactile learning in humans is similar to that of primates [95].

C. Selective Attention and Somatosensory Stimulation

The term attention is used to describe many different phenomena. A dichotomy that is commonly used to classify attentional processes is the one between global and selective attention. The concept of global attention is similar to the concepts of arousal and vigilance [149]. Its relevance to functional imaging studies of somatosensory perception is marginal and therefore global attention will not be discussed further.

Several different cognitive theories exist about the way selective attention is organized (for reviews, see Refs. [150–153]). Selective attention has been seen as a mechanism whose function is to filter irrelevant from relevant stimuli for perception; such filters may operate at early or later stages in the chain of neural events that lead to perception [154,155]. Others [150] put less emphasis on the filtering functions of attention and see it as a facilitatory mechanism that gives (perceptual) prominence to attended or cued stimuli like the beam of a spotlight which highlights a target. It has been argued [153] that such a model implies the existence of a separate, anatomically specific, circuit that controls attention [156,157]. A further theory proposes selective attention as a mechanism that is necessary, and therefore functionally closer, to selection for action [158]. In its anatomical formulation, this model is called the premotor theory of attention [153,159] and postulates that facilitation of perception to attended stimuli is the result of the activation of circuits responsible for motor preparation. Such a model [153] is very much against the concept of attention as a central processing (amodal) system, as predicted by cognitive psychologists [160].

Further discussion of these theories appears elsewhere in this book. This brief introduction puts into context this review of functional imaging experiments on somatosensory perception. However, functional anatomical studies of attention to sensory stimuli have been used to support one or other of the above theories. Indeed, the studies on selective and divided visual attention by Corbetta et al. [161] have been interpreted in different ways. Posner et al. [157] have seen the results as strongly supportive of his theories of selective attention, while Rizzolatti and Berti [153] see the Corbetta et al. data as clear evidence against the concept of an autonomous and unitary (anatomical) system for attention.

There seems to be little controversy about the fact that association cortices have neurons with "attentional" properties. Neurophysiological studies in primates have shown that attentional association cortices (e.g., posterior parietal cortex) show increased firing when an animal is attending to a location where a visual stimulus may appear, even before the generation of saccades toward a stimulus location [162,163]. Something similar occurs in area 7b, where increased firing is observed when an animal is attending to a tactile stimulus [110].

More controversial is the behavior of primary somatosensory cortex in relation to attention. In Hyvärinen's [164] experiment, microelectrode recordings were performed in awake monkeys that were instructed to (a) attend and respond to vibratory stimuli delivered to the hand or (b) to ignore the same stimulation. Only a small proportion (16%) of neurons in area SI had enhanced responses to vibrotactile stimuli because of attention. In particular, the proportion of "attentive" neurons was highest in area 1 and minimal in area 3b, where the thalamic input is more direct. A laminar analysis of the location of the cells studied showed that the attentive neurons were located in layers I, II, and VI, suggesting the involvement of nonspecific noradrenergic or nicotinic cholinergic terminals, rather than specific thalamo-cortical afferents to layer IV.

In a more recent experiment on one monkey by Hsiao et al. [165], a different paradigm that involved active distraction of the monkey during a baseline condition was used. In an experimental condition the monkey was instructed to detect, by touch, letters presented with an embossed rotating cylindrical drum. The monkey responded to a given letter whenever it appeared on a screen at the same time. In a baseline task, the monkey was stimulated with the same rotating drum, but this time it had to detect the dimming of a spotlight on a screen. Under these circumstances, Hsiao et al. [165] found that the number of activated neurons in SI during the experimental condition was 80%. Hsiao *et al.* attributed the different outcome of their experiment (80% activated neurons in SI as opposed to 16% activated neurons of Hyvärinen *et al.* [164]) to active distraction in the baseline condition. No assessment of the laminar distribution of activated neurons is available in Hsiao's paper [165].

In humans, the study of neural mechanisms underlying enhanced signal processing due to attention has been a focus of few somatosensory functional imaging experiments. Meyer *et al.* [166] studied whether attention can modulate the activity of primary somatosensory cortex during vibratory stimulation. The authors tested the hypothesis that SI may show increased activation because of attentional set. In their experiment, eight subjects were scanned during (1) rest, (2) simple vibratory stimulation to the fingertips, (3) vibratory stimulation to the fingertips while subjects were instructed to detect a change in frequency and pressure, (4) vibratory stimulation to the fingertips while subjects performed an arithmetic task, (5) an arithmetic task only. During task 3 no actual changes were made to the stimuli so that any change of activity due to this task could be attributed to attentional phenomena. As expected, vibratory stimulation, compared with rest, revealed activation of SI. While no significant additional activation of SI was observed in task 3 compared with task 2, a significant difference was observed in the "attention" task compared to task 4, the distractor task. The authors speculated that their data were consistent with those of Hyvärinen *et al.* [164]. The analysis of data for this study was constrained to area SI, so that no information is available about any contribution of other areas to the attentional set in task 3.

Two further experiments have studied the functional correlates of attentional set in the absence of actual somatosensory stimulation. Such studies may have relevance for understanding how the brain increases the neural signal to noise ratio. Unfortunately, the results are in profound disagreement. In a nontomographic xenon-133 study, Roland [167] investigated perfusion changes due to anticipation of somatosensory stimulation. Subjects were instructed to direct their attention toward the tip of an index finger and to count the number of touches received over a 50-sec period of scanning. No touches were actually delivered. An activation was described by Roland in the contralateral hand somatosensory area, in the middle and inferior frontal gyrii and in association somatosensory cortex corresponding to the intraparietal sulcus. A similar increase in the face area was observed when subjects attended to touches to the right upper lip.

Roland [115] suggests that activation of the SI complex during attention to an anticipated stimulus cannot be due to an increase in the number of action potentials. He proposed that activation in the hand area could be due to increases of local excitatory postsynaptic (EPSPs) potentials. Such increases would put pyramidal cells in area SI in a readiness state so that even a few stimuli from the periphery would trigger neuronal firing.

In a more recent paper Drevets *et al.* [168] have monitored changes of brain activity in SI and SII while expecting a somatosensory stimulus. Three experiments are reported with expected stimulation of the toe (experiment 1), the index and middle finger (experiment 2) and the face (experiment 3). The expected stimuli were a light touch with a Von Frey's hair for experiment 1, an electric shock for experiment 2, and contact with a threatening animal (snake or tarantula) for experiment 3. As in Roland's experiment, no actual stimulation was delivered. However, contrary to the activation of SI seen by Roland [167], specific parts of SI, representing the body parts to which expected stimuli were to be applied, showed neither activations nor deactivations. In addition, highly significant deactivations were seen in parts of the primary somatosensory cortex outside the area of representation of the body to which the expected stimuli were to be applied. For example, when expecting electric shocks to the index and middle fingers, there were deactivations in the mouth and foot areas of SI. This finding is interpreted by Drevets and colleagues as a mechanism of signal enhancement based on inhibition of background activity. Similar gating of sensory cortical activity has been observed in animal models. Drevets (1995) also suggests that this background inhibition may be a basis for the poorer perceptual performance with stimuli that occur in locations other than those where subjects are focusing their attention.

Drevets *et al.* [168] also report detecting a lateral premotor activation during experiment 2 at the level of the hand area. They suggest that this activation may represent an anticipatory premotor response/plan to the expected painful stimulus. They also argue that the activation seen by Roland [167] with a nontomographic technique may represent activation of premotor rather than somatosensory cortex.

On the basis of these preliminary studies it is clearly premature to attempt any correlation of human physiological data and cognitive models of attention. Further studies are needed to address the issue of which of the cognitive models finds greater support in human physiology. Drevets' [168] study is useful in making the point that functional imaging will provide new challenges to existing models of attention. His data could be used to support more than one theory of attention. Inhibition of somatosensory maps at unattended locations could be seen as the operation of a filter mechanism; premotor activation could be viewed as support for a selection for action theory. If both filtering and premotor mechanisms are important for attention, a model that blends them into an integrated new model would probably have better explanatory value than each alone.

Finally, it is important to mention a study on sustained attention by Pardo *et al.* [106]. Subjects monitored short pauses in a volley of suprathreshold touches to a left or right toe. Other subjects monitored changes in luminance of a spotlight. A dominance for these forms of sustained attention was demonstrated for the right hemisphere in prefrontal and parietal cortex, whatever the side of tactile stimulation or type of stimulation modality (tactile or visual). Surprisingly, activity in primary somatosensory cortex did not change significantly. A right hemisphere dominance for sustained attention may help to explain the prevalence of hemianaesthesic symptoms due to damage to the right hemisphere [66].

VI. BRAIN MAPPING STUDIES OF THE VESTIBULAR SYSTEM AND ITS INTERACTIONS WITH MENTAL REPRESENTATIONS OF THE BODY

A. The Vestibular System and the Perception of Body and Space: Normality and Pathological Findings with Reference to Unilateral Neglect and Hemianaesthesia

The vestibular system plays a crucial role in monitoring the position of the head in space. This function is essential for proper posture and balance and to keep a given direction of gaze while the head is moving. The peripheral receptors of the vestibular system are located in the membranous inner ear which consists of two otolith organs, the utricule and the saccule, and three semicircular canals which are perpendicular one to the other and oriented to describe three orthogonal planes with reference to the pyramid of the temporal bone. The utricle and the saccule are sensitive to linear acceleration and gravity. The receptors of the semicircular canals are sensitive to angular accelerations of the head in space. The vestibular receptors convey information to four distinct vestibular nuclei in the brain stem and to the cerebellum through the vestibular portion of the eighth cranial nerve. The vestibular nuclei in the brain stem are connected with the nuclei that control the extraocular muscles. These anatomical connections allow the vestibular system to play a special role in visual fixation on a target in space while the head is moving. A review of the anatomy and physiology of vestibular receptors, nerve, and nuclei is outside the scope of this chapter. For an overview on this subject, see Kelly [169].

Any unusual stimulation of the vestibular system, such as caloric stimulation with cold water in the external ear, induces in normal people a degree of dizziness and vertigo, a tonic deviation of gaze towards the stimulated side and profound spatial misperception [170]. The last symptom is evident if subjects are asked to point towards the centre of space with their eyes closed. Under conditions of cold caloric stimulation, pointing is shifted towards the stimulated side.

Conversely, the same stimulation may transiently reverse the unilateral neglect syndrome. Neglect is a quite common neuropsychological condition mostly associated with right hemispheric lesions, mainly characterised by an inability or difficulty to attend and respond to stimuli coming from contra-lesional space [171]. These difficulties cannot be ascribed to sensory or motor deficits. A patient suffering from unilateral neglect frequently has the head and/or gaze rotated to the right side of space. A common test used to reveal visuo-spatial neglect is Albert's line cancellation test [172] in which subjects are asked to cross out lines distributed on a sheet of paper. A patient with unilateral neglect, when challenged with Albert's test, is unable to cross out stimuli on the left side of the display. Other typical symptoms of unilateral neglect are the inability to read the left side of a word or to draw the left side of objects (for a review, see Halligan and Marshall [173]). Unilateral neglect is also associated with other cognitive symptoms; anosoagnosia (denial of illness) for left hemiplegia or hemianopia; somatoparaphrenia, a delusional disturbance usually characterised by the feeling of nonbelonging of the left paralysed limb; hemisomatoagnosia, the inability to touch a paralysed hand with the healthy hand (for a review, see Bisiach and Berti [174]).

In addition, neglect patients may show a representational (or mental imagery) deficit for left sided space that can be easily revealed by asking patients to describe from memory a well known place from a particular view-point [175]. Finally, unilateral neglect is also associated with more basic neurological deficits such as hemiplegia and hemianaesthesia.

Different theories of neglect postulate impairments at different signal processing levels; integration of sensory inputs [176], attentional processing [171,177,178], inner representation of space [174], and premotor planning [159].

In 1985 Rubens was the first to show the positive effect of cold caloric vestibular stimulation (CVS) on a group of neglect patients [179]. The dramatic effect of CVS was shown with the Albert line cancellation test. Following cold CVS to the left ear, patients significantly improved and crossed out left sided stimuli that were previously neglected. The effect lasted for about 5 min. It is noteworthy that he also observed a worsening of the syndrome following similar stimulation in the right ear. Rubens' interpretation of the phenomenon was that vestibular stimulation could transiently overcome spatial neglect on the basis of the peripheral oculo-vestibular reflex that provokes eye deviation towards neglected space.

However, further studies have shown that CVS may also induce a temporary remission of cognitive symptoms that cannot be easily ascribed to a lack of visual exploration, for example, hemisomatoagnosia, anosoagnosia, somatoparaphrenia, and deficits in mental imagery tasks [180–182]. In addition, CVS may transiently improve basic neurological deficits such as tactile hemianaesthesia [183]. Following an observation made on a single case, Vallar and colleagues (1993) explored the effect of left cold CVS systematically in a group of right brain damaged patients with left tactile hemianaesthesia, the majority of whom also had left unilateral neglect [184]. The authors replicated their original observation of significant improvement of left tactile imperception immediately after left CVS. The same effect was present in two patients who showed no other signs of unilateral neglect. A control group of left brain damaged patients was also studied. No positive effect was reported on right hemianaesthesia after right cold CVS with the remarkable exception of two patients suffering from right unilateral neglect. These results concur to suggest that an attentional component may underlie left tactile imperception and that CVS can transiently modulate this cognitive aspect of conscious perception. It is also important to note that hemianaesthesia was associated with a variety of lesions, all of which can also be associated with unilateral neglect. However, in right brain damaged patients there was no lesion site that prevented an ameliorating effect of vestibular stimulation. This observation allowed us to predict that the interaction between CVS and symptoms associated with neglect must occur in a distributed neural system, parts of which are spared by the lesion, rather than in a single critical brain area, and therefore that there should be multiple vestibular projections above the brain stem. In addition, as CVS can modulate cognitive symptoms (*e.g.*, somatoparaphrenia), we also predicted that these projections should reach the cerebral cortex. To summarise, there is a rich pattern of interactions between activity in the vestibular system, body and space perception in normal subjects, and the symptoms of unilateral neglect.

The neurophysiological bases of such interactions were unexplored until recently. We will review here the results of a series of our own functional neuroimaging experiments that were performed (a) to identify the central vestibular projections in humans, (b) to study the overlap of such projections with the central projections of the somatosensory system, and (c) to characterise the interaction between these two systems in a patient with left hemianaesthesia.

B. The Positron Emission Tomography Activation Technique: Special Issues Relating to Vestibular Stimulation Experiments

Categorical activation studies are performed by comparing the distribution of perfusion during control and experimental conditions. There are different ways of delivering the radiotracer used to measure blood flow. Understanding of these differences is fundamental to interpreting the results of a PET activation study. Each method has a particular time window within which brain activity can be recorded. There are three main techniques: the autoradiographic fast-bolus technique [185,186], the slow-bolus technique [187], and the build-up infusion technique [188]. The first method is probably mostly sensitive to stimulation occurring from the moment of tracer injection to when the activity recorded by the scanner reaches its peak, *i.e.,* approximately 10 sec after the initial arrival of the radiotracer in the brain. The build-up infusion technique allows delivery of stimuli for 2 minutes while radioactivity is progressively accumulating in the brain [107,188]. The slow-bolus method, which was used in the experiments described below, has a 30-sec window for the detection of brain events, which starts from the arrival of the radiotracer in the brain, until activity peaks. It has been shown that stimulation occurring before the arrival of radiotracer in the head, or after activity peaks, does not contribute significantly to the differential signals recorded in scans [187]. In vestibular stimulation experiments, 30 sec of stimulation with cold water was stopped 10 sec before the beginning of scanning which coincided with arrival of radioactivity in the head. Therefore, tactile and nociceptive components of caloric stimulation did not contaminate the scan signal as the method is blind to brain activity occurring before the arrival of blood flow tracer in the brain [187]. The scan thus captured brain activity caused only by vestibular symptoms that come on after a short delay from the start of caloric stimulation and persist for 1 minute or so after it ceases [170].

C. Identification of the Cerebral Vestibular Projections in Humans

Penfield [189] produced vertiginous sensations following the stimulation of superior temporal cortex near primary auditory cortex. This isolated observation suggested the existence of a vestibular cortex. Using functional imaging techniques an early attempt to identify the cerebral projections of the vestibular system was made by Friberg and colleagues [190]. They used a nontomographic xenon-133 inhalation technique. In that study a significant activation was observed in the temporal region, but, given the limitations of the technique no better mapping of brain activity was achieved. In order to better characterise the cerebral vestibular projections in humans we performed a series of activation experiments combined with MRI information to optimise anatomical localisation [108,191].

Six right handed normal males underwent 12 scans, 6 immediately after left cold caloric vestibular stimulation and 6 in the absence of such stimulation. During scanning subjects' eyes were closed and they were asked to point with the right index finger towards the centre, left, or right side of space, as instructed by the examiner. Pointing was paced by the examiner at a rate of 18 movements for each scan. The frequency of pointing was the same across nonstimulated and stimulated conditions. After each movement subjects returned to a resting position, with the right hand on the middle of the sternum. A protractor was fixed to the scanner bed to measure the angle of pointing. Measures of pointing angle from the centre were used to detect significant shifts induced by CVS.

CVS was performed by pouring 30 cm³ of iced water into the external ear since this is the most effective way of inducing a remission of symptoms associated with unilateral neglect. The procedure was discontinued 10 sec before radioactivity arrived in the brain. The effects of vestibular stimulation were assessed in all subjects immediately after each scan. A slow phase of nystagmus towards the left was detected clinically. Subjects also reported different degrees of dizziness and vertigo. None of the volunteers experienced pain during stimulation. A significant deviation of pointing angle was found (pointing in the absence of CVS, 0.717 cm towards the right of the midline; pointing after CVS, 7.75 cm towards the left; Wilcoxon Signed Rank Test, $P = 0.014$).

To be sure that the activations induced by left CVS were related to specific central modulation of a distributed vestibular system and not to a nonspecific attentional effect due to the strongly lateralised stimulus, we performed a second experiment. We investigated the central effects of CVS further by stimulating the right ear in six subjects. The expected rightward slow phase of nystagmus was seen in all of them. A significant shift towards the right side of space was evident during the pointing task (pointing in the absence of CVS = 0.350 cm towards the right; pointing after CVS = 5.25 cm towards the right; Wilcoxon Signed Rank Test, $P = 0.023$).

The results of these two experiments (group analyses) are presented in Fig. 9. Left CVS induced activation in the right temporo-parietal junction, in posterior insula, transverse temporal gyrus, putamen, anterior cingulate cortex, and in right primary sensory cortex (SI). Stereotactic anatomical coordinates for these regions and their assigned Brodmann areas are reported elsewhere [108]. CVS in the right ear induced activation of the same anatomical structures but in the left hemisphere (Fig. 9). There was also significant activation of the right insula. Analysis of data from single subjects confirmed the accuracy of anatomical assignations made on the basis of group analyses [108].

D. Identification of the Cerebral Vestibular Projections in Humans: Further Studies

In our experiments subjects performed a pointing task during both the vestibular and the nonvestibular scans [108]. Observation of a significant shift of pointing direction towards a stimulated side constituted behavioural evidence of spatial misperception induced by CVS. In order to exclude the possibility that results were biased by an intrinsic interaction between CVS and the pointing task, a further experiment was carried out in three normal volunteers in which left CVS was compared with rest. The CVS procedure was the same as previously and subjects' eyes were closed. A slow phase of nystagmus towards the left was seen after each vestibular scan. Subjects reported that vestibular scans were associated with dizziness and vertigo. Six scans were collected per condition and the order of the two experimental conditions was counterbalanced. Activations due to left CVS were very similar to those previously described (Fig. 10), bilaterally distributed in the insula/temporal cortex and putamen, though the number of activated voxels above threshold was three times greater in the right than the left hemisphere. In this data set we were also able to see an activation focus in right ventral premotor cortex, cerebellar vermis, and the mesial aspect of the left posterior thalamus.

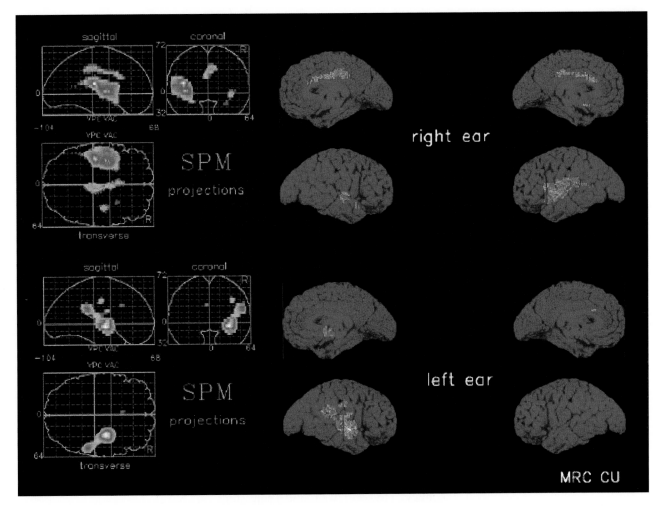

Figure 9 Cerebral regions activated by right and left cold caloric vestibular stimulation (CVS). (Left) The locations of activations associated with cold CVS are shown as integrated projections along sagittal, coronal, and transverse views of the brain. The axial extent of the data set is defined by lines in the sagittal view. Stereotactic coordinates for the activated areas and their significance levels are published elsewhere [104]. (Right) The same areas of activation are rendered onto the lateral and mesial surfaces of the cortex of the brain used by Talairach and Tournoux [118] to illustrate the distribution of the major sites of activation. The magnitude of activation in the cingulate cortex appears to be greater for cold CVS in the right ear than that seen in the left. However, the spatial extent of this activation was comparable at a slightly lower significance threshold ($P < 0.001$).

E. Central Vestibular Projections: Cross-Correlation of Functional Imaging Studies with Nonhuman Primate Data

In monkeys, the brain area that has been most consistently involved with the vestibular system is retroinsular cortex (parieto-insular vestibular cortex-PIVC) to which anatomical vestibular projections have been found [192] and in which neurons that behave like polymodal vestibular units have been demonstrated [193,194]. Our data implicate this area in man also.

A vestibular projection has also been reported in macaque parietal area 2 at the tip of the intraparietal sulcus [195] and in the anterior parietal area

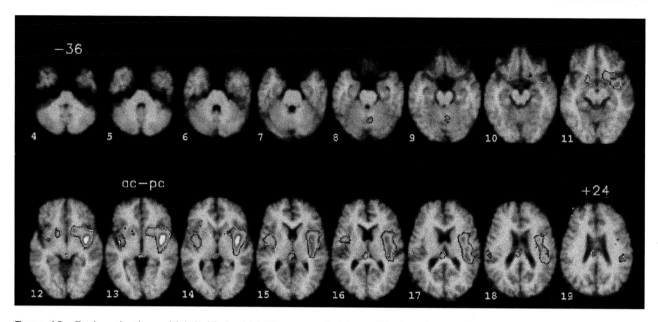

FIGURE 10 Brain activations with left sided cold CVS compared with rest. The locations of activations associated with left cold CVS are shown as SPM{*t*} maps (coloured areas) overlapped on an MRI template from all subjects in transaxial slices in stereotactic anatomical space. Only voxels over $P < 0.05$ threshold for significance, corrected for multiple comparisons, are displayed. Numbers refer to the distance in millimetres of the transaxial images from the intercommissural (ac–pc) plane. Slice thickness is 4 mm. The description of the anatomical location of the activated areas is given in the text.

3aV [196], which is located in the central sulcus. In addition vestibular fields have been described in parietal area 7 of the macaque inferior parietal lobule [197]. Our data do not permit identification of separate homologues for every parietal vestibular area described in monkeys. However, we found a consistent focus of activation in primary somatosensory cortex near the central sulcus (stereotactic coordinates—right SI: $x = 36$, $y = -12$, $z = 36$; and left SI: $x = -40$, $y = -20$, $z = 24$) (see Fig. 9). Given the relationship to the central sulcus, we propose that the primary somatosensory cortex activation may correspond to area 3aV. We also suggest that a consistent focus of activation seen in the supramarginal gyrus [Brodmann area (BA) 40] corresponds to the vestibular field in area 7b described by Faugier-Grimaud and Ventre [197] as human BA 40 is, for other reasons, a good candidate homologue for macaque area 7b (for a discussion, see Passingham [198, pp. 245–246].

Our experiments also show that other areas contribute to the vestibular cortical network. In the first place, the cortex of the posterior half of the superior temporal gyrus (BA 22/42) and transverse temporal gyrus (BA 21/41) are areas where neurophysiological stimulation in man can evoke vertiginous sensations [189]. The presence of vestibular neurons in these regions is also confirmed by the lesion mapping study of Brandt *et al.* [80]. Recently Grüsser and co-workers [199] reported that the anterior cingulate projects directly into the brainstem vestibular nuclear complex, and Munari and co-workers have observed vertiginous sensations after electrocortical stimulation of the anterior cingulate in epileptic patients during stereotactic surgery (C. Munari, personal communication). We found a consistent activation focus in the anterior cingulate cortex. Finally, in the CVS *versus* rest contrast, we also observed activation of ventral premotor cortex in BA 6. This finding is corroborated by recent observations in the squirrel monkey made by Guldin *et al.* [200]. An entire group of thalamic nuclei that receives vestibular projections has been identified in the squirrel monkey [201]. Different vestibular cortical areas receive inputs from discrete nuclei of the ventro-posterior complex and from the medial pulvinar. The results of a neurosurgical retrospective study suggest the existence of a vestibulo-thalamic projection in man [202]. A consistent thalamic signal was not found in our experiments. However, thalamic signals were seen occasionally in single subjects [108] notably in a posterior medial thalamic vestibular area that appears to be in the pulvinar. This result would be consistent with observations of vestibular syndromes in patients with thalamic lesions (for a short review, see the discussion in Brandt *et al.*, [80]).

Our results also consistently implicate the putamen as a projection site of the vestibular system. We are not aware of previous experiments in the monkey demonstrating vestibular projections to the putamen (see, however, the following section).

F. Central Vestibular Projections: Cross-Correlation of Functional Imaging Studies with Human Lesional Studies

The transient nature of vestibular symptoms has contributed to a long-standing belief that there are no projections of the vestibular system to cerebral cortex. Nevertheless, Brandt *et al.* [80] performed a lesion mapping study in patients with altered perception of verticality, a sign of static vestibular dysfunction in the roll plane. Consistent with our functional imaging findings in normal subjects they found areas of maximum overlap of lesions in the insula and putamen (Fig. 3 in Brandt *et al.* (1994); areas indicated in black). Although the function of the putamen is unclear, observations in patients with Parkinson's disease (which is associated with atrophy of the putamen) suggest a role for this structure in the control of movement and posture. The putamen receives inputs from sensorimotor cortex and the visual system [203] and is involved in a number of anatomically defined motor circuits. Our results suggest that it may well receive inputs from the vestibular system also and thus have a specific role in directing movement through space. Finally, activation of the putamen has been reported in a recent fMRI study of the vestibular pathways using caloric vestibular stimulation [204].

G. Where Is the Primary Vestibular Area and What Is the Function of Other Vestibular Areas?

While experiments performed in man have shown a network of cortical areas that can be compared with those receiving vestibular projections in primates, identification of any hierarchy amongst these areas is beyond our current data. Microelectrode recordings in the primate brain suggest that neurons in all the areas fire not only in response to vestibular stimuli, but also in response to somatosensory and optokinetic stimuli (see Guldin *et al.* [200]). Friberg *et al.* [190] proposed that the postacoustic superior temporal cortex is the primary human vestibular area [190]. Maybe this proposal was based on the fact that only one area was resolved using the planar xenon-133 scanning technique used. Clearly, this suggestion is not supported by more recent data in which the pattern of activation is far more complex.

There are technical limitations that prevent us from addressing the hierarchy issue in man with current functional imaging techniques. Neither PET nor fMRI have sufficient temporal or spatial resolution. In theory, good temporal resolution would allow tracking of activity from a primary vestibular area to associative areas. Noninvasive physiological techniques such as magnetoencephalography (MEG) have sufficient time resolution, but MEG lacks the necessary spatial resolution. If ways could be found to combine the information from PET (or fMRI) and MEG, this issue may become more tractable.

On the other hand, there are anatomical criteria that could be used to address this problem in primates. By analogy with visual cortex, there are patterns of cortical layer organisation associated with forward projections from primary to associative areas and reverse projections from associative to primary sensory cortex [28,29]. If analogues could be found in the vestibular cortices of primate brains, a pivotal primary vestibular cortex might be identifiable. Some evidence along these lines has been found in the squirrel monkey by Guldin *et al.* [200], who suggest that a feedforward pathway may exist from area 3aV to area Ri (the squirrel monkey analogue of macaque PIVC). Even these anatomical criteria may not be straightforward as discussed by Guldin *et al.* [200].

In summary, a hypothesis generated from a synthesis of the clinical and functional mapping data is that the human network of cortical vestibular areas can be accessed in parallel, by multiple vestibular afferent pathways, with or without subcortical relays or feedback.

Definitive attributions of discrete computational functions to the various human vestibular areas is also not possible from the present data. Brandt *et al.* [80] associated lesions of a large number of perisylvian areas to the misperception of verticality in the roll plane. This is a transient symptom with recovery that suggests that other areas can compensate for the spatial misperception. Activation studies in which CVS is combined with spatial awareness tasks could, in principle, contribute to the issue of functional specialisation within vestibular cortices. We are not aware of any such studies for the moment.

H. Deactivations during Caloric Vestibular Stimulation

In all our CVS experiments we observed a rich pattern of deactivations (see also Fig. 5 in Bottini *et al.* [191]). Relative deactivations were mostly localised to extrastriate visual cortex of the occipital and temporal lobes and were larger ipsilateral to the side of cold CVS. It is noteworthy that in the left hemisphere relative deactivation was found in an area of the human V5 complex that is involved in visual motion detection [107,205]. The stereotactic coordinates of this area ($x = -44$, $y = -72$, $z = -8$; Z score 4.46 for left CVS) are very close to coordinates reported by Watson *et al.* [107] as the most posterior location of area V5 ($x = -40$, $y = -72$, $z = -4$). Figure 11 illustrates deactivations during left cold CVS in comparison with rest.

Relative deactivations associated with CVS have also been reported by Wenzel *et al.* [206]. They described deactivations of the whole occipital cortex that was maximal in primary visual cortex. This observation is somewhat at variance with our own data, based on three independent observations, which point to more significant deactivations in extrastriate cortex following CVS. There is no obvious explanation for this difference; one possibility is the data

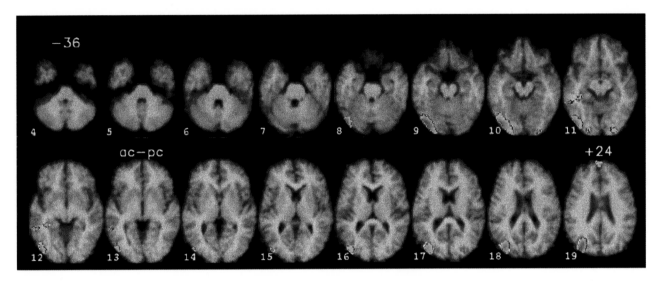

FIGURE 11 Cerebral regions deactivated by right and left cold CVS. Brain areas with significant deactivations associated with left cold CVS (compared with rest) are displayed according to the conventions of Fig. 10 ($P < 0.05$ corrected for multiple nonindependent comparisons).

analysis method used. Wenzel *et al.* [206] used the technique of Worsley *et al.* [207] that assesses regional significance of rCBF changes by using a pooled error-variance estimate from the entire scanned brain volume. However, as discussed by Friston [208], error variance is not homogeneous across brain regions so that the use of pooled estimates may lead to erroneous estimates of the statistical significance of rCBF changes. An illustration of this possibility is given in Fig. 1 of Bottini *et al.* [191].

Whatever the regional magnitude of deactivations induced by CVS, their interpretation is a relatively controversial issue [209–211]. Jenkins *et al.* (1993) found large relative deactivations in visual association areas during a motor learning task and interpreted these as a manifestation of a decrease in attentional resources allocated to brain structures irrelevant to their task [212]. A similar interpretation of deactivations was proposed by Kawashima *et al.* [213]. Frith *et al.* [209] and Friston *et al.* [210] provided an alternative explanation for deactivations that they detected in the superior temporal gyrus during a verbal fluency task. They suggest that the superior temporal gyri are activated or deactivated depending on whether access to word representations is by external stimulation (*e.g.*, hearing words) or due to intrinsic generation (*e.g.*, generating words).

These two interpretations are not mutually exclusive. In principle, deactivations in one experimental condition may simply represent activations in the condition arbitrarily defined as control, relative to that designated the experimental condition. Despite ambiguities concerned with interpretations of deactivations, it is interesting that most deactivations associated with CVS were in extrastriate visual cortex, usually lateralized to the hemisphere ipsilateral to cold CVS stimuli. The lateralization of deactivation suggests that a specific neurobiological mechanism is involved. It is also interesting that deactivations included, amongst others, visual area V5. Our subjects were scanned with their eyes closed, and therefore we do not have a behavioural measure to associate with the deactivation in the visual cortex. It can be speculated, however, that such deactivations reflect a compensatory intrinsic mechanism; reduced firing in visual motion detection areas may contribute to the stability of the visual scene during nystagmus induced by CVS. Such a mechanism may be so strong as to operate even with the eyes closed (nystagmus induced by CVS is not suppressed by keeping the eyes closed).

Direct evidence for such a mechanism comes from a recent experiment by Paus *et al.* [214]. Volunteers lay in the dark and moved their eyes at different rates during a series of scans. Activity in the frontal eye fields was positively correlated with the rate of eye movements. However, in visual cortex and visual association areas activity was negatively correlated with rate of eye movements. This result implies that each eye movement was accompanied by reduced activity in visual areas and provides a physiological basis for saccadic suppression as well as for the reductions we observed in association with nystagmus. Attribution of functional significance to deactivations due to CVS requires explicit investigation of interactions between vestibular activations and visual perception.

I. Modulation of Conscious Tactile Perception by Caloric Vestibular Stimulation

A considerable part of our interest in the functional anatomy of the vestibular system was motivated by an interaction between CVS and symptoms associated with the neglect syndrome, including hemianaesthesia (touch imperception), that can itself be manifest without other neglect symptoms. The modulation, by CVS, of touch imperception suggests that vestibular and touch projections may, to some extent, overlap in the brain. This hypothesis was tested explicitly in the following experiment [98].

Four normal adult right-handed males underwent 12 scans. Two subjects received light, short tactile stimuli of the left hand during 6 scans and no stimulation during the remainder. After each scan, subjects explicitly confirmed that they had consistently perceived tactile stimuli. The area stimulated was the center of the fourth metacarpal space of the left hand because this stimulus was previously used in an experiment showing transient remission of tactile imperception following CVS in brain damaged patients [183]. The other two subjects had left CVS before 6 (3 touch and 3 control) of their 12 scans. The order of the experimental and control scans was counterbalanced in both experiments to avoid habituation and order effects.

To assess anatomical overlap between touch and vestibular pathways we computed a combined [main] effect of the experimental procedures compared to the common baseline. The pattern of activations shared by touch and vestibular stimulation are presented in Fig. 12. Significant activation foci were detected in the right putamen, insula, retro-insular and somatosensory area II, ventral premotor cortex, and inferior parietal cortex in the supramarginal gyrus. We propose [94] that these brain regions constitute conjoint projection sites for touch and afferent vestibular pathways.

We subsequently studied a patient with touch selective hemianaesthesia who achieved temporary remission from left cold CVS. He is a right-handed, 65-year-old man with a right hemispheric stroke. At onset he showed left tactile imperception (hemianaesthesia) and a hemiparesis. Four weeks after the stroke, he was still densely hemianesthetic without signs of spatial neglect. Left CVS was tried at the bedside. Awareness for tactile stimuli, tested on

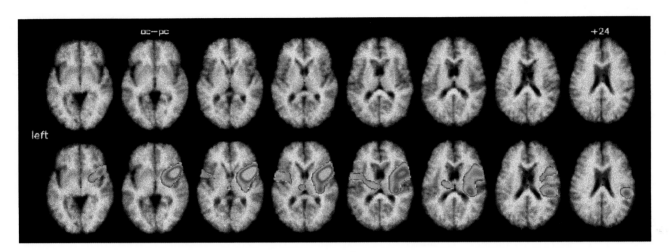

FIGURE 12 Areas of overlap between touch and vestibular projections. The top row illustrates average MRI maps from all normal subjects in transaxial slices in stereotactic anatomical space. The locations of activations associated with both touch stimulation and vestibular stimulation are shown as *t* maps in the second row (white areas), overlapped on the same MRI template. Numbers refer to the distance in millimetres of the transaxial images from the intercommissural (ac–pc) plane. Slice thickness is 4 mm. A description of the anatomical location of the activated areas is given in the main text.

the left hand, recovered transiently for about 30 min. The temporal profile of this recovery is illustrated in Fig. 13.

His brain lesion, demonstrated on a CT scan, involved a large portion of his right primary somatosensory and motor areas, supramarginal gyrus, and possibly, somatosensory area II. The coincident distribution of the functional lesion was confirmed by the rCBF-PET scans. At +48 to +52 mm above the bicommissural plane, where many place the cortical field of the hand in primary somatosensory cortex [99], there was marked hypoperfusion (Fig. 14). This observation raised a possibility that transient recovery of tactile perception could be due to a modulatory effect of CVS in a brain region other than area S1.

Alternating rest and touch PET scans were performed as in normal subjects. However, scans 4 to 9 were carried out under the influence of the effects of left CVS with recovery of conscious tactile perception (Figs. 13B–13C). Scans 10–12 were performed when conscious touch perception had again disappeared.

To examine the neurophysiological basis of recovered conscious touch perception we looked for positive interactions between networks associated with touch and vestibular stimulation, manifesting as a modulation of touch-induced regional activity by concurrent caloric vestibular stimulation. Such positive interactions were demonstrated by treating the experiment as a 2 × 2 factorial design (touch, + and −; CVS, + and −). Conscious compared with unconscious touch processing ([conscious touch *versus* rest, with caloric stimuli] − [touch imperception *versus* rest, without caloric stimuli]) was associated with maximal activations in right putamen and insula. Stereotactic anatomical locations of these foci were almost identical to a subset of those observed to receive conjointly vestibular and touch afferents in normal subjects [98]. We also found a positive interaction in the right basal prefrontal cortex that

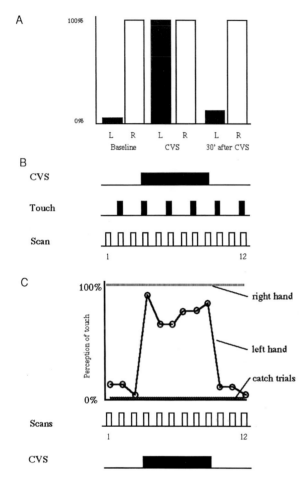

FIGURE 13 Behavioural profile before PET scanning, scanning procedure, and behavioural profile during the PET experiment in patient RF. (A) Bedside examination of touch perception in both hands. A dense left hemianaesthesia was found which remitted immediately after left cold CVS and reappeared 30 min later. The histograms report percentages of correct responses for light touch stimuli in the left (L) and in the right (R) hand. (B) Schedule of the 12 PET scans performed in patient RF. (C) Percentage of touch perception in both hands and performance on catch trials was assessed during the interval between scans. A dramatic recovery from left hemianesthesia was observed following CVS. Touch perception in the right hand was always at ceiling. Scan 10 was performed only after the patient became hemianaesthetic again.

did not correspond to any of the joint somatosensory–vestibular projections (Fig. 14).

J. Neurophysiological Interactions between the Vestibular System and Brain Areas Devoted to Body and Space Representation: A Summary

The different vestibular areas that we identified largely coincide with those brain areas that are believed to form a distributed network that subserves the representation and exploration of body and space [156,171]. Such a network

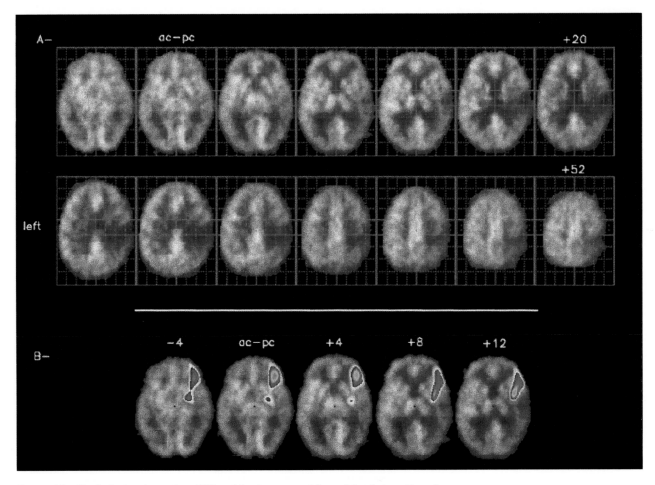

FIGURE 14 Brain lesion in patient RF and brain areas with positive interactions between touch and vestibular stimulation. The functional brain lesion of patient RF is illustrated with averaged rCBF maps transformed into a standard stereotactic space (first two rows). Abnormal asymmetry of rCBF is evident (from plane +8 mm to plane +52 mm from the ac–pc plane) in right putative somatosensory area II, primary somatosensory area, and supramarginal gyrus. The functional lesion was due to an ischaemic stroke involving the same areas as seen on CT scan. The third row illustrates brain areas where a positive interaction between touch and cold CVS was found: right putamen, insula, and basal prefrontal cortex.

requires a vestibular input that can be integrated with visual and proprioceptive inputs to give a nonambiguous representation of orientation and movement and provide a continuous readout of the position of a body in the environment. We believe that our results suggest that the vestibular system projects simultaneously to most of the major sites in this network. The implication is that there are multiple representations of body and space within the network.

The explicit contribution of these areas to body and spatial representation is suggested by the behavioural effects observed in our subjects, who were biased to point towards the side of cold CVS. Such spatial bias was associated with strongly asymmetrical activation of the central vestibular projection areas.

Can we make any deduction about how the modulation of neglect by vestibular signals occurs? Clinical reports indicate that unilateral focal lesions at any of the major sites in the vestibular network can disrupt perception of space and lead to a syndrome of unilateral neglect. Our results suggest that these disturbances occur because a unilateral lesion anywhere in the network will lead to long-term asymmetry of activation similar to the short-term asymmetry that is induced by CVS in healthy volunteers.

The CVS-induced transient improvement of neglect occurs wherever the initial anatomical lesion is [65,184]. This result is consistent with our suggestion that there are parallel inputs from the vestibular system into a cortical network subserving the representation of body and space. As a result, vestibular stimulation will activate whatever remains of the network in the right hemisphere. We speculate that such modulation will lead to symmetrical activation across the two hemispheres and the patient will be able to attend normally to surrounding space for as long as the effects of vestibular stimulation last.

The CVS effect also applies to conceptual space associated with visual images and the internal image of the patient's own body as shown by our experiment on hemianaesthesia. Accordingly, we consider touch imperception to be a result of distorted body representation. Recovery of touch imperception in a patient with a lesion in primary somatosensory cortex suggests that sensory body representations must exist in other areas, such as SII, the insula, and putamen, for example. An undamaged subset of these representations, retaining subcortical afferents, was able to mediate crude tactile perception when an appropriate modulation was introduced that had sufficient anatomical specificity to reduce the representational distortion produced by a lesion.

K. Hierarchical Organisation of Somatosensory Cortices and Perception of Touch: Does This Concept Apply to Humans?

Our findings on our patient, together with behavioural observations in brain damaged patients [45], have implications for an understanding of the anatomical bases of conscious perception and in particular of the role of primary sensory cortices (see Cowey and Stoerig [215] and Barbur *et al.* [216] for a discussion of the role of primary sensory (visual) cortex in conscious perception). Transient recovery of conscious awareness of touch was associated with modulatory activity generated by vestibular stimulation in a set of touch areas that normally also receive vestibular stimuli, as shown by the joint-projections experiment in normal subjects. At variance to what is proposed by neurophysiological studies in the monkey [74], our data would suggest a parallel access of somatosensory inputs to the cortex rather than serial access from area SI to other somatosensory areas. We suggest that primary somatosensory cortex has no primacy for conscious tactile perception in humans, rather, multiple sensory representations of the body exist in the brain and any of these can contribute to perception. This would be more evidence for the contention of Barbur *et al.* [216] that *"... each (cortical) area is capable of contributing directly and explicitly to ... perception in relation to its capacities..."*

VII. FUNCTIONAL IMAGING STUDIES OF SOMATOSENSORY SYSTEMS: ANY NOVEL FINDINGS? A GENERAL CONCLUSION

Ars longa, vita brevis is a Latin maxim that seems particularly appropriate to functional imaging studies of somatosensory functions, especially if one thinks of the sophisticated knowledge that anatomists and physiologists acquire with invasive studies in monkeys and the relative youth of functional imaging. Nevertheless, 10 years of research with functional neuroimaging have provided some interesting results. For example, the localisation of human area SII or the physiological interactions, and their distribution, between attention and conscious somatosensory perception. There have also been innovative studies concerning the functional anatomy of pain perception. Many of these findings relate to issues about which there was no previous information. The future can only get better. Functional imaging has reached maturity to the extent that data can be compared and combined between and from different laboratories; acquisition and processing of the data are largely standardized and the magnitude of the samples on which observations need to be made defined so that there is considerable reproducibility of results [217]. This is a recent achievement that invites repetition of some of the earlier experiments. Future work is likely to expand our understanding of functional segregation in the perceptual somatosensory domain and of multimodal integration associated with normal and abnormal body and space representations and motor action.

References

1. D. H. Ingvar. Patterns of brain activity revealed by measurements of regional cerebral blood flow. *In* "Brain Work" (D. H. Ingvar and N. A. Lassen, Eds.), pp. 397–413. Munksgaard, Copenhagen, 1975.
2. P. T. Fox, H. Burton, and M. E. Raichle. Mapping human somatosensory cortex with positron emission tomography. J. Neurosurg. **67,** 34–43 (1987).
3. R. J. Seitz and P. E. Roland. Vibratory stimulation increases and decreases the regional cerebral blood flow and oxidative metabolism: a positron emission tomography PET study. *Acta Neurol. Scand.* **86,** 60–67 (1992).
4. S. M. Rao, J. R. Binder, T. A. Hammeke, P. A. Bandettini, J. A. Bobholz, and J. A. Frost. Somatotopic mapping of the human primary motor cortex with functional magnetic resonance imaging. *Neurology* **45,** 919–924 (1993).
5. V. B. Mountcastle. Central nervous mechanism in sensation. *In* "Medical Physiology" (V. B. Mountcastle, Ed.), Vol. I, pp. 327–605. Mosby, St. Louis, 1980.
6. A. Brodal, "Neurological Anatomy in Relation to Clinical Medicine." Oxford Univer. Press, Oxford, 1981.
7. J. H. Kaas. Somatosensory system. *In* "The Human Nervous System" (G. Paxinos, Ed.), pp. 813–844. Academic Press, San Diego, 1990.
8. J. H. Martin. Coding and processing of sensory information. *In* "Principles of Neural Science" (E. R. Kandel, J. H. Schwartz, and T. M. Jessel, Eds.), pp. 329–340. Elsevier Science, New York, 1991.
9. J. H. Martin and T. M. Jessel. Modality coding in the somatic sensory system. *In* "Principles of Neural Science" (E. R. Kandel, J. H. Schwartz, and T. M. Jessel, Eds.), pp. 341–352, Elsevier Science, New York, 1991.
10. R. Melzack and P. D. Wall. On the nature of cutaneous sensory mechanisms. *Brain* **83,** 331–356 (1962).
11. E. Zander and G. Weddel. Observations on the innervation of the cornea. *J. Anat. London* **85,** 68 (1951).
12. R. D. Adams and M. Victor. "Principles of Neurology." McGraw-Hill, New York, 1989.
13. M. Frey-von. Beiträge zur Sinnesphysiologies der Haut. Königliche Sächsische Gesellschaft der Wissenschaften. Leipzig. *Ber. Verh. Math. Phys. Kl.* **47,** 166–184 (1895).
14. H. E. Turebjörk, Å. B. Vallbo, and J. L. Ochoa. Intraneural microstimulation in man. Its relation to specificity of tactile sensations. *Brain* **110,** 1509–1529 (1987).

15. C. Ohye. Thalamus. *In* "The Human Nervous System" (G. Paxinos, Ed.), pp. 439–468. Academic Press, San Diego, 1990.

16. G. F. Poggio and V. B. Mountcastle. The functional properties of ventrobasal thalamic neurons studied in unanesthetized monkeys. *J. Neurophysiol.* **26,** 775–806 (1963).

17. D. P. Friedman and E. A. Murray. Thalamic connectivity of the second somatosensory area and neighboring somatosensory fields of the lateral sulcus in the macaques. *J. Comp. Neurol.* **252,** 348–373 (1986).

18. H. Burton. Second somatosensory cortex and related areas. *In* "Cerebral Cortex. Sensory Motor Areas and Aspects of Cortical Connectivity" (E. G. Jones and A. Peters, Eds.) Vol. V, pp. 31–98, Plenum, New York, 1986.

19. K. Brodmann, "Vergleichende Lokalisationslehre der Grosshirnrinde." J. A. Barth, Leipzig, 1909.

20. C. Vogt and O. Vogt. Allgemeinere Ergebnisse unserer hirnforschung. *J. Psychol. Neurol.* **25,** 279–462 (1919).

21. A. W. Campbell, "Histological Studies on the Localization of Cerebral Function." Cambridge Univ. Press, Cambridge, England, 1905.

22. J. C. Marshall, C. N. Woolsey, and P. Bard. Cortical representation of tactile sensibility as indicated by cortical potentials. *Science* **85,** 388–390 (1937).

23. M. M. Merzenich, J. H. Kaas, M. Sur, and C.-S. Lin. Double representation of the body surface within cytoarchitectonic Areas 3b and 1 in "S1" in the Owl monkey (Aotus trivirgatus). *J. Comp. Neurol.* **181,** 41–74 (1978).

24. J. H. Kaas, R. J. Nelson, M. Sur, C. S. Lin, and M. M. Merzenich. Multiple representations of the body within primary somatosensory cortex in primates. *Science* **204,** 521–523 (1979).

25. J. H. Kaas. What, if anything, is SI? Organization of first somatosensory area of cortex. *Physiol. Rev.* **63,** 206–231 (1983).

26. R. J. Nelson, M. Sur, D. J. Felleman, and J. H. Kaas. Representations of the body surface in postcentral parietal cortex of Macaca fascicularis. *J. Comp. Neurol.* **199,** 29–64 (1980).

27. A. E. Wood. What, if anything, is a rabbit? *Evolution* **11,** 417–425 (1957).

28. J. H. R. Maunsell and D. C. V. Essen. The connections of the middle temporal visual area MT and their relationship to a cortical hierarchy in the macaque monkeys. *J. Neurosci.* **3,** 2563–2586 (1983).

29. S. Zeki and S. Shipp. The functional logic of cortical connections. *Nature* **335,** 311–317 (1988).

30. M. F. Shanks, R. C. A. Pearson, and T. P. S. Powell. The ipsilateral cortico-cortical connexions between the cytoarchitectonic subdivisions of the primary somatic sensory cortex in the monkey. *Brain Res. Rev.* **9,** 67–88 (1985).

31. M. Sur. Receptive fields of neurons in area 3b and 1 of somatosensory cortex in monkeys. *Brain Res.* **198,** 465–471 (1980).

32. D. N. Pandya and L. A. Vignolo. Interhemispheric projections of the parietal lobe in the rhesus monkey. *Brain Res.* **15,** 49–65 (1969).

33. E. A. Karol and D. N. Pandya. The distribution of the corpus callosum in the Rhesus monkey. *Brain* **94,** 471–486 (1971).

34. H. P. Killackey, H. J. Gould, C. G. Cusick, T. P. Pons, and J. H. Kaas. The relation of corpus callosum connections to architectonic fields and body surface maps in sensorimotor cortex of New and Old World monkeys. *J. Comp. Neurol.* **219,** 384–419 (1983).

35. K. Zilles. Cortex. *In* "The Human Nervous System" (G. Paxinos, Ed.), pp. 757–802. Academic Press, San Diego, 1990.

36. T. Allison, G. McCarthy, C. C. Wood, T. M. Parcey, D. P. Spenar, and P. P. Williamson. Human cortical potentials evoked by stimulation of median nerves. I. Cytoarchitectonic areas generating SI activity. *J. Neurophysiol.* **62,** 711–722 (1988).

37. S. C. Gandevia, D. Burke, and B. B. McKeon. The projections of muscle afferents from the hand to the cerebral cortex in man. *Brain* **107**, 1–13 (1984).

38. E. Kaukoranta, M. Hamalainen, J. Sarvas, and R. Hari. Mixed and sensory nerve stimulations activate different cytoarchitectonic areas in human primary somatosensory cortex I. *Exp. Brain Res.* **63**, 60–66 (1986).

39. C. N. Woolsey, T. C. Erickson, and W. E. Gilson. Localization in somatic sensory and motor areas of human cerebrum as determined by direct recording of evoked potentials and electric stimulation. *J. Neurosurg.* **51**, 476–506 (1979).

40. W. W. Sutherling, M. F. Levesque, and C. Baumgartner. Cortical sensory representation of the human hand. Size of finger regions and non-overlapping digit somatotopy. *Neurology* **42**, 1020–1028 (1992).

41. W. J. Penfield and E. Boldrey. Somatic motor and sensory representation in the cerebral cortex of man as studied by electrical stimulation. *Brain* **60**, 389–443 (1937).

42. O. Hikosaka, M. Tanaka, M. Sokamoto, and Y. Iwamura. Deficits of manipulative behaviors induced by local injections of muscimol in the first somatosensory cortex of the conscious monkey. *Brain Res.* **325**, 375–380 (1985).

43. M. Carlson. Characteristics of sensory deficits following lesions of Brodmann's areas 1 and 2 in the post-central gyrus of Macaca Mulatta. *Brain Res.* **204**, 424–430 (1981).

44. S. Corkin, B. Milner, and M. Rasmussen. Somatosensory thresholds contrasting effects of postcentral gyrus and posterior parietal-lobe excisions. *Arch. Neurol Chicago* **23**, 41–58 (1970).

45. P. E. Roland. Somatosensory detection in patients with circumscribed lesions of the brain. *Exp. Brain Res.* **12**, 43–94 (1987).

46. J. Hyvärinen. Posterior parietal lobe of the primate brain. *Physiol. Rev.* **62**, 1060–1129 (1982).

47. A. Galaburda and F. Sanides. Cytoarchitectonic organization of the human auditory cortex. *J. Comp. Neurol.* **190**, 597–610 (1980).

48. T. P. Pons, P. E. Garraghty, C. G. Cusick, and J. H. Kaas. The somatotopic organization of area 2 in macaque monkeys. *J. Comp. Neurol.* **248**, 313–335 (1985).

49. R. C. A. Pearson and T. P. S. Powell. The projection of the primary somatic sensory cortex upon area 5 in the monkey. *Brain Res. Rev.* **9**, 89–97 (1985).

50. F. H. Duffy and J. L. Burchfiel. Somatosensory system organizational hierarchy from single units in monkey area 5. *Science* **172**, 273–275 (1979).

51. Y. M. Iwamura, A. Iriki, and M. Tanaka. Bilateral hand representation in postcentral somatosensory cortex. *Nature* **369**, 554–556 (1994).

52. H. Sakata, Y. Takaoka, and A. Kawarasaki. Somatosensory properties of neurons in superior parietal cortex area 5 of the rhesus monkey. *Brain Res.* **64**, 85–102 (1973).

53. T. L. Peele. Acute and chronic parietal lobe ablations in monkeys. *J. Neurophysiol.* **7**, 269–286 (1944).

54. P. D. Nixon, P. Burbaud, and R. E. Passingham. Control of arm movement after bilateral lesions of area 5 in the monkey (Macaca mulatta). *Exp. Brain Res.* **90**, 229–232 (1992).

55. D. N. Levine, K. J. Kaufman, and J. P. Mohr. Innacurate reaching associated with a superior parietal lobe tumor. *Neurology* **28**, 556–561 (1978).

56. R. Balint. Seelenlähmung des "Schauens", Optische Ataxie, Raümlike Störung der Aufmerksamkeit. *Monatschr. Psichiatr. Neurol.* **25**, 51–81 (1909).

57. W. J. Penfield and H. Jasper, "Epilepsy and the Functional Anatomy of the Human Brain." Little Brown, Boston, 1954.

58. R. J. Caselli. Ventrolateral and dorsomedial somatosensory association cortex damage produces distinct somesthetic syndromes in humans. *Neurology* **43**, 762–771 (1993).

59. C. J. Robinson and H. Burton. Somatic submodalities distribution within the

second somatosensory (SII), 7b, retroinsular, postauditory and granular insular of M. fascicularis. *J. Comp Neurol.* **192,** 93–108 (1980a).

60. C. J. Robinson and H. Burton. Somatotopographic organization in the second somatosensory area of M. fascicularis. *J. Comp Neurol.* **192,** 43–67 (1980b).

61. L. Bianchi. The functions of the frontal lobe. *Brain* **18,** 497–522 (1895).

62. K. Welch and P. Stuteville. Experimental production of unilateral neglect in monkeys. *Brain* **81,** 341–347 (1958).

63. R. E. Passingham and G. Ettlinger. A comparison of cortical functions in man and the other primates. *Int. Rev. Neurobiol.* **16,** 233–299 (1974).

64. J. F. R. Fleming and E. C. Crosby. The parietal lobe as an additional motor area. The motor effects of electrical stimulation and ablation of cortical area 5 and 7 in monkeys. *J. Comp. Neurol.* **103,** 485–512 (1955).

65. G. Vallar. The anatomical basis of spatial hemineglect in humans. *In* "Unilateral Neglect, Clinical and Experimental Studies" (I. H. Robertson and J. C. Marshall, Eds.), pp. 27–59. Lawrence Earlbaum Associates, Howe, 1993.

66. R. Sterzi, G. Bottini, M. G. Celani, E. Righetti, M. Lamassa, S. Ricci, and G. Vallar. Hemianopia, hemianaesthesia, and hemiplegia after right and left hemisphere damage. A hemispheric difference. *J. Neurol. Neurosurg. Psychiatry* **56,** 308–310 (1993).

67. G. Vallar and D. Perani. The anatomy of unilateral neglect after right hemisphere stroke lesions. A clinical CT/scan correlation study in man. *Neuropsychologia* **24,** 609–622 (1986).

68. A. R. Damasio. Aphasia. *N. Engl. J. Med.* **326,** 531–539 (1992).

69. T. Shallice and G. Vallar. The impairment of auditory-verbal short-term storage. *In* "Neuropsychological Impairments of Short-Term Memory" (G. Vallar and T. Shallice, Eds.) Cambridge Univ. Press, New York, 1990.

70. E. D. Adrian. Afferent discharges to the cerebral cortex from peripheral sense organs. *J. Physiol. London* **100,** 159–191 (1941).

71. C. N. Woolsey and G. H. Wang. Somatic areas 1 and 2 of the cerebral cortex of the rabbit. *Abstr. Fed. Proc.* **4,** 79 (1945).

72. C. N. Woolsey. "Second" somatic receiving areas in the cerebral cortex of cat, dog and monkey. *Fed. Proc.* **2,** 55–56 (1946).

73. D. P. Friedman, E. A. Murray, J. B. O'Neill, and M. Mishkin. Cortical connections of somatosensory fields of the lateral sulcus of macaques. Evidence for a cortico-limbic pathway for touch. *J. Comp. Neurol.* **252,** 323–347 (1986).

74. T. P. Pons, P. E. Garragthy, D. P. Friedman, and M. Mishkin. Physiological evidence for serial processing in somatosensory cortex. *Science* **237,** 417–420 (1987).

75. R. E. Bennett, D. G. Ferrington, and M. Rowe. Tactile neuron classes within second somatosensory area SII of cat cerebral cortex. *J. Neurophysiol.* **43,** 292–309 (1980).

76. E. A. Murray and M. Mishkin. Relative contributions of area SII and area 5 to tactile discrimination. *Behav. Brain Res.* **11,** 67–83 (1984).

77. W. J. Penfield and T. Rasmussen, "The Cerebral Cortex of Man." Macmillan, New York, 1950.

78. H. Lüders, R. P. Lesser, D. S. Dinner, J. F. Hahn, V. Salanga, and H. H. Morris. The second sensory area in humans, evoked potentials and electrical stimulation studies. *Ann. Neurol.* **17,** 177–184 (1985).

79. W. Guldin and O.-J. Grüsser. The anatomy of vestibular cortices of primates. *In* "Le cortex vestibulaire" (M. Collard, M. Jeannerod, and Y. Christen, Eds.), pp. 17–26. Irvin, Paris, 1996.

80. T. Brandt, M. Dieterich, and A. Danek. Vestibular cortex lesions affect the perception of verticality. *Ann. Neurol.* **35,** 403–412 (1994).

81. J. D. Greenspan and J. A. Winfield. Reversible pain and tactile deficit associated with a cerebral tumor compressing the posterior insula and parietal operculum. *Pain* **58,** 29–39 (1992).

82. E. J. Mufson, M. M. Mesulam, and D. N. Pandya. Insular interconnections with the amygdala in the rhesus monkey. *Neuroscience* **6,** 1231–1248 (1981).

83. M. M. Mesulam and E. J. Mufson. Insula of the old world monkey. I. Architectonics in the insulo-orbito-temporal component of the paralimbic brain. *J. Comp. Neurol.* **212,** 1–22 (1982).

84. M. M. Mesulam and E. J. Mufson. The insula of reil in man and monkey. Architectonics connectivity and function. *In* "Cerebral-Cortex. Sensory-Motor Areas and Aspects of Cortical Connectivity" (E. G. Jones and A. Peters, Eds.), vol. V, pp. 179–226. Plenum, New York, 1986.

85. R. J. Schneider, D. P. Friedman, and M. Mishkin. A modality-specific somatosensory area within the insula of the rhesus monkey. *Brain Res.* **621,** 116–120 (1993).

86. R. Desimone, T. D. Albright, C. G. Gross, and C. Bruce. Stimulus-selective properties of inferior temporal neurons in the macaque. *J. Neurosci.* **3,** 2051–2062 (1984).

87. E. G. Jones and D. P. Friedman. Projection pattern of functional components of thalamic ventro-basal complex on monkey somatosensory cortex. *J. Neurophysiol.* **48,** 521–544 (1982).

88. G. Bottini, S. F. Cappa, R. Sterzi, and A. Vignolo. Intramodal somesthetic recognition disorders following right and left hemisphere damage. *Brain* **118,** 395–399 (1995).

89. T. Manzoni, R. Caminiti, G. Spidalieri, and E. Morelli. Anatomical and functional aspects of the associative projections from somatic area SI to SII. *Exp. Brain Res.* **34,** 453–470 (1979).

90. H. Burton and C. J. Robinson. Responses in the first or second somatosensory cortical area in cats during transient inactivation of the other ipsilateral area with lidocaine hydrochloride. *Somatosens. Res.* **4,** 215–236 (1987).

91. P. E. Garraghty, S. L. Florence, W. N. Tenhula, and J. H. Kaas. Parallel thalamic activation of the first and second somatosensory areas in prosimian primates and tree shrews. *J. Comp. Neurol.* **311,** 289–299 (1991).

92. T. P. Pons, P. E. Garragthy, and M. Mishkin. Lesion-induced plasticity in the second somatosensory cortex of adult macaques. *Proc. Natl. Acad. Sci. USA* **85,** 5279–5281 (1988).

93. T. P. Pons, P. E. Garragthy, and M. Mishkin. Serial and parallel processing of tactual information in somatosensory cortex of rhesus monkeys. *J. Neurophysiol.* **68,** 518–527 (1992).

94. P. E. Garraghty, T. P. Pons, and J. H. Kaas. Ablations of areas 3b (SI proper) and 3a of somatosensory cortex in marmosets deactivate the second and parietal ventral somatosensory areas. *Somatosens. Mot. Res.* **7,** 125–135 (1990).

95. M. Mishkin. Analogous neural models for tactual and visual learning. *Neuropsychologia* **17,** 139–149 (1979).

96. H. Burton, K. Sathian, and S. Dian-Hua. Altered responses to cutaneous stimuli in the second somatosensory cortex following lesions of the postcentral gyrus in infant and juvenile macaques. *J. Comp. Neurol.* **291,** 395–414, (1990).

97. H. Q. Zhang, G. M. Murray, A. B. Turman, P. D. Mackie, G. T. Coleman, and M. J. Rowe. Parallel processing in cerebral cortex of the marmoset monkey: Effect of reversible SI inactivation on tactile responses in SII. *Neurophysiol.* **76,** 3633–3655 (1996).

98. G. Bottini, E. Paulesu, R. Sterzi, E. Warburton, R. J. S. Wise, G. Vallar, R. S. J. Frackowiak, and C. D. Frith. Modulation of conscious experience by peripheral sensory stimuli. *Nature* **376,** 778–781 (1995).

99. H. Burton, T. O. Videen, and M. E. Raichle. Tactile-vibration-activated foci in insular and parietal-opercular cortex studied with positron emission tomography mapping the second somatosensory area in humans. *Somatosens. Mot. Res.* **10,** 297–308 (1993).

100. R. C. Coghill, J. D. Talbot, A. C. Evans, E. Meyer, A. Gjedde, M. C. Bushnell,

and G. H. Duncan. Distributed processing of pain and vibration by the human brain. *J. Neurosci.* **14,** 4095–4108 (1994).

101. S. T. Grafton, R. P. Woods, and J. C. Mazziotta. Within-arm somatotopy in human motor areas determined by positron emission tomography imaging of cerebral blood flow. *Exp. Brain Res.* **95,** 172–176 (1993).

102. P. Remy, M. Zilbovicius, A. Leroy-Willig, A. Syrota, and Y. Samson. Movement- and task-related activations of motor cortical areas a positron emission tomographic study [see comments]. *Ann. Neurol.* **36,** 19–26 (1994).

103. J. G. Colebatch, M. P. Deiber, R. E. Passingham, K. J. Friston, and R. S. J. Frackowiak. Regional cerebral blood flow during voluntary arm and hand movements in human subjects. *J. Neurophysiol.* **65,** 1392–1401 (1991).

104. C. I. Moore, A. Gehi, A. R. Guimerea, S. Corkin, B. R. Rosen, and C. E. Stern. Somatotopic mapping of cortical areas SI and SII using fMRI. *NeuroImage* **3,** S333 (1996).

105. M. Matelli, G. Rizzolatti, V. Bettinardi, M. C. Gilardi, D. Perani, G. Rizzo, and F. Fazio. Activation of precentral and mesial motor areas during the execution of elementary proximal and distal arm movements a PET study. *Neuroreport* **4,** 1295–1298 (1993).

106. J. V. Pardo, P. T. Fox, and M. E. Raichle. Localization of a human system for sustained attention by positron emission tomography. *Nature* **349,** 61–64 (1991).

107. J. D. G. Watson, R. Myers, R. J. S. Frackowiak, J. V. Hajnal, R. P. Woods, J. C. Mazziotta, S. Shipp, and S. Zeki. Area V5 of the human brain: Evidence from a combined study using positron emission tomography and magnetic resonance imaging. *Cereb. Cortex* **3,** 79–94 (1993).

108. G. Bottini, R. Sterzi, E. Paulesu, G. Vallar, S. F. Cappa, F. Erminio, R. E. Passingham, C. D. Frith, and R. S. J. Frackowiak. Identification of the central vestibular projections in man a positron emission tomography activation study. *Exp Brain Res.* **99,** 164–169 (1994).

109. K. J. Friston, A. P. Holmes, K. J. Worsley, J. B. Poline, C. D. Frith, and R. S. J. Frackowiak. Statistical parametric maps in functional imaging. A general linear approach. *Human Brain Mapping* **3,** 189–210 (1995).

110. C. J. Robinson and H. Burton. Organization of somatosensory receptive fields in cortical areas 7b, retroinsular, postauditory, granular insular of M. fascicularis. *J. Comp Neurol.* **192,** 69–92 (1980c).

111. L. Fogassi, V. Gallese, L. Fadiga, G. Luppino, M. Matelli, and G. Rizzolatti. Coding of peripersonal space in inferior premotor cortex area F4. *J. Neurophysiol.* **76,** 141–157 (1996).

112. J. Hyvärinen, H. Sakata, W. H. Talbot, and V. B. Mountcastle. Neuronal coding by cortical cells of the frequency of oscillating peripheral stimuli. *Science* **162,** 1130–1132 (1968).

113. V. Ibañez, M. P. Deiber, N. Sadato, C. Toro, J. Grissom, R. P. Woods, J. C. Mazziotta, and M. Hallett. Effect on stimulus rate on regional cerebral blood flow after median nerve stimulation. *Brain* **118,** 1339–1351 (1995).

114. N. Sadato, V. Ibañez, M. P. Deiber, G. Campbell, M. Leonardo, and M. Hallett. Frequency-dependent changes of regional cerebral blood flow during finger movements. *J. Cereb. Blood Flow Metab.* **16,** 23–33 (1996).

115. P. E. Roland, "Brain Activation." Wiley-Liss, New York, 1993.

116. P. T. Fox and C. N. Applegate. Right-hemispheric dominance for somatosensory processing in humans. *Soc. Neurosci. Abstr.* **14,** 760 (1988).

117. J. C. Hsieh, O. Hagermark, M. Stahle-Backdahl, K. Ericson, L. Eriksson, S. Stone-Elander, and M. Ingvar. Urge to scratch represented in the human cerebral cortex during itch. *J. Neurophysiol.* **72,** 3004–3008 (1994).

118. J. Talairach and P. Tournoux., "A Co-planar Stereotactic Atlas of the Human Brain." Thieme Verlag, Stuttgart, 1988.

119. H. Head and G. Holmes. Sensory disturbances from cerebral lesions. *Brain* **34,** 102–254 (1911).

120. D. Albe-Fessard, K. J. Berkley, L. Kruger, H. J. Ralston, and W. D. Willis. Diencephalic mechanisms of pain sensation. *Brain Res. Rev.* **9,** 217–296 (1985).

121. D. R. Kenshalo-Jr. and O. Isensee. Responses of the primate SI cortical neurons to noxious stimuli. *J. Neurophysiol.* **50,** 1479–1496 (1983).

122. J. Talairach, P. Tournoux, and J. Bancaud. Chirurgie parietale de la douleur. *Acta Neurochirurgica* **8,** 153–250 (1960).

123. W. H. Sweet. Cerebral localization of pain. *In* "New Perspectives in Cerebral Localization" (R. A. Thompson and J. R. Green, Eds.), pp. 205–242. Raven Press, New York, 1982.

124. D. R. Kenshalo Jr., D. A. Thomas, and R. Dubner. Primary somatosensory cortical lesions reduce the monkey's ability to discriminate and detect noxious thermal stimulation. *Brain Res.* **454,** 378–382 (1991).

125. E. L. Foltz and L. E. J. White. Pain relief by frontal cingulotomy. *Neurosurgery* **19,** 89–100 (1962).

126. B. A. Vogt, D. N. Pandya, and D. L. Rosen. Cingulate cortex of the rhesus monkey. I. Cytoarchitecture and thalamic afferents. *J. Comp. Neurol.* **262,** 256–270 (1987).

127. J. D. Talbot, S. Marrett, A. C. Evans, E. Meyer, M. C. Bushnell, and G. Duncan. Multiple representations of pain in human cerebral cortex. *Science* **251,** 1355–1358 (1991).

128. A. K. Jones, W. D. Brown, K. J. Friston, L. Y. QI, and R. S. Frackowiak. Cortical and subcortical localization of response to pain in man using positron emission tomography. *Proc. R. Soc. London B* **244,** 39–44 (1991).

129. D. R. Kenshalo Jr., D. A. Thomas, and R. Dubner. Primary somatosensory cortical lesions reduce the monkey's ability to discriminate and detect noxious thermal stimulation. *Soc. Neurosci. Abstr.* **17,** 1206 (1991).

130. K. L. Casey, S. Minoshima, K. L. Berger, R. A. Koeppe, T. J. Morrow, and K. A. Frey. Positron emission tomographic analysis of cerebral structures activated specifically by repetitive noxious heat stimuli. *J. Neurophysiol.* **71,** 802–807 (1994).

131. S. W. Derbyshire, A. K. Jones, P. Devani, K. J. Friston, C. Feinmann, M. Harris, S. Pearce, J. D. Watson, and R. S. Frackowiak. Cerebral responses to pain in patients with atypical facial pain measured by positron emission tomography. *J. Neurol. Neurosurg. Psychiatry* **57,** 1166–1172 (1994).

132. S. W. Derbyshire, A. K. P. Jones, S. Clarke, D. Townsend, F. Gyulai, L. Firestone, M. Mintun, and M. Jayson. Cerebral responses to laser pain stimulus measured using positron emission tomography. *NeuroImage* **3,** S327 (1996).

133. J. C. White. Cardiac Pain. Anatomic pathways and physiologic mechanisms. *Circulation* **16,** 644–655 (1957).

134. A. Malliani, M. Pagani, and F. Lombardi. Visceral *versus* somatic mechanisms. *In* "Textbook of Pain" (P. D. Wall and R. Melzack, Eds.), pp. 128–140. Churchill Livingstone, New York, 1989.

135. S. T. Meller and G. F. Gebhart. Visceral pain, a review of experimental studies. *Neuroscience* **48,** 501–524 (1992).

136. S. D. Rosen, E. Paulesu, C. D. Frith, R. S. Frackowiak, G. J. Davies, T. Jones, and P. G. Camici. Central nervous pathways mediating angina pectoris. *Lancet* **344,** 147–150 (1994).

137. R. R. Terreberry and E. J. Neafsey. Rat medial frontal cortex, a visceral motor region with a direct projection to the solitary nucleus. *Brain Res.* **278,** 245–249 (1983).

138. K. M. Hurley, H. Herbert, M. M. Moga, and C. B. Saper. Efferent projections of the inferolimbic cortex of the rat. *J. Comp. Neurol.* **308,** 249–276 (1991).

139. S. D. Rosen, E. Paulesu, P. Nihoyannopoulos, D. Tousoulis, R. S. Frackowiak, C. D. Frith, T. Jones, and P. G. Camici. Silent ischemia as a central problem: regional brain activation compared in silent and painful myocardial ischemia. *Ann. Intern. Med.* **124,** 939–949 (1996).

140. M. Krams, M. J. Mayston, L. Harrison, R. S. J. Frackowiak, and R. E. Passingham.

Passive finger movements in normals. A PET study. *NeuroImage* **3,** S393 (1996).

141. P. D. Cheney and E. E. Fetz. Corticomotorneural cells contribute to long latency stretch reflexes in Rhesus monkey. *J. Physiol. London* **349,** 249–272 (1984).

142. M. D. Ginsberg, J. Y. Chang, R. E. Kelley, F. Yoshii, W. W. Barker, and G. I. T. E. Boothe. Increases in both cerebral glucose utilization and blood flow during execution of a somatosensory task. *Ann. Neurol.* **23,** 152–160 (1988).

143. B. O'Sullivan, P. Roland, and R. Kawashima. A PET study of somatosensory discrimination. Microgeometry *versus* macrogeometry. *Eur. J. Neurosci.* **6,** 137–148 (1994).

144. A. Ledberg, B. T. O'Sullivan, S. Kinomura, and P. E. Roland. Somatosensory activations of the parietal operculum of man. A PET study. *Eur J. Neurosci.* **7,** 1934–1941 (1995).

145. P. E. Roland, B. T. O. Sullivan, R. Kawashima, and A. Ledberg. Somatosensory perception of microgeometry and macrogeometry activate different somatosensory association areas. *NeuroImage* **3,** S338 (1996).

146. P. E. Roland and E. Mortensen. Somatosensory detection of microgeometry, macrogeometry and kinesthesia in man. *Brain Res. Rev.* **12,** 1–42 (1987).

147. E. A. Murray and M. Mishkin. Severe tactual as well as visual memory deficits follow combined removal of amygadala and hippocampus in monkeys. *J. Neurosci.* **4,** 2565–2580 (1984).

148. P. E. Roland, L. Eriksson, L. Widen, and S. Stone-Elander. Changes in regional cerebral oxidative metabolism induced by tactile learning and recognition in man. *Eur. J. Neurosci.* **1,** 3–18 (1988).

149. B. Seltzer and M. M. Mesulam. Confusional states and delirium as disorders of attention. *In* "Handbook of Neuropsychology" (F. Boller and J. Grafman, Eds.), Vol. 1, pp. 165–174. Elsevier Science, Amsterdam, 1988.

150. M. I. Posner. Cumulative development of attentional theory. *Am. Psychol.* **37,** 168–179 (1982).

151. R. Parasuraman and D. R. Davies, "Varieties of Attention." Academic Press, New York, 1984.

152. C. Umiltà. Orienting of attention. *In* "Handbook of Neuropsychology" (F. Boller and J. Grafman, Eds.), Vol. I, pp. 175–193, Elsevier Science, Amsterdam, 1988.

153. G. Rizzolatti and A. Berti. Neural mechanisms of spatial neglect. *In* "Unilateral Neglect, Clinical and Experimental Studies" (I. H. Robertson and J. C. Marshall, Eds.), pp. 87–105. Lawrence Erlbaum Associates, Howe, 1993.

154. D. E. Broadbent. Task combination and selective intake of information. *Acta Psychol.* **50,** 253–290 (1982).

155. J. A. Deutsh and D. Deutsh. Attention: Some theoretical considerations. *Psychol. Rev.* **87,** 272–300 (1963).

156. M. M. Mesulam. A cortical network for directed attention and unilateral neglect. *Ann. Neurol.* **10** (1981).

157. M. I. Posner and S. E. Petersen. The attention system of the human brain. *Annu. Rev. Neurosci.* **13,** 25–42 (1990).

158. A. Allport. Selection for action some behavioural and neurophysiological considerations of attention and action. *In* "Perspectives on Perception and Action" (H. Heuer and A. F. Saunders, Eds.). Lawrence Erlbaum, Hillsdale NJ, 1987.

159. G. Rizzolatti and R. Camarda. Neural circuits for spatial attention and unilateral neglect. *In* "Neurophysiological and Neuropsychological Aspects of Spatial Neglect" (M. Jeannerod, Ed.), pp. 289–313. Elsevier Science, Amsterdam, 1987.

160. T. Shallice. "From Neuropsychology to Mental Structure." Cambridge University Press, 1988.

161. M. Corbetta, F. M. Miezin, S. Dobmeyer, G. L. Shulman, and S. E. Petersen. Selective and divided attention during visual discrimination of shape color and speed functional anatomy by positron emission tomography. *J. Neurosci.* **11,** 2383–2402 (1991).

162. M. C. Bushnell, M. E. Goldberg, and D. L. Robinson. Dissociation of movement and attention neuronal correlations in posterior parietal cortex. *Soc. Neurosci. Abstr.* **4,** 621 (1978).

163. M. C. Bushnell, M. E. Goldberg, and D. L. Robinson. Behavioral enhancement of visual responses in monkey cerebral cortex. I. Modulation in posterior parietal cortex related to selective visual attention. *J. Neurophysiol.* **46,** 755–772 (1981).

164. J. Hyvärinen, A. Poranen, and Y. Jokinen. Influece of attentive behavior on neuronal responses to vibration in primary somatosensory cortex of the monkey. *J. Neurophysiol.* **43,** 870–882 (1980).

165. S. S. Hsiao, D. M. O'Shaughnessy, and K. O. Johnson. Effects of selective attention on spatial form processing in monkey primary and secondary somatosensory cortex. *J. Neurophysiol.* **70,** 444–447 (1993).

166. E. Meyer, S. S. Ferguson, R. J. Zatorre, B. Alivisatos, S. Marrett, A. C. Evans, and A. M. Hakim. Attention modulates somatosensory cerebral blood flow response to vibrotactile stimulation as measured by positron emission tomography. *Ann. Neurol.* **29,** 440–443 (1991).

167. P. E. Roland. Somatotopical tuning of postcentral gyrus during focal attention in man. A regional cerebral blood flow study. *J. Neurophysiol.* **46,** 744–754 (1981).

168. W. C. Drevets, H. Burton, T. O. Videen, A. Z. Snyder, J. R. Simson, and M. E. Raichle. Blood flow changes in human somatosensory cortex during anticipated stimulation. *Nature* **373,** 249–252 (1995).

169. J. P. Kelly. The sense of balance. *In* "Principle of Neural Science" (E. R. Kandel, J. H. Schwartz, and T. M. Jessel, Eds.), pp. 500–511. Elsevier Science, New York, 1991.

170. H. F. Lidvall. Vertigo and nystagmus responses to caloric stimuli repeated at short intervals. *Acta Oto-Laryng* **53,** 33–44 (1962).

171. K. M. Heilman, D. Bowers, E. Valenstein, and R. T. Watson. Hemispace and hemispatial neglect. *In* "Neurophysiological and Neuropsychological Aspects of Spatial Neglect" (M. Jeannerod, Ed.), pp. 115–150. Elsevier Science, Amsterdam, 1987.

172. M. L. Albert. A simple test of visual neglect. *Neurology* **23,** 658–664 (1973).

173. P. W. Halligan and J. C. Marshall. The history and clinical presentation of neglect. *In* "Unilateral Neglect, Clinical and Experimental Studies" (J. C. Marshall and I. Robertson, Eds.), pp. 3–25. Lawrence Erlbaum Associates, Howe, 1993.

174. E. Bisiach and A. Berti. Dyschiria. An attempt to its systematic explanation. *In* "Neurophysiological and Neuropsychological Aspects of Spatial Neglect" (M. Jeannerod, Ed.), pp. 183–201. Elsevier, Amsterdam, 1987.

175. E. Bisiach and C. Luzzatti. Unilateral neglect of representational space. *Cortex* **14,** 129–133 (1978).

176. D. Denny-Brown, J. S. Meyer, and S. Horenstein. The significance of perceptual rivalry resulting from parietal lesions. *Brain* **75,** 433–471 (1952).

177. M. Kinsbourne. Mechanisms of unilateral neglect. *In* "Neurophysiological and Neuropsychological Aspects of Spatial Neglect" (M. Jeannerod, Ed.), pp. 69–86. Elsevier Science, Amsterdam, 1987.

178. K. M. Heilman, R. T. Watson, and E. Valenstein. Neglect and related disorders. *In* "Clinical Neuropsychology" (K. M. Heilman and E. Valenstein, Eds.), pp. 243–293. Oxford Univ. Press, New York, 1985.

179. A. B. Rubens. Caloric stimulation and unilateral visual neglect. *Neurology* **35,** 1019–1024 (1985).

180. S. F. Cappa, R. Sterzi, G. Vallar, and E. Bisiach. Remission of hemineglect and anosognosia during vestibular stimulation. *Neuropsychologia* **25,** 775–782 (1987).

181. E. Bisiach, M. L. Rusconi, and G. Vallar. Remission of somatoparaphrenic delusion through vestibular stimulation. *Neuropsychologia* **29,** 1029–1031 (1991).

182. G. Geminiani and G. Bottini. Mental representation and temporary recovery from unilateral neglect after vestibular stimulation. *J. Neurol. Neurosurg. Psychiatry* **55,** 332–333 (1992).

183. G. Vallar, R. Sterzi, G. Bottini, S. F. Cappa, and M. L. Rusconi. Temporary remission of left hemianaesthesia following vestibular stimulation: A sensory neglect phenomenon. *Cortex* **26,** 123–131 (1990).

184. G. Vallar, G. Bottini, M. L. Rusconi, and R. Sterzi. Exploring somatosensory hemineglect by vestibular stimulation. *Brain* **116,** 71–86 (1993).

185. J. C. Mazziotta, S. C. Huang, M. E. Phelps, R. E. Carson, N. S. M. Donald, and K. Mahoney. A non-invasive positron computed tomography technique using oxygen-15 labelled water for the evaluation of neurobehavioral task batteries. *J. Cereb. Blood Flow Metab.* **5,** 70–78 (1985).

186. M. E. Raichle. Circulatory and metabolic correlates of brain function in normal humans. *In* "Handbook of Physiology. The Nervous System. Higher Functions of the Brain" (V. B. Mouncastle, F. Plum, and S. R. Geiger, Eds.), Vol. V, pp. 643–674. American Physiological Society, Bethesda, MD, 1987.

187. D. A. Silbersweig, E. Stern, C. D. Frith, C. Cahill, L. Schnorr, S. Grootoonk, T. Spinks, J. Clark, R. S. J. Frackowiak, and T. Jones. Detection of thirty-second cognitive activations in single subjects with positron emission tomography: A new low dose H215O regional cerebral blood flow three-dimensional imaging technique. *J. Cereb. Blood Flow Metab.* **13,** 617–629 (1993).

188. A. A. Lammerstma, V. J. Cunninham, M. P. Deiber, J. D. Heather, P. M. Bloomfield, J. Nutt, R. S. J. Frackowiak, and T. Jones. Combination of dynamic and integral methods for generating reproducible CBF images. *J. Cereb. Blood Flow Metab.* **9,** 461–470 (1989).

189. W. J. Penfield. Vestibular sensation and the cerebral cortex. *Ann. Otol. Rhinol. Laring.* **66,** 691–698 (1957).

190. L. Friberg, T. S. Olse, P. E. Roland, O. B. Paulson, and N. A. Lassen. Focal increase of blood flow in the cerebral cortex of man following vestibular stimulation. *Brain* **108,** 609–623 (1985).

191. G. Bottini, E. Paulesu, C. D. Frith, and R. S. J. Frackowiak. Functional anatomy of the human vestibular cortex. *In* "Le Cortex Vestibulaire" (M. Collard, M. Jeannerod, and Y. Christen, Eds.), pp. 27–48. Irvinn, Paris, 1996.

192. O. J. Grüsser, M. Pause, and U. Schreiter. Neuronal responses in the parieto-insular vestibular cortex of the alert Java monkeys (Macaca fascicularis). *In* "Physiological and Pathological Aspects of Eyes Movements" (A. Roucoux and M. Crommelink, Eds.), pp. 251–270. W. Junk, The Hague, 1982.

193. O. J. Grüsser, M. Pause, and U. Schreiter. Localization and responses in the parieto-insular vestibular cortex of awake monkeys (Macaca fascicularis). *J. Physiol.* **430,** 537–557 (1990).

194. S. Akbarian, K. Berndl, O. J. Grusser, W. Guldin, M. Pause, and U. Schreiter. Responses of single neurons in the parietoinsular vestibular cortex of primates. *Ann. NY Acad. Sci.* **545,** 187–202 (1988).

195. M. Fredrickson, U. Figge, P. Scheid, and H. H. Kornhuber. Vestibular nerve projection to the cerebral cortex of the Rhesus monkey. *Exp. Brain Res.* **2,** 318–327 (1966).

196. L. M. Odkvist, D. W. F. Schwartz, J. M. Fredrickson, and R. Hassler. Projection of the vestibular nerve to the area 3a arm field in the squirrel monkey. *Exp. Brain Res.* **21,** 97–105 (1974).

197. S. Faugier-Grimaud and J. Ventre. Anatomic connections of inferior parietal cortex area 7 with subcortical structures related with vestibulo-ocular function in a monkey (Macaca facicularis). *J. Comp. Neurol.* **280,** 1–14 (1989).

198. R. E. Passingham, "The Frontal Lobes and Voluntary Action." Oxford Univ. Press, Oxford, 1993.

199. O. J. Grüsser, S. Akbarian, and W. O. Guldin, "Physiology and Anatomy of the Inner Cortical Vestibular Circuit of the Primate Brain." Presented at the 15th Annual Meeting of the European Neuroscience Association, Münich, 1992.

200. W. O. Guldin, S. Akbarian, and O. J. Grusser. Cortico-cortical connections and

cytoarchitectonics of the primate vestibular cortex. A study in squirrel monkeys (Saimiri sciureus). *J. Comp. Neurol.* **326,** 375–401 (1992).

201. S. Akbarian, O. J. Grusser, and W. O. Guldin. Thalamic connections of the vestibular cortical fields in the squirrel monkey (Saimiri sciureus). *J. Comp. Neurol.* **326,** 423–441 (1992).

202. P. A. Hawrylyshyn, A. M. Rubin, R. R. Tasker, L. W. Organ, and J. M. Fredrickson. Vestibulothalamic projections in man—A sixth primary sensory pathway. *J. Neurophysiol.* **2,** 394–401 (1978).

203. E. T. Rolls and S. Johnstone. Neurophysiological analysis of striatal functions. *In* "Neuropsychological Disorders Associated with Subcortical Lesions" (G. Vallar, S. F. Cappa, and C. W. Wallesch, Eds.), pp. 61–97. Oxford Univ. Press, Oxford, 1992.

204. E. Lobel, D. L. Bihan, A. Leroy-Willig, and A. Berthoz. Searching for the vestibular cortex with functional MRI. *NeuroImage* **4,** S351 (1996).

205. S. Zeki, J. D. G. Watson, C. J. Lueck, K. J. Friston, C. Kennard, and R. S. J. Frackowiak. A direct demonstration of functional specialisation in human visual cortex. *J. Neurosci.* **11,** 641–649 (1991).

206. R. Wenzel, P. Bartenstein, M. Dieterich, A. Danek, A. Weindl, S. Minoshima, S. Ziegler, M. Schwaiger, and T. Brandt. Deactivation of human visual cortex during involuntary ocular oscillations. A PET activation study. *Brain* **119,** 101–110 (1996).

207. K. J. Worsley, A. C. Evans, S. Marrett, and P. Neelin. A three dimensional statistical analysis for rCBF activation studies in human brain. *J. Cereb. Blood Flow Metab.* **12,** 900–918 (1992).

208. K. J. Friston. Statistical parametric mapping: ontology and current issues. *J. Cereb. Blood Flow Metab.* **15,** 361–70 (1995).

209. C. D. Frith, K. J. Friston, P. F. Liddle, and R. S. J. Frackowiak. A PET study of word finding. *Neuropsychologia* **29,** 1137–1148 (1991).

210. K. J. Friston, C. D. Frith, P. Liddle, and R. S. J. Frackowiak. Investigating a network model of word generation with positron emission tomography. *Proc. R. Soc. London B* **244,** 101–106 (1991).

211. E. Paulesu, J. Harrison, S. Baron-Cohen, J. Watson, J. Heather, R. S. J. Frackowiak, and C. D. Frith. The physiology of coloured hearing. A positron tomography study of colour word synaesthesia. *Brain* **118,** 661–676 (1995).

212. I. H. Jenkins, D. J. Brooks, P. D. Nixon, R. S. J. Frackowiak, and R. E. Passingham. The functional anatomy of motor sequence learning studied with positron emission tomography. *J. Neurosci.* **14,** 3775–3790 (1993).

213. R. Kawashima, B. T. O'Sullivan, and P. E. Roland. A PET study of selective attention in man, cross-modality decreases in activity in somatosensory and visual tasks. *J. Cereb. Blood Flow Metab.* **13** (Suppl. 1), S502 (1993).

214. T. Paus, S. Marrett, A. C. Evans, and K. Worsley. Imaging motor-to-sensory discharges in the human brain: an experimental tool for the assessment of functional connectivity. *Neuroimage* **4,** 78–86 (1996).

215. A. Cowey and P. Stoerig. Reflections on blindsight. *In* "The Neuropsychology of Consciousness" (D. Milner and M. Rugg, Eds.), pp. 11–37. Academic Press, London, 1992.

216. J. L. Barbur, J. D. G. Watson, R. S. J. Frackowiak, and S. Zeki. Conscious visual perception without V1. *Brain* **116,** 1293–1302 (1993).

217. J.-B. Poline, R. Vandenberghe, A. P. Holmes, K. J. Friston, and R. S. J. Frackowiak. Reproducibility of PET activation studies: lessons from a multi-center European experiment. *NeuroImage* **4,** 34–54 (1996).

218. J. H. Kaas and T. P. Pons. The somatosensory system of primates. *In* "Comparative Primate Biology" (H. P. Steklis and J. Erwin, Eds.), vol. 4. Liss, New York, 1988.

219. T. P. Pons and J. H. Kaas. Connections of area 2 of somatosensory cortex with

the anterior pulvinar and subdivisions of the ventroposterior complex in macaque monkeys. *J. Comp. Neurol.* **240,** 16–36 (1985).

220. E. G. Jones, J. D. Coutler, and S. H. C. Hendry. Intracortical connectivity of architectonic fields in the somatosensory, motor and parietal cortex of monkeys. *J. Comp. Neurol.* **181** (1978).

221. E. G. Jones and T. P. S. Powell. An anatomical study of converging sensory pathways within the cerebral cortex of the rhesus monkey. *Brain* **93,** 793–820 (1970).

222. D. P. Friedman, E. G. Jones, and H. Burton. Representation pattern in the second somatic sensory area of the monkey cerebral cortex. *J. Comp. Neurol.* **192,** 21–42 (1980).

223. V. B. Mountcastle, J. C. Lynch, A. Georgopulos, H. Sakata, and C. Acuna. Posterior parietal association cortex of the monkey: Command functions for operations within extrapersonal space. *J. Neurophysiol.* **38,** 871–908 (1975).

224. H. J. Gould and J. H. Kaas. The distribution of commissural terminations in somatosensory areas I and II of the grey squirrel. *J. Comp. Neurol.* **196,** 489–504 (1981).

225. E. G. Jones and S. H. C. Hendry. Distribution of callosal fibers around the hand representations in monkey somatic sensory cortex. *Neurosci. Lett.* **19,** 167–172 (1980).

226. E. G. Jones and T. P. S. Powell. Connections of the somatic sensory cortex of the rhesus monkey II. Contralateral cortical connexions. *Brain* **92,** 717–730 (1969).

227. R. J. Nelson. Responsiveness of monkey primary somatosensory cortical neurons to peripheral stimulation depends on "motor-set." *Brain Res.* **304,** 143–148 (1984).

228. T. P. S. Powell and V. B. Mountcastle. Some aspects of the functional organization of the cortex of the postcentral gyrus of the monkey. A correlation of findings obtained in a single unit analysis with cytoarchitecture. *Bull. Johns Hopkins Hosp.* **105,** 133–162 (1959).

229. J. Tanji and S. P. Wise. Submodality distribution in sensorimotor cortex of unanesthetized monkey. *J. Neurophysiol.* **45,** 467–481 (1981).

230. M. Randolph and J. Semmes. Behavioral consequences of selective subtotal ablations in the postcentral gyrus of Macaca mulatta. *Brain Res.* **70,** 55–70 (1974).

231. J. Talairach, G. Zikla, P. Tournoux, A. Prosalentis, M. Bordas-Ferrer, L. Covello, M. Iacob, and E. Mempel, "Atlas d'Anatomie Stéréotaxique du Télencéphale: Études Anatomo-Radiologiques." Masson & Cie, Paris, 1967.

232. K. M. Stephan, G. R. Fink, R. E. Passingham, D. Silbersweig, A. O. Caballos-Baumann, C. D. Frith, and R. S. J. Frackowiak. Functional anatomy of the mental representation of upper extremity movements in healthy subjects. *J. Neurophysiol.* **73,** 373–386 (1995).

CHAPTER ELEVEN

FUNCTIONAL ORGANISATION OF THE MOTOR SYSTEM

I. COMPONENTS OF THE MOTOR SYSTEM

This chapter considers the way in which the motor system is organised. It draws on two sorts of information. Our knowledge of the anatomical connections comes from experiments with macaque monkeys. Our knowledge of the functions of different areas in the human brain comes from experiments with functional brain imaging. It is important to note that this chapter is not a general review of the literature on functional imaging of the motor system. It is written to make sense of PET data that we have collected in recent years.

Figure 1 shows the components of the motor system in schematic form. The figure is greatly simplified. First, it omits the parts of the motor system that are involved in directing movements of the eyes. Second, it does not include all the nuclei involved in the direction of limb movements, for example the subthalamic nucleus and the red nucleus. Third, it omits the parietal areas which provide cortico-cortical inputs into the motor system. The figure is given for the human brain, but it contains some details that have been demonstrated in the macaque monkey brain. Further work is needed to compare the anatomical organisation of the premotor areas in the human and macaque frontal cortex.

A. Frontal Cortex

For the limb system, the frontal cortex can be divided into three main strips. The first strip is area 4, the motor cortex (MI). In front of this lies area 6; and the most anterior strip is the dorsal prefrontal cortex (areas 9 and 46).

Figure 1 further subdivides area 6 on the medial and lateral surface into an anterior and a posterior strip. In the macaque brain Matelli *et al.* [1,2] have subdivided the medial area 6 on the basis of cytochrome oxidase staining. They distinguish a posterior area F3 and an anterior area F6. The posterior area F3 corresponds to the supplementary motor area proper (SMA) and the anterior area F6 to the pre-SMA [3].

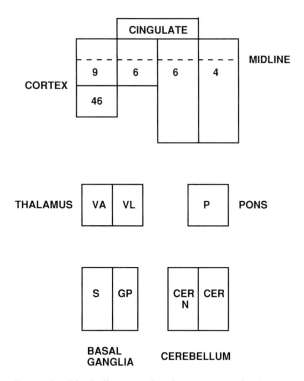

FIGURE 1   Block diagram of major structures in the motor system. Numbers are Brodmann areas; VA, anterior nucleus of ventral thalamus; VL, lateral nucleus of ventral thalamus [12]; S, striatum; GP, globus pallidus; CER N, cerebellar nuclei; CER, cerebellum.

Zilles *et al.* [4] also subdivide medial area 6 on the basis of cytoarchitecture and receptor densities in the human brain. In the atlas of Talairach and Tournoux [5] the division is marked by the VCA line. This is the line drawn vertically through the anterior commissure, and at 90° to the AC–PC line connecting the anterior and posterior commissure. There is also functional evidence suggesting that the VCA line divides an anterior and posterior area on the medial surface of the human brain [6,7].

On the lateral surface the situation is less clear. In the macaque brain Matelli *et al.* [1,2] distinguish an anterior part of the dorsal area 6 which they label F7 and a posterior dorsal area which they label F2. The posterior part includes the lateral premotor area PMd; part of this may send projections to motor cortex [8]. On the basis of cytoarchitecture and receptor anatomy, Zilles (personal communication) has identified an anterior area with a posterior border roughly 0.5 mm in front of the VCA line. However, it has not been established whether this area corresponds to lateral F7 in the macaque brain.

In the macaque brain Matelli *et al.* [1] also distinguish between dorsal and ventral parts of the lateral premotor cortex. The ventral part (F5, F4) includes the postarcuate area PMv identified by Strick [9] as sending direct projections to the motor cortex. The distinction between dorsal and ventral lateral area 6 is not shown in Fig. 1.

There are also cingulate premotor areas on the medial surface. The medial premotor cortex (SMA) includes the convexity cortex of area 6 on the medial surface. Tanji [3] includes some of the cortex in the upper bank of the cingulate sulcus. However, Dum and Strick [10] argue that under the posterior SMA there is a separate representation of the body in the upper bank of the cingulate sulcus, and they classify this as a cingulate premotor area (CMAd). They also identify other cingulate premotor areas in the cingulate sulcus (CMAv, CMAr).

Area 32 lies on the medial surface of the frontal lobe. This is not shown in Fig. 1. It is not clear whether area 32 should be treated as medial prefrontal cortex or cingulate cortex. In the human brain, part of area 32 lies dorsal to the cingulate cortex area 24. This part differs in cytoarchitecture from area 32 in the macaque brain [11].

B. Subcortical Areas

There are two major subcortical components, the basal ganglia and the cerebellum. In the basal ganglia the cortical input is directed to the striatum, and the outputs are sent from the globus pallidus. In the cerebellum, the cortical inputs are directed via the pontine nuclei to the vermis and lateral cerebellar cortex, and the outputs originate from the deep nuclei, the dentate, interpositus, and fastigial.

The basal ganglia and cerebellum influence the frontal cortex via the ventral nuclei of the thalamus. The bulk of the basal ganglia projections are to an anterior division of the thalamus: this anterior division is termed the VA nucleus by Ilinsky and Kultas-Ilinsky [12] and it includes the VA and VLa nuclei of Jones [13]. The bulk of the dentate and interpositus nucleus projection are to a posterior division: this is the VL nucleus of Ilinsky and Kultas-Ilinsky [12] and the VLp nucleus of Jones [13]. Both the anterior and the posterior divisions of the ventral nuclei project to all the frontal cortical strips [14].

The whole of this distributed system can be imaged with the PET scanner. Figure 2 shows the areas that are activated when subjects are scanned while

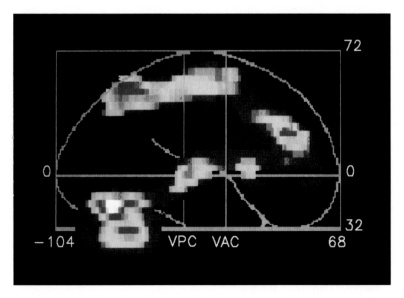

FIGURE 2 SPM of activation for the comparison NEW *vs* BASE. This lateral view shows the activation in the left and right hemisphere at all mediolateral points.

they learn a sequence of finger movements [15]. The comparison is with a baseline condition in which the subjects make no movements. The scan shows activity in motor cortex, the premotor areas and prefrontal cortex, in the somatosensory cortex and the parietal association areas which project to the frontal lobes, and in the cerebellum, basal ganglia, and the ventral thalamic nuclei through which the cerebellum and basal ganglia influence the frontal lobes.

II. FRONTAL CORTICAL OUTPUTS

There are direct outputs to the spinal cord from the motor cortex, from the posterior part of area 6 that lies in front of it, and from cortex in the cingulate sulcus. On the medial surface there are several distinct regions which send pyramidal projections, the posterior part of medial area 6 (SMA) and CMAr and CMAd within the cingulate sulcus [10,16]. There are also pyramidal projections from PMd and PMv within lateral area 6 [8,16,17]. All of the areas that project to the cord also project to motor cortex.

One might assume that these areas all differ in their specialised contribution to movement. The analogy is with the many visual areas outside the striate cortex which differ in their contribution to perception. However, it does not follow that, because these areas project to the cord, they must be specialised for different aspects of the execution of movement. It is important to distinguish between those pyramidal projections which synapse directly onto the motor neurones and those that terminate on "premotor" cell groups in the cord.

We have scanned three subjects while they make repetitive movements with their fingers, arm or leg [18]. The scans for individual subjects show many frontal areas: motor cortex, the dorsal lateral premotor cortex, the SMA, three areas in the cingulate sulcus—tentatively taken to correspond to CMAr, CMAd, and CMAv [10]—an opercular part of premotor area 6, and an insular area. All these areas are known in macaques to project to the spinal cord [16,17,19,20]. Figure 3 shows for one subject the loci of maximal activation for movements of the fingers, shoulder, and leg.

Functional imaging should prove valuable in comparing the contributions of these different premotor areas. One issue, for example, is the degree to which the activation is related to the different parameters of movement. Jenkins *et al.* [21] studied the relation between the rate or frequency at which subjects moved a joystick and the changes in cortical activation. They found a significant relation in the motor cortex and the SMA (Figs. 4a,4b). This contrasts with the lack of any significant relation in the dorsal prefrontal cortex (Fig. 4e), an area which sends no projections directly either to motor cortex or to the spinal cord.

Dettmers *et al.* [22] studied the relation with force under near isometric conditions. The subjects were required to apply pressure to a static dynamonitor and were given auditory feedback so as to enable them to apply different forces. There was a clear correlation with force exerted for the motor cortex (Fig. 5). There was also a significant correlation for the SMA (posterior medial premotor cortex) and the posterior part of the anterior cingulate cortex.

If an area contributes to the execution of movement, it should be more active when subjects actually execute movements than when they are just

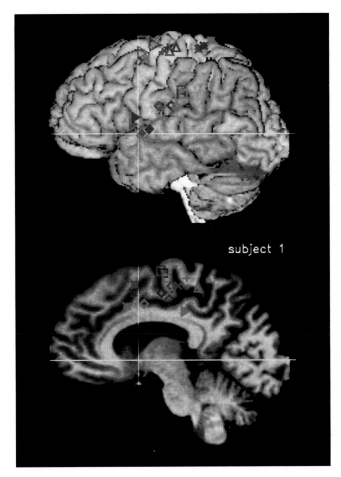

FIGURE 3 Data for a single subject showing location of peaks when subject repetitively moved one side. Red, hand, blue, shoulder; green, leg. On the lateral surface, motor cortex (MI, +); lateral premotor (PMd, ▼, ×); ventral opercular premotor (6, ▼); insula (▽); primary sensorimotor (SI, △); secondary sensorimotor (SII, ◇); inferior anterior parietal (□); superior parietal area 5 (*). On the medial surface, motor cortex (+); supplementary motor cortex (SMA, □); cingulate motor area (CMAr, *); cingulate motor area (CMAd, ×); cingulate motor area (CMAv, ▼); primary sensorimotor (SI, △). For PMd and CMAd there are two peaks for each body part, but they are conservatively grouped as part of one area. (The acronyms are defined and referred to in the text.)

preparing to do so. Stephan *et al.* [23] compared two conditions. In one the subjects were required to prepare to make one of four movements (PREP), and in the other they repeatedly executed each of the movements (EXEC). When the subjects actually performed the movements (EXEC *vs* PREP) there was more activation in the motor cortex, SMA (posterior medial premotor cortex), posterior part of the anterior cingulate cortex, and posterior part of the lateral premotor cortex (Fig. 6).

These data provide functional evidence that it is the more posterior regions within the frontal lobe that are most directly linked with motor execution. This is what one would have inferred from the anatomical evidence that these regions send direct projections to the cord.

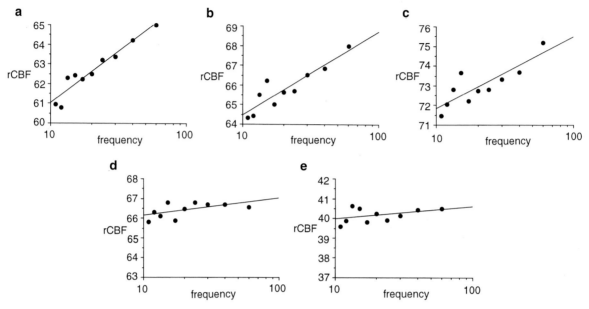

FIGURE 4 rCBF plotted against log frequency (rate) for five areas: a, primary motor cortex (MI); b, SMA; c, right cerebellar vermis; d, putamen; e, dorsal prefrontal cortex (areas 46/9). The line gives the least squares regression through the data points [data from 21].

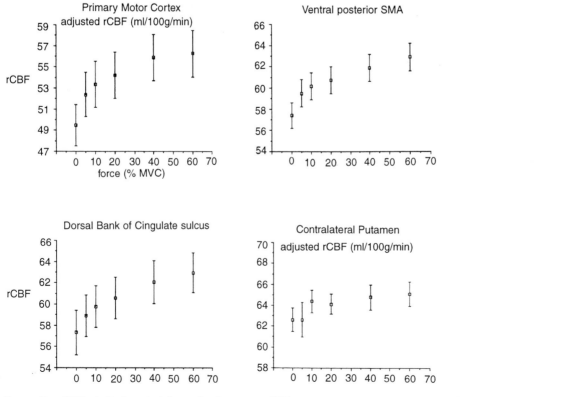

FIGURE 5 rCBF plotted against force for four areas [22].

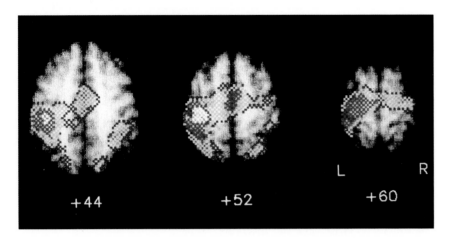

FIGURE 6 Activation for the comparison of executing movements (EXEC) *vs* preparing to move (PREP). Transverse sections showing left motor cortex (MI) and SMA [23].

III. MEDIO/LATERAL ORGANISATION OF FRONTAL CORTEX

A. Anatomy

Motor cortex receives inputs in parallel from both the lateral and the medial premotor areas (area 6). However, there are connections between the lateral and medial area 6 [24]. This means that in the normal brain we would not expect the two areas to function independently.

It has been shown that in the macaque brain there are independent maps of the body in both lateral and medial area 6 [8,10,17]. In the human brain it is possible to identify several areas on the medial and lateral surface of the frontal lobe in which there is activation when a subject moves the leg, shoulder, or fingers [18] (Fig. 3).

B. Functional Organisation

It has been claimed that in the macaque brain there is a difference in the specialisation of the lateral and medial premotor areas (area 6) [25–27]. Monkeys with lateral premotor lesions are impaired at relearning a visual conditional task on which the responses are specified by visual cues, whereas monkeys with medial (SMA) lesions are not [27]. Monkeys with medial (SMA) lesions are impaired at relearning a motor sequence task without external cues, whereas monkeys with lateral premotor lesions are unimpaired [26–28]. In 1993, Passingham [27] argued that these data support the hypothesis that the lateral premotor cortex is especially involved when external cues tell the subject what to do, and the medial premotor cortex (SMA) is especially involved when there are no external cues to tell the subject what to do.

The claim was based on studying the effects of lesions in the lateral or medial premotor cortex (SMA). However, the studies were performed before anatomical and physiological studies had shown that there were various sub-areas within the lateral and medial premotor cortex. The lesions removed both PMd and PMv on the lateral surface and both the pre-SMA and the

SMA on the medial surface. Functional imaging studies have an advantage in that it is possible to distinguish the activation of these different areas and thus allow hypotheses about more specific areas. The following account contrasts PMd with the SMA proper.

PET studies have not appeared to support the hypothesis that PMd is especially involved when there are external cues and the SMA when there are no external cues. Two findings are difficult to account for on this hypothesis. First, we have tested subjects on a "free-selection" task (FREE) on which they decide afresh on each trial which of four movements to make. A comparison was made with a "repetitive task" (REP) on which they repeat the same movement on each trial. For this comparison (FREE *vs* REP) we found activation in the dorsal lateral premotor cortex as well as in the SMA proper [29]. Yet the subject's actions were not determined by external cues.

Second, Jenkins *et al.* [30] required the subjects to vary the intervals at which they raised a finger. In one condition no external cues were given, and the subjects made their own decisions as to when to make the movement (SELF). In the other condition the subjects reponded to tones (EXT). As in the earlier experiment by Jahanshahi *et al.* [31] the computer stored the times at which the subjects raised their finger in the first condition (SELF) and played back the tones at the identical intervals in the condition with external cues (EXT). However, the two studies differ in that in the earlier study [31] there was little variability in the intervals, whereas in the later study [30] the subjects varied the intervals from 1 to 9 sec around a mean interval of 4.46 sec.

We found that the activation of the medial premotor cortex was much more extensive when the subjects decided on the intervals than when they responded to the tones (SELF *vs* EXT) (Fig. 7). Zeffiro *et al.* [32] have made the same comparison, and have briefly reported the same finding. Remy *et al.* [33] failed to find activation of the SMA when subjects flexed and extended their fingers at their own pace. However, the task differs in that the subjects made the movements at a regular pace and did not have to vary the intervals and make decisions on each occasion.

However, we also found more activation of the dorsal lateral premotor cortex when subjects decided when to respond (SELF *vs* FREE) [30]. Yet, as for the free-selection task, the movements on the self-paced task are not determined by external cues. Thus for both tasks, the data are not as predicted by the hypothesis that the lateral premotor cortex is especially involved when the movements are guided by external cues. There are more conclusive data to suggest that the hypothesis needs emendation. While it can accomodate the finding that cells are active in both PMd and the SMA during tasks with or without external cues, it cannot predict that cells in PMd will be more active than cells in SMA when a task is performed without external cues. Yet Jenkins *et al.* [15] found that during learning of a motor sequence, the dorsal lateral premotor cortex was activated more than the SMA (Fig. 21).

To resolve the issue we have recently used PET to compare directly the learning of a visual conditional task and a motor sequence task [Toni *et al.*, in preparation]. The subjects were scanned for four periods during learning of each task. In the first period they learned the task for the first time and in the second they continued learning. Before the third period they were given more practice, and again before the fourth, so that the task was overlearned by the end of scanning.

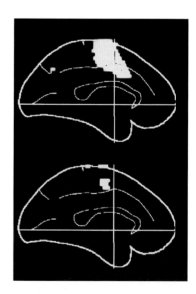

FIGURE 7 Activation of the SMA for self-initiated movements (SELF *vs* REST) (top) but little activation for externally triggered movements (EXT *vs* REST) (bottom). The range in intervals for self-initiated movements was from 1 to 9 sec [data from 30].

The subjects learned the sequence by trial and error, as described by Jenkins *et al.* [15], except that visual nonsense shapes were used as pacing cues, and the feedback cues were a "tick" on the screen if the response was correct and a "cross" if it was incorrect. The four fingers of the right hand lay on keys, and at each pacing cue the subject moved one of them. The subject learned the sequence by using the feedback cues. The visual conditional task was learned in the same way, except that the pacing cues now also served to tell the subjects which response to make. Each nonsense shape specified a particular finger. This task is formally the same task as that used by Mitz *et al.* [34].

We found that the lateral premotor cortex was equally activated during learning of either task (periods 1 and 2). This is not as predicted by the hypothesis. There was, however, a difference between the two tasks in periods 3 and 4, when the task had become overlearned. There was significant activation in the SMA for the motor sequence but not for the visual conditional task (Fig. 8). For both tasks there was an increase in activation of the anterior cingulate cortex around the level of the VCA line (Fig. 8). Mitz *et al.* [34] also reported an increase in activation of cingulate cortex as subjects learned a visual conditional task.

These data suggest a revised version of the hypothesis. During new learning of either task, performance can be described as closed loop. On both tasks the subjects must pay attention to the outcomes and on the visual conditional task the subjects must pay attention to the visual cues. However, during overlearned performance of the motor sequence performance is open loop. The subjects know in advance what movements to make and need no longer pay attention to the outcomes. Performance of the visual conditional task never becomes open loop since subjects must always respond to the particular visual cue that is presented on any trial.

It is now clear that the dorsal lateral premotor cortex is involved in the learning of associations, whether these are associations between one movement and another (sequence) or the associations between movements and external cues (visual conditional). However, there is a suggestion that the SMA is more involved in open loop performance, as when a motor sequence has become overlearned. In such circumstances the movements are known in advance and can be performed without reference to external information.

The revised hypothesis will account for the other PET data. On the free-selection task the series of moves are not predetermined; the subjects have to keep in mind the moves they made on previous trials so as to achieve a random series of responses over trials. The same is true for the self-paced task; the subjects must keep in mind the intervals between responding on previous trials so as to achieve the target of a mean interval with variation around it.

The revised hypothesis can also account for the lesion data. In the experiments reviewed above [27] the monkeys were tested on retention of motor sequence and visual conditional tasks that had been prelearned before surgery. The human PET data suggest that during prelearned performance the SMA is involved more for the motor sequence than for the visual conditional task. It is also the case that studies of single unit activity during motor sequences have been carried out in monkeys that have previously been overtrained on the sequences [3]. The hypothesis makes the prediction that a lateral premotor lesion would impair the learning of a motor sequence task.

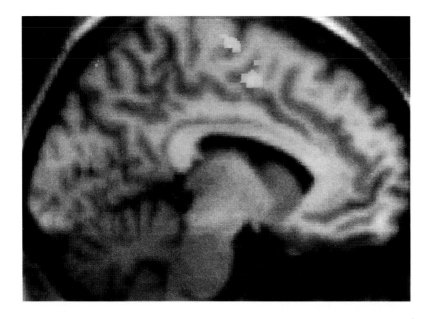

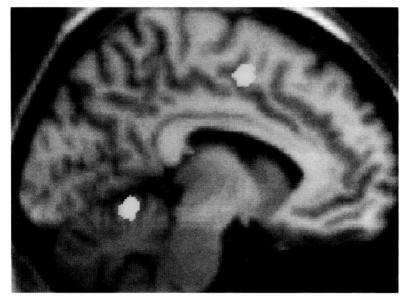

FIGURE 8   Activation of the SMA for overlearned sequence (top) but not for over-learned visual conditional (bottom). There is activation in the anterior cingulate cortex for both (unpublished data from I. Toni *et al.*).

C. Comparing the Effects of Lesions and Recording

There is, however, a difference between the effects of lesions and the results of recording in the two areas. The effects of lesions suggest a more radical difference between the lateral premotor cortex and the SMA than is suggested by a comparison of activity in the two areas. The differences obtained in PET are differences of degree only. In the recent study by Toni *et al.* (in preparation), we found that for the visual conditional task the SMA was not activated at a robust significance level ($P < 0.001$) when the task had been overlearned, but there was a trend for activation in this region.

The differences in unit activity between the lateral premotor cortex and the SMA are also differences of degree. Mushiake *et al.* [35] recorded the activity of single cells in monkeys while the animals performed sequence tasks. In one condition, lights told the monkeys which buttons to press (visual sequence). In the other condition, the monkeys performed the sequence from memory, with no external cues to tell them what to do (remembered sequence). Figure 9 shows the activity of cells in premotor cortex (PMv) and the SMA. There was a tendency for the activity of cells in the lateral premotor cortex to be more active when visual cues told the animal what to do, and for the activity of cells in the SMA to be greater when the sequence was performed without external cues.

However, many of the cells in both areas were active during both tasks. Similarly, other studies show that there are many cells in the lateral premotor cortex that become active when monkeys make self-initiated movements [36] and that there are many cells in the SMA that become active when monkeys perform a visually cued conditional task [37].

PET and single unit recordings are taken when the brain is intact; thus the medial and lateral premotor areas are interconnected. The lesion experiment removes one of the areas and observes how far the other area can cope with the relevant task. No recordings have been taken from the lateral or medial premotor areas when the other has been removed. It is quite possible that some of the functional properties of cells in one area are derived from the

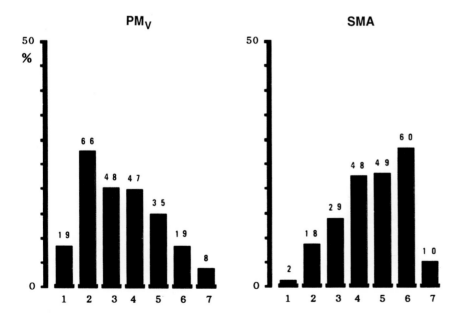

FIGURE 9 Distribution of cells in lateral premotor cortex (PMv) and SMA classified according to the degree to which they were active in association with the visually guided sequence (VS) or the sequence performed from memory (MS). 1, Exclusively related to VS; 2, predominantly related to VS; 3, more related to VS than MS; 4, equally related to VS and MS; 5, more related to MS; 6, predominantly related to VS; 7, exclusively related to MS. The ordinate shows the percentage of cells, and the numbers above the histograms show the number of cells [35].

other area. If this is so, one would predict that each area would lose these derived properties if the other area was lesioned. Consider, for example, the data shown in Fig. 9. If the medial premotor cortex (SMA) was removed, there might be fewer cells in the lateral premotor cortex that fired on the memory guided sequence.

We have therefore used functional imaging to study patients with pathology. Patients with Parkinson's disease are poor at making self-generated movements. In the early stages of illness the loss of dopamine is found mainly in the lateral putamen [38], and we have found less activation of the SMA than in normal control subjects [31,39]. Yet we found either no change [39], or only a small change [31] in the activation of the lateral premotor cortex. The results suggest that the lateral premotor cortex is unable to subserve normal self-generated movements in the absence of a normally functioning SMA.

D. Conclusions

This section has compared the dorsal premotor cortex and the SMA. Lesion data suggest that visual cues influence the motor system via the premotor cortex, whereas the supplementary motor cortex is specialised for the direction of movements that do not depend on external cues. The data from functional brain imaging suggest that the dorsal premotor cortex is activated when a task is learned and the task is closed loop; and that this is true even if the task is a sequence task. They also provide tentative evidence that the SMA is particularly activated when a sequence task can be performed in open loop mode. The dissociations found in imaging are nonetheless much less clear cut than the dissociations suggested by the lesion experiments. It has been suggested that this may be because in the normal brain the two areas are functionally interconnected, whereas lesions indicate the competence of one area when the other has been removed.

IV. ANTERIOR/POSTERIOR ORGANISATION OF FRONTAL CORTEX

A. Anatomy

There is an anterior-posterior organisation of the frontal cortex. Figure 10 shows the strips of frontal cortex identified in Fig. 1. These are oriented vertically. This figure omits the cingulate cortex which lies on the medial surface below medial area 6 (Fig. 1).

1. Thalamic Input

The thalamic inputs to these strips have been recently described for the macaque by Matelli and Luppino [40,41], using the nomenclature of Olszewski [42]. Motor cortex and the posterior parts of area 6 (F3, F2, F5) send pyramidal outputs to the cord, and these areas receive an input from the ventral thalmic nuclei VLo and VPLo. In turn VLo receives a projection from the putamen via the GPi (globus pallidus, pars interna) [43], and VPLo receives a projection from the dentate and interpositus nuclei of the cerebellum [44]. Thus both basal ganglia and cerebellum can influence the posterior frontal strips (area 4, and F2 and F3).

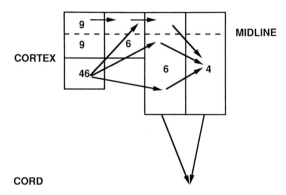

Figure 10   Strips of frontal cortex. Numbers give Brodmann areas.

The general pattern of projections to the anterior parts of area 6 is different. On the medial surface the anterior part receives an input from VApc and MD (mediodorsal nucleus) and from nucleus X. In turn, the caudate nucleus is thought to influence VApc and MD via projections to the dorsal GPi [45,46], and the lateral dentate sends projections to nucleus X [44]. On the lateral surface, Matelli and Luppino [41] suggest that the caudo-ventral part of F7 also receives a limb input from VApc and nucleus X.

Both MD and VApc also project to the prefrontal cortex that lies more anteriorly [47]. However, it has recently been shown that the cerebellum can also influence prefrontal cortex through a projection from the ventral dentate via VLc [48].

This account is oversimplified. However, the thalamic inputs support the suggestion that more posterior parts of area 6 may be more directly involved in the execution of movement than the anterior parts, which share some common inputs with the more anterior dorsal prefrontal cortex [41].

2. Cortico-Cortical Projections

The cortico-cortical projections between these strips are shown in Fig. 10. There are no direct projections from the dorsal prefrontal cortex either to motor cortex or to the spinal cord. The dorsal prefrontal cortex can influence motor cortex only via the intervening strips of area 6 or anterior cingulate cortex or via subcortical projections.

In the macaque monkey it has been shown that prefrontal area 46 is interconnected with several areas that send direct projections to the motor cortex. On the medial surface these include the cingulate areas CMAr and CMAv on the medial surface [50], not shown in Fig. 10. However, it is also interconnected with the anterior part of the medial area 6 (F6) [49,50], and Bates and Goldman-Rakic [49] state that there is a similar connection from area 9. Luppino *et al.* [51] have suggested that there is a connection between the anterior and posterior part of medial area 6.

On the lateral surface of the macaque brain, prefrontal area 46 is also interconnected with the ventral premotor area PMv and the rostral part of PMd [50]. There are also projections to F7 (not shown on the figure) [50]; it is not clear whether these are directed mainly to the supplementary eye field in medial F7 or whether they are also directed to that part of caudal F7 that receives a thalamic projection from VApc.

B. Area 6

1. Preparation for Movement

It was shown above that there is more activation of area 4 and the posterior part of medial area 6 when subjects actually execute movements rather than simply prepare to make a self-selected movement (EXEC *vs* PREP) [23] (Fig. 6). In the same experiment it was found that there was more activation of the anterior part of medial area 6 when subjects prepared for movement compared with executing actual movements (PREP *vs* EXEC) [23] (Fig. 11). This result suggests that the anterior strip of medial area 6 is less concerned than the posterior strip with the details of movement execution. It has also been reported in monkeys that the cells that are active during preparation for a response are more concentrated in the pre-SMA than in the SMA [52].

Deiber *et al.* [53] also scanned subjects while they prepared to make movements. However, the paradigm differed in that the movements were visually cued. The authors did not find more activation of either medial or lateral premotor cortex when subjects prepared for and then executed a movement, compared with a condition in which they executed the movements as soon as the visual cued appeared. It may be that this comparison is not a sensitive one, since the movements were executed in both conditions. Kawashima *et al.* [54] used a different paradigm: they scanned subjects only during the period of preparation. They reported activation in the lateral premotor cortex and distinguish between anterior and posterior activations.

2. Selection of Movement

There are two ways in which subjects can prepare for movement. First, they can get ready for movement in general. Second, they can get ready to perform a specific movement. In the latter case they select a movement and then prepare to perform it.

We have compared a selection with a nonselection condition. In one condition we required subjects to select between four movements each time

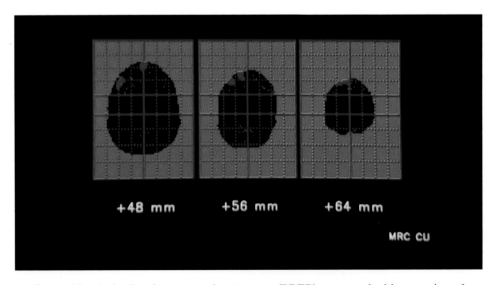

FIGURE 11 Activation for preparation to move (PREP) compared with execution of the movement (EXEC). Transverse sections showing activation in the pre-SMA (in front of the VCA line) (Stephan, personal communication).

that they heard a pacing tone. The pacing tones were played once every 3 sec. This free-selection task (FREE) has been referred to previously: the subjects had a free choice over which movements to make. This condition was contrasted with a "repetitive condition" (REP) in which the subjects were required to make the same movement on all trials. In the studies by Deiber *et al.* [29] and Playford *et al.* [39] the subjects moved a joystick in one of four directions, whereas in the recent study by Jueptner *et al.* [55] they selected between movements of the four fingers.

For the selection condition (FREE *vs* REP) there is activation on the medial surface anterior to the VCA line. Deiber *et al.* [29] and Playford *et al.* [39,56] reported activation that they assigned to the anterior SMA (peak $z = +52$). However, Jueptner *et al.* [55] only found an activation anterior to the VCA line that they assign to the anterior cingulate cortex (area 32).

On the lateral surface, there is activation of premotor cortex for the same comparison (FREE *vs* REP). Deiber *et al.* [29] reported activation in front of the VCA line (for peak, $y = +10$). Jueptner *et al.* [55] found activation that extended up to the VCA line on the left; on the right there was a peak 4 mm in front of the VCA line.

In the study by Jueptner *et al.* [55] there was no significant activation of the lateral or medial area 6 when subjects performed the nonselection task (REP *vs* BASE). However, it can be objected that the free-selection condition differs from the repetitive condition in two respects: in free selection the subjects select, but they also move all four fingers over the trials, whereas in the repetitive condition they move only one. Deiber *et al.* [29] therefore compared free-selection with other tasks in which all four movements were made. They still found significant activation of the lateral premotor cortex. In the more recent studies by Jueptner *et al.* subjects were scanned while they freely selected between four finger movements (55) or performed a prelearned sequence of the four finger movements (57). When performing the free-selection task, the subjects made a new selection between movement one each trial, whereas when performing the prelearned sequence, the responses were predetermined. The lateral premotor cortex was strongly activated during free selection (FREE *vs* BASE), but during the prelearned task (PRE *vs* BASE) the activation lay more posteriorly, on the border with motor cortex.

These findings support the view that area 6 plays a role in the selection of movement [27]. There are suggestions that activations can be seen around or in front of the VCA line. However, the findings are not fully consistent in how far forward they place the activations within medial and lateral area 6.

C. Dorsal Prefrontal Cortex (Areas 9/46)

The dorsal prefrontal cortex forms the most anterior strip of the frontal cortex. It receives a heavy input from the parietal cortex [58]. It can influence movement via its connections with area 6 (Fig. 10). The dorsal prefrontal cortex is not concerned with the parameters of movement. Activation of the dorsal prefrontal cortex does not depend on the rate at which the movements are performed [21] (Fig. 4e).

1. Decision Making

Like the anterior strip of area 6, the dorsal prefrontal cortex is activated when subjects select between movements (FREE *vs* REP) [29,55]. Figure 12 shows activation of the dorsal prefrontal cortex and medial frontal cortex,

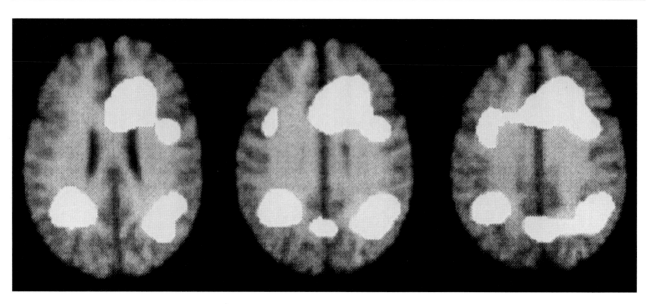

FIGURE 12 Activation of the dorsal prefrontal cortex and anterior cingulate cortex when comparing free-selection with a repetitive condition (FREE *vs* REP). Activations are also shown in parietal cortex. Transverse sections at $z = +28$ (left), $+32$ (middle), and $+36$ (right) [data from 55].

area 32, when subjects select between movements of the fingers [55]. Frith *et al.* [59] also found activation of the dorsal prefrontal and anterior cingulate cortex when subjects made new decisions as to which finger to move.

The dorsal prefrontal cortex is activated not only while subjects decide which actions to perform but also while they decide when to make them. Jahanshahi *et al.* [31] required subjects to decide when to raise a finger. The subjects varied the time around a mean interval of 3.4 sec (SELF). In the other condition they responded to tones (EXT). Thus in the first condition (SELF) the subjects made a series of decisions. In the other condition (EXT) there were no new decisions to make; the subjects simply acted as instructed by the tones. The dorsal prefrontal cortex was the only area that was very significantly more active when the subjects made decisions (SELF *vs* EXT) (Fig. 13).

These studies suggest that the dorsal prefrontal cortex is activated when subjects make decisions as to what to do or when to do it. However, in both studies the subjects were required to produce a random series, and to do so they presumably referred to previous moves. The studies do not therefore distinguish two possibilities, that the dorsal prefrontal cortex is involved in decision making *per se* or that it is involved when decisions are made on the basis of working memory.

2. Imagination

The dorsal prefrontal cortex is also activated when subjects make decisions in their head. We required subjects to make repeated decisions as to which way to move a joystick [60]. They performed the free-selection task but without actually moving the joystick. Their task was to decide on the direction and to imagine moving the joystick (IMAG). When a comparison was made with a resting condition, the dorsal prefrontal cortex was

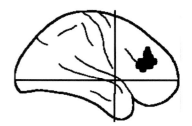

FIGURE 13 Activation of the right dorsal prefrontal cortex (black) when comparing self-initiated with externally triggered movements (SELF *vs* EXT). The mean interval was 3.4 sec and the SD was 0.42 sec [31].

more active when the subjects did the task in imagination (IMAG *vs* REST) [60].

D. Conclusions

There is an anterior–posterior organisation of the frontal cortex. It has been shown in the macaque that there are direct outputs to the cord from the motor cortex (area 4) and from posterior regions within area 6. There are no such direct projections from the most anterior strip (prefrontal cortex) and the more anterior regions within area 6.

The more posterior regions play a role in the execution of movement. There is more activation in area 6 when subjects select between movements. The anterior part of medial area 6 appears to play a role in preparation for movement. The most anterior strip (dorsal prefrontal cortex) is involved in the process by which subjects decide which movement to make or when to make it.

V. CORTICAL/SUBCORTICAL ORGANISATION

A. Anatomy

There are interconnections between the neocortex and the two major subcortical structures, the basal ganglia and the cerebellum. The connections from the frontal lobe are shown in Fig. 14.

The cerebellum receives an input via the pontine nuclei from the sensorimotor areas, that is premotor areas 6, motor cortex (MI, area 4), somatosensory cortex (SI, areas 3,2,1), and parietal areas 5 and 7 [61]. There is also a projection from the dorsal but not the ventral prefrontal cortex; it has been reported that this is less heavy [61], but further research is needed to estimate the size of this projection. There are also projections from the superior temporal sulcus in the temporal lobe [62], but there appear to be few from the lateral and ventromedial convexity cortex of the temporal lobe [61]. The bulk of the projections come from areas that are known to play a role in somatosensory or motor function.

The projections to the basal ganglia differ in that all areas of the neocortex other than the primary sensory areas send projections to them. These areas include all the temporal lobe and both dorsal and ventral prefrontal cortex.

Both the basal ganglia and the cerebellum send projections to the ventral thalamus. There are projections to each of the frontal strips from both the basal ganglia and cerebellar territory of the ventral thalamus [40,41] (Fig. 15). A projection from the cerebellar territory to caudal area 9 was originally suggested on the basis of physiological experiments [63]. It has recently been shown by using tracers that the dentate nucleus can influence prefrontal area 46 via the thalamic nucleus VLc [48].

B. Functional Organisation

1. Attention to Action

PET can be used to distiguish the contributions of cortical and subcortical areas. In a recent study we taught subjects a sequence of finger movements.

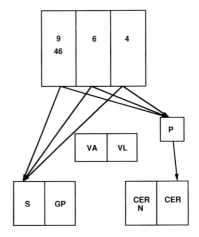

Figure 14 Block diagram showing projections from frontal strips to the basal ganglia and cerebellum. Numbers, Brodmann areas; VA, anterior nucleus of ventral thalamus; VL, lateral nucleus of ventral thalamus [12]; S, striatum; GP, globus pallidus; P, pons; CER, cerebellum; CER N, cerebellar nuclei.

We then trained them until the task had become automatic so that the subjects no longer had to attend to what they were doing. The task and training were the same as for an earlier experiment described by Jenkins *et al.* [15]. In the follow-up study we included an "attention" condition (ATT) [57]. In this condition the subjects performed the prelearned sequence that they had over-learned, but they were instructed to attend to what they were doing The instruction was that after each movement they should think about the next one.

We compared the activation for the "attention" condition with that for the prelearned task performed automatically (ATT *vs* PRE). At a high significance level there was an increase in activation of the dorsal prefrontal cortex and the anterior cingulate area 32 [57] (Fig. 16). The most statistically robust increases were in the cortex. There was a trend for activation in the caudate nucleus and cerebellum (ATT *vs* PRE) but the activation was not significant at a high level of significance ($P < 0.001$).

These results are consistent with the naive view that it is cortical rather than subcortical structures that are involved in performance of which we are conscious. Both the dorsal prefrontal cortex and the anterior cingulate area 32 are activated when subjects make decisions as to what to do (FREE *vs* REP) (Fig. 12). The findings for the attention condition suggest that they are involved when decisions are conscious, in the sense that the subject pays attention to them and thinks about them (see Chapters 9 and 14). Evidence that this may be so comes from a study by Watkins and Passingham [described in Ref. 64] in which the attention of subjects was distracted by requiring them to generate verbs in response to nouns that were presented on a screen. If they were required to do this during new learning of a sequence, they made many errors on the sequence. However, if required to do this during over-learned performance, they made few errors on the sequence. These results

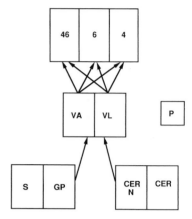

FIGURE 15 Block diagram showing projections from basal ganglia and cerebellum to frontal strips. Numbers, Brodmann areas; VA, anterior nucleus of ventral thalamus; VL, lateral nucleus of ventral thalamus [12]; S, striatum; GP, globus pallidus; P, pons; CER, cerebellum; CER N, cerebellar nuclei.

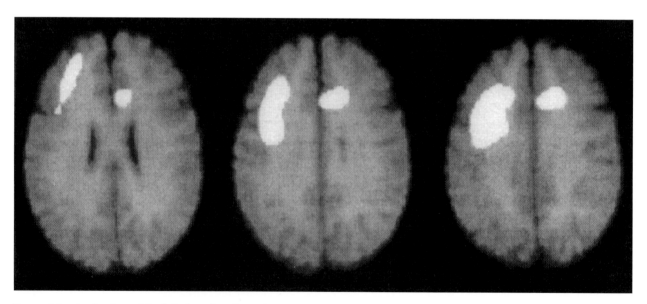

FIGURE 16 Activation of the left dorsal prefrontal cortex and right anterior cingulate cortex when comparing the condition in which subjects were required to attend to performance of an overlearned sequence with a condition in which they performed the overlearned sequence without attending (ATT *vs* PRE). Transverse sections at $z = +28$ (left), $+32$ (middle), and $+36$ (right) [57].

show that during new learning subjects must attend to what they are doing. Passingham [64] argues that the interference occurs because verb generation and new learning of the sequence make competing demands on the prefrontal and/or anterior cingulate cortex. However, when the motor task has become automatic, it can be performed by subcortical motor structures and related cortical motor areas (see Changes in Organisation below). The tasks can be performed without attention. The dorsal prefrontal and/or anterior cortex are no longer committed, and the subject can pay conscious attention to other tasks.

2. Implicit Motor Learning

There is other evidence that subcortical motor areas are involved in processing of which the subjects are unaware. Grafton *et al.* [65] and Doyon *et al.* [66] have tested subjects on the serial reaction time task under conditions of implicit learning. The subjects respond to four locations on a screen, pressing each one when it lights up. Unbeknown to them, the locations light up in a long sequence that repeats throughout the task. It can be shown that learning takes place because the response times of the subjects decrease over trials, even though the subjects remain unaware that they are learning. Grafton *et al.* [65] took special care to ensure that the subjects were unaware that there was a sequence: the subjects were required to carry out a counting task at the same time.

There are changes in subcortical structures during implicit learning. Grafton *et al.* [65] found changes in activation of the putamen that were correlated with learning. Doyon *et al.* [66] found that there was more activity in the ventral striatum and in the cerebellar nuclei when subjects performed the learned sequence compared with a control task in which the presentation of the location was random and there was no sequence. Rauch *et al.* [67] also report activation in the caudate nucleus when subjects learned a sequence by implicit learning. These studies support the view that there are changes in subcortical structures though the subjects are not aware that they are learning. However, it is not the case that the changes are confined to subcortical structures. Changes have also been reported in the motor cortex and SMA during implicit learning [65]. The final common path is through these cortical areas.

3. Explicit Motor Learning

We have studied motor learning when subjects learn explicitly and by trial and error. The learning task has been referred to in a previous section; it is described by Jenkins *et al.* [15]. In the version used by Jueptner *et al.* [55] the four fingers of the right hand lie on keys, and at each pacing tone the subject moves one of them. During the scan the subject learns a sequence by using feedback from a computer. Whenever the subject moves a finger, one of two tones is presented to tell the subject whether the move is correct at that point in the sequence. When the subjects learn this task they have to make new decisions, attend to what they are doing, and remember the moves that are correct.

We compared new learning of this task (NEW) with a condition in which the subjects had to make new decisions and attend to what they were doing, but in which no learning occurred. This condition was the "free selection" task (FREE) described on page 250. Here the subjects move a finger at each pacing tone, but there is no sequence to learn.

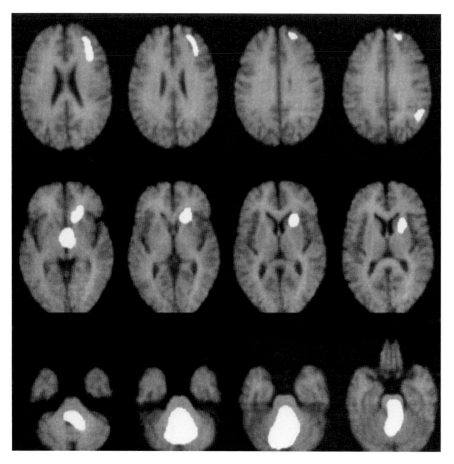

Figure 17 Activation of the right dorsal prefrontal cortex (top), right caudate and globus pallidus (middle), and cerebellum (bottom) when comparing the new learning condition with the free-selection condition (NEW *vs* FREE). Transverse sections at $z = 24$ (left), $z = +28$, $z = +32$, and $z = +36$ (right) [57].

Figure 17 shows that when new learning was compared with free selection (NEW *vs* FREE) there was activation in the right dorsal prefrontal cortex, the caudate nucleus and the cerebellum. Grafton *et al.* [65] and Doyon *et al.* [66] also found that the prefrontal cortex was activated when subjects learned motor sequences and were aware that there was a sequence to learn. It is known that the dorsal prefrontal cortex is activated when subjects hold past responses in memory, and regulate their responses on this basis [68].

The study by Jueptner *et al.* [55] suggests that the basal ganglia and cerebellum may play a role in motor memory, motor preparation, or motor learning. However, it does not distinguish experimentally between the contributions made by these two subcortical structures. The reason is that the new learning task differs in several respects from the free selection task. For example, during new learning, but not free-selection, the subjects must remember the previous moves, remember the outcomes, and correct their responses on the basis of these outcomes.

4. Comparison of Basal Ganglia and Cerebellum

Experiments are now needed to distinguish the contributions of the cerebellum and basal ganglia to motor memory and learning. Friston *et al.*

[69] required subjects to practice simple finger movements while they were being scanned. There were changes of activation in the cerebellum but not the basal ganglia as subjects practiced the task. In this study, unlike the studies by Jenkins *et al.* [15] and Jueptner *et al.* [55,57] subjects knew the sequence before scanning. Since the moves were known, the change in activity may be related to how the moves were performed.

In a more recent study [70] we have scanned subjects during visual tracking. Every 3 sec a line appeared on a screen, and the subjects had to keep a mouse pointer at the end of the line as it slowly contracted. In a prior condition the subjects drew a line every 3 sec with the mouse pointer with no visual cues as to where to draw it. The lines that appeared in the visual tracking or "copying" condition (COPY) were identical to the lines that the subjects drew in the prior drawing (DRAW) condition.

The cerebellar vermis and the left cerebellar nuclei and hemisphere were activated more in visual tracking than in drawing (COPY *vs* DRAW) (Fig. 18). However, there was no difference in activation between the two tasks for the basal ganglia; they were activated equally in both. Grafton *et al.* [71] have shown that during initial acquisition of a visual tracking task, the cerebellar activation is related to the degree of the learning. The study by Jueptner *et al.* [70] suggests that the activation can be related not just to the movements made, but specifically to the use of visual information to correct errors.

These studies point to a specialised role for the cerebellum in learning of skilled movements. There is additional evidence that cerebellar activity may be more closely related to the execution of movement than is activity in the basal ganglia. There is a significant and close relation between cerebellar activation and the rate [21] and force [22] of movement, but this is not the case for activation in the putamen (Figs. 4,5). Furthermore, microstimulation of the cerebellar territory of the ventral thalamus evokes movement, but microstimulation of the basal ganglia territory does not [72].

When subjects learn motor sequences by trial and error [15,57] there are two changes. First, the subjects learn which keys to press at any particular point in the sequence. Second, the subjects learn to perform the movements smoothly and quickly. Figure 19 compares the response times to the pacing tones during new learning (NEW) and during performance of a sequence that has previously been overlearned for 75 min (PRE) [57]. While the subjects are learning their response times are long and variable. When they are performing a sequence automatically their response times are short and less variable. It is possible that the basal ganglia are more involved in learning and remembering what moves to make, and that the cerebellum is more involved in learning to make the moves smoothly and quickly. However, for the moment this hypothesis remains untested.

C. Conclusions

This section has been concerned with comparisons between cortex and subcortex. It has been shown that the dorsal prefrontal and anterior cingulate cortex are activated when subjects pay attention to their actions, but not when they perform the same movements automatically. Evidence has also been reviewed which indicates that these areas are not activated when subjects learn motor tasks implicitly, that is they are not aware of learning. These anterior frontal

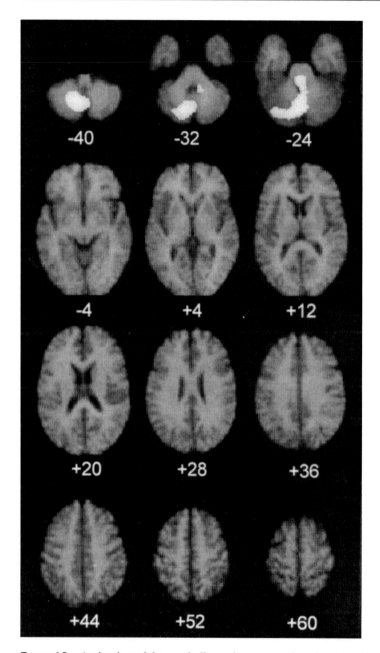

FIGURE 18　Activation of the cerebellum when comparing visual tracking or "copying" of lines with free drawing of lines (COPY *vs* DRAW). Transverse sections with heights (*z*) given below [70].

areas appear to be involved when subjects make "conscious" decisions concerning action.

Though changes can be demonstrated in the basal ganglia and cerebellum during motor learning, there are few studies that compare the roles of these two structures. It is a challenge for functional imaging to look for ways of characterising the different functions of the cortico-basal ganglia and the cortico-cerebellar paths.

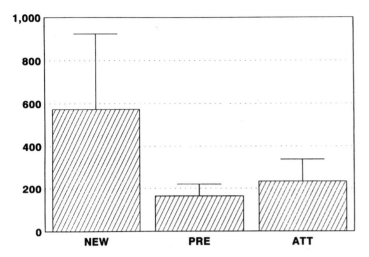

FIGURE 19 Mean and SD for response time in new learning (NEW), performance of the prelearned sequence (PRE), and the attention condition (ATT). Ordinate gives RT in milleseconds.

VI. CHANGES IN ORGANISATION

The previous sections have described the basic organisation of the motor system. This section considers the changes in organisation that occur over time.

A. Cortex

In two studies [15,57] we have mapped the activation of different cortical areas when subjects learn new motor sequences. The activation for this condition has been compared with the activation when subjects perform a motor sequence that they have overlearned until they can perform it automatically. There is a dramatic contraction in the activity from new learning to automatic performance (Fig. 20).

In both studies the prefrontal cortex was extensively activated during new learning (NEW *vs* PRE) (Fig. 20). However, when the subjects performed an automatic sequence, the prefrontal cortex was not significantly activated above the levels of global flow (Fig. 20). In other words, the most anterior cortical strip was activated when subjects had to make decisions during new learning, but not when they no longer had to make new decisions as to what to do.

A similar change was also reported by Raichle *et al.* [73] in a study on verbal associative learning. The prefrontal cortex was strongly activated when subjects produced new verbs that were appropriate for nouns, but not when they repeated the same verbs on successive repetition of the same list of nouns.

Changes can also be detected in more posterior strips when comparing new learning (NEW) and performance of the prelearned sequence (PRE). In the study by Jenkins *et al.* [15], for new learning the activation in the lateral premotor cortex extended in front of the VCA line (for peak, $y = +10$) (NEW *vs* PRE) (Fig. 21). In the study by Jueptner *et al.* [57] there was also activation in the dorsal premotor cortex, extending on the right to the level of the VCA line (for peak on right, $y = +4$) (NEW *vs* PRE).

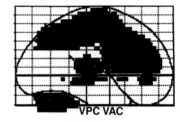

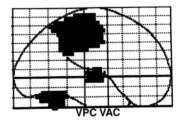

FIGURE 20 SPM diagrams showing activation during new learning compared with the baseline (NEW *vs* BASE) (top), and during performance of the overlearned sequence compared with the baseline (PRE *vs* BASE) (bottom). This lateral view shows the activation in the left and right hemisphere at all mediolateral points [data from 57].

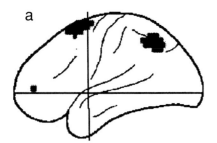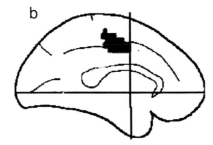

FIGURE 21 Activation of the lateral premotor cortex (a) when comparing new learning of a sequence with overlearned performance of the sequence (NEW *vs* PRE) and activation of the SMA and anterior cingulate cortex (b) when comparing overlearned performance of the sequence with new learning of a sequence [data from 15].

Jenkins *et al.* [15] also compared automatic performance with new learning [PRE *vs* NEW]. They reported that it was the posterior part of the medial premotor cortex (SMA) that was more activated during automatic performance (for peak, $y = -12$) (Fig. 21). In the study by Jueptner *et al.* [57], for automatic performance the peak on the lateral surface lay on the border between area 6 and motor cortex (PRE *vs* BASE). In the medial premotor cortex (SMA) the activation also lay posteriorly (for peak, $y = -16$) (PRE *vs* BASE). These data suggest a retraction of activity in the cortex as a motor task is learned. The more anterior cortex is activated only when the task is nonroutine.

B. Basal Ganglia

The different cortical strips are all interconnected with the basal ganglia. Alexander *et al.* [74] have suggested that there are a series of loops arranged in parallel. Hoover and Strick [43] have used a virus as a retrograde tracer so as to visualize the series of connections through the basal ganglia and ventral thalamus to the motor cortex, SMA and arcuate premotor area (PMv). There is controversy about the extent to which there is significant overlap between the various cortico-subcortical loops (27,75).

There are two principles of organisation in the cortical projections to the basal ganglia. First, each cortical area projects to a strip that runs throughout the anterior/posterior extent of the striatum [45]. Second, each cortical area sends the bulk of its projections to the part of the striatum that is closest to it. This has been demonstrated for the visual projections from occipito-temporal cortex [76]. It also appears to hold for other areas. For example, in the macaque the prefrontal cortex lies slightly more medially than the motor and premotor areas, and it projects heavily to the medial part of the striatum (caudate nucleus and medial putamen) [45]. The motor and premotor areas lie more laterally, and they project mainly to lateral striatum, that is to the putamen. The premotor areas lie anterior to the motor cortex, and the bulk of their projections terminate more anteriorly in the striatum [45,77].

Just as it is possible to detect changes in activation of the various frontal strips when subjects learn motor tasks, so one can detect changes in the site of maximum activation of the striatum [55,57]. When a comparison is made between the learning of a new sequence of finger movements and automatic performance (NEW *vs* PRE), there is more activation of the caudate nucleus

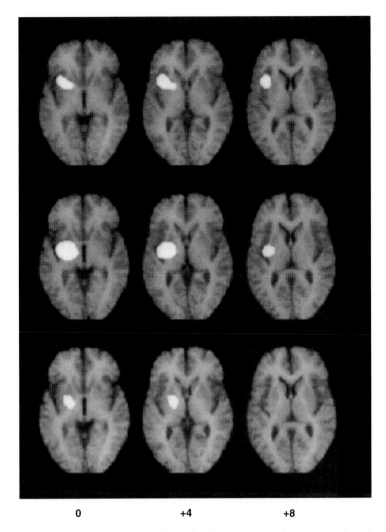

0   +4   +8

FIGURE 22 Activation anteriorly in the putamen when comparing the free-selection task with the baseline condition (FREE *vs* BASE; above); activation more posteriorly in the putamen when comparing overlearned performance of a sequence with baseline (PRE *vs* BASE; middle), and activation posteriorly in the putamen when comparing the repetitive task with baseline (REP *vs* BASE; below) [data from 55 and 57].

[57]. When subjects select between movements, there is activation anteriorly in the putamen (FREE *vs* REST) [55] (Fig. 22, top). When subjects perform a motor sequence automatically, there is activation more posteriorly in the putamen (PRE *vs* REST) [57] (Fig. 22, middle). The activation is similar to that for repeated movement of the same finger (REP *vs* REST) [55] (Fig. 22, bottom).

The results provide suggestive evidence that the changes in cortical strips during learning are paralleled by changes in the activation of the different loops between frontal cortex and basal ganglia. When a complex motor task becomes automatic, more posterior loops are involved, just as they are when a subject performs a simple repetitive task for which no practice is needed.

C. Conclusions

When subjects learn a new sequence or select between movements, anterior cortical areas are activated (prefrontal cortex, medial frontal area 32, anterior area 6). These areas are not activated in performance of a task that has been overlearned or performance of a repetitive task which does not require practice. There appears to be a similar pattern in the basal ganglia. The caudate is activated when a new sequence is learned, but not when the sequence is overlearned.

Our findings suggest that more anterior cortical areas are engaged only when the the task is nonroutine, for example when the subjects must make new decisions. Such decisions may require attention, memory of recent information, or preparation for future responses. In such circumstances, cortical areas are activated that are less directly linked with the motor cortex. This means that the circuitry is less direct, and this has a cost in terms of response time. Figure 18 shows that subjects take slightly, but significantly, longer to respond when required to attend to performance of a prelearned motor sequence (ATT) than when they perform the task automatically (PRE).

VII. GENERAL CONCLUSIONS

This chapter has suggested that several trends or gradients can be discerned in the organisation of the motor system. The system consists of interconnected networks of cells with distinct but overlapping sets of functional properties.

A. Neighbouring Populations of Cells

It is a common finding of single unit recording that there are similarities in the functional properties of cells in different regions. For example, cells with "set activity" or "preparatory activity" have been found in all the regions of frontal cortex including motor cortex and in the basal ganglia [78–80]. Alexander and Crutcher [81,82] made comparisons between the globus pallidus, the medial premotor cortex (SMA), and motor cortex. They were struck by the fact that it was possible to detect cells with the same functional properties in each of these areas.

However, it is also possible to demonstrate gradients over neighbouring areas. Take, for example, the medial and lateral premotor cortex (area 6). Single cell recording shows that many of the cells in these two areas share the same functional properties, but that there are differences in the distribution of these properties [35] (Fig. 9). Johnson *et al.* (83) have also recorded single units from 8 sites, moving rostrally from motor cortex to the anterior border of the lateral premotor cortex. They found that the percentage of cue related cells and set related cells increased the more anterior the recording sites.

Differences in the proportions of cell types can occur because each region differs in its set of inputs and outputs. For example, unlike the SMA, the lateral premotor cortex receives inputs from many regions of parietal cortex that are visually responsive [83]. Another example is provided by the cortico-cortical inputs into the premotor and prefrontal cortex: the dorsal lateral premotor cortex receives an input from parietal area 5, whereas the dorsal prefrontal cortex does not; by contrast, the parietal area 7a projects to the dorsal prefrontal cortex but not to the lateral premotor cortex [58].

Areas may also differ not in having unique inputs but in the size of any particular input. An example is provided by the thalamocortical inputs into the anterior and posterior parts of the medial premotor cortex [40,41]. The nucleus VLo sends a heavier projection to the posterior part (F3) than to the anterior part (F6). By contrast, the nucleus VApc sends a heavier projection anteriorly (F6) than posteriorly (F3).

Functional brain imaging records the activity of populations of cells, and thus it can be used to compare the functional properties of neighbouring areas. For example, we know that when monkeys prepare to make movements more cells are active before movement in the anterior than in the posterior medial premotor cortex (SMA) [52]. Using PET, we [23] have shown that there is greater activity in the posterior part of area 6 (SMA) when one contrasts execution with preparation (EXEC *vs* PREP) (Fig. 6) and greater activity in the anterior part of area 6 when the opposite contrast is made (PREP *vs* EXEC) (Fig. 11).

B. Changes over Time

The brain is not a static system. The relative activity of different regions is not the same from moment to moment, and there are changes in the activity of areas as a consequence of learning.

PET is not the method of choice when considering changes in activity over short times. The temporal resolution of PET is very limited and only crude comparisons are possible. The issue of changes in organisation with time will best be studied by other techniques such as fMRI with a better temporal resolution. Nonetheless PET can be used to compare different stages of learning. We have compared initial learning of a sequence and the late stage of learning at which the task is automatic [15,57]. Similarly, Roland *et al.* [84] have compared early, middle, and later stages in the learning of a complex finger sequence. Grafton and colleagues [71] have studied different stages of the learning of visually guided motor tracking.

Several studies have reported a retraction in the activation of areas as the tasks become overlearned [15,57,73]. We do not know how these changes occur. There are many paths, both direct and less direct, *via* which information can influence the executive motor system. Given the premium on speed of response, it is possible that there is competition between these paths, such that the more direct paths win out. Alternatively, it may be that there are central executive areas which control the degree to which other areas are activated. Whichever suggestion is correct, we will understand the mechanism only by carrying out research on other animals, since it is only in animal brains that we can intervene so as to demonstrate causal relations.

The issue underlines two points that have been made here and elsewhere in this book concerning functional imaging. The first is that functional brain imaging is just one of the methods of neuroscience. These studies should be integrated with studies using other methods, such as those of anatomy and physiology. The second point is that functional brain imaging concerns populations of cells, differences in the distribution of the functional properties of different areas, and changes in the activity of different areas over time. Human brain mapping is not the new phrenology.

References

1. W. Matelli, G. Luppino, and G. Rizzolatti. Pattern of cytochrome oxidase activity in frontal agranular cortex of the macaque monkey. *Behav. Brain Res.* **18,** 125–136 (1985).

2. M. Matelli, G. Luppino, and G. Rizzolatti. Architecture of superior and mesial area 6 and the adjacent cingulate cortex in the macaque monkey. *J. Comp. Neurol.* **311,** 445–462 (1991).

3. J. Tanji. The supplementary motor area in the cerebral cortex. *Neurosci. Res.* **19,** 251–268 (1994).

4. K. Zilles, G. Schlaug, S. Geyer, G. Luppino, M. Matelli, M. Qu, A. Schleicher, and T. Schormann. Anatomy and transmitter receptors of the supplementary motor areas in the human and non-human primate brain. *In* "The Supplementary Sensorimotor Area" (H. O. Luders, Ed.), pp. 29–44. Raven Press, New York, 1996.

5. J. Talairach and P. Tournoux. "Co-Planar Stereotaxic Atlas of the Human Brain," Thieme, Stuttgart, 1988.

6. R. E. Passingham. Functional specialisation of the SMA in monkey and man. *In* "The Supplementary Sensorimotor Area" (H. O. Luders, Ed.), pp. 105–116. Raven Press, New York, 1996.

7. R. E. Passingham. The status of the premotor areas: Evidence from PET scanning. *In* "Neural Control of Movement" (W. R. Ferrell and U. Proske, Eds.), pp. 167–178. Plenum, New York (1995).

8. K. F.Muakkassa and P. L. Strick. Frontal lobe inputs to primate motor cortex: Evidence for four somatotopically organized "premotor areas." *Brain Res.* **177,** 176–182 (1979).

9. P. L. Strick. How do the basal ganglia and cerebellum gain access to the cortical motor areas? *Behav. Brain Res.* **18,** 107–124 (1985).

10. R. P. Dum, and P. L. Strick. Cingulate motor areas. *In* "Neurobiology of Cingulate Cortex and Limbic Thalamus" (B.A. Vogt and M. Gabriel, Eds.), pp. 415–441. Birkhauser, Boston, 1993.

11. B. A. Vogt, E. A. Nimchinsky, C. J. Vogt, and P. R. Hof. Human cingulate cortex: Surface features, flat maps and cytoarchitecture. *J. Comp. Neurol.* **359,** 490–506 (1995).

12. I. A. Ilinsky and K. Kultas-Ilinsky. Sagittal cytoarchitectonic maps of the *Macaca mulatta* thalamus with a revised nomenclature of the motor-related nuclei validated by observations of their connectivity. *J. Comp. Neurol.* **262,** 331–364 (1987).

13. E. G. Jones. "The Thalamus," Plenum, New York, 1985.

14. M. Matelli and G. Luppino. Cortical projections of motor thalamus. *In* "Thalamic Networks for Relay and Modulation" (D. Mietciacchi, M. Molinari, G. Miacchi, and E. G. Jones, Eds.), pp. 165–174. Pergamon, Oxford, 1994.

15. I. H. Jenkins, D. J. Brooks, P. D. Nixon, R. S. J. Frackowiak, and R. E. Passingham. Motor sequence learning: A study with positron emission tomography. *J. Neurosci.* **14,** 3775–3790 (1994).

16. R. P. Dum and P. L. Strick. The origin of corticospinal projections from the premotor areas in the frontal lobe. *J. Neurosci.* **11,** 667–689 (1991).

17. S-Q He, R. P. Dum, and P. L. Strick. Topographic organisation of corticospinal projections from the frontal lobe: motor areas on the medial surface of the hemisphere. *J. Neurosci.* **13,** 952–980 (1993).

18. G. R. Fink, R. S. J. Frackowiak, U. Pietrzyk, and R. E. Passingham. Multiple non-primary motor areas in the human cortex. *J. Neurophysiol.,* in press.

19. Galea and I. Darian Smith. Multiple corticospinal neuron populations in the macaque monkey are specified by their unique cortical origins, spinal terminations and connections. *Cereb. Cortex* **4,** 166–194 (1995)

20. K. Toyoshima and H. Sakai. Exact cortical extent of the origins of the corticospinal tract (CST) and the quantitative contribution to the CST in different cytoarchitec-

tonic areas. A study with horseradish peroxidase in the monkey. *J. Hirnforsch* **23,** 257–169 (1981).

21. I. H. Jenkins, R. E. Passingham, R. S. J. Frackowiak, and D. J. Brooks. The effect of movement rate on cerebral activation. *Mov. Dis.* **9** (Suppl. 1), P486 (1994).

22. C. Dettmers, G. Fink, R. N. Lemon, K. M. Stephan, R. E. Passingham, D. Silbersweig, A. Holmes, M. C. Ridding, D. J. Brooks, and R. S. J. Frackowiak. The relation between neuronal activity and force in the motor areas of the human brain. *J. Neurophysiol.* **74,** 802–815 (1995).

23. K. M. Stephan, G. R. Fink, R. E. Passingham, D. Silbersweig, A. Ceballos-Baumann, C. D. Frith, and R. S. J. Frackowiak. Functional anatomy of the mental representation of upper extremity movements in healthy subjects. *J. Neurophysiol.* **73,** 373–386 (1995).

24. H. Barbas, and D. N. Pandya. Architecture and frontal cortical connections of the premotor cortex (area 6) in the rhesus monkey. *J. Comp. Neurol.* **256,** 211–228 (1987).

25. G. Goldberg. Supplementary motor area structure and function: Review and hypotheses. *Behav. Brain Res.* **8,** 567–588 (1985).

26. R. E. Passingham. Two cortical systems for directing movements. *In* "Motor Areas of the Cerebral Cortex," (R. Porter, Ed.), CIBA Symposium 132, pp. 151–164, Wiley, Chichester, 1987.

27. R. E. Passingham. "The Frontal Lobes and Voluntary Action," Oxford Univ. Press, Oxford, 1993.

28. U. Halsband. Higher disturbances of movement in monkeys (*Macaca mulatta*). *In* "Motor Control" (G. N. Gantchev, B. Dimitev, and P. C. Gatev, Eds.), pp. 79–85, Plenum, New York, 1987.

29. M-P. Deiber, R. E. Passingham, J. G. Colebatch, K. J. Friston, P. D. Nixon, and R. S. J. Frackowiak. Cortical areas and the selection of movement: A study with positron emission tomography. *Exp. Brain Res.* **84,** 393–402.

30. I. H. Jenkins, M. Jahanshahi, R. G. Brown, M. Jueptner, C. D. Marsden, R. E. Passingham, and D. J. Brooks. "Self Initiated *versus* Externally Triggered Movements. II. The Effect of Stimulus Predictability on Regional Cerebral Blood Flow and Movement-Related potentials." Submitted for publication.

31. M. Jahanshahi, I. H., Jenkins, R. G. Brown, C. D. Marsden, R. E. Passingham, and D. J. Brooks. Self-initiated *versus* externally-triggered movements. I. An investigation using regional cerebral blood flow and movement-related potentials in normals and Parkinson's disease. *Brain* **118,** 913–933 (1995).

32. T. A. Zeffiro, C. Kertzmann, C. Peilzzari, and M. Hallet. The role of the supplementary motor area in the control of self-paced movements: A PET study. *Soc. Neurosci. Abstr.* **17,** 443.3 (1991).

33. P. Remy, M. Zilbovicius, A. Lery-Willig, A. Syrota, and Y. Samson. Movement- and task-related activations of motor cortical areas: A positron emission tomographic study. *Ann. Neurol.* **36,** 19–26 (1994).

34. A. R. Mitz, S. P. Wise, and T. A. Zeffiro. Regional cerebral blood flow changes during conditional motor learning in the human motor cortex. *Soc. Neurosci. Abstr.* **19,** 496.9 (1993).

35. H. Mushiake, M. Inase, and J. Tanji. Neuronal activity in the primate premotor, supplementary, and precentral motor cortex during visually guided and internally determined sequential movements. *J. Neurophysiol.* **66,** 705–718 (1991).

36. R. Romo and W. Schultz. Neuronal activity preceding self-initiated or externally timed arm movements in area 6 of monkey cortex. *Exp. Brain Res.* **67,** 656–662 (1987).

37. Tanji, K. Taniguchi, and T. Saga. The supplementary motor area: Neuronal responses to motor instructions. *J. Neurophysiol.* **43,** 60–68 (1980).

38. D. J. Brooks, V. Ibanez, G. V. Sawle, N. Quinn, A. J. Lees, C. J. Mathias, R. Bannister, C. D. Marsden, and R. S. J. Frackowiak. Differing patterns of striatal

18F-Dopa uptake in Parkinson's disease, multiple systems atrophy, and progressive supranuclear palsy. *Ann. Neurol.* **28,** 549–555 (1990).

39. E. D Playford, I. H. Jenkins, R. E. Passingham, J. Nutt, R. S. J. Frackowiak, and D. J. Brooks. Impaired mesial frontal and putamen activation in Parkinson's disease: A positron emission tomography study. *Ann. Neurol.* **32,** 151–161 (1992).

40. M. Matelli and G. Luppino. Cortical projections of motor thalamus. *In* "Thalamic Networks for Relay and Modulation" (D. Mietciacchi, M. Molinari, M. Miacchi, and E. G. Jones, Eds.), pp. 165–174. Pergamon Press, Oxford, 1994.

41. M. Matelli and G. Luppino. Thalamic input to mesial and superior area 6 in the macaque monkey. *J. Comp. Neurol.* **372,** 59–87 (1996).

42. J. Olszewski. "The Thalamus of the Macaca Mulatta," Karger, Basel, 1952.

43. J. E. Hoover and P. L. Strick. Multiple output channels in the basal ganglia. *Science* **259,** 819–821 (1993).

44. P. J. Orioli and P. L. Strick. Cerebellar connections with the motor cortex and the arcuate premotor area: An analysis employing retrograde transneuronal transport of WGA-HRP. *J. Comp. Neurol.* **288,** 612–626.

45. L. D. Selemon and P. S. Goldman-Rakic. Longitudinal topography and interdigitation of corticostriatal projections in the rhesus monkey. *J. Neurosci.* **5,** 776–794 (1985).

46. J. L. DeVito and M. E. Anderson. An autoradiographic study of efferent conneciptons of the globus pallidus in *Macaca mulatta. Exp. Brain Res.* **46,** 107–117 (1982).

47. H. Barbas, T. H. Haswell Henion, and C. R. Dermon. Diverse thalamic projections to the prefrontal cortex in the rhesus monkey. *J. Comp. Neurol.* **313,** 65–94 (1991).

48. F. A. Middleton and P. L. Strick. Anatomical evidence for the cerebellar and basal ganglia involvement in higher cognitive function. *Science* **266,** 458–461 (1994).

49. J. F. Bates and P. S. Goldman-Rakic. Prefrontal connections of medial motor areas in the rhesus monkey. *J. Comp. Neurol.* **336,** 211–228 (1993).

50. M-T. Lu, J. R. Preston, and P. L. Strick, Interconnections between the prefrontal cortex and the premotor areas in the frontal lobe. *J. Comp. Neurol.* **341,** 375–392 (1994).

51. G. Luppino, M. Matelli, and G. Rizzolatti. Cortico-cortical connections of two electrophysiologically identified arm representations in the mesial agranular frontal cortex. *Exp. Brain Res.* **82,** 214–218 (1990).

52. Y. Matsusaka, H. Aizawa, and J.Tanji. Motor area rostral to the supplementary motor area (presupplementary motor area) in the monkey: Neuronal activity during a learned motor task. *J. Neurophysiol.* **68,** 653–662 (1992).

53. M-P. Deiber, V. Ibanez, N. Sadato, and M. Hallett. Cerebral structures participating in motor preparation in humans: A positron emission tomography study. *J. Neurophysiol.* **75,** 233–247 (1996).

54. R. Kawashima, P. E. Roland, and B. T. O'Sullivan. Fields in human motor areas involved in preparation for reaching, actual reaching, and visuomotor learning: A positron emission tomography study. *J. Neurosci.* **14,** 3462–3474 (1994).

55. M. Jueptner, C. D. Frith, D. J. Brooks, R. S. J. Frackowiak, and R. E. Passingham, The anatomy of motor learning. II. Subcortical structures and learning by trial and error. *J. Neurophysiol.* **77,** 1325–1337 (1996).

56. D. Playford. "The Pathophysiology of Idiopathic Torsion Dystonia Studied with Positron Emission Tomography," Unpublished MD thesis, University of London, 1993.

57. M. Jueptner, K. M. Stephan, C. D. Frith, D. J. Brooks, R. S. J. Frackowiak, and R. E. Passingham. The anatomy of motor learning. I. The frontal cortex and attention to action. *J. Neurophsyiol.* **77,** 1313–1324 (1996).

58. C. Cavada and P. S. Goldman-Rakic. Posterior parietal cortex in rhesus monkeys: II Evidence for segregated corticocortical networks linking sensory and limbic areas with the frontal lobe. *J. Comp. Neurol.* **28,** 422–445 (1989).

59. C. D. Frith, K. Friston, P. F. Liddle, and R. S. J. Frackowiak. Willed action and

the prefrontal cortex in man: A study with PET. *Proc. R. Soc. London B* **244,** 241–246 (1991).

60. A. O. Ceballos Baummann, C. D. Marsden, R. E. Passingham, K. M. Stephan, R. S. J. Frackowiak, and D. J. Brooks. Cerebral activation with performing and imagining movements in idiopathic torsion dystonia (ITD): A PET study. *Neurology* **44,** 837S (1994).

61. M. Glickstein, J. G. May, and R. E. Mercier. Corticopontine projections in the macaque: The distribution of labelled cortical cells after large injections of horse-radish peroxidase in the pontine nuclei. *J. Comp. Neurol.* **235,** 343–359 (1985).

62. J. D. Schmahmann and D. N. Pandya. Projections to the basis pontis from the superior temporal sulcus and superior temporal region in the rhesus monkey. *J. Comp. Neurol.* **308,** 224–248 (1991).

63. K. Sasaki, H. Jinnai, H. Gemba, S. Hashimoto, and N. Mizuno. Projections of the cerebellar dentate nucleus onto the frontal association cortex in monkeys. *Exp. Brain Res.* **37,** 193–198 (1979).

64. R. E. Passingham. Attention to action. *Phil. Trans. R. Soc. B* **351,** 1423–1432 (1996).

65. S. T. Grafton, E. Hazeltine, and R. Ivry. Functional mapping of sequence learning in normal humans. *J. Cogn. Neurosci.* **7,** 497–510 (1995)

66. J. Doyon, A. M. Owen, M. Petrides, V. Sziklas, and A. C. Evans. Functional anatomy of visuomotor skill learning examined with positron emission tomography. *Eur. J. Neurosci.* **8,** 637–648 (1996).

67. S. L. Rauch, C. R. Savage, N. M. Alpert, H. D. Brown, T. Curran, A. Kendrick, A. J. Fischman, and S. M. Kosslyn. Functional neuroanatomy of implicit sequence learning studied with PET. *Hum. Brain Mapping (suppl.1)* 409.

68. M. Petrides, B. Alivisatos, A. C. Evans, and E. Meyer. Dissociation of human mid-dorsolateral from posterior dorsolateral forntal cortex in memory processing. *Proc. Natl. Acad. Sci. USA* **90,** 873–877 (1993).

69. K. J. Friston, C. D. Frith, R. E. Passingham, P. F. Liddle, and R. S. J. Frackowiak. Motor practice and neurophysiological adaptation in the cerebellum: A positron tomographic study. *Proc. R. Soc. London B* **248,** 223–228 (1992).

70. M. Jueptner, I. H. Jenkins, D. J. Brooks, R. S. J. Frackowiak, and R. E. Passingham. The sensory guidance of movement: A comparison of the cerebellum and basal ganglia. *Exp. Brain Res.* **112,** 462–469 (1996).

71. S. T. Grafton, R. P. Woods, and M. Tyszka. Functional imaging of procedural motor learning: Relating cerebral blood flow with individual subject performance. *Hum. Brain Mapping* **1,** 221–234 (1994).

72. R. C. Miall, S. Price, R. E. Passingham, J. L. Winter, and J. F. Stein. Electrical stimulation of complex movements from the ventro-lateral but not the ventro-anterior nucleus of the macaque thalamus. *XXXIIth Int. Congr. Union Physiol. Sci.* **248.15/P** (1993).

73. M. E. Raichle, J. A. Fiez, T. O. Videen, A. K. MacLeod, J. V. Pardo, P. T. Fox, and S. E. Petersen. Practice-related changes in human brain functional anatomy during non-motor learning. *Cereb. Cort.* **4,** 8–26 (1994).

74. G. E. Alexander, M. D. Crutcher, and M. R. DeLong. Basal ganglia-thalamocortical circuits: Parallel substrates for motor, oculomotor, "prefrontal" and "limbic" functions. *Progr. Brain Res.* **85,** 119–146 (1991).

75. L. D. Selemon and P. S. Goldman-Rakic. Parallel processing in the basal ganglia: Up to a point. *Trends Neurosci.* **14,** 58–59 (1991).

76. J. Saint-Cyr, L. G. Ungerleider, and R. Desimone. Organisation of visual cortical inputs to the striatum and subsequent outputs to the pallido-nigral complex in the monkey. *J. Comp. Neurol.* **298,** 129–156 (1990).

77. H. Kunzle. H. Projections from the primary somatosensor cortex to basal ganglia and thalamus in the monkey. *Exp. Brain Res.* **30,** 481–492 (1977).

78. E. Evarts, Y. Shinoda, and S. P. Wise. "Neurophysiological Approaches to Higher Brain Functions," Wiley, New York, 1984.

79. W. Schultz and R. Romo. Role of primate basal ganglia and frontal cortex in the

internal generation of movements. I. Preparatory activity in the anterior striatum. *Exp. Brain Res.* **91,** 363–384 (1992).

80. R. Romo, E. Scarnati, and W. Schultz. Role of primate basal ganglia and frontal cortex in the internal generation of movements. II. Movement-related activity in the anterior striatum. *Exp. Brain Res.* **91,** 385–395 (1992).

81. G. E. Alexander and M. D. Crutcher. Preparation for movement: Neural representations of intending direction in three motor areas of the monkey. *J. Neurophysiol.* **64,** 133–149 (1990).

82. M. D. Crutcher and G. E. Alexander. Movement-related neuronal activity selectively codning either direction or muscle pattern in three motor areas of the monkey. *J. Neurophysiol.* **64,** 151–163 (1990).

83. P. B. Johnson, S. Ferraina, L. Biachni, and R. Caminiti. Cortical networks for visual reaching: Physiological and anatomical organisation of frontal and parietal lobe arm regions. *Cereb. Cort.* **6,** 102–119 (1996).

84. P. E. Roland, B. Gulyas, and R. J. Seitz. Structures in the human brain participating in visual learning, tactile learning, and motor learning. *In* "Memory, Organisation and Locus of Change" (L. R. Squire, N. M. Wienberger, G. Lynch, and J. L. McGaugh, Eds.), pp. 95–113. Oxford Univ. Press, Oxford, 1991.

CHAPTER TWELVE

The Cerebral Basis of Functional Recovery

I. INTRODUCTION

This chapter begins with a definition of human cerebral plasticity that is predicated on the concept of long-term alteration in patterns of behaviour related activity in distributed brain systems. The theme is developed to show how such a concept and the mechanisms it implies can be investigated using noninvasive functional imaging. A discussion of functional reorganisation following brain injury, which is associated with spontaneous recovery from motor, cognitive, and perceptual deficits, is presented from a perspective of activity in large-scale neuronal populations.

Noninvasive functional brain monitoring techniques present an experimental opportunity for measuring changes in connectivity and functional segregation that accompany and underpin behavioural change or functional improvement after brain injury. The experimental questions such methods address relate to neural interactions and activity at the level of large scale neuronal populations. In the literature plasticity means different things to different workers. We define it operationally in this chapter as reorganisation of distributed patterns of normal task-associated brain activity that accompany action, perception, and cognition and that compensate impaired function resulting from disease or brain injury. Our results allow for very few conjectures about the molecular or cellular mechanisms responsible for such reorganisation.

It is a clinical fact that loss of function following acute brain injury, for whatever reason, is often followed by some degree of functional improvement [1]. Such recovery may be dramatic and cannot be explained completely by trivial mechanisms, such as the resolution of acute inflammation following stroke or head injury, because it often continues beyond any immediate recovery in the acute phase. Following stroke substantial recovery may continue for months after onset. Explanations based on alternative pathways, novel cognitive strategies, or takeover of function by contralateral homologous cortex are common, heuristically valuable, but not explanatory in the absence of empirical evidence [2,3]. At a more basic level, axonal sprouting, alterations of synaptic strengths, and synaptic reorganization are proposed, largely by analogy with experimental observations *in vitro* and in rodent models of brain damage [4–6]. The relevance of such mechanisms to human brains remains to be determined. It has been reliably established that human brains show considerable plastic change during development [7,8], though they are often considered essentially hard wired by maturity. Nevertheless, laying down of new memories, learning of motor skills, and similar normal behaviours implies that changes of brain connectivity continue into adulthood. As yet, a coherent, system-level, anatomical description of brain mechanisms associated with normal and compensatory change are difficult to formulate. An empirical science of adaptive functional change in normal and lesioned human brain is urgently required. Noninvasive functional imaging provides a means for collecting data to generate system-level descriptions, theories, and hypotheses.

Plasticity implies enduring changes of neural function with time, in other words, an adaptation of activity (often activity that is correlated across brain areas) with repeated behaviour or following injury. Behaviour related plasticity can be monitored by repeated determinations of the distribution of neural activity during sequential repetitions of a task of interest. Comparison of patterns of activation as a function of time (repetitions) identifies areas of brain in which time-related modification of activity occurs [9,10]. This idea has been applied in experiments designed to investigate changes of brain function that accompany the aquisition of motor skills (see Chapter 11).

II. BRAIN INJURY AND MOTOR RECOVERY

A central tenet of brain activation methodology is that typical brain activation patterns can be associated with clearly defined cerebral processes and mental states. This aim is achieved by a combination of judiciously chosen tasks and experimental designs [11] (categorical, parametric, factorial—see Chapter 8). A rest task is rarely informative even as a control, except when it serves as a reference state for determining whether relative changes found in comparisons of more specified and hence informative tasks are due to differential activations, deactivations, or a mixture of both. Nevertheless, between-group comparisons at rest can be informative, especially when patient populations are compared to normal subjects [12]. The disturbance of normal patterns of resting brain activity caused by small, restricted cerebral lesions can be large and in some instances unsuspected.

It is remarkable that brain activity is reflected with such apparent coherence by an integrated measure of local synaptic activity, *i.e.*, perfusion. This remarkable fact suggests that at a system level the brain is well-behaved in the sense that the available physiological responses are limited and predictable. There are two facts that help to explain such well-behaved responsivity at the level of neuronal populations: (a) most cortico-cortical connections are glutamatergic and hence excitatory, and (b) over 80% of intrinsic cortical synapses are of type 1, which are usually implicated in excitatory activity [13]. Thus, as a reasonable approximation, the signals recorded by functional imaging (or more precisely, perfusion mapping) can be regarded as largely representative of excitatory cortico-cortical traffic in the brain.

A. Effects of Circumscribed Lesions on Resting Activity

A comparison of resting state brain activity in a group of patients who had recovered from contralateral paralysis due to internal capsule lesions and that of an age matched normal control group showed extensive differences in both the lesioned and unlesioned hemispheres [12]. In the lesioned hemisphere relative deactivation occurs in presumed component areas of the cerebral motor system. In addition to very low activity centred on the internal capsule (the site of the lesion) there was deactivation of dorso-lateral prefrontal cortex (DLPFC), premotor and parietal cortex, including insular and opercular regions, contralateral cerebellum, and nuclei in the midbrain and pons ipsilateral to the lesioned hemisphere (Fig. 1). These results suggest that, although the various areas subserving motor function are segregated and autonomous,

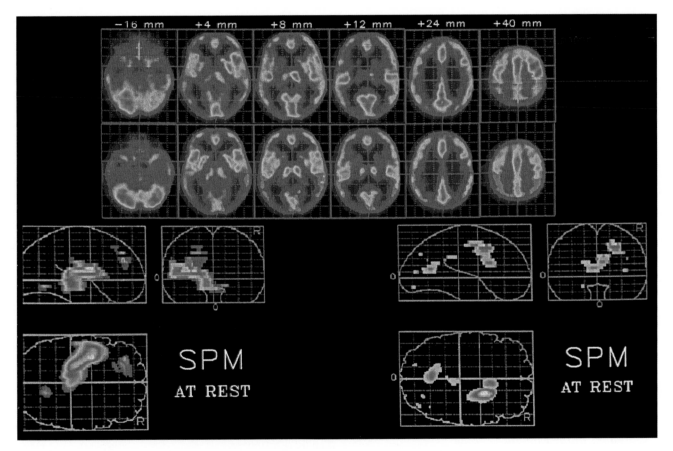

Figure 1 This figure shows transaxial maps of perfusion in the upper two rows. The first row represents the mean cerebral perfusion in a group of patients all suffering from a lesion in the internal capsule that had led to paralysis of the contralateral limbs with subsequent very substantial recovery. In the second row is the group mean perfusion in an age matched normal control population. The statistical parametric maps show the sagittal, coronal and transaxial views of the results of a comparison of the patient and normal populations at rest. The areas in colour show significant deactivations in patients compared to normal subjects. The right set of SPMs indicate in colour those areas of the brain where there is relative activation in the patient population compared to that seen in the normal group. It is clear that there is substantial reorganisation of resting activity following a relatively small lesion in white matter.

alterations of activity in and between components of the motor system may have far reaching effects on other components of that system. The causes for these disturbances of functionally interdependent regions are presumably anatomical disconnections due to white matter tract lesions. Such lesions can themselves be visualised and identified by appropriate MR scanning. For example, degeneration of the human pyramidal tract following capsular infarction has been identified in life [14,15].

In unlesioned, contralateral cerebral hemispheres in such patients relative hyperactivity was documented in posterior cingulate, ventral premotor cortex and in the caudate nucleus. The significance of such unexpected changes in hemispheres contralateral to those harbouring internal capsule lesions is, as yet, poorly understood and indeed the observations probably require replication. One suggestion is that they may be due to a loss of inhibition by the lesioned hemisphere, or to relative augmentation of activity in cortices that, at least in the nonhuman primate, contain representations of movements of both sides of the body. In summary, there is a profound redistribution of resting state activity in both hemispheres associated with recovered motor function, despite the discrete, unilateral, location of the lesion in white matter that is responsible for initial motor paralysis. By our working definition this finding suggests plastic change of the cerebral organisation of function that is demonstrable at considerable distances from the site of the original lesion. Furthermore, the plastic changes apparently occur exclusively in brain areas that constitute components of the cerebral motor system.

B. Plasticity and the Motor System

Some degree of spontaneous recovery accompanies many cases of motor paralysis caused by stroke. Recovery can sometimes be complete but, as already noted, the mechanisms and biological basis are largely unknown. Experimentation is complicated by the fact that motor-associated brain activity is modifiable by many variables, a majority of which are still uncharacterised. It is difficult to envisage what useful information about the cerebral basis for motor recovery could be obtained by comparing task-associated distributions of brain activity in normal subjects with those obtained in patients who cannot perform an activating task properly. This is because the degree of activation is a complex function of many factors including performance. As a first approach to this problem, therefore, we have studied completely recovered patients because performance of a motor task can then be equalised across patient and control groups.

1. Lesions of the Internal Capsule

A comparison of brain activity associated with paced, sequential, repetitive opposition movements of fingers to thumb with that at rest, using the unaffected and recovered hands separately, was performed [16]. In a group of patients with recovered, predominantly capsular strokes a number of features were found. First, the normal lateralized pattern of cortical and subcortical activity associated with the task became bilateral. The cerebellum was also bilaterally activated. Second, there were additional activations when a recovered limb was moved that were restricted to known (or putative) motor-associated brain areas. Third, among regions activated there were areas that normally participate in freely selected, complex sequential movement

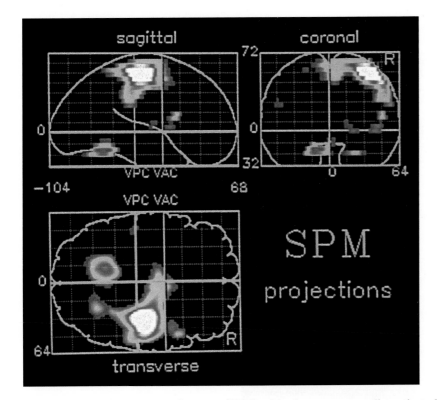

FIGURE 2 Statistical parametric maps (SPM) of brain areas normally activated (in comparison with rest) by a paced, sequential, left handed, finger-to-thumb opposition task. Activation is centred on motor, premotor, immediately adjacent parietal and supplementary motor cortices on the right, and in the contralateral cerebellum on the left. The SPMs are presented as projections through the brain seen from side (sagittal), back (coronal), and top (transverse) views. The right side of the figure represents the right side of the brain and the frontal pole is on the right of the transverse section. Highly significant changes of activity between active and resting states are shown in color, coded to represent levels of significance (white, greatest significance).

tasks involving the whole limb, but not in simple repetitive tasks performed distally, such as the one used in these experiments (Figs. 2 and 3).

The bilateral nature of activations elicited by simple finger movements in patients with recovery from hemiplegia begs a question: how does this pattern differ from that found in normal subjects when more complex movements are made? In other words, are the findings explained in terms of reorganisation or are the patients just trying harder? Bilateral activations with upper limb movement have been reported with functional imaging using both PET and fMRI techniques [17]. Indeed, it has been suggested that use of a nondominant hand results in bilateral activation, whereas use of a dominant hand results in uniquely contralateral cerebral activations. We carried out a number of studies to characterize with greater precision such responses in terms of the various performance variables.

2. Generating Force Pulses with the Fingers

We performed a set of studies in normal subjects whilst they exerted repetitive force pulses by pressing on a Morse key with an index finger. The force pulses were kept constant by visual and auditory feedback in the first

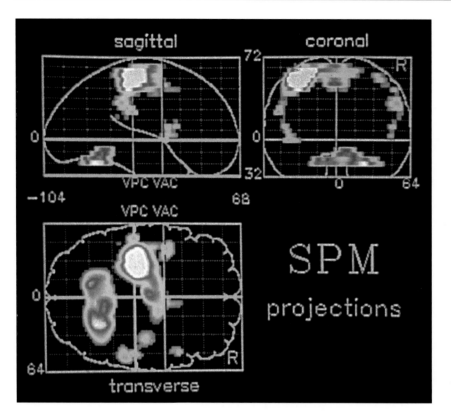

FIGURE 3 The pattern of activation found in patients with lesions of the left internal capsule who recover from any resultant paralysis of the right arm. The pattern is obtained by comparing activity during a paced, sequential, right sided, finger-to-thumb opposition task with rest. Activation is bilateral. The prominent activation seen in left (contralateral) motor cortex reflects local and afferent activity onto pyramidal cells of area M1. The lesion is in motor output fibres of the internal capsule. Both cerebellar hemispheres are activated and there is also some activation in ipsilateral motor cortex. There are also activations in insular areas, both premotor and parietal cortices and in the supplementary motor area and anterior cingulate cortices. This pattern should be compared with Fig. 2 and was obtained from the same patients; the viewing conventions are similar.

instance, but subjects rapidly became able to maintain a high degree of precision with minimal feedback [18]. Four discrete brain regions showed highly correlated activity with the degree of force exerted. Force was calibrated in terms of each individual's maximal exertable force in order to normalise results across subjects. The first region was located in the arm representation area of the contralateral primary somatosensory and motor cortex [19]. The second region was situated on the left mesial surface of the brain, posterior to the anterior commissure, encompassing the first gyrus dorsal to the cingulate sulcus thought to be homologous with the posterior part of the supplementary motor area. The third region was found in the dorsal bank of the posterior cingulate sulcus and the fourth was in the right cerebellar hemisphere ipsilateral to the used limb. Comparisons of all scans collected whilst force pulses were being exerted with rest scans indicated significant activation of the cerebellar vermis, the contralateral putamen, both insular cortices, both ventrolateral premotor areas, both parietal opercular regions and contralateral ventral posterior and dorsal posterior supplementary motor areas. Of interest was a prominent deactivation of ipsilateral primary sensorimotor cortex when low forces were applied. Our conclusions were that the motor system could be considered in terms of two broad functional divisions; an executive component and other, nonexecutive components, in which activity was only indirectly related to performance parameters of the task, in our case the exertion of repetitive identical force pulses of different size. A second conclusion was that bilateral activations of the nonexecutive division were possible with unilateral tasks in normal subjects.

3. Generating a Constant Force with the Fingers

We repeated this experiment during exertion of unilateral sustained (as opposed to phasic) forces [20]. Our aim was to determine whether there were any differences in cerebral activation during prolonged exertion of a static force compared to repeated dynamic force pulses. Subjects pressed a Morse key continuously for different periods of time at a constant 20% of maximal voluntary contraction. The activations were at least as extensive as those during exertion of repetitive dynamic force pulses. Interestingly, despite a considerable sense of fatigue and increased effort no compensatory changes of activity were detected in motor or sensory related cerebral structures. There was a significant correlation between activity in ipsilateral dorsolateral prefrontal cortex and the duration of key press. The basal ganglia were also prominently activated during this task but not by dynamic force pulses. These results suggested to us that sustained exertion was an active process modulated, at least in part, by mechanisms involving the basal ganglia. This result in particular may be of relevance to current debates about the "mysterious" functions of the basal ganglia.

C. Interhemispheric Modulation of Motor Cortical Activity

We then explored the striking observation of deactivation in ipsilateral sensorimotor cortex at low forces by performing combined functional imaging, electromyographic (EMG) and transcranial magnetic stimulation studies [21]. From surface EMG recordings from multiple muscles of both hands, forearms, and arms we noted that key presses at low force pulses (less than 10% of maximal voluntary contraction (MVC)) resulted exclusively in activation of hand muscles. At 20% of MVC and larger more proximal muscles and proximal muscles of the contralateral limb were also activated, often without clinically observable evidence of movement. Activation in proximal muscles tended to be tonic rather than phasic. Phasic responses were present in more distal muscles of the limb performing the key press task.

Activations were seen in contralateral primary motor cortex. Changes in activity were logarithmically related to increases of force indexed as percentage of maximal voluntary contraction. In ipsilateral primary motor cortex an initial and marked deactivation was followed by a similar logarithmic increase such that activity in motor cortex was equivalent at rest and at 20% of maximal voluntary contraction, rising to levels at 60% of MVC that were similar to those found at under 10% MVC in the contralateral hemisphere. This differential pattern of changing activity in the two hemispheres in response to a task with graded performance parameters was associated with striking findings using transcranial magnetic stimulation. The stimulus threshold was determined as a percentage of the strength of magnetic pulse needed to just elicit a recognisable electromyographic response in contralateral limbs at rest. The pulses were applied with subjects exerting brief tonic contractions of the index finger against resistance at the same force levels used in the functional imaging studies. In a hemisphere contralateral to a moving limb the threshold for stimulation fell progressively with increasing forces. The EMGs were recorded from biceps muscles and were easily recognisable against a background of tonic activity seen when higher forces were exerted. In contrast, there was no significant change of magnetic threshold with increasing force when magnetic stimulation was applied to ipsilateral motor cortex (to the moving limb) except possibly for a slight decrease in threshold at 60% of MVC (Figs. 4 and 5). These findings, taken together, suggest that as finger movements become more complex or stronger, proximal muscles are automatically activated in order to stabilise the necessary joints. Such stabilising activity may also involve axial and ipsilateral arm muscles. This physiological response explains, in all likelihood, the discrepant unilateral or bilateral activations reported with hand movements in previous functional imaging studies. In a finger opposition task involving tapping of fingers one against another without excessive force, it remains likely that bilateral patterns of cerebral activation obtained from moving recovered fingers are representative of significant reorganisation. The fact that similar movements of the normal side in such patients evoke unilateral activity is further evidence in support of such a conclusion.

There remains one caveat that we have to address. Resting state studies indicate that reorganisation of activity affects unlesioned as well as lesioned hemispheres. It is therefore not entirely valid to compare results from normal and recovered sides in patients, given that the cerebral physiology underlying function on the normal side is itself different to normal. Indeed, there are clinical observations that suggest mild, often covert involvement of ipsilateral muscles in patients with cerebral lesions [22]. We therefore repeated our experiments in a group of normal subjects and a new group of patients. The findings were reproduced, indicating no signficant disease by activation interaction when patients used their normal limbs [12].

Whereas bilateral activations of the motor system characterised movements of the recovered limb, ipsilateral primary motor cortex (MI) was activated in only half [23]. Activation of MI ipsilateral to the recovered side was invariably associated with mirror movements of the unaffected limb, making it impossible to decide whether MI activation represents an epiphenomenon or a causal component of normal spontaneous recovery. In summary, the changes in both resting and activated brain function are remarkable for their extent and witness to a considerable capacity for plastic change in the lesioned brain, at least when that lesion occurs in corticofugal fibres.

D. Partial Motor Recovery

Extension of similar studies to people with partial motor recovery has been very difficult. In an attempt to solve problems arising from the confounding effect of differential performance in patients and normal control subjects we thought of restricting our studies, in the first instance, to motor imagery alone, thus eschewing activation effects due to motor execution [24]. The rationale behind this idea is that removal of any necessity to perform a motor act will eliminate potential confounds arising from residual partial or complete paralysis. The experiments cited above have already suggested that the motor system may be functionally divided into executive and preexecutive divisions. The latter is presumably responsible for initiating, sequencing, monitoring

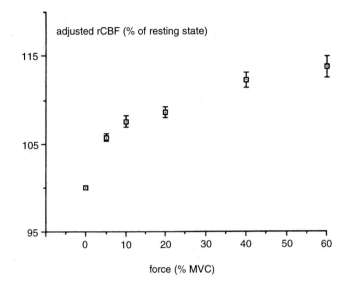

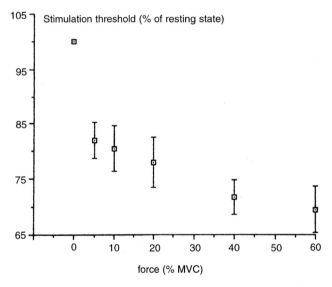

Figure 4 There is a relationship between perfusion and isometric force exerted between thumb and little finger expressed as a percentage of maximum voluntary contraction (MVC). In the contralateral hemisphere there is an exponential increase of perfusion with force exerted that is associated with a progressive decline in the strength of magnetic impulse required to elicit an electromyographic response in the arm contralateral to the stimulated motor cortex. Transcranial magnetic stimulation was performed whilst subjects exerted isometric forces between the thumb and the index finger identical to those exerted during scanning. The progressive decrease of threshold to magnetic stimulation mirrors increasing cortical excitability and is associated with activation.

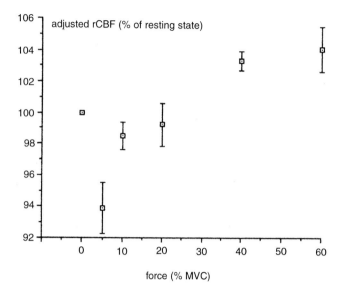

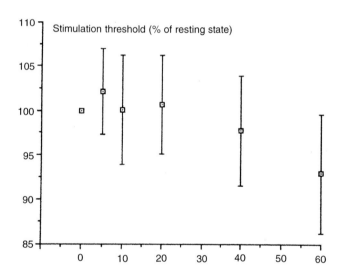

FIGURE 5 The results in this figure should be compared with those in Fig. 4. They show an initial deactivation followed by activation in ipsilateral motor cortex when isometric forces are exerted between thumb and index finger. In this case there is no significant change of magnetic stimulation needed to elicit electromygraphic activity in the unused and immobile arm. This result strongly supports the idea that the initial deactivation identified when force is exerted by the fingers is associated with electrophysiological inhibition of ipsilateral motor cortex.

and selecting of movement parameters (see Chapter 11). As a first attempt at reducing the problem we argue that it is reasonable to assess the effects of lesions in each of these systems separately. The ideal would be to examine groups of patients with lesions at identical (functional) anatomical sites. This ideal is hardly practical because of the vagaries of vascular supply to different regions in different individuals and to the logistical problems of collecting sufficient numbers of patients with (near) identical lesions. The strategy of examining single patients, though reasonable, does not permit generalisation across a population.

1. Motor Imagery

We performed studies of subjects performing paced random joystick movements in self-selected sequences in which the joystick was constrained to move only in the four cardinal directions from a central position. The randomness of movement was monitored. We used this task because we had previously shown that it activated virtually the complete motor system when compared with rest [25]. A preliminary experiment showed that dorsolateral prefrontal cortex and anterior parts of the anterior cingulate were specifically activated in association with initiation and selection of movements [26]. We therefore designed an experiment with an intention task (preparation of motor set) as the base level. The second task was imagining joystick movements and the third was their actual execution. The results confirmed a distinction between an executive motor system composed of (1) primary motor and somatosensory cortices, (2) dorsal parts of the medial and lateral premotor cortex, (3) adjacent posterior cingulate areas, and (4) rostral parts of left superior parietal cortex. These areas acting in concert with the remainder of the motor system (and, importantly, not alone) were responsible for motor execution [24].

A group of areas lying outside the central executive division comprising (1) medial and lateral premotor areas, (2) anterior cingulate areas, (3) ventral opercular premotor areas, and (4) parts of superior and inferior parietal areas were all activated when the same movements were imagined (see Fig. 3 in Chapter 14). These motor imagery activated areas were all activated bilaterally by this highly complex movement that involved both proximal and distal muscles. These data taken together suggest that imagined movements can be viewed as a special form of motor behaviour distinct from preparing to move and are presumably associated with selection of actions and multisensory integration. The neural substrate of imagining a movement differs from that involved in its execution most notably by an absence of activation in primary sensorimotor cortex in the central sulcus and immediately adjacent premotor, cingulate, and parietal structures.

2. Patient Studies—Imagery

We have performed two preliminary studies in patients with residual hemiparesis. They both undertook the same attentional, imagery, and execution tasks just described for normal subjects. In one patient with a mild residual motor deficit there was clear activation of parietal cortex, medial frontal areas, and anterior cingulate cortex; those areas activated by motor imagery in normal subjects (Fig. 6). In a second patient with a lesion in the ventral premotor operculum and insula and little useful recovery there was some minor activation in the supplementary motor area but no other activation was recorded elsewhere in the brain (Fig. 7). These, as yet unpublished, findings raise a number of interesting questions. The execution of a normal volitional movement requires much more than activation of pyramidal cells in primary motor cortex. Is it possible that opercular regions play a critical, possibly integrative, role between pre- and postcentral components of the cerebral motor apparatus? Our evidence suggests that there are profound effects on the capacity to recover if areas involved in motor initiation, planning, and sequencing are dysfunctional. Indeed, if these areas are activated and motor cortical activity is attenuated the motor deficit is mild. Are there significant

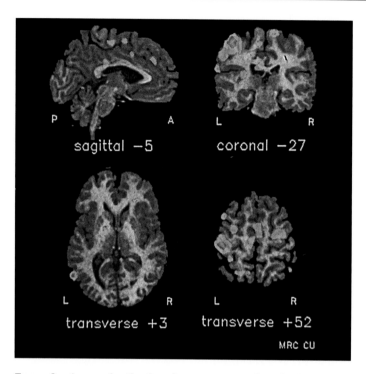

FIGURE 6 Areas of activation shown on coronal, sagittal, and transverse views of the MRI anatomical scan of a patient with a mild paresis of the right hand following a stroke. The patient is imagining a paced, freely selected joystick movement into four possible positions. Areas in the parietal cortex, medial frontal areas, and anterior cingulate cortex have been activated.

and sufficient direct corticofugal pathways in the human motor system to sustain some volitional activity without recourse to motor cortex? These are pure speculations with our presently impoverished data set.

3. Patient Studies—Force Activity Correlations

We have also carried out parametric studies in such patients using graded force exertion and normalising data to maximal voluntary contraction [27]. In three patients we find a binomial relationship between activity and forces in contralateral motor cortex, a pattern quite different to that found in normal volunteers where the relationship is always logarithmic (Fig. 8). In these three patients there was an initial steep rise of activity at low forces, a plateau, and then a second steep increase at 50% MVC (which was itself, on average, much lower than normal). In addition, ipsilateral ventral posterior supplementary motor and both parietal areas showed some force correlated activity that was not a feature of normal subjects. There was, however, considerable intersubject variability in the patterns of response, but correlated activity was always confined to motor areas. These data suggest that recruitment of preexisting cortico-cortical and possibly parallel cortico-spinal pathways plays a prominent role in functional reorganisation. Whether the marked increase of activity at forces greater than 50% MVC has any relationship to an overwhelming sense of increased effort that patients report at that level remains a matter for conjecture.

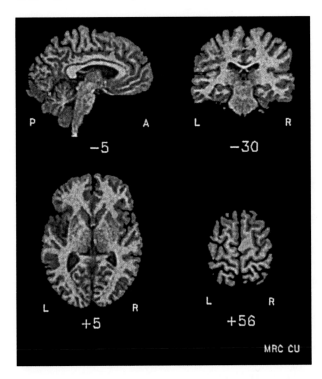

Figure 7 Patient with a severe paresis of the right arm following a stroke in the region of the left insular and inferior premotor cortex. Imagining the movements made by the patient in Fig. 6 results in very little cerebral activity except in a small mid-line frontal region.

E. Motor Output Zones

During recovery, individual patients with capsular infarcts show different types of motor cortical activation [23]. Under certain circumstances, recovery is accompanied by little change in the extent of motor cortex activated. In other circumstances the motor output zone, located in part at the site of representation of fingers and thumb, is greatly enlarged, spreading ventrally into the representation of the face and rostro-caudally into premotor and parietal cortex. We have speculated that a reason for such differences may be found in the anatomical location of lesions in subcortical white matter [28]. An analysis of a group of eight patients with lesions in the internal capsule who showed motor recovery showed that those with lesions in the posterior half of the posterior limb of the internal capsule (that interrupt output from MI) result in motor output zone enlargement, whilst the others did not. Tract tracing studies in primates indicate a topographic organisation of the output from motor associated cortical zones in the internal capsule. Thus, (a) fibres arising in medial frontal structures tend to pass through the anterior half of the internal capsule, (b) those arising in the premotor cortex, especially around the principal sulcus, pass through the genu and anterior half of the posterior part of the internal capsule, whereas (c) those from the motor cortex itself pass through the posterior half of the posterior limb. Thus it is lesions in the posterior portion of the posterior limb of internal capsule that disrupt output from MI. How does this fact help us to understand any resulting motor output zone enlargement?

One possibility is that interruption of MI axons in the internal capsule results in a loss of recurrent inhibition mediated through glutamatergic collaterals and GABA-ergic interneurons feeding back onto surrounding pyramidal cells [29]. We have sought evidence to support this suggestion by investigating patients with other forms of pyramidal tract disease. There are two varieties of motor neurone disease that are of interest in relation to testing our hypothesis about the basis for motor output zone enlargement in patients with internal capsule lesions. The common variety involves degeneration of both upper and lower motor neurons. A much rarer form, known as progressive muscular atrophy, results in pure degeneration of the lower motor neurons. In both cases there is muscular atrophy and patients can be matched for degree of weakness. It turns out that the motor output zone is enlarged if upper motor neurons degenerate, but not if they are unaffected [30]. Degeneration is only partial at the stage of disease in which movements of a joystick are still possible. This finding provides added evidence that a reason for enlargement of the motor output zone may indeed be failure of recurrent inhibition. It is still unclear whether the phenomenon of motor output zone enlargement is a useful component of recovery.

In summary the data reviewed so far show that the relationship between activation determined by functional imaging and cortical excitability needs to be carefully examined before interpretations in terms of inhibitory and excitatory influences are drawn. It should be possible to modulate neuronal excitability or activity in areas such as motor cortex by using physical or pharmaceutical means. It may then be possible to determine whether modulation of enlarged motor output zones is beneficial or detrimental to function.

III. PLASTICITY IN SENSORY SYSTEMS

A. Plasticity Secondary to Deafferentation

A reorganisation of somatosensory maps has been demonstrated in patients with upper limb amputations using a variety of noninvasive techniques [31,32]. We have examined patients with both traumatic and congenital amputations moving their stumps [33]. Paced shoulder movements were associated with activation in contralateral primary motor and somatosensory cortex of both groups of amputees. In traumatic amputees activations were present over a wider area and were of a significantly greater magnitude in the cortex contralateral to an amputation. On the other hand, in congenital amputees activations were also present over a somewhat wider area in contralateral primary motor and sensory cortices but in magnitude and extent were not significantly different from those elicited in the opposite hemisphere by movements of the normal arm. Abnormal activations were present in the cortex contralateral to an amputation in those with a traumatic cause, even during movements of the ipsilateral, intact arm. Abnormal ipsilateral primary motor and sensory responses were not seen during movement of the intact arm in the congenital group (Figs. 9 and 10).

Transcranial magnetic stimulation showed that abnormal activations in cortex contralateral to an amputation in traumatic amputees were associated with increased excitability [33]. There were no such changes in cortex contralateral to stumps of congenital amputees. This finding suggests that reorganisa-

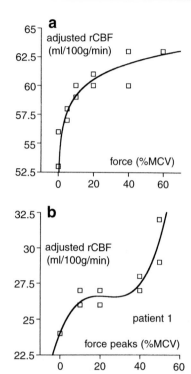

FIGURE 8 (a) A graph relating the relationship between perfusion and repetitive predetermined force pulses exerted by an index finger on a Morse key to levels expressed as a percentage of maximum voluntary contraction (MVC). The relationship is nonlinear and logarithmic. (b) The same relationship in a patient with moderate residual motor impairment after a stroke. The maximum voluntary contraction is significantly less than in normal subjects. However, when changes of perfusion are plotted against forces exerted an initial nonlinear relationship is seen up to 30% MVC, when a steep increase in perfusion occurs for quite modest further increases in exerted forces. We speculate that this altered relationship, which has been replicated in a number of patients, may represent a physiological concomitant of effort.

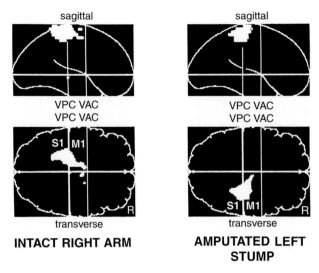

FIGURE 9 Statistical parametric maps of congenital amputees performing shoulder movements with intact right arms or with amputated left stumps. Sagittal and transaxial projections are shown. S1 and M1 refer to the primary somatosensory and motor cortices. There are significant activations mapped onto contralateral M1/S1 and supplementary motor area during movement of both intact and amputated upper limbs.

tion may be mediated by different mechanisms depending on whether deafferentation occurs during early development or in adult life (see later).

A further finding in traumatic amputees was activation of posterior parietal cortex and inferior parietal lobule opposite to a stump during movements of both amputated and intact arms. Posterior parietal cortical responses

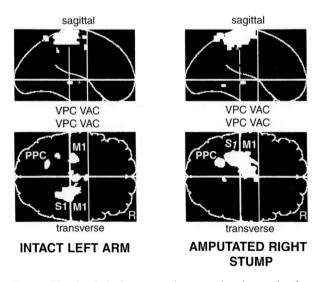

FIGURE 10 Statistical parametric maps showing activation with shoulder movements in patients with traumatic amputations to contrast with those of congenital amputees shown in Fig. 9. PPC is the superior posterior parietal cortex. The activations map onto contralateral M1/S1, supplementary motor area, and PPC in these patients with movement of both amputated and intact sides. The PPC is not activated in the congenital group (see Fig. 9).

were not present in congenital amputees. By analogy with magnetic stimulation results these studies may indicate increased excitability of parietal cortex in traumatic amputees that may be related to sensory symptoms, such as phantom perceptions. It is possible that such perceptions may be related to impaired inhibition in primary sensory and posterior parietal cortices that mediate sensory representations, or maps of the missing body parts.

B. Sensory Interactions and Perceptual Deficits

An intriguing result relating to recovery of sensory function is that reported more extensively in Chapter 10. In a patient with hemianaesthesia based on a neglect syndrome it was possible transiently to reverse the sensory deficit by ipsilateral (left) vestibular stimulation [34]. Prior to stimulation forced choice detection tasks were performed at chance level. In this instance the behavioural evidence suggests that input through one sensory pathway can modulate afferent signals in another sensory channel to generate perceptions in that separate modality. This behavioural model directly addresses questions of sensory integration in the context of a neglect syndrome and perhaps also tells us something about sensory attentional mechanisms. Scanning with and without sensory stimuli, in the presence and absence of vestibular stimulation, allowed detection of areas where an interaction between activity in the two sensory systems occurred, lending support to the idea that these neural interactions are responsible for perception. In at least two areas that received common vestibular and somato-sensory projections there was direct evidence of interactions and, in addition, a third fronto-orbital area showed activity dependent on somatosensory activation in the presence of vestibular stimuli. This observation may suggest that though sensory channels are, in general, kept segregated throughout their passage through the brain, significant interactions leading to considerable modification of sensory behaviour can occur as a result of integrative mecha-nisms that seem to depend on prefrontal mechanisms.

C. Long Term Changes after Visual System Lesions

Long-term recovery after critical lesions in unique informative patients has been another model we have used to investigate spontaneous plastic changes in cerebral activity. These patients are described in greater detail from a physiological perspective in Chapter 9. A particularily informative case is that of a patient with traumatic infarction of the left primary visual cortex who exhibited the phenomenon of residual vision [35]. After an indetermi-nate period of time the characteristics of visual loss and his residual capacities changed in that he was now aware of and able to discriminate the direction of specific types of moving stimuli in his "blind" visual field. That this capacity was conscious was testified to by his ability to accurately and verbally report what was going on. The question arose, how was this recovery possible? Unilateral visual motion stimuli resulted in activation of the prestriate area (V5) associated with perception of visual motion, despite the total absence of activation of primary visual cortex (V1). Interpretation of this finding, once again, rests heavily on the prevailing anatomical data. Accessory retino-prestriate pathways are described that bypass area V1 [36]. They pass through the pulvinar of the thalamus and terminate directly on prestriate cortex. Recent evoked potential data suggest that conduction in these pathways is remarkably fast and results in retinally derived signals reaching V5 before V1 [37]. This fact raises interesting issues in relation to models of feedforward modulation of V1 activity by functionally segregated prestriate areas. Another issue raised by the patient's visual behavior relates to an anatomical basis for the conscious component of his performance. Clearly, in his case activity in the prestriate cortex, divorced from afferent or feedback connections with V1, is sufficient in itself to generate a percept (albeit a degraded one). Finally, there remain questions as to how the residual visual functions and behavioral phenomena come about with such a time course. Of importance to general theories invoking plasticity and recovery of function in human brain is the fact that reorganisation involves, as in the motor and somataesthetic systems, only anatomical regions that are part of the system in which the lesion occurs.

An equally intriguing observation has been made in an unique patient with dyskinetopsia who demonstrates, psychophysically, residual perception of very slow visual motion [38]. This patient has large ischemic lesions in the posterior temporo-occipital cortices that contain human area V5. Activation with visual motion stimuli results in activations in superior parietal cortex and dorsal occipital regions that ordinarily contain human area V3. This finding again suggests that recovery is mediated by functional substitution by an anatomically distant area within the same sensory system. Some activation of these dorsal regions also occurs in normal subjects stimulated with visual motion. Hence, to date, in simple sensory input and motor output systems, a response to injury associated with recovery of behaviour does not imply acquisition of new functional characteristics by cerebral areas that are not already involved in some way in the system mediating that impaired function.

An example of the acquisition of new functional characteristics by a brain area is afforded by recent data suggesting that blind patients who are proficient Braille readers use occipital cortex for interpreting Braille symbols [39]. This finding is challenging and affords hope that perhaps whole functional areas can be remodelled to sustain new behavioural functions. If true, there may also be a theoretical implication suggesting a common, possibly modular, organization to cortex that is pluripotent with functional segregation dependent on the afferent/efferent characteristics of the region. This is not a new idea, but one for which strong evidence has not been forthcoming in man. The wholesale takeover of functions of one brain region by another seems to be the only example of such major functional takeover in the imaging literature to date. Our own studies (submitted) challenge this conclusion since our results indicate a quite different pattern of activation in those subjects who have never perceived light and those who became blind in infancy or childhood [40]. Thus, in a situation in which neuronal connections in primary visual cortex could not have been modified because of a total absence of any afferent visual signals V1 does not become pluripotent. On the other hand, some exposure to visual signals before blindness results in activation of V1 by Braille reading. Why this should be so is a matter for conjecture at present. We favour the idea that activity in V1 may be reflecting visual imagery processes, though yet other explanations need to be considered [41,42]. The general notion we favour is that wholesale takeover of an area by a completely new function (*e.g.*, somatoaesthesia in V1) is not likely.

IV. RECOVERY AND DISTURBED COGNITION

Recovery of higher cognitive function has been the object of little study to date given the complexities of multifaceted functions such as language and memory. Most patients rendered aphasic by a cerebral infarct show some recovery of language function that continues, as in the motor and visual systems, for months and sometimes years. Hence, there is evidence for potential plasticity within language as well as motor and sensory networks. This is an important issue because it speaks to the fact that deficits in functions that demand complex integration can be compensated. All the results to date implicate system specific reorganisation. If recovery occurs in higher order functions these may also be embodied in discrete systems. Explanations for mechanisms of language recovery most commonly cited are that functional viability is regained in periinfarct tissue or that homologous regions in the right hemisphere are recruited to take over impaired function in the left (dominant) hemisphere. We have tested explicitly the validity of such explanations by functional imaging studies of partially recovered aphasic patients.

A. Language Recovery

Weiller and his colleagues [43] have shown that patients recovering from Wernicke's aphasia activate right hemisphere language areas more strongly than normal subjects. These results were interpreted as evidence that the right hemisphere has some potential to take over functions of the damaged left hemisphere. However, the six recovered aphasic patients were studied as a single group. Such an experimental approach decreases any likelihood of detecting periinfarct activation (that will vary substantially between patients), whilst increasing the likelihood of detection of right hemisphere activation, especially if patients who recover language function come from a subpopulation of normal subjects who have bilateral representation of language functions.

We have completed two studies of language recovery [44,45]. Both considered the activation profiles of individual patients. In the first we investigated recovered aphasic patients (ML and JM) performing the same pair of language tasks as for the patients of Weiller described above [43]. The experimental task was verb generation in response to a heard target word and the baseline task was rest with eyes closed. Processing differences between these tasks include a full complement of language functions from phonological analysis, through semantic processing to phonological retrieval [44,45]. The second study investigated reading responses of an aphasic patient (HK) who had made a partial recovery. HK is unable to generate words in response to a target but has regained some ability to read words aloud. His performance was not sufficient for us to scan him during a task that required explicit verbal responses because it would have been impossible to equate task performance with normal subjects (see above). However, since he had excellent comprehension of visual words, we scanned him reading words compared with viewing false font with instructions to press a response key whenever he saw a target. Activation differences were then attributed to the (implicit) word processing functions available to him [46]. The rationale for this experimental design is described in detail in Chapter 13.

For each study there were nine normal control subjects. Analysis of individual activation profiles in the first study revealed that four subjects activated bilateral language areas with verb generation and also that four normals in the second study activated bilateral language areas when viewing words. Figures 11 and 12 demonstrate activation profiles of patients relative to normal subjects. In the first study (Fig. 11) recovery of function in ML is associated with periinfarct activation in the damaged left hemisphere with no activation of right hemisphere regions. Similarly, JM activated periinfarct tissue but in addition she activated her right superior temporal gyrus. This activation was the same as that of four, bilaterally responding, normal subjects. We suggest, as a working hypothesis, that right hemisphere activation is consistent with JM having bilaterally organised language function prior to her stroke.

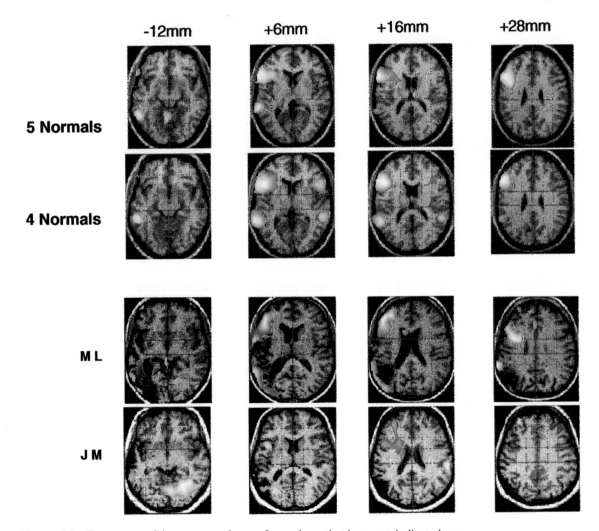

FIGURE 11 Four rows of images are shown. In each, activations are indicated as coloured areas on transaxial MRI anatomical scans of the patients and normal subjects. Planes parallel to the intercommissural line are shown at distances below and above as indicated by the numbers at the top of each row. The normal subjects are divided into two groups: one contains five normal subjects who individually show predominantly unilateral activation by language tasks; the other contains the average of the four subjects who activated both sides of the brain with the same language task. Patient ML shows predominantly unilateral and significant peri-infarct activation. Patient JM shows bilateral activation that includes posterior temporal areas among others.

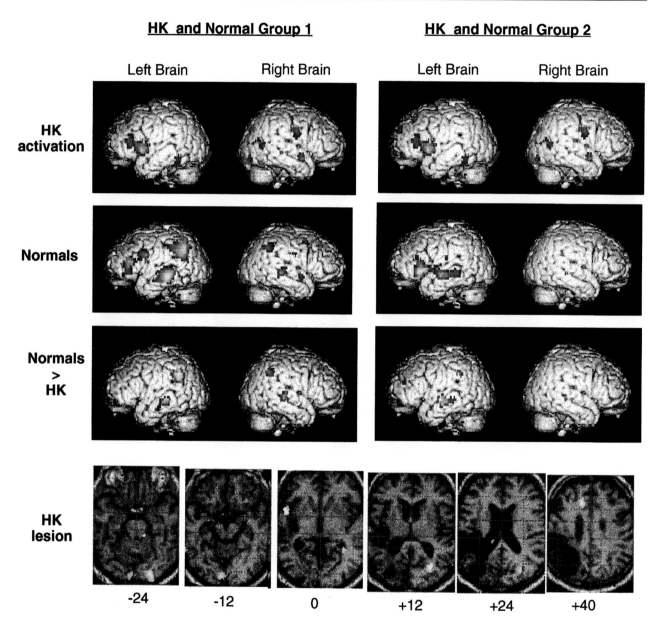

FIGURE 12   This figure compares the activation in patient HK when exposed to visually presented words. His MRI anatomical scan is shown at the bottom to indicate the extent of his left temporo-parietal lesion. (The numbers represent distance above and below the intercommissural line.) Above, activations are shown projected onto the surfaces of the right and left hemispheres. On the left are the results compared to the bilaterally activating normal group (see Fig. 11). On the right the comparison is with the unilaterally activated normal group. Activations in HK are shown on the top row, those in normals in the second row, and those areas where there is significantly greater activation in normal subjects than HK in the third row. Note the impaired activation in dominant temporal and inferior parietal cortex in HK.

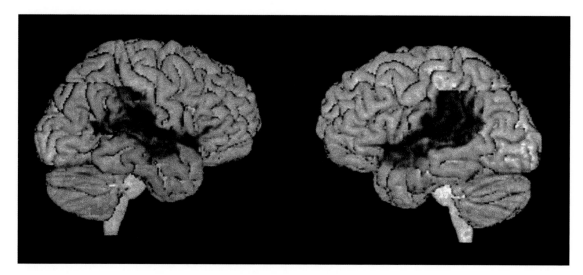

FIGURE 13   Anatomical MRI scans showing bilateral superior temporal and inferior parietal lesions in a case of cortical deafness.

Only studies of patients before and after stroke are likely to confirm such a hypothesis, and such a scenario will arise only rarely and by chance. Nevertheless, if the hypothesis is correct, and people with bilateral language function are more likely to recover from aphasia following left hemisphere infarcts, then recovered aphasics will activate the right hemisphere during language tasks more than a heterogeneous group of normal subjects.

The results of the second study demonstrate that in response to visually presented words HK activates left prefrontal regions normally but shows deactivation (relative to control groups) in left temporal and parietal regions. Decreased activation in left temporo-parietal regions is associated with HK's poor phonological skills. Interestingly, HK also activates some of the right hemisphere language areas engaged by subjects with bilateral activation in relation to language (Fig. 12, group 1). Our interpretation must, once again, remain speculative; however, it is tempting to suggest that the right-sided activations could reflect normal right hemisphere function, resulting in good comprehension associated with limited speech production [47].

Our conclusions from these preliminary studies are that recovery of language functions depends on the viability of periinfarct tissue and the state of premorbid lateralisation of function in a patient. We have additionally demonstrated periinfarct activation in another functional imaging study of a word deaf patient with bilateral perisylvian strokes who recovered some ability to recognize environmental sounds [48] (Fig. 13). The patient was scanned at rest and while passively listening to and then categorising environmental sounds. During passive listening relative to rest, he activated periinfarct tissue in normal bilateral auditory processing regions. During sound categorisation, relative to passive listening, normal subjects activate only left hemisphere regions but our patient also activated some right hemisphere areas, suggesting, again, some bilateral organisation of language function before his strokes.

V. SUMMARY AND CONCLUSIONS

The hope is that by describing patterns of compensation, hypotheses about mechanisms for these changes will be generated not only at systems but also at molecular and cellular levels. Clearly, knowledge of such mechanisms will provide an opportunity to modulate or manipulate them. That in turn could provide means for speeding up or promoting processes that lead to improved recovery. Imaging methods are able to test directly such therapeutic strategies by conjoint behavioral and therapeutic challenge and by demonstrating proposed mechanisms of change (see Chapter 16). An example that suggests that such a program is feasible is provided by a demonstration of the failure to activate supplementary motor area during a free choice sequential motor task in Parkinson's disease, and the subsequent demonstration of its reversibility by the coadministration of a dopaminergic agonist [49]. The realisation that functional recovery from Parkinson's disease can be achieved with human fetal mesencephalic engraftment into the diseased striatum was functionally proven by PET scanning with [^{18}F]-dopa as a tracer [50]. A similar interaction between the placement of graft and supplementary motor area activity during a motor task could be shown with perfusion scans before and after operation.

In summary, there is considerable evidence for profound long-lasting changes in patterns of cerebral activation in patients with cerebral lesions. The mechanisms for such large-scale changes are poorly understood and are best framed at present in terms of alterations in patterns of firing of large-scale neuronal networks that are imposed by alterations in local inputs and/or outputs. The degree to which alterations of inputs and outputs, both from and to the outside world and within the cerebral structure of the relevant functional network, are possible is probably restricted by hard-wired anatomical constraints that limit the extent to which any compensation can occur. In certain instances it may be that normally minor pathways take on crucial input roles or that top–down influences activate functionally segregated brain areas in specific networks by alternate routes.

References

1. T. E. Twitchell. The restoration of motor function following hemiplegia in man. *Brain* **74,** 443–480 (1951).
2. P. D. Wall. The presence of ineffective synapses and the circumstances that unmask them. *Philos. Trans. R. Soc. London B.* **278,** 361–372 (1977).
3. S. G. Waxman. Functional recovery in diseases of the nervous system. *In* "Advances in Neurology" (S. G. Waxman, Ed.), Vol. 47, pp. 1–7. Raven Press, New York, 1988.
4. E. G. Merrill and P. D. Wall. Plasticity of connections in the adult nervous system. *In* "Neuronal Plasticity" (C. W. Cottman, Ed.), pp. 97–111. Raven Press, New York, 1978.
5. W. W. Chambers, C. N. Liu, and G. P. MacGough. Anatomical and physiological correlates of plasticity in the central nervous system. *Brain Behav. Evol.* **8,** 675–694 (1973).
6. B. Kolb. "Brain Plasticity and Behaviour," pp. 1–194. Lawrence Erlbaum, Mahwah, NJ, 1995.
7. H. T. Chugani, M. E. Phelps, and J. C. Mazziotta. Positron emission tomography study of human brain functional development. *Ann. Neurol.* **22,** 487–497 (1987).
8. P. R. Huttenlocher. Synaptic density in human frontal cortex—Developmental changes and effects of ageing. *Brain Res.* **163,** 195–205 (1979).
9. S. Grafton, J. C. Mazziotta, S. Presty, K. J. Friston, R. S. J. Frackowiak, and M. E. Phelps. Functional anatomy of human procedural learning determined with regional cerebral blood flow and PET. *J. Neurosci.* **12,** 2542–2548 (1992).

10. K. J. Friston, C. D. Frith, R. D. Passingham, P. F. Liddle, and R. S. J. Frackowiak. Motor practice and neurophysiological adaptation in the cerebellum: a PET study. *Proc. R. Soc. London B.* **243,** 223–228 (1992).

11. R. S. J. Frackowiak and K. J. Friston. Functional neuroanatomy of the human brain: Positron emission tomography—A new neuroanatomical technique. *J. Anat.* **184,** 211–225 (1994).

12. C. Weiller, F. Chollet, K. J. Friston, R. J. S. Wise, and R. S. J Frackowiak. Functional reorganization of the brain in recovery from striatocapsular infarction in man. *Ann. Neurol.* **31,** 463–472 (1992).

13. G. M. Shepherd and K. Koch. Introduction to synaptic circuits. *In* "The Synaptic Organisation of the Brain" (G. M. Shepherd, Ed.) pp. 3–31. Oxford Univ. Press, New York, Oxford, 1990.

14. A. Danek, M. Bauer, and W. Fries. Tracing of neural connections in the human brain by magnetic resonance imaging in vivo. *Eur. J. Neurosci.* **2,** 112–115 (1990).

15. W. Fries, A. Danek, and T. N. Witt. Motor responses after transcranial electrical stimulation of cerebral hemispheres with a degenerated pyramidal tract. *Ann. Neurol.* **29,** 646–650 (1991).

16. F. Chollet, V. DiPiero, R. J. S. Wise, D. J. Brooks, R. J. Dolan, and R. S. J. Frackowiak. The functional anatomy of motor recovery after ischaemic stroke in man. *Ann. Neurol.* **29,** 63–71 (1991).

17. S. G. Kim, J. Ashe, A. P. Georgopoulos, H. Merkle, J. M. Ellermann, R. S. Menon, S. Ogawa, and K. Ugurbil. Functional imaging of human motor cortex at high magnetic-field. *J. Neurophysiol.* **69,** 297–302 (1993).

18. C. Dettmers, G. R. Fink, R. N. Lemon, K. M. Stephan, R. E. Passingham, D. Silbersweig, A. Holmes, M. C. Ridding, D. J. Brooks, and R. S. J. Frackowiak. Relation between cerebral activity and force in the motor areas of the brain. *J. Neurophysiol.* **74,** 802–815 (1995).

19. J. G. Colebatch, M. P. Deiber, R. E. Passingham, K. J. Friston, and R. S. J. Frackowiak. Regional cerebral blood flow during voluntary arm and hand movements in human subjects. *J. Neurophysiol.* **65,** 1392–1401 (1991).

20. C. Dettmers, R. N. Lemon, K. M. Stephan, G. R. Fink, and R. S. J. Frackowiak. Cerebral activation during the exertion of sustained static force in man. *NeuroReport* **7,** 2103–2110 (1996).

21. C. Dettmers, M. C. Ridding, K. M. Stephan, R. N. Lemon, J. C. Rothwell, and R. S. J. Frackowiak. Comparison of regional cerebral blood flow with transcranial magnetic stimulation at different forces. *J. Appl Physiol.* **81,** 596–603 (1996).

22. J. G. Colebatch and S. C. Gandevia. The distribution of muscular weakness in upper motor neurone lesions affecting the arm. *Brain* **112,** 749–763 (1989).

23. C. Weiller, S. C. Ramsay, R. S. J. Wise, K. J. Friston, and R. S. J. Frackowiak. Individual patterns of functional reorganization in the human cerebral cortex after capsular infarction. *Ann. Neurol.* **33,** 181–189 (1993).

24. K. M. Stephan, G. Fink, R. E. Passingham, D. Silbersweig, A. O. Ceballos-Baumann, C. D. Frith, and R. S. J. Frackowiak. Functional anatomy of mental representation of upper extremity movements. *J. Neurophysiol.* **73,** 373–386 (1995).

25. M. P. Deiber, R. E. Passingham, J. G. Colebatch, K. J. Friston, P. D. Nixon, and R. S. J. Frackowiak. Cortical areas and the selection of movement: A study with PET. *Exp. Brain Res.* **84,** 392–402 (1991).

26. C. D. Frith, K. J. Friston, P. F. Liddle, and R. S. J. Frackowiak. Willed action and the prefrontal cortex in man. *Proc. R. Soc. London B* **244,** 241–246 (1991).

27. C. Dettmers, K. M. Stephan, R. N. Lemon, and R. S. J. Frackowiak. Reorganization of the executive motor system after stroke. *Cerebrovasc. Dis.* **7,** 187–200 (1997).

28. W. Fries, A. Danek, K. Scheidtmann, and C. Hamburger. Motor recovery following capsular stroke—role of descending pathways from multiple motor areas. *Brain* **116,** 369–382 (1993).

29. S. Gosh, and R. Porter. Morphology of pyramidal neurons in monkey motor cortex

and the synaptic actions of their intracortical axon collaterals. *J Physiol.* **400,** 593–615 (1988).

30. J. J. M. Kew, D. J. Brooks, R. E. Passingham, J. C. Rothwell, R. S. J. Frackowiak, and P. N. Leigh. Cortical function in progressive lower motor neurone disorders and amyotrophic lateral sclerosis: A comparative PET study. *Neurology* **44,** 1101–1110 (1994).

31. L. G. Cohen, S. Bandinelli, T. W. Findley, and M. Hallett. Motor reorganisation after upper limb amputation in man. *Brain* **114,** 615–627 (1991).

32. T. P. Pons, P. E. Garraghty, A. K. Ommaya, J. H. Kaas, E. Taub, and M. Mishkin. Massive cortical reorganization after sensory deafferentation in adult macaques. *Science* **252,** 1857–1860 (1991).

33. J. J. M. Kew, M. C. Ridding, J. C. Rothwell, R. E. Passingham, P. N. Leigh, S. Sooriakumaran, R. S. J. Frackowiak, and D. J. Brooks. Reorganisation of cortical blood flow and transcranial magnetic stimulation maps in human subjects after upper limb amputation. *J. Neurophysiol.* **72,** 2517–2524 (1994).

34. G. Bottini, E. Paulesu, R. Sterzi, E. Warburton, R. J. S. Wise, G. Vallar, R. S. J. Frackowiak, and C. D. Frith. Modulation of conscious experience by peripheral sensory stimuli. *Nature* **376,** 778–780 (1995).

35. J. L. Barbur, J. D. G. Watson, R. S. J. Frackowiak, and S. Zeki. Conscious visual perception without V1. *Brain* **116,** 1293–1302 (1993).

36. W. Fries. The projection of the lateral geniculate nucleus to the prestriate cortex of the macaque monkey. *Proc. R. Soc. London B* **213,** 73–80 (1981).

37. D. H. Ffytche, C. N. Guy, and S. Zeki. The parallel visual motion inputs into areas V1 and V5 of human cerebral cortex. *Brain* **118,** 1375–1394 (1995).

38. S. Shipp, B. M. De Jong, J. Zihl, R. S. J. Frackowiak, and S. Zeki. The brain activity related to residual motion vision in a patient with bilateral lesions of V5. *Brain* **117,** 1023–1038 (1994).

39. N. Sadato, A. Pascual Leone, J. Grafman, V. Ibanez, M. P. Deiber, G. Dold, and M. Hallett. Activation of the primary visual cortex by Braille reading in blind subjects. *Nature* **380,** 526–528 (1996).

40. C. Buechel, C. J. Price, R. S. J. Frackowiak, and K. J. Friston. Different activation patterns in the visual cortex of late and congenitally blind subjects. Submitted for publication.

41. P. C. Fletcher, C. D. Frith, S. C. Baker, T. Shallice, R. S. J. Frackowiak, and R. J. Dolan. The mind's eye—precuneus activation in memory-related imagery. *NeuroImage* **2,** 195–200 (1995).

42. G. Bottini, R. Corcoran, R. Sterzi, E. Paulesu, P. Schenone, P. Scarpa, R. S. J. Frackowiak, and C. D. Frith. The role of the right hemisphere in the interpretation of the figurative aspects of language. A positron emission tomography activation study. *Brain* **117,** 1241–1254 (1994).

43. C. Weiller, C. Isensee, M. Rijntjes, W. Huber, S. Muller, D. Bier, K. Dutschka, R. P. Woods, J. Noth, and H. C. Diener. Recovery from Wernicke's aphasia: A positron emission tomographic study. *Ann Neurol.* **37,** 723–732 (1995).

44. E. Warburton, R. J. S. Wise, C. J. Price, C. Weiller, U. Hadar, S. Ramsay, and R. S. J. Frackowiak Studies with positron emission tomography of noun and verb retrieval in norml subjects. *Brain* **119,** 159–180 ((1996).

45. E. Warburton, C. J. Price, K. Swinburn, and R. J. S. Wise. Mechanisms of Recovery from Aphasia: Evidence from Positron Emission Tomography. Submitted for publication.

46. C. J. Price, R. J. S. Wise, and R. S. J. Frackowiak Demonstrating the implicit processing of visually presented words and pseudowords. *Cereb. Cortex* **6,** 62–70 (1996).

47. K. Patterson and B. Besner Is the right hemisphere literate? *Cogn. Neuropsychol.* **1,** 315–341 (1984).

48. A. Engelien, D. Silbersweig, E. Stern, W. Huber, W. Doring, C. Frith, and R. S. J. Frackowiak The functional anatomy of recovery from auditory agnosia.

A PET study of sound categorisation in a neurological patient and normal controls. *Brain* **118,** 1395–1409 (1995).

49. I. H. Jenkins, W. Fernandez, E. D. Playford, A. J. Lees, R. S. J. Frackowiak, R. E. Passingham, and D. J. Brooks. Impaired activation of the supplementary motor area in Parkinson's disease is reversed when akinesia is treated with apomorphine. *Ann Neurol.* **32,** 749–757 (1992).

50. O. Lindvall, P. Brundin, H. Widner, S. Rehncrona, B. Gustavii, R. S. J. Frackowiak, K. Leenders, G. Sawle, J. C. Rothwell, C. D. Marsden, and A. Björklund. Intracerebral grafts of fetal dopamine neurons survive and improve motor function in idiopathic Parkinson's disease. *Science* **247,** 574–577 (1990).

CHAPTER THIRTEEN

FUNCTIONAL ANATOMY OF READING

I. INTRODUCTION

The aim of this chapter is to discuss investigations of the functional neuroanatomy of reading. The study designs are based on information processing models that subdivide reading into a series of processing stages [1–4]. According to these models, reading involves (i) visual processing of the seen word to reveal the pattern of visual features (perception of form), (ii) orthographic letter processing to reveal the component letters of the word and their order (*e.g.*, H+O+R+S+E), (iii) semantic processing to reveal the meaning of words, and (iv) phonological processing to reveal the sounds of words.

In the model shown in Fig. 1, a distinction is made between lexical and sublexical orthography. Lexical orthography (sometimes referred to as the word form system [1] or the visual input lexicon [5]) involves familiar letter combinations that represent whole words and has direct links to whole word semantic and phonological descriptions. Sublexical orthography involves subword letter combinations for which there are no corresponding semantic descriptions but unlike other visual stimuli, the subcomponents of written words have phonological correspondences that can be assembled into whole word phonology, providing indirect access to semantics. Irrespective of whether phonology is 'addressed directly' or 'assembled via sublexical pathways', the individual speech sounds must be sequenced in the correct order with appropriate coarticulation and stress and formulated into motor plans (the execution of phonology) prior to articulation and the generation of sound.

Evidence that these subcomponents are associated with different regions of the brain comes from patients who, following damage to a particular region of the brain, are selectively impaired with one component of the reading system whilst other components are left unimpaired. For example, one type of dyslexic patient may be unable to access any semantic or phonological information from visually presented words despite having normal vision and spelling; another type can access some semantic information but incorrect phonological codes are formulated (reading, for instance, the word YACHT

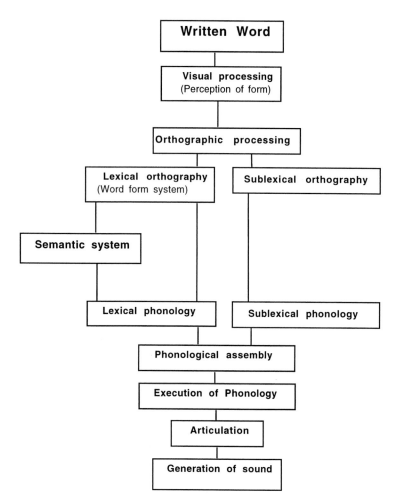

FIGURE 1   An information processing model of reading.

as "ship"). In a third variety of acquired dyslexia, YACHT will be read aloud as "yatched," suggesting virtually the reverse of the previous pattern, *i.e.*, good ability to assemble phonology from print (by sublexical pathways), but failure to access the correct semantic code via addressed phonology. See Ellis and Young [6] and Shallice [4] for recent descriptions of various patterns of reading disorder.

These findings imply that the subcomponents of reading are located in different regions of the brain. By relating the site of focal brain damage to the impaired behaviour, neuropsychological studies have attempted to associate function with structure. Deficits in speech production have been associated with damage to Broca's area in the left inferior frontal gyrus and deficits in speech comprehension have been associated with damage to Wernicke's area in the posterior half of the left superior temporal gyrus [7]. In the reading domain, deficits in accessing visual word forms for reading and spelling have been associated with damage to the left angular gyrus [8–10], deficits in spelling by sound have been associated with damage to the supramarginal gyrus and the insula medial to it [10], and impairments in semantic processing have been associated with damage to the left basal temporal lobe [11]. Despite these advances, the functional anatomy of reading has not been revealed fully by lesion studies because of the inherent limitations of the approach. The primary limitation is that studies are reliant on damaged brains. This has a number of drawbacks because (i) patients with distinct lesions and specific functional impairments are rare; in the majority of cases, lesions are large or multiple and patients have more than one functional deficit; (ii) following brain damage, performance may not reflect normal word processing because patients may attempt to compensate for their deficits by using abnormal word processing strategies; and (iii) the loss of function may not be a consequence of damage to an anatomically discrete subcomponent, but a remote effect of interruption to the pathways to or from that subcomponent. Given these limitations, there is great potential for advancing our knowledge of reading processes by imaging the normal human brain in action. This more recent approach is still in the early stages of discovery but current work is already confirming and extending the findings of neuropsychological studies.

It is now 8 years since the publication of the first language activation study with positron emission tomography [12]. During the ensuing years, there have been many changes in methodological design and analysis. In all cases the experiments rely on contrasting the distribution of brain activity under different conditions, but whilst the initial studies relied entirely on simple cognitive subtraction, experimental designs have subsequently been elaborated to include factorial designs, parametric designs, and recently cognitive conjunctions (see Chapter 8). In order to keep a perspective on how results have changed with changing methodology, a selection of experiments related to reading will be discussed in historical order and will be categorised according to the type of methodology used.

II. COGNITIVE SUBTRACTIONS

Virtually all language experiments to date have been based on cognitive subtraction. Stimulus conditions are chosen on the assumption that the activation task engages one more component of the word processing model than the control task and that the increased activation associated with that additional component will be revealed by categorical comparison of scans obtained during the different tasks. This is best illustrated by the pioneering studies of Petersen *et al.* [12,13].

A. The Pioneering Studies

The first language activation study reported by Petersen *et al.* [12] investigated the anatomical areas engaged by visual and auditory word processing by comparing the cerebral blood flow distribution during different word tasks within a three-level subtractive hierarchy. The first level of the reading hierarchy was silent word viewing and comparison of blood flow in this task with blood flow when viewing a fixation point (the baseline task) was intended to isolate sensory input and involuntary word form processing. The second level of the hierarchy was reading aloud and comparison of blood flow to that during silent word viewing (the first level of the reading hierarchy) aimed at isolating speech output processes. The third level of the hierarchy was a verb generation task (saying an appropriate verb in response to a seen noun) and comparison of flow in this task to that during reading aloud (the second level

WORDS	PSEUDOWORDS	LETTER STRINGS	FALSE FONT
cave	vace	vsnc	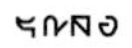 ꙮᴎᴚꙨ
tree	reet	tnnr	\ᴧꙨꙨ
sand	nads	nsvd	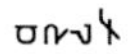 ᴛᴎᴧᴋ
ring	girn	gnxr	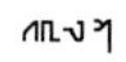 ᴨᴛᴧᴧ

FIGURE 2 Examples of words, pseudowords, consonant letter strings, and false font stimuli.

of the hierarchy) aimed at isolating semantic processing. The results revealed that involuntary word processing engaged the striate and extrastriate visual cortex, speech output processes engaged bilateral motor areas, and the supplementary motor cortex (SMA) and a left premotor area and semantic processing engaged the left dorsolateral prefrontal cortex (DLPFC) and the anterior cingulate.

In a subsequent functional imaging study by Petersen *et al.* [13], the areas activated during visual word processing were investigated further by comparing brain activity during silent viewing of false font (strings of unfamiliar letter-like characters; see Fig. 2), consonant letter strings (*e.g.*, JVJFC), pseudowords (*e.g.*, FLOOP), and real words. The brain activity during silent viewing of each stimulus type was compared to that seen in visual fixation. Words have legitimate word forms with semantic and phonological representations; related activity was detected in the left medial extrastriate visual cortex and a left prefrontal area. Pseudowords have legitimate word forms from which phonological but not semantic associations can be determined; related activity was detected in the left medial extrastriate cortex but not in the left prefrontal cortex. Consonant letter strings and false font do not have stored word associations and did not activate either the left medial extrastriate cortex or the left prefrontal cortex. These results were interpreted as evidence that the left medial extrastriate cortex is activated by legitimate word forms and is the site of the visual word form system whilst the left prefrontal region is associated with semantic processing. No area of activation was associated with the phonological processing that ensues from viewing words and pseudowords.

The first reading activation study to follow up the work of Petersen *et al.* [12,13] was reported by Howard *et al.* [14] and investigated differences of regional brain activity between reading aloud and saying "crime" to strings of false font stimuli. The repetitive phonological response "crime" to each presentation of false font was intended to control for the articulation involved in reading aloud. In addition to viewing words and false font, subjects repeated heard words and said "crime" in response to hearing reversed words. The sounds of reversed words have the same auditory complexity as the sounds of words, but with little or no perceptible phonology. The prediction was that in comparison to their respective baselines, heard and seen words would activate (i) two unique activation foci that could be related to the visual and auditory input lexicons (the word form systems), (ii) a third activation focus common to both tasks if automatic semantic processing causes significant changes of brain activity in the real word tasks, and (iii) activation in

Wernicke's area during word reading if phonological recoding is involved in reading. However, the results were not clear cut; both reading and repeating activated areas within the left temporal cortex that, though separable, were very close to each other. Also, there were no other common areas that could be attributed to semantics. In particular, there was no activity in the left frontal region that Petersen et al. [13] associated with semantics (see above). Although Howard et al. [14] considered the possibility that the left temporal cortex is involved in lexical, semantic, and phonological processing, they argued that the activations reflected the auditory and visual input lexicons because the peaks of the auditory and visual signals were separable. Activity in the left medial extrastriate cortex did not change significantly in the visual word *versus* false font comparison; therefore, there was no evidence to support the Petersen et al. [13] claim that the left medial extrastriate cortex is the site of the visual word form system. In summary, Howard et al. [14] attributed activation in the left middle temporal cortex to the visual word form system but found no activity related to semantic or phonological processing.

That neither the Petersen et al. [12,13] nor the Howard et al. [14] studies were able to attribute brain areas to all the component reading processes means that both were revealing only part of what would be expected. The most likely explanation for this difference is that inherent limitations in the sensitivity of the techniques used and differences in the design of the two studies weighted the results to show different subcomponents of the reading process.

B. Developments in Scanning and Analysis Techniques

In the past 4 years the sensitivity of the cameras and techniques used have improved dramatically with the introduction of 3D image acquisition and development of new data analysis techniques. These changes have had a corresponding effect on the results of recent studies. Now when viewing words is contrasted to viewing false font, widespread activation of bilateral language areas is detected, including activation of the left inferior prefrontal regions reported by Petersen et al. [13] and the left posterior temporal cortex activated by Howard et al. [14] (Fig. 3). Other areas engaged by reading are the left inferior parietal cortex, the right posterior temporal cortex, both sensorimotor cortices, and the supplementary motor area [15–18]. Activity during silent viewing in the sensorimotor cortex and the SMA suggests that there is subvocal outflow to the muscles responsible for articulation even when subjects are not instructed to speak. Such implicit processing of words, beyond the demands of a task, is consistent with the psychological literature which has demonstrated that visual presentation of words automatically activates lexical, semantic, and phonological processes even when subjects are engaged in an irrelevant task [19–23].

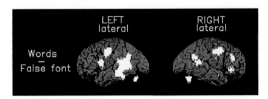

Figure 3 Areas of activation when viewing words is contrasted to viewing false font stimuli.

Although areas activated during reading tasks are now more consistent with lesion studies and previous neuroimaging studies that explicitly explored activation of semantic and phonological processing using auditory tasks [24,25], the interpretation of the function of each active area becomes more complex when there are multiple differences between conditions and multiple areas of activation. In terms of information processing models the differences between viewing words and false font include (i) orthographic letter processing, (ii) semantic processing, (iii) phonological processing, and (iv) execution and articulation of phonology. Our challenge is to design tasks that isolate the different components from one another. Some obvious approaches have been attempted, which are discussed below.

C. Reading Aloud—Reading Silently

Although phonological and semantic processes are activated implicitly when subjects read silently (see above), phonological recoding may be stronger during reading aloud, which is dependent on explicit activation of phonological codes. This rationale was adopted in the original study by Petersen *et al.* [12] that detected greater activation in the region of the left sylvian fissure in association with reading aloud. However, as discussed above, the early studies were not as sensitive as more recent studies and many regions of activation could have been missed. In a recent study by Bookheimer *et al.* [18], the superior temporal regions and the supramarginal gyrus were found to be more active during reading aloud than during reading silently. Bookheimer *et al.* [18] associate these regions with assembling sublexical phonology because they argue that reading aloud activates both lexical and sublexical phonology whilst reading silently involves only lexical phonology. There are two problems with this interpretation. First, psychological studies are not consistent with the view that reading silently activates only whole word phonology. Van Orden *et al.* [22] have demonstrated that sublexical phonology from pseudowords (*e.g.*, SUTE) interferes with silent comprehension tasks and argue that word identification in silent reading proceeds from spelling to sound to meaning. Second, a direct comparison of reading aloud and reading silently is confounded by differences in articulation and auditory processing in response to the generation of sound during reading aloud [17,26] and these processes were not controlled in the Bookheimer *et al.* study [18]. When the differences between conditions are limited to the generation of sound and auditory processing of own voice (by contrasting reading aloud to a condition when subjects silently articulate the words) activation of the superior temporal and supramarginal gyri, as seen in the Bookheimer *et al.* study, returns [17]. Overall, these data indicate that a contrast between reading aloud and reading silently is dominated by differences in articulation and the sound of own voice which has been shown to activate the superior temporal and supramarginal gyri.

D. Real Words—Pseudowords

Studies attempting to isolate semantic processing from reading tasks [13,16] have contrasted activation associated with reading known words with activation associated with reading pronounceable pseudowords (that have no direct semantic representation). In the Petersen *et al.* study [13] activation in the inferior regions of prefrontal cortex (BA 44/BA 45) was reported for words relative to fixation but not for pseudowords relative to fixation. This result leads to the conclusion that the left prefrontal activation is associated with semantic processing but such a conclusion is based on two assumptions. The first assumption is that the pronounceability of the words and pseudowords is matched. The second assumption is that real words will activate semantic representations more strongly than pseudowords. The first assumption does not hold true because familiar words can address phonology directly via whole word orthography, whereas pseudowords rely on assembling subword phonology. Neither assumption is supported by our results [16]. We found greater activation during pseudoword presentation than real word presentation in the inferior temporal, inferior frontal, and supramarginal gyri (Fig. 4).

Our results [16] suggest that pseudowords may activate semantic and phonological processes more strongly than real words because the phonological code is unfamiliar and because an unsuccessful search for (missing) semantic representations is initiated. This hypothesis can be interpreted in terms of connectionist models of word processing that propose that activation of feature, letter, and word representations, consistent with the input, accumulate simultaneously (rather than in a discrete fashion within an hierarchy) [2]. Active word and letter representations inhibit competing responses at all levels of the system until a single interpretation emerges. For pseudowords, there are no connections to specific representations to inhibit competing responses and the system takes longer to converge on an interpretation, thereby creating more activity in the word recognition network relative to when the stimuli are familiar words. Contrasting activation during word and pseudoword presentation is therefore confounded by the dilemma of whether we are measuring activation associated with accessing stored representations (for word processing) or activity associated with a search for missing representations (for pseudoword processing).

In both the example of reading aloud relative to reading silently and that of reading real words relative to reading pseudowords, the application of cognitive subtraction has been unsuccessful because even when subjects are not instructed to process words, the mere presence of a lexical stimulus in the visual field engages word processing areas. One possible way around this problem is to use a technique first reported by Corbetta *et al.* [27], where the contrast of activity is between tasks that selectively maximize engagement of particular cognitive functions. For example, in auditory word processing tasks Demonet *et al.* [25] contrasted a semantic monitoring task with a phoneme monitoring task and found differential activation in several language

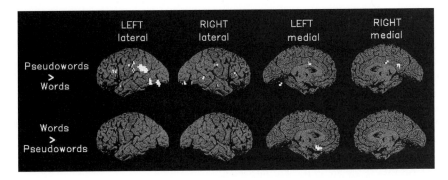

Figure 4   Areas of differential activation for real words and pseudowords.

processing areas. Attempts to use this approach in reading studies are discussed below.

E. Orthographic Word Processing

To maximize orthographic processing, a task that does not rely on semantic and phonological processing is needed. The one study to date that attempted to isolate orthographic processing in this way used a lexical decision task [15], which involved distinguishing between visually presented letter strings that were real words from those that corresponded to nonwords. Activation during lexical decision was contrasted with activation during reading aloud and visual feature decision on false font with the hypothesis that lexical decision places greater demands on orthographic word processing. Relative to both reading aloud and feature decision, the areas more active for lexical decision were the left premotor and prefrontal cortices and the SMA, regions that have been consistently activated in tasks thought to involve inner speech and subvocal articulation [24,28–30]. Rather than indicate the site of orthographic processing the results suggest that subjects were adopting a phonological strategy to perform a lexical decision task, "sounding out" the words and pseudowords, and basing their decisions on the phonological characteristics of the stimulus rather than on lexical orthography.

F. Semantic Processing

Several studies have investigated semantic processing of visually presented words using semantic monitoring tasks that require subjects to monitor words for a semantic attribute (*e.g.*, is it a living thing?) or decide whether two or more simultaneously or sequentially presented words are semantically related. In nearly all cases, activation during the semantic tasks is contrasted to activation during decision tasks that require subjects to attend to orthographic or phonological characteristics. When the control is orthographic decision, subjects make decisions on a perceptual attribute of the word, for example the presence of a target letter [31] or the letter case of the stimuli [32,33]. In the Kapur *et al.* study [31] activity in the whole brain was assessed on a voxel by voxel basis and activation during semantic decisions was greater than during orthographic decisions in left inferior prefrontal cortex. The Demb *et al.* [32] and Gabrielli *et al.* [33] studies applied regions of interest to the prefrontal cortices only, that were again more strongly activated during a semantic decision than an orthographic decision task. However, no activation in the inferior prefrontal cortices has been detected when semantic decision is contrasted to phonological decision on nonwords (a decision on the sound structure of the stimuli). For instance, in a functional MRI study by Shaywitz *et al.* [34] with regions of interest in the temporal, frontal and extrastriate regions, activation during semantic decisions (deciding whether two visually presented words had similar meanings) was contrasted with activation during phonological decisions (deciding whether two visually presented words rhymed). Increased activation was detected in bilateral temporal cortices. Similarly, in a PET study that measured activation across the whole brain on a voxel by voxel basis [35], we have contrasted semantic decisions on visually presented words with phonological decisions on the same stimuli. The semantic task involved deciding whether visually presented words were living or nonliving items. The phonological task involved deciding whether the name of a visually presented word had two syllables or not. Both tasks involve implicit semantic processing and phonological retrieval. Nevertheless, the living/nonliving decision requires subjects to attend explicitly to semantic attributes of a word and the syllable judgement requires subjects to attend explicitly to phonological attributes of words.

Areas that were more active during semantic decisions than during phonological decisions were located in extrasylvian temporal regions with strongest activation in the left anterior temporal lobe, the left posterior temporal cortex at the junction with the angular gyrus, and the left caudate nucleus (Fig. 5). No activation changes in the left prefrontal regions were detected. The implication from this study and that of Shaywitz *et al.* [34] is that differences in prefrontal activation between the semantic and orthographic decision tasks reported by Kapur *et al.* [31], Demb *et al.* [32], and Gabrielli *et al.* [33] may relate to differences in phonological processing demands. This is consistent with psychological experiments which have shown that phonological activation influences semantic decision tasks [22,23]. For example, when subjects are instructed to respond only to exemplars of a given category, they incorrectly accept words or nonwords that sound like category exemplars (*e.g.*, ROWS as a flower; SUTE as an article of clothing). Second, in the lexical decision task reported above, increased activation relative to visual decisions and reading aloud is detected in brain regions associated with inner speech and subvocal articulation even though the task is not dependent on phonological codes [15]. Psychological and functional neuroimaging studies therefore support the hypothesis that phonology is involved in semantic decisions. When phonologi-

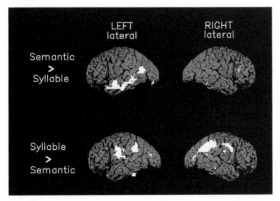

DESIGN:

	2 SYLLABLES	1 SYLLABLE	3 SYLLABLES
ANIMATE	carrot	horse	cucumber
INANIMATE	table	chair	photograph

RESULTS:

FIGURE 5 Areas of activation when semantic decision (is it animate?) is contrasted to phonological decision (does it have two syllables?).

cal processing is controlled, semantic decisions activate extrasylvian temporal regions [34,35]. The same temporal regions are engaged when semantic processing is enhanced during sentence comprehension tasks [36,37], word generation [38–40], and semantic decisions on auditory words when phonological processes are controlled [25,30].

G. Phonological Processing

There have been a few attempts to isolate phonological processes during reading using phonological tasks on visually presented words. The most commonly used task is deciding whether pairs of simultaneously presented words rhyme or whether sequentially presented words rhyme with a given target. Rhyming tasks have been contrasted with passive word viewing [41], spatial orientation decision on letters [42], and orthographic decision on consonant strings [34]. Irrespective of the baseline, activation associated with rhyming is detected in the left posterior temporal and left inferior prefrontal regions (although the left inferior prefrontal region was not assessed by Petersen *et al.* [41]). Despite the consistency of these results, the studies do not allow the determination of the precise functions of activated areas because differences between activation and control tasks involve short-term memory as well as phonological retrieval. The left inferior prefrontal signal may relate to a phonological rehearsal strategy used to hold two phonological codes in memory whilst they are matched for sound structure [28]. Nevertheless, the left inferior prefrontal cortex is classically associated with deficits in speech production which accords well with the results of rhyming studies.

   Phonological processing has many components. This chapter is primarily concerned with retrieving the names associated with letter strings, which may involve lexical or sublexical processes. When a syllable judgement (deciding whether a word had two syllables) was contrasted with a semantic judgement [35], syllable judgments enhanced activation relative to semantic judgements in bilateral supramarginal gyri, the left precentral sulcus, and the left cuneus (Fig. 5). These areas are strikingly similar to those reported by Demonet *et al.* [25,30] and Paulesu *et al.* [28], who associated supramarginal activation with the phonological store component of verbal short-term memory. In a syllable judgment task subjects are forced to attend to sublexical phonology in order to parse words into syllables. Possibly, sublexical activation is maintained in the phonological store whilst a decision is made.

H. Summary of Findings from Studies Based on Pure Cognitive Subtraction

Studies designed and analysed using pure cognitive subtraction have successfully identified multiple distributed areas involved in reading. The regions identified in the left hemisphere are consistent with findings from neuropsychological studies that have clearly established the importance of left posterior temporal and left inferior frontal regions for language processing [7,42]. In addition to reconfirming the left hemisphere areas involved in reading, functional imaging studies indicate that right hemisphere temporal and prefrontal regions are also activated [15,17]. The right hemispheric involvement is surprising given that dyslexia is frequently observed when left perisylvian regions are damaged but is seldom observed when right perisylvian regions are damaged. At this point we can conclude only that right hemisphere regions are activated but they do not always achieve normal word processing when the left hemisphere is damaged (although the left hemisphere can process words independently when the right hemisphere is damaged).

The functions of the activated regions have been only partially determined using cognitive subtraction experiments. Visual and visual association areas are activated when reading is contrasted to rest [17,18] but not in contrast to false font [15], indicating a role in visual processing. Activation of Heschl's gyri during reading aloud indicates that we process the sound of our own voice; and activation in motor, premotor, and cerebellar regions during reading silently is consistent with subvocal articulation and regulation of respiration even when no verbal response is required [15]. Despite this success, attempts to dissociate lexical, semantic, and phonological components of the reading system using cognitive subtraction methodology have, so far, produced largely inconsistent and unconvincing interpretations. The reason is that the studies have been based on assumptions and hypotheses that have not held true. For example, the expectation that there is more neuronal activity in functionally specialised areas when a task demands the explicit involvement of a pertinent function than when it does not is invalidated by greater activation of reading areas during presentation of pseudowords than during presentation of real words. Further, the difficulty of selecting control tasks that engage all but the process of interest is not limited to passive viewing tasks. In complex monitoring tasks (*e.g.*, semantic and phonological decisions) that aim to maximise activation of a particular process, task specific strategies are engaged that are difficult to equate in the control conditions. The clearest example of this is the activation in motor and premotor areas when subjects make lexical decisions in contrast to reading aloud; a result that illustrates that subjects are resorting to a phonological strategy to perform the task even though the decision could, theoretically, be made at the level of orthography.

III. COGNITIVE CONJUNCTIONS

Cognitive conjunctions are an extension to the cognitive subtraction paradigm. While cognitive subtraction looks for activation differences between a pair of tasks that share all but the component of interest, cognitive conjunctions look for a commonality of activation differences (*i.e.*, subtractions) between two pairs of tasks that share only the component of interest. Figure 6 illustrates this difference.

Figure 6a represents a cognitive subtraction hierarchy. Subtracting activity during task A from that during task B aims to reveal process 3, and subtracting activity during task B from that during task C aims to reveal process 4. Figure 6b represents a cognitive conjunction design. The process of interest (PX) is revealed by finding common areas of difference for each task pair. The advantage of cognitive conjunction design is that although it is initially dependent on subtraction, it is not dependent on selecting a baseline condition that is closely matched to the activation tasks. The activation and baseline could share no cognitive components (*e.g.*, when the control condition

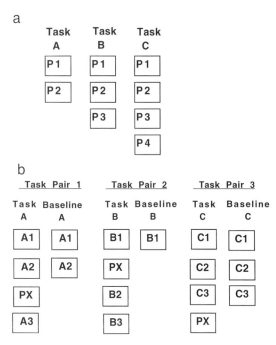

FIGURE 6 (a) An example of a design based on cognitive subtraction with three different tasks. Task 1 engages process 1 and process 2 (P1 and P2), task 2 engages a third process (P3) which is revealed by subtracting task 1 from task 2. Task 3 engages a fourth process (P4) which is revealed by subtracting task 2 from task 3. (b) An example of a design based on cognitive conjunction with three different task pairs. Each task pair has an activation task and a baseline task and the difference between activation and baseline tasks always entailes the process of interest (PX).

is rest); alternatively, the analysis can capitalize on one initial subtraction by incorporating controls that remove stimulus specific processes such as sensory input or output.

A. Isolating the Neural Correlates of Phonological Retrieval Using Cognitive Conjunctions: Multimodal Naming Experiments

We have used cognitive conjunctions to investigate the neural correlates of phonological retrieval during reading. The design of the experiments relies on finding tasks that activate phonological retrieval but do not activate other reading processes such as lexico-semantic processing. Examples of such tasks are letter naming, colour naming, and object naming (Fig. 7).

In isolation, letter, colour, or object naming will activate areas specific to letter, colour, and object processing, respectively, but in combination with reading a conjunction analysis isolates only regions that are activated by all conditions and these regions can be associated with common processing components. To limit common processing to phonological retrieval, activation during each naming task was measured relative to control conditions involving early visual analysis and articulation of one prespecified word. Strings of false font controlled for visual processing of words, single false font controlled for visual processing of letters, coloured nonsense patterns controlled for visual processing of colours, and the control for object naming was object viewing (see top sections of Figs. 8 and 9). Two experiments were conducted, one group of subjects read high frequency, monosyllabic, unrelated words (condition 1), named single letters (condition 2), and said a prespecified word in response to the visually matched controls for words (condition 3) or letters (condition 4). Similarly, a second group of subjects named objects (condition 1), named colours (condition 2), and said a prespecified word to the visually matched controls for objects (condition 3) and shapes (condition 4).

The conjunction analysis identifies areas of common activation across tasks and subjects using a series of orthogonal contrasts. Each contrast is based upon independent observations of task pairs and therefore the probability that any one brain region will be activated by chance in all contrasts is exceedingly small. The results of a conjunction analysis in our naming studies demonstrated that areas in common to reading, object naming, colour naming, and letter naming were the left frontal operculum (in the vicinity of Broca's area) with separate activations in the anterior insula and precentral sulcus, left posterior basal temporal lobe (BA 37), and medial cerebellum (see Fig. 10). These regions are associated with processing components common to all naming tasks, *i.e.*, the retrieval and execution of phonology. The results are consistent with those found in rhyming tasks (see section IG) and demonstrate that the left inferior prefrontal activations are also consistent with the neuropsychologi-

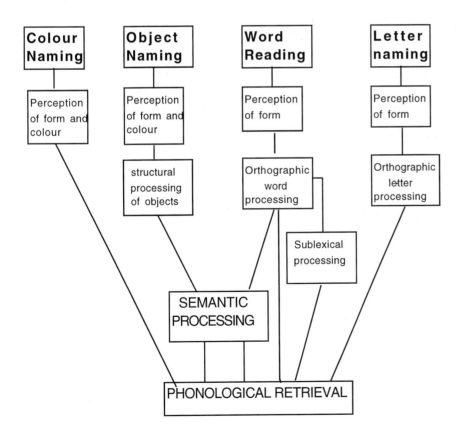

FIGURE 7   An information processing model for naming visual stimuli (colours, objects, words, and letters) showing the convergence on phonological retrieval.

DESIGN:

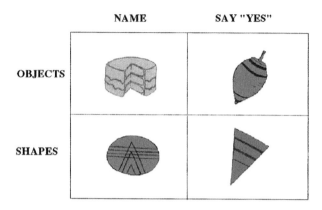

RESULTS:

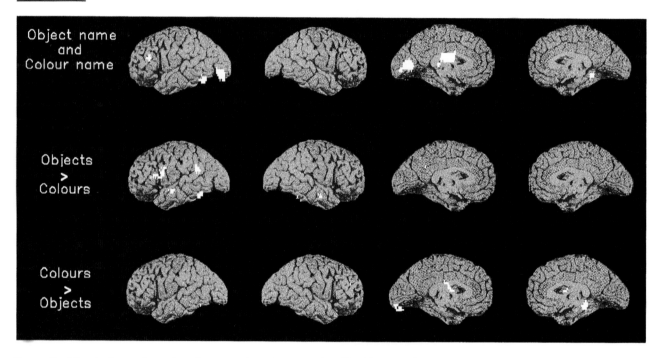

FIGURE 8 The design and results of an experiment contrasting (i) object naming to viewing the same objects and saying "Yes" and (ii) colour naming relative to viewing coloured shapes and saying "Yes." The results show (a) common areas of activation for object and colour naming; (b) areas that were more active for object naming (relative to viewing the same objects) than colour naming (relative to viewing the coloured shapes); and (c) areas that were more active for colour naming (relative to viewing and coloured shapes) than object naming (relative to viewing the same objects).

cal literature because damage to Broca's area and the left posterior temporal lobe result in modality independent naming deficits.

Cognitive subtraction and cognitive conjunction designs can be elaborated further to distinguish areas that are task specific by analysing the interaction term. This can be achieved if the experimental design is factorial.

<u>**DESIGN:**</u>

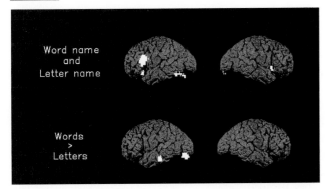

<u>**RESULTS:**</u>

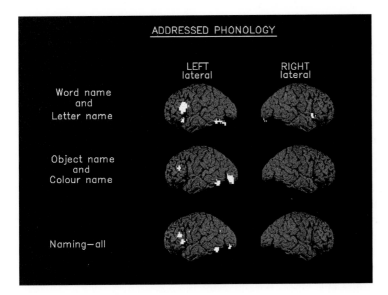

FIGURE 9   The design and results of an experiment contrasting (i) reading relative to viewing false font stimuli and saying "Yes" and (ii) letter naming relative to viewing false font stimuli and saying "Yes." The results show common areas of activation for reading and letter naming and areas that were more active for reading real words (relative to false font control) than naming letters (relative to false font control).

FIGURE 10   Areas of common activation for naming (i) words and letters (relative to controls—see Figure 9); (ii) objects and colours (relative to controls—see Figure 8); and (iii) words, letters, objects, and colours.

IV. FACTORIAL DESIGNS

In designs based purely on cognitive subtraction or cognitive conjunction, there may be only one variable (or factor) that has several different levels. For instance, the study reported by Petersen *et al.* [13] had one variable with five different levels relating to the type of stimuli viewed: visual fixation, false font, consonant letter strings, pseudowords, and real words. The cognitive subtraction analysis identifies differences in activation between different levels and associates these with the differences in psychological processes between levels. A cognitive conjunction analysis on the same design identifies commonalities in activation (relative to visual fixation) between levels and associates these to shared psychological processes (early visual processing in the Petersen *et al.* design). In factorial designs, there are two or more variables (or factors) and the different levels of each factor are matched. This is the case in the naming experiments reported above which had two factors (stimulus type and task) with two levels of stimulus type (objects and colours or words and letters) and two levels of task (naming and control).

Factorial designs have several important advantages over one factor subtraction designs. First, they allow greater generalisability of the results because the level effects can be specified for each factor (as in pure subtraction) or generalised for all factors. Second, and most important, when the effect of one factor level varies according to the level of another factor, experiments based on factorial designs allow us to verify the significance of this difference with the interaction term. For instance, in the naming experiments described above, the effect of naming (naming *vs* control) on brain activation varies with the stimulus type and the significance of differential activations can be revealed by the interaction between naming and stimulus type (see below). A third advantage of factorial designs is economy of subjects because, for the same degree of power, fewer subjects are required for one "two variable factorial design" than for two "one way designs" (since the effects of one variable across the levels of the other variable can be averaged in a factorial design).

A. Isolating the Neural Correlates of Semantic Processing Using Factorial Designs

In the naming experiments described above, cognitive conjunctions identified brain regions associated with phonological retrieval, a process common to object, word, colour, and letter naming. Interactions between stimulus type and task should reveal activations specific to different naming routes. For instance, the interaction between object naming (*vs* object control) and colour naming (*vs* colour control) revealed that the left anterior basal temporal lobe and left angular gyrus were more active for object naming (see Fig. 8). These areas correspond to those found in the experiment described in Section IF which contrasted semantic decisions on visually presented words with syllable decisions on the same words (see Fig. 5). The interaction between object naming and colour naming therefore indicates a clear role for the anterior and posterior temporal regions in semantic processing. Interestingly, the interaction between reading words and letter naming did not show activation differences in the anterior and posterior temporal regions, only in the left medial extrastriate cortex and a small part of the mid-inferior temporal gyrus (BA 20) (Fig. 9). Reduced activation in extrasylvian temporal regions during reading relative to semantic decisions or object naming indicates that semantic processing was not strongly activated when subjects were reading monosyllabic, high frequency, unrelated words.

B. Are There Common Semantic and Phonological Processing Systems for Words and Pictures?

A recent study of ours [44] contrasted semantic processing of words and pictures using a factorial design and cognitive conjunctions. There were two factors in the design—modality and task, with two levels of modality (words or pictures) and two levels of task (semantic decision and actual size decision) (Fig. 11).

Conjunctions revealed (i) increased activation for words relative to pictures irrespective of task (visual and semantic) in the left supramarginal gyrus (Fig. 11a), (ii) increased activation for pictures relative to words irrespective of task in the right inferior occipital gyrus (Fig. 11b), and (iii) increased activation for the semantic task relative to the visual task irrespective of modality (words and pictures) in posterior and anterior regions of the ventral surface of the left middle and inferior temporal cortex, the left inferior frontal gyrus, the junction between the left superior occipital gyrus (BA 19) and left angular gyrus (BA 39), and the right cerebellum (Fig. 11c). Interaction between stimulus modality (words *vs* pictures) and task (semantic *vs* visual) revealed that (i) the left inferior occipital gyrus was specifically involved in semantic decisions on pictures (Fig. 11d), whereas (ii) a region in the left anterior temporal cortex was specifically involved in semantic decisions on words. There was also increased activation in the inferior frontal cortex for semantic judgements on words relative to pictures (Fig. 11e).

As discussed above (Section I), psychological and neuroimaging data demonstrate that phonological processing is enhanced during semantic decisions on words. The commonality between the areas activated for words and pictures, particularly those in the left posterior inferior temporal cortex (BA 37) and the left inferior frontal gyrus (BA 45), suggest that phonological processes were also activated during semantic decisions on pictures. Overall our results indicate that words and pictures share many common semantic and phonological processing regions [44]. In relation to the findings from the multimodal naming experiment described above (Fig. 8) and the contrast between semantic and phonological processing (Fig. 5), the left anterior temporal cortex, the left mid-inferior temporal cortex, and the left angular gyrus relate to semantic processing whilst the ventral surface of the left posterior temporal and the left inferior frontal gyrus relate to processes shared with phonological decision. To clarify these conclusions, sections from Figs. 5, 8, and 11 are redisplayed together in Fig. 12.

C. Sublexical Processing

The results of the experiment reported by Vandenberghe *et al.* [44] demonstrate that irrespective of task, activation in the left supramarginal gyrus is greater for word processing than for picture processing. Studies by Bookheimer *et al.* [18] and Mennard *et al.* [45] also show increased left supramarginal activation for words relative to pictures. As illustrated in Figs. 1 and 7, cognitive components specific for word processing include orthographic processing and sublexical phonology. An association of the left supramarginal gyrus with

DESIGN:

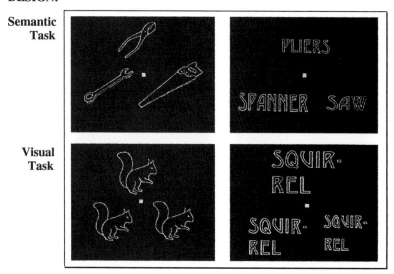

RESULTS:

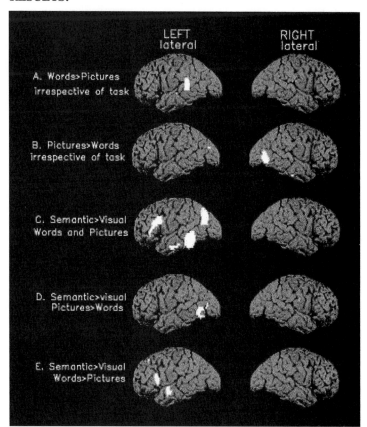

FIGURE 11 A factorial design with two factors: task (semantic decision or visual decision) and modality (pictures or words). The results show (A) areas that were more active for words than pictures (visual decision on words relative to visual decision on pictures and also semantic decision on words relative to semantic decision on pictures); (B) areas that were more active for pictures than words (visual decision on pictures relative to visual decision on words and also semantic decision on pictures relative to

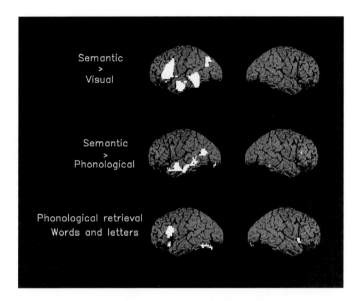

FIGURE 12 Areas activated for semantic decision relative to visual decision (top); semantic decision relative to phonological decision (middle row); and phonological retrieval relative to saying "Yes" to the same stimuli (bottom).

sublexical processing fits with (i) neuropsychological studies showing that damage to this region results in a deficit spelling from sound [10] and (ii) neuroimaging data showing that the left supramarginal gyrus is more strongly activated when reading pseudowords (which depend on sublexical phonology) than when reading real words (see Section I). Similarly, supramarginal activations are stronger during syllable judgements (which depend on sublexical segmentation of words) than during semantic judgements which do not rely on sublexical information. A role for the left supramarginal gyrus in sublexical phonology is also consistent with the association of this region with a short-term phonological store [28,46] that may be required to hold sublexical segments of words whilst assimilation of the segments takes place.

If these conclusions are correct, then the presence or absence of supramarginal activation should indicate whether sublexical phonology is involved in different tasks or indeed different subjects. In most reading studies, there is parietal activation which extends across the supramarginal gyrus [15–18,45]. However, we did not see supramarginal activation in a study in which reading high frequency, monosyllabic, unrelated words was contrasted to letter naming (see Section III.A and Fig. 10). In this paradigm, short, monosyllabic, familiar words were chosen in order to match articulation requirements as closely as possible between letter naming and word naming conditions. The result is consistent with the notion that short familiar words address phonology directly

semantic decision on words); (C) areas that were more active for semantic decision than visual decision for both words and pictures; (D) areas where activation was greater for semantic decision on pictures (relative to visual decision on pictures) than semantic decision on words (relative to visual decision on words); (E) areas where activation was greater for semantic decision on words (relative to visual decision on words) than semantic decision on pictures (relative to visual decision on pictures).

via the left posterior basal temporal lobe and suggests that sublexical phonology and supramarginal activation may be more relevant to reading longer, less familiar words. The next study investigates this prediction.

D. The Effect of Altering Word Length and Frequency on Activation Due to Reading

In a factorial design, the effect of word length on reading aloud was manipulated with word frequency. There were three levels of word length (three-letter one-syllable words, five-letter two-syllable words, and seven-letter three-syllable words)—and two levels of frequency; high frequency (familiar) words and low frequency (less familiar) words. In addition to the word conditions, false font strings matched to the words for number of characters were included into the design in order to identify the reading areas. The design of the experiment and the results can be seen in Fig. 13.

The results show (i) that when all the words are contrasted to strings of false fonts there is activation of the left supramarginal gyrus (not seen when short monosyllabic words were contrasted with false font; sections IIA and IIIA), and (ii) that for low frequency words, activation in the left supramarginal gyrus, the left inferior frontal gyrus, and the left inferior temporal gyrus (BA 20) increases as word length increases. Thus, as predicted, supramarginal activation and the involvement of sublexical processing is greatest for long, less familiar words. However, there was also increased activation in the inferior temporal (BA 20) and inferior frontal cortices for long, low frequency words. These areas have been associated respectively with semantics and "addressed phonology" (see Sections IIA and III), suggesting that long words put greater demands on both lexical and sublexical processing.

E. The Left Medial Extrastriate Cortex and Orthographic Processing

Activation of the left medial extrastriate cortex during word processing was first reported by Petersen et al. [12]. The association is consistent with neurological studies that link damage to the medial extrastriate cortex with pure alexia. However, damage to the medial extrastriate also impairs performance in naming colours, letters, and objects [47]. If there is a portion of the medial extrastriate cortex that is specific to word forms, we would expect to see differences in activation here for words relative to picture processing. Such differences have not been detected [18,44,45]. Furthermore, although reading activates the left medial extrastriate more than letter naming; colour naming activates a similar region more strongly than object naming (see Fig. 9). These results fit with the theories of De Renzi et al. [47] and Oxbury et al. [48], who suggest that category specific visual naming deficits following occipital infarcts relate to the severity of damage with reading and colour naming performance being most sensitive to damage and object naming least sensitive.

If the medial extrastriate cortex is related to modality independent visual analysis that is not specific to words, why is there no readily apparent region that we can associate with orthographic letter processing? There are several possible explanations. One option is that different regions of the extrastriate cortex are specialised for processing different types of visual

DESIGN:

	3 LETTERS	5 LETTERS	7 LETTERS
HIGH FREQUENCY	car	music	hospital
LOW FREQUENCY	jaw	baton	mercury
FALSE FONT	ꓘ𝘕𝘷𝘈	∠𝘕\𝘈ˠ	ꕯΛ𝘜↓𝘯\𝘕ˠ

RESULTS:

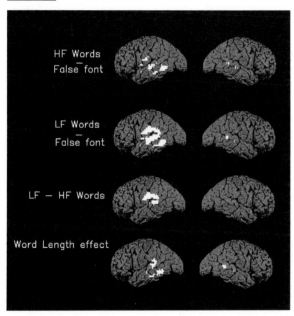

FIGURE 13 The design and results of an experiment investigating the effect of word length (3-, 5-, or 7-letter words) on activation in response to reading high- and low-frequency words relative to visually matched false font. The results show areas that were activated for (i) high-frequency (HF) words relative to false font; (ii) low-frequency words (LF) relative to false font; (iii) low-frequency words relative to high-frequency words; and (iv) the effect of increasing word length from 3-letter words to 7-letter words.

stimuli but the spatial resolution of the PET studies reported have prevented dissociation of the regions. Another option is that the anatomical substrates of orthographic word processing overlap with other features of word processing. For instance, orthographic word descriptions may not be distinct from semantic processing areas which would explain why orthographic and semantic processing do not generally dissociate following brain damage. Future neuroimaging studies with high spatial resolution should help to differentiate these options.

F. Summary of Findings from Cognitive Conjunctions and Factorial Designs

By focusing on similarity of activation rather than differences in activation, the experiments based on cognitive conjunction designs have led to the following conclusions. Phonological processes common for naming words, objects, colours, and letters (addressed phonology) engage the left posterior inferior temporal lobe (BA 37) and left Broca's area. Semantic processes common to semantic decision tasks on words and objects engage a distributed network of areas in posterior and anterior regions of the ventral surface of the left middle and inferior temporal cortices, the left inferior frontal gyrus, the junction between the left superior occipital gyrus (BA 19) and left angular gyrus (BA 39) and the right cerebellum.

Modality specific effects can be distinguished from modality independent effects with factorial designs which have shown that a region of the left anterior temporal cortex is involved in semantic decisions on words but not objects and the mid portion of the left inferior temporal gyrus and the left medial extrastriate cortex are specifically involved in naming words but not letters. Finally, a factorial study with word length and frequency as variables has demonstrated that activation of the supramarginal gyrus increases with long and unfamiliar words. To clarify the role of the supramarginal gyrus in sublexical processing, Fig. 14 illustrates (i) word specific processing from the Vandenberghe *et al.* [44] study (Section III), (ii) increased activation for pseudowords relative to words (Section I), and (iii) increased activation with increasing word length of low frequency words (Section III).

In the word length study, false font stimuli were included in the design to reveal areas involved in processing words irrespective of baseline. Without false font stimuli the design could be construed as parametric in addition to

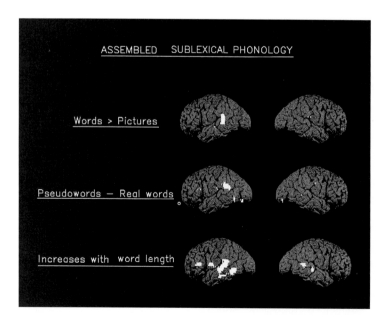

FIGURE 14 Areas where activation is enhanced for tasks that maximize sublexical processing: (i) reading words relative to naming pictures; (ii) reading pseudowords relative to real words; and (iii) increasing word length on low-frequency words.

factorial. The advantages of parametric studies to the investigation of reading are the subject of the next section.

V. PARAMETRIC DESIGNS

In all the experiments reported so far brain activation has been measured by contrasting activity in the activation state with control tasks. Another approach is to measure activation changes as a presentation or stimulus parameter is varied, for example, variations in rate of presentation of the stimuli, duration of the stimuli, word length, word frequency, or word imageability. The advantage of this approach is that no baseline control task need be selected and only changes in the parameter of interest are measured. An illustration of how this approach can inform us of functional segregation is the finding that when subjects listen to words at varying rates of presentation the response in the left posterior temporal and left inferior frontal regions differs from that in bilateral anterior regions of the temporal lobes. Activation in both anterior regions of the temporal lobes is directly correlated with stimulus rate but this effect is not seen in the left posterior temporal and left inferior frontal regions [26,49].

A. The Effect of Altering Rate of Word Presentation on Activation Due to Reading

The effect of altering stimulus rate from 20 words per minute (wpm) to 60 wpm on brain activation during reading aloud has recently been investigated [17]. As stimulus rate increased activation of regions associated with visual analysis (bilateral posterior fusiform gyri) and response generation (cerebellum, SMA, and bilateral precentral gyri) increased. There was also a positive correlation with rate in the primary auditory cortices—around Heschl's gyri—which is attributed to subjects processing the sound of their own voices and consistent with the response obtained when subjects listen to another's voice [49]. Finally, there was a positive correlation between activity and rate in the left middle frontal cortex. These effects in visual, motor, and auditory areas are consistent with stimulus rate influencing regions involved in stimulus analysis or response generation. The effect in the left middle frontal cortex may also be associated with response generation given that this area is involved in retrieving phonology (see Section II.A).

A negative correlation of activation and rate was detected in bilateral posterior temporal and inferior parietal regions and no effects of stimulus rate were found in the lingual gyrus, the frontal opercula, or the right middle temporal or right middle frontal gyri. The contrasting response in these areas to those associated with stimulus analysis and response generation demonstrates functional segregation of the different regions. Of particular interest is the response of the lingual gyrus, independent of rate, that indicates the function in this area for reading is upstream to that of the surrounding posterior fusiform gyrus (see also Section III).

B. The Effect of Altering Stimulus Duration on Activation Due to Reading

We have now completed a number of studies investigating the effect of exposure duration on brain activation due to reading. The first indication that duration might be an important variable came from a comparison of data from Petersen *et al.* [12,13]—who presented words for 150 msec—and Howard *et al.* [14]—who presented words for 1000 msec. To assess the effect of these different durations on brain activation we contrasted words presented for 150 msec with the same words presented for 1000 msec during lexical decision, reading aloud, reading silently, and silent articulation [15,17]. For each task, there were highly significant differences in activation associated with reading at the different durations. As expected, activation in areas associated with early visual analysis was greatest with longer word durations (1000 msec) than shorter durations (150 msec) but contrary to expectation there was decreased activation in temporal and frontal word processing areas with longer word durations [17]. A possible explanation for this deactivation in word recognition areas is that sustained inhibition of word processing occurs if a word remains in the visual field after processing is complete [15]. The combined effect over the 90-sec scanning time is that decreases will counteract increases, thereby reducing the detected activation.

In two follow-up studies we have investigated the effect of stimulus duration in more detail. The first of these studies investigated how activation in word processing areas varied with durations of 150, 300, 450, 600, and 750 msec. The second study investigated how activation in word processing areas varied with durations of 150, 750, 1000, and 1250 msec. As with the previous studies, there were strong and highly significant increases of activation in visual areas as duration of word presentation increased. In temporal and parietal regions, however, small changes of duration, between 150 and 750 msec, revealed some interesting effects that inform us of the time course of activation in the different regions. For example, in ventral temporal regions (inferior and middle temporal cortex) activation fell steeply from a maximum at 150 msec whilst in posterior temporal and inferior parietal regions activation remained at a maximum level for the first 500 msec or more before falling. This effect was confirmed in the study contrasting 150-, 750-, 1000-, and 1250-msec presentations. Between, 150 and 750 msec the greatest deactivation was detected in the middle temporal cortex, whilst between 750 and 1000 msec the strongest deactivations were detected bilaterally in the inferior parietal lobes. These results suggest that activation in the dorsal temporal and parietal regions has a more prolonged time course that outlives activation in ventral temporal regions.

C. Summary of Parametric Designs: The Effect of Rate and Duration on Brain Activation during Reading

Several new findings have emerged from parametric studies. First, the contrasting responses of different brain regions to varying presentation conditions illustrate their physiological and functional segregation. For instance, whilst the posterior fusiform gyri are strongly affected by stimulus load, activation of the lingual gyrus is independent of either stimulus rate or duration. This finding indicates that the role of the medial extrastriate cortex is indeed upstream to that in the surrounding fusiform gyri. Second, the linear activation response in the primary auditory cortices with increased stimulus rate when subjects read aloud illustrates that in these regions we process our own voice in a qualitatively similar way to other heard voices. Third, the different time course of decreased activation in ventral and dorsal temporal regions demonstrates that dorsal temporal activation outlives ventral temporal activation.

Finally, the deactivation in word processing areas with increased presentation duration and the differential effects in different regions with different tasks [15] is consistent with an hypothesis that as a word remains in the visual field, activation in response to words is counteracted by subsequent deactivation of word processing areas.

VI. SUMMARY OF FINDINGS WITH NORMAL SUBJECTS

The current status of functional neuroimaging studies of reading support the following formulation.

A. Visual/Orthographic Processing

Presentation of visual stimuli (such as words, letter strings, false fonts, and objects) activate striate and extrastriate visual cortex in the posterior occipital lobe. The response in the posterior fusiform gyri is directly related to stimulus input, suggesting a role in sensory processing, while the responses in the medial occipital gyri is independent of stimulus presentation. A specialised role for the medial extrastriate cortex is supported by the enhancement of activation in this area when subjects must distinguish between stimuli (*e.g.*, when naming). However, at present, activation in the medial extrastriate cortex does not appear to be specific to word processing because the area is also activated by objects and meaningless shapes. Further studies with higher spatial resolution are needed to determine whether the region is subdivided into category specific processing areas, including an area specialised for orthographic processing.

B. Retrieval and Execution of Phonology

When subjects retrieve phonology to read words or name letters, pictures, or colours, the left posterior inferior temporal cortex (BA 37) and the left inferior frontal cortex (BA 45) are activated, suggesting a role for these areas in retrieving and executing phonology that is modality independent. Modality specific processes for reading words involve sublexical processing and a modality specific area for seen words in the left supramarginal gyrus [44]. Studies have also shown that this area is particularly active when subjects read pseudowords (that relies on sublexical processing) and long unfamiliar real words (that put greater demands on both lexical and sublexical processing). Furthermore, neuropsychological data have shown that damage to the supramarginal gyrus impairs spelling from sound [10].

C. Word Recognition/Semantic Processing

The more anterior regions of the ventral extrasylvian temporal cortex and the posterior inferior parietal cortex in the vicinity of the angular gyrus are particularly engaged when subjects retrieve the meaning of words during sentence processing and semantic decision tasks. These findings are consistent with those from neuropsychological studies that associate the left ventral temporal cortex with semantic processing [11] and the angular gyrus with knowledge of words for reading and spelling [8]. For instance, following damage to the angular gyrus, spelling is dependent on sublexical sounds [10].

D. Articulation

Finally, articulation enhances activation in both sensorimotor cortices, the left thalamus, and the cerebellum. There is also activation of bilateral superior temporal gyri when subjects articulate aloud which has been related to subjects processing the sound of their own voice [17].

VII. CONCLUSION

We have now reached a stage where the neural correlates of reading revealed by neuroimaging studies are mainly consistent with established neuropsychological findings. With an established basis of normal function, neuroimaging studies can progress to unravel (i) how the different areas respond to different types of words and word combinations, (ii) the relationship between left and right hemisphere processing, (iii) the variability between and within subjects, and (iv) the compensatory behaviour of patients suffering from brain damage.

References

1. J. C. Marshall and F. Newcombe. Patterns of paralexia: A psycholinguistic approach. *J. Psycholinguistic Res.* **2**, 175–199 (1972).
2. J. L. McClelland and D. E. Rumelhart. An interactive activation model of context effects in letter perception. 1. An account of basic findings. *Psychol. Rev.* **88**, 375–407 (1981).
3. K. E. Patterson and C. Shewell. Speak and spell: Dissociations and word class effects. *In* "The Cognitive Neuropsychology of Language" (M. Coltheart, G. Sartori, and R. Job, Eds.). Erlbaum, London, 1987.
4. T. Shallice. "From Neuropsychology to Mental Structure." Cambridge Univ. Press, New York, 1988.
5. J. Morton and K. E. Patterson. A new attempt at an interpretation, or, an attempt at a new interpretation. *In* "Deep Dyslexia" (M. Coltheart, K. E. Patterson, and J. C. Marshall, Eds.). Routledge, London, 1980.
6. A. W. Ellis and A. W. Young. "Human Cognitive Neuropsychology." Erlbaum, London, 1988.
7. S. E. Blumstein. The neurobiology of the sound structure of language. *In* "The Cognitive Neurosciences" (M. S. Gazzanigia, Ed.), pp. 915–929. MIT Press, Cambridge, MA.
8. J. Dejerine. Sur un cas de cécite verbale avec agraphie, suivi d'autopsie. *Mém. Soc. Biol.* **3**, 197–201 (1891).
9. H. Hecaen and H. Kremlin. Neurolinguistic research on reading disorders resulting from left hemisphere lesions: Aphasic and "pure" alexia. *In* (H. Whitaker and H. A. Whitaker, Eds.), Vol. 2, pp. 269–329. New York Academy Press, 1976.
10. D. P. Roeltgen and K. M. Heilman. Lexical agraphia. Further support for the two strategy hypothesis of linguistic aphasia. *Brain* **107**, 811–827 (1984).
11. J. R. Hodges, K. Patterson, S. Pxbury, and E. Funnell. Semantic dementia: Progressive fleunt aphasia with temporal lobe atrophy. *Brain* **115**, 1783–1806 (1992).
12. S. E. Petersen, P. T. Fox, M. I. Posner, M. Mintun, and M. E. Raichle. Positron emission tomographic studies of the cortical anatomy of single word processing. *Nature* **331**, 585–589.
13. S. E. Petersen, P. T. Fox, A. Z. Synder, and M. E. Raichle. Activation of extrastriate and frontal cortical areas by words and word-like stimuli. *Science* **249**, 1041–1044 (1990).

14. D. Howard, K. Patterson, R. Wise, W. D. Brown, K. Friston, C. Weiller, and R. S. J. Frackowiak. The cortical localisation of the lexicons: positron emission tomography evidence. *Brain* **115,** 1769–1782 (1992).

15. C. Price, R. Wise, J. Watson, K. Patterson, D. Howard, and R. Frackowiak. Brain activity during reading: The effects of task and exposure duration. *Brain* **117,** 1255–1269 (1994).

16. C. J. Price, R. J. S. Wise, and R. S. J. Frackowiak. Demonstrating the implicit processing of visually presented words and pseudowords. *Cereb. Cortex* **6,** 62–70 (1996).

17. C. J. Price, C. J. Moore, and R. S. J. Frackowiak. The effect of varying stimulus rate and duration on brain activity during reading. *Neuroimage* **3,** 40–52 (1996).

18. S. Y. Bookheimer, T. A. Zeffiro, T. Blaxton, W. Gaillard, and W. Theodore. Regional cerebral blood flow during object naming and word reading. *Hum. Brain Mapping* **3,** 93–106 (1995).

19. S. J. Lupker. Relatedness effects in word and picture naming: Parallels, differences and structural implications. *In* "Progress in the Psychology of Language" (A. W. Ellis, Ed.), Vol. 1, pp. 109–142. Lawrence Erlbaum, London, (1985).

20. C. M. Macleod. Half a century of research on the Stroop effect: An integrative review. *Psychol. Bull.* **109,** 163–203 (1991).

21. J. H. Neely. Semantic priming effects in visual word recognition: A selective review of current findings and theories. *In* "Basic Processes in Reading: Visual Word Recognition" (D. Besner and G. W. Humphreys, Eds.) Lawrence Erlbaum, Hillsdale, NJ. (1991).

22. G. C. Van Orden, J. C. Johnston, and B. L. Hale. Word identification in reading proceeds from spelling to sound to meaning. *J. Exp. Psychol. Learning Mem. Cog.* **14,** 371–386 (1988).

23. V. Coltheart, K. Patterson, and J. Leahy. When a ROWS is a ROSE: Phonological effects in written word comprehension. *Q. J. Exp. Psychol.* **47A,** 917–955 (1994).

24. R. Wise, F. Chollet, U. Hadar, K. Friston, E. Hoffner, and R. Frackowiak. Distribution of cortical neural networks involved in word comprehension and word retrieval. *Brain* **114,** 1803–1817 (1991).

25. J-F. Démonet, F. Chollet, S. Ramsay, D. Cardebat, J-D. Nespoulous, R. Wise, A. Rascol, and R. S. J. Frackowiak. The anatomy of phonological and semantic processing in normal subjects. *Brain* **115,** 1753–1768 (1992).

26. C. J. Price, R. J. S. Wise, E. A. Warburton, C. J. Moore, D. Howard, K. Patterson, R. S. J. Frackowiak, and K. J. Friston. Hearing and saying: The functional neuroanatomy of auditory word processing. *Brain* **119,** 919–931 (1996).

27. M. Corbetta, F. M. Miezin, S. Dobmeyer, G. L. Shulman, and S. E. Peterson. Selective and divided attention during visual discrimination of shape, colour. And speed: Functional anatomy by positron emission tomography. *J. Neurosci.* **11,** 2383–2402 (1991).

28. E. Paulesu, C. D. Frith, and R. S. J. Frackowiak. The neural correlates of the verbal component of working memory. *Nature* **362,** 342–344 (1993).

29. C. D. Frith, K. J. Friston, P. F. Liddle, and R. S. J. Frackowiak. A PET study of word finding. *Neuropsychologia* **29,** 1137–1148 (1991).

30. J-F. Démonet, C. Price, R. Wise, and R. S. J. Frackowiak. A PET study of cognitive strategies in normal subjects during language tasks: Influence of phonetic ambiguity and sequence processing on phoneme monitoring. *Brain* **117,** 671–682 (1994).

31. S. Kapur, R. Rose, P. F. Liddle, R. B. Zipursky, G. M. Brown, D. Stuss, S. Houle, and E. Tulving. The role of the left prefrontal cortex in verbal processing: Semantic processing or willed action? *NeuroReport* **5,** 2193–2196 (1994).

32. J. B. Demb, J. E. Desmond, A. D. Wagner, C. J. Vaidya, G. H. Glover, and J. D. E. Gabrieli. Semantic encoding and retrieval in the left inferior prefrontal cortex: A functional MRI study of task difficulty and process specificity. *J. Neurosci.* **15,** 5870–5878 (1995).

33. J. D. E. Gabrielli, J. E. Desmond, J. B. Demb, A. D. Wagner, M. V. Stone, C. J. Vaidya, and G. H. Glover. Functional magnetic resonance imaging of semantic memory processes in frontal lobes. *Psychol. Sci.* **7,** 278–283 (1996).

34. B. A. Shaywitz, S. E. Shaywitz, K. R. Pugh, R. T. Constable, P. Skudlarski, R. K. Fulbright, R. A. Bronen, J. M. Fletcher, P. Skudlarski, L. Katz, and J. C. Gore. Sex differences in the functional organisation of the brain for language. *Nature* **373,** 607–609 (1995).

35. C. J. Price, C. J. Moore, G. W. Humphreys, and R. J. S. Wise. Segregating semantic from phonological processes during reading. Submitted for publication.

36. G. Bottini, R. Corcoran, R. Sterzi, E. Paulesu, P. Schenone, P. Scarpa, R. S. J. Frackowiak, and C. D. Frith. The role of the right hemisphere in the interpretation of figurative aspects of languge. *Brain* **117,** 1241–1253 (1994).

37. P. C. Fletcher, C. D. Frith, P. M. Grasby, T. Shallice, R. S. J. Frackowiak, and R. J. Dolan. Brain systems for encoding and retrieval of auditory-verbal memory. *Brain* **118,** 401–416 (1995).

38. M. E. Raichle, J. A. Fiez, T. O. Videen, A. K. Macleod, J. V. Pardo, P. T. Fox, and S. E. Peterson. Practice-related changes in human brain fuctional anatomy during non-motor learning. *Cereb Cortex* **4,** 8–26 (1994).

39. B. A. Shaywitz, K. R. Pugh, R. T. Constable, S. E. Shaywitz, R. A. Bronen, R. K. Fulbright, D. P. Shankweiler, L. Katz, J. M. Fletcher, P. Skudlarski, and J. C. Gore. Localization of semantic processing using functional magnetic resonance imaging. *Hum. Brain Mapping* **2,** 149–158 (1995).

40. E. Warburton, R. J. S. Wise, C. J. Price, C. Weiller, U. Hadar, S. Ramsay, and R. S. J. Frackowiak. Noun and verb retrieval by normal subjects: studies with positron emission tomography. *Brain* **119,** 159–179 (1996).

41. S. E. Petersen, P. T. Fox, M. I. Posner, M. Mintun, and M. Raichle. Positron emission tomographic studies of the processing of single words. *J. Cog. Neurosci.* **1,** 153–170 (1989).

42. J. Sergent, E. Zuck, M. Lévesque, and B. MacDonald. Positron emission tomography study of letter and object processing: Empirical findings and methodological considerations. *Cereb. Cortex* **2,** 68–80 (1992).

43. R. A. McCarthy and E. K. Warrington. "Cognitive Neuropsychology: A Clinical Introduction." Academic Press, San Diego, 1989.

44. R. Vandenberghe, C. Price, R. Wise, O. Josephs, and R. S. J. Frackowiak. Functional anatomy of a common semantic system for words or pictures. *Nature* **383,** 254–256 (1996).

45. M. T. Menard, S. M. Kosslyn, W. L. Thompson, N. M. Alpert, and S. L. Rauch. Encoding words and pictures: A positron emission tomography study. *Neuropsychologia* **34,** 185–194 (1996).

46. E. Paulesu, U. Frith, M. Snowling, A. Gallagher, J. Morton, R. S. J. Frackowiak, and C. D. Frith. Is developmental dyslexia a disconnection syndrome? Evidence from PET scanning. *Brain* **119,** 143–157 (1996).

47. E. De Renzi, A. Zambolin, and G. Crisi. The pattern of neuropsychological impairment associated with left posterior cerebral artery territory infarcts. *Brain* **110,** 1099–116 (1987).

48. J. M. Oxbury, S. M. Oxbury, and N. K. Humphrey. Varieties of colour anomia. *Brain* **92,** 847–860 (1969).

49. C. Price, R. Wise, S. Ramsay, K. Friston, D. Howard, K. Patterson, and R. Frackowiak. Regional response differences within the human auditory cortex when listening to words. *Neurosci. Lett.* **146,** 179–182 (1992).

CHAPTER FOURTEEN

HIGHER COGNITIVE PROCESSES

I. INTRODUCTION

Attention, imagery, will, and emotion are all examples of higher cognitive processes. We know about these processes largely through introspection. It is only through introspection that we know what it is like to attend to something, to want something, or to be happy. In the major psychiatric disorders, such as depression and schizophrenia, there is something amiss with these higher order functions. The range of experiences that patients with these conditions manifest include an inability to attend, a loss of will, a dramatic change of mood, or intrusive images and hallucinations. Again we know about these abnormal experiences only because that is what patients with these conditions tell us. This intimate relationship between higher cognitive processes and consciousness raises special problems for the study of brain function that underlie these processes.

Our knowledge of how most cognitive processes relate to brain function has been, to a considerable extent, dependent upon studies in animals other than man. Studies of higher cognitive processes in animals are always limited precisely because animals cannot report their experiences. Consequently, there can never be a satisfactory animal model of psychotic phenomena such as hallucinations or the experience of alien control. For these reasons functional brain imaging is enormously important in the study of higher cognitive function. In many cases studies based upon these methodologies have provided the first glimpse of the brain processes that underlie these unique and largely subjective human experiences. In this chapter we shall not simply write a section on each of a series of topics, but attempt to place "higher cognitive processes" in the broader context of conscious experience. It is therefore inevitable that we shall touch on (but not solve) the problem of how a mental entity, consciousness, can emerge from a physical entity, the brain.

II. COGNITION

A. What Is Cognition?

There are many different definitions, but a consensus would associate cognition with knowledge or, in one modern terminology, information processing. How and where is information represented in the brain? How does this information, coded as neural firing patterns, control behaviour? These are the sorts of questions that cognitive neuroscience seeks to answer and many of the previous chapters in this book address exactly these problems.

What is higher order cognition? It is obvious that there are different levels of difficulty/complexity associated with cognitive processes, but this distinction is very hard to define. Much of the literature in cognitive psychology is devoted to finding a rationale for making the distinction. Low order cognitive processes are characterised as automatic or routine, while higher order processes always contain a novel element and are characterised as requiring controlled, strategic, or executive processes [1]. A parallel account of this distinction is that of modular and nonmodular systems [2]. These accounts distinguish low order processes that are obligatory and automatic from high order processes that are conscious and under voluntary control. It is clear that the distinction cannot be made solely in terms of the complexity of the computations required. Understanding speech and reading are both difficult problems in computational terms, but both tasks can be carried out routinely and with little effort. Speech recognition is thus an example of a complex skill for which appropriate specialised mechanisms have evolved within the brain [3]. Reading, in contrast, is a skill that develops within the span of a few years in most individuals. This fact serves to emphasise that almost any difficult task can become an easy one (in the sense of automatic) with sufficient practice (see Chapter 11), even though the inherent complexity of the task remains the same. Perhaps the best distinction between high level and low level cognition is in terms of the subjective degree of "mental effort" required for any particular task.

B. The Relevance of Consciousness

Another important distinction is that, for tasks requiring higher level cognition, we have to think about what we are doing, whereas for routine low level tasks we need not think about what we are doing. In other words, high level cognition is associated with phenomenological consciousness; we do not simply carry out the task, we have a sense of our own agency in executing the task, we are aware of the associated sensations and the specific choices we are making. While phenomenal consciousness seems always to be associated with high level cognitive processes, no one has yet produced a satisfactory account of whether phenomenological consciousness is a necessary component of such processes [4].

In addition to direct perception of the world about us, there are two major components of phenomenological consciousness; will and mood. In our phenomenological consciousness we have the impression that we choose between various possible future or ongoing actions: Shall I press the right button or the left button? Shall I carry on with this incredibly boring task or shall I make an excuse and leave? Indeed it may well be the need to choose between a number of different options with incomplete knowledge about outcome that makes such tasks seem effortful.

The other major component of our phenomenological consciousness concerns mood and affect. This "colouring" of our experience seems to have a major role in the selection of action. We are constantly having to balance short-term pain against long-term pleasure (or *vice versa*). When we are depressed it seems that nothing is worth doing. When it is a beautiful day or when we are in love all actions seem effortless. No account of consciousness that ignores these components of phenomenological experience can be entirely satisfactory [5]. In this chapter we shall discuss brain imaging studies that address these various aspects of consciousness.

III. HOLDING THINGS IN MIND

A. Active Memory

A key feature of consciousness is our ability to represent things in our minds even in the absence of direct perception of such things. This holding in mind can be maintained over time periods of seconds or even minutes if necessary. Following Fuster, we call this active memory because of the perceptible amount of mental effort that is required to keep things continuously in mind [6]. If we permit a lapse of concentration then the likelihood of subsequently retrieving this relevant information is diminished. This ability, therefore, enables us to bridge short temporal discontinuities between perception and action. The process is thought to be critical for behavioural flexibility, internal monitoring of behavioural responses, and ongoing guidance of action [6].

One theoretical model for the active maintenance of spatial material is that developed by Baddeley [7]. He postulated a slave system, the visuo-spatial "scratch pad" as responsible for spatial working memory with maintenance of material in this slave system being dependent on an interaction with a central executive. From studies of neurological patients the dorsolateral prefrontal cortex emerges as a plausible anatomical substrate for this central executive system.

Because of its active nature, this type of memory storage can easily be disrupted. There are essentially two ways in which this disruption can occur. First, the memory can be disrupted by doing something complex. Second, the memory can be disrupted by doing anything involving the same kind of material. For instance, we might think about something sufficiently complex that it uses up all our "conscious capacity" with the result that the material in active memory is lost. However, a simple competing task (*i.e.*, one needing little thought) can also interfere if it involves the same process (or codes) required for the material being actively stored. In cognitive terms, then, active memory involves at least two components (i) a general system for "holding in mind" material (the central executive) and (ii) the process or code to be held in mind which can involve any modality (the slave system) [7].

Neurophysiological accounts modeled on the cognitive approach outlined emphasise interactions between DLPFC (the central executive) and task specific posterior areas (the slave systems) [8]. These models have been derived principally from studies in nonhuman primates. Primate studies usually involve tasks that require a delay between a perception (the cue) and an action (the response) as in delayed response, delayed matching to sample, or delayed nonmatching to sample tasks. In primates the dorsolateral prefrontal cortex is the region most closely associated with this active memory function. Thus, circumscribed lesions to the dorsolateral prefrontal or ventrolateral prefrontal cortex impair performance on delay tasks irrespective of the nature or content of what is held in mind [6].

Functional imaging studies in normal human subjects have investigated the neural basis of maintaining an active representation over varying time intervals. Delayed spatial recognition tasks have been reported as leading to activation in a wide network of brain regions that include the right inferior frontal, premotor, parietal and occipital cortex [9]. In tasks involving spatial working memory bilateral DLPFC activations, with right hemisphere predominance, have been observed [10]. However, the tasks utilised in these studies have invariably involved cognitive operations additional to that of maintaining a representation.

To study the brain regions involved purely in "the maintenance of a representation" we measured neural activity during the delay period of either a spatial delayed response (DR) or a delayed matching (DM) task. The tasks used were formally similar to those used in studies of nonhuman primates. The tasks required subjects to fixate on a central cross prior to the scan. A stimulus, an open circle 1 cm in diameter (DR task) or a rectangular shape (DM), was displayed for 200 msec approximately 5 sec before the scanning window. Throughout the delay period of 45 sec subjects were required to fixate the cross and hold in mind the relevant representation. Responses were made subsequent to the scan and involved pointing to the location of the stimulus in the DR (see Fig. 1) or matching the rectangle to one of two choice shapes in the DM. The control conditions required subjects to fixate a central cross throughout the 45-sec scanning period and subsequently to touch the centre of a circular target that appeared at a pseudorandom location (DR) or to touch a rectangle (DM). The crucial element of our study was that stimuli were presented, and responses made, outside the scanning window in each condition. The sole requirement during scanning was either active representation of spatial location in the DR task or attributes of shapes in the DM task. In both tasks the representation also necessarily embodied a future action that occurred outside the window of the scan, in the form of preparation for a motor response to a predetermined location (DR task) or to an unspecified location (DM task), respectively.

For both conditions a widespread pattern of cortical activation was observed (Fig. 2). Bilateral dorsolateral prefrontal cortex (DLPFC) activations were common to the delay period of both tasks. However, the pattern of activation was greater on the right in the DR task and on the left in the DM task. Active representation of spatial location in the DR task was associated with coactivation of medial and lateral parietal cortices and also extrastriate visual cortex. Active representation of shape in the DM task was associated with co-activation of the medial and lateral parietal cortices and the inferior temporal cortex. During both tasks activations were also observed in regions that are associated with motor preparation and response. Activation of anterior cingulate, inferior frontal, lateral premotor, and rostral inferior parietal cortex was observed in the DR condition, a task in which it is possible to prepare for a movement to a predetermined location. In the DM task a different pattern of activation in motor areas was observed with the predominant activation being centred on the rostral SMA. This difference between tasks can be attributed to the fact that motor preparation in the DM task was for an action to an undetermined location. Comparisons of activity in the DM *versus* the DR condition revealed focal activations specific to the spatial memory condition in the right DLPFC, inferior frontal cortex and SMA and bilaterally in premotor cortex, anterior inferior parietal cortex, medial parietal cortex, occipital cortex, and the occipito-temporal junction. Activations specific to the shape memory condition were localised to the left rostral SMA and the middle and inferior temporal gyri bilaterally [11].

The findings from this study are remarkably consistent with the extensive animal literature based upon delay type tasks. Consistent with this literature

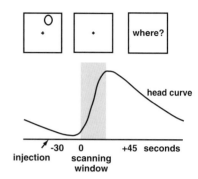

FIGURE 1. The experimental paradigm for studying active memory. In the study of active memory for location and shape the task was timed so that the critical scanning window (the 30 sec coinciding with the rising phase of the head curve when the radioactive tracer is entering the brain) coincided with the active memory stage. The presentation of the target to be remembered occurred just before scanning and the response, indicating where the target had been, occurred after the active phase of scanning was complete. During the scan the volunteer was fixating the cross and "holding in mind" where the target had been.

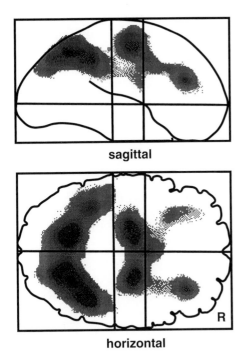

sagittal

horizontal

Figure 2. The brain activity associated with active memory. The brain regions active while the volunteers are holding a spatial location in mind are shown using the "glass brain" convention. All areas of activity are shown looking through the brain from two view points, from the side and from above. Bilateral activity can be seen in the parietal cortex, in premotor cortex, and in prefrontal cortex.

we observed prefrontal cortex (DLPFC) activation in both tasks that required holding a representation in mind. This convergence of data from animal and human studies indicates that the neural substrate for the active maintenance of a representation, of either a shape or of a spatial location, is the DLPFC. The one finding that is divergent from the animal literature is a degree of hemispheric specialisation for different types of representations.

Another striking feature of the data is that the location of the coactivated posterior brain regions is dependent upon the nature of the representation. In the DR task the predominant coactivation involved posterior medial and lateral parietal cortex. In the DM task parietal activation was again observed but, in addition, there was also a focus of activity in the inferior temporal cortex. These findings are again consistent with observations in primate studies that have indicated relative functional specialisation in the parietal cortex for spatial representations and inferior temporal cortex for object representations. The data strongly suggest that the nature or content of a maintained representation is less dependent on prefrontal activation, but is conditional on which particular regions are coactivated with the DLPFC. Analogous observations in primates indicate that working memory is a function of sustained activity, not only in DLPFC, but also in the relevant distributed neural system [12]. The role of DLPFC in maintaining sustained activity in the network remains to be explained. For example, it may be the case that the prefrontal cortex actively modulates neuronal activity in multiple cortical regions through bidirectional anatomical pathways.

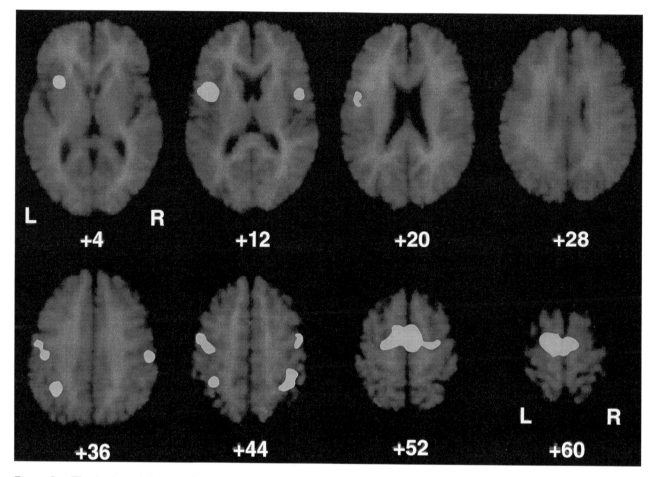

FIGURE 3. The brain activity associated with imagined hand movements. Significant activity when imagined movement is compared with preparation to move is shown as grey areas superimposed on horizontal slices of the average structural MRI for the group. The numbers refer to the distance in millimeters from the reference slice containing the anterior and posterior commissures. Activity is seen in the supplementary motor area (+52, +60), in the parietal cortex (+36, +44), and in the insula (+12).

B. Imagination

The results of this experiment are largely confirmatory of animal studies. However, there are now data from related tasks that cannot be performed with animals where very similar patterns of brain activity can also be found with tasks that would not normally be thought to involve memory. For example, we asked volunteers to imagine making a series of hand movements (in order to move a joystick in four different directions) [13]. Brain activity associated with this task was contrasted with what occurred when actually making movements and with preparing to make movements. Imagining making the movements was associated with activity in parietal cortex and PMC in locations strikingly similar to those found in the active memory task for spatial location (Fig. 3). In cognitive terms the two tasks are similar in that volunteers have to hold in mind movements in particular directions. However, the critical difference is that in the memory task it was an external stimulus that indicated a direction of movement to be held in mind, whereas in the imagination task a direction of movement was self-generated. The implication of these results is that the brain uses identical mechanisms and systems for handling representations of movement and spatial location irrespective of whether these are given externally or are self-generated. It is therefore appropriate to discuss in this section not only active memory tasks, but also studies of imagery.

In the study by Stephan *et al.* there was no activity in frontal cortex when imagining movements was compared with the control task [13]. This is because the control task, preparing to make a movement, was also associated with frontal activity. In a very similar study by Ceballos-Baumann *et al.* frontal activity was observed in the motor imagery task when this was compared with rest [14]. These results imply that the same frontal activity is required for holding one movement in mind for an extended time period or a series of movements in mind for a short time. In contrast, posterior areas display an increment of activity each time an imaginary movement is "performed." Indeed, it has been proposed that frontal activity is associated with holding in mind the instructions for doing a task, while posterior activity is concerned with "actual" task performance [15].

In the early, exploratory studies it was often observed that there was greater frontal activity associated with imagining doing something than actually doing it [16]. We agree with the general conclusion that frontal activity is a critical component of motor imagery which we believe is due to the fact that in order to imagine something we have to "hold it in mind," while there are many things we can do in reality without holding an action in mind. William James (1890, Chap. 26) called these ideo-motor acts. *"Wherever movement follows unhesitatingly and immediately the notion of it in the mind. We are then aware of nothing between the conception and the execution"* [17]. Examples come from studies of learning. We have shown that, in the early stages of learning (when we have to think about what we are doing), there is considerable frontal activity (Chapter 11). Once a task has become routine (after much practice) we no longer have to think about what we are doing and frontal activation is no longer apparent (relative to rest). However, if we are asked to think about what we are doing in this routine task, then the frontal activity reappears (interestingly the performance gets slightly worse). Of necessity, in order to imagine doing even the most routine of tasks we have to hold in mind what we are doing. Thus it seems likely that all imagery will be associated with frontal activity.

C. Selective Attention

One major attribute of consciousness is its selectivity. We choose what is to be the focus of our attention as in the classic example of the "cocktail party" situation. From among 10 different conversations we can select one to listen to. This is a form of voluntary attention in which perceptual processes are modified from a higher level (top–down processing). It is quite distinct from the involuntary or reflexive process by which our attention is grabbed by a salient stimulus, such as our name, occurring in another conversation. In this case our attention has been modified by perception (bottom–up processing).

Corbetta and colleagues studied selective voluntary attention by presenting volunteers with a complex array of stimuli that could vary in shape, colour, or motion [18,19]. On each scan volunteers were asked to attend selectively to one of these features. Thus, the perceptual input was invariant across scans but volunteers attended to different aspects of the display. The results showed that attention activated brain areas specialised for processing an attended feature. When volunteers attended to colour there was increased activity in the lingual gyrus close to an area we have identified as the human homologue of V4. When volunteers attended to motion brain activity increased in the vicinity of a region specialised for motion, human V5. The same phenomenon of modulation in early visual processing streams is observed when volunteers are asked to attend to either local or global features of a complex stimulus [20]. Even though the stimulus across experimental conditions is the same, attention to the global features is associated with increased activation in the right lingual gyrus (human V3) while attention to local features is associated with increased activity in the left inferior occipital gyrus (human V2; Fig. 4).

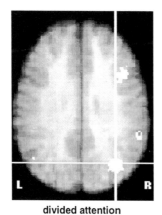

divided attention

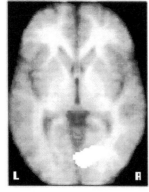

globally directed attention

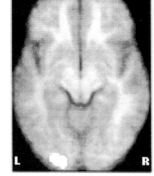

locally directed attention

FIGURE 4. The effects of attention on the early visual processing of global and local features. (Top left) An example of the stimuli used: a large L composed of small Ds. (Bottom left) The activity in the right lingual gyrus (V3) when attending to global features (the large letter). (Bottom right) The activity in the left inferior occipital gyrus (V2) when attending to local features (the small letters). (Top right) Activity at the left temporo-parietal-occipital junction associated with switching attention to either the global or the local level.

These results are consistent with claims for lateralised hemispheric differences during global and local processing of visual stimuli derived from studies of patients with lesions [21,22]. However, the most striking implication of this result is that selective attention is producing top–down modulation of brain areas relatively early in the visual processing stream (V2 and V3). An important question therefore is what is the source of this top–down modulation? We attempted to identify the source by systematically varying the number of switches between local and global levels across a series of 12 scans. Activity in a number of right hemisphere areas, including the temporo-parietal-occipital junction, was associated with sustained attention at one level. This result is consistent with lesion data that implicate this region in high level attentional processing. What was also notable in this experiment was bilateral prefrontal activity.

The precise mechanism by which early visual processing areas are modulated by selective attention remains unknown. A tonic increase of activity in a target area might occur in anticipation of a stimulus. Alternatively, there could be a phasic modulation such that each stimulus elicited a larger response in a target area. Conceptually, it is possible to disentangle these two alternatives by presenting stimuli at a series of different rates. Preliminary studies suggest that there is tonic modulation in an area that is the target for top–down processing where changes in activity occur in anticipation of any stimulus [23].

If our preliminary result is confirmed, then we can conceive of this sort of voluntary action or attention as another form of active memory: anticipatory set for a future stimulus. Thus, there is not only anticipatory set for a response we are about to make but also for a stimulus we expect to perceive. The enhancement of activity in posterior modular systems is directly related to the anticipatory set and has clear parallels with the prefrontal–posterior interactions observed in working memory tasks. It is widely believed that attention depends upon a widely distributed brain system that includes both the anterior cingulate cortex and the thalamus [24], but this system has yet to be fully delineated experimentally as has the question of supramodal or modality specific attentional systems.

D. Mental Imagery and the Contents of Consciousness

We have shown that the brain areas concerned with active memory, mental imagery, and selective attention are essentially the same. In all cases information derived from an external cue, or from the person's own imagination, has to be kept in mind. The location of the activity depends upon the type of information that has to be kept in mind and, for information held over more than a few seconds, seems to require an interaction with a prefrontal system. Some writers have equated the contents of active memory with the contents of consciousness. However, we are clearly conscious even when we simply perceive the world around us and are not actively engaged in holding anything in mind. Is it possible to distinguish the process underlying phenomenological consciousness from those additional processes that are engaged when we manipulate the information held in mind in various ways? In the following section we consider a paradigm in which we have tried to study phenomenological consciousness in isolation.

colour-word synaesthesia

photograph   **fish**

police   judge

kind   **cut**

FIGURE 5. The phenomenon of colour–word synaesthesia. People with colour–word synaesthesia have an experience of colour when they hear a word. The figure shows the colours experienced with various words for one of our volunteers. The colour is determined largely by the first letter, rather than the first sound of the word. The experience of colour is not located at any particular point in space.

1. Synaesthesia

A small proportion of people, who are otherwise normal, report the experience of synaesthesia. In this condition stimulation in one sensory modality gives rise to a sensation, or "obligatory imagery," in another modality [25,26]. Many different modalities can be linked in this way. Musical chords can give an experience of colour, textures sensed by touch can give an experience of shape. In perhaps the most common form the sounds of words are associated with the visual experience of colour. This experience of colour is involuntary and does not seem to be learned since synaesthetes report that they have had such experiences for as long as they can remember [27]. The colour experience associated with a particular word is very consistent across time and seems to be determined by the first letter of the word (*e.g.*, philosophy is pink). In most cases the colour experience elicited by a word is not localised in space, suggesting that the area of the brain that gives rise to this experience is not retinotopically organised (Fig. 5).

We compared six synaesthetes with six matched controls who did not have colour experiences when hearing words [28]. Subjects were scanned in two conditions. In the control condition (hearing random tones) the experiences of the two groups were the same. In the experimental condition (hearing random word lists) the groups differed only insofar as the synaesthetes had a subjective experience of colour. There was no difference between the groups in terms of sensory input or motor output. Thus any difference in brain activity observed between the groups is concerned solely with differences in phenomenological consciousness. There were a number of areas where the synaesthetes showed significantly greater activation than controls (Fig. 6). Two of these areas were in association cortex known to be associated with high level processing of colour; namely the posterior inferior temporal cortex [19,29] and the parietal–occipital junction [30]. The precise function of these areas in the high level processing of colour cannot be deduced from these findings. This study of synaesthesia does provide support for the view that phenomenological consciousness is dependent on activity in brain areas associated with representing the kind of information that provides the content of our conscious awareness. However, this activity is not sufficient for phenomenological consciousness and it

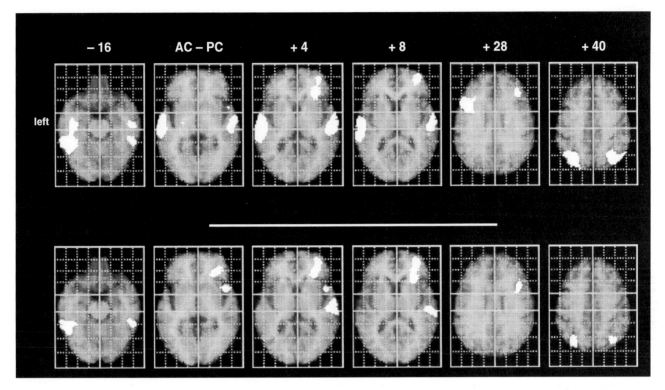

FIGURE 6. The brain experience associated with the experience of synaesthesia. (Top) The brain activity associated with hearing words (*vs* tones) is shown for our volunteers with synaesthesia. Areas of significant activity are shown in white superimposed on horizontal slices showing brain structure. The numbers refer to the distance in mm from the reference slice containing the anterior and posterior commissures. (Bottom) The extra activity seen in the synaesthetes, but not in the controls. These extra regions included the posterior inferior temporal cortex bilaterally (-16), and the parietal–occipital junction bilaterally ($+40$).

seems likely that there must also be an interaction with nonspecific activity in prefrontal areas.

E. Failure to Be Able to Hold Things in Mind

The implications of the results we have discussed so far are that, underlying our ability to hold things in mind, there is an extended brain system with two major components. One component of this system concerns the content, what we are holding in mind. Divergent, largely posterior, locations in the brain are associated with different contents. The second major component is that which operates to activate or maintain the representation in mind in the absence of a sensory input. This component involves activity in prefrontal cortex and its operation is much less contingent on the nature or content of the representation.

There is much evidence that damage to posterior brain areas can eliminate certain contents from our consciousness. In other words, after specific damage we can no longer hold certain things in mind. A patient with damage to primary visual cortex is no longer aware of parts of the visual world. However, such a patient may still be able to use visual information to guide behaviour [31]. One such patient studied in our laboratory was able to detect rapid movement of large objects across the visual field and reported that he was aware of movement. A brain imaging study revealed that this detection of motion was associated with activity in the visual motion area, V5, even though primary visual cortex, V1, was absent [32]. This result emphasises the principle that there are many parallel routes by which neural signals are available to, and influence, high level brain function.

A dramatic demonstration of this idea is provided by a patient with the condition of hemianaesthesia. We studied a case in which a right hemisphere stroke was associated with a loss of sensation in the left arm [33]. One result of the lesion was that the patient could not report being touched on his left arm. As in cases described previously this patient demonstrated the phenomenon whereby a loss of feeling could, temporarily, be reversed by stimulation of the vestibular system on the side opposite the lesion (*i.e.*, ice-cold water in the left ear; see Fig. 13 in Chapter 10). In normal volunteers this manipulation distorts the perception of the position of the body in space and biases attention towards the contralateral side of the body. The vestibular system sends inputs to a number of brain areas that are probably concerned with representations of the position of the body in space and that are also stimulated by simple touch [34]. In our patient several of these areas were no longer functioning as a result of damage from the stroke (supramarginal gyrus, premotor cortex, SII). However, two areas that are part of this system were still intact (putamen, insula).

Unilateral brain damage produces long-term asymmetry of activity in those brain areas into which the vestibular and touch systems share afferent projections. Accordingly touch imperception can be viewed as the result of a distorted body representation generated by a distributed neural system whose activity is set at a low level in anatomically spared regions and at zero in those areas directly damaged. It was precisely in the spared areas that activation by touch could be observed, but only in the presence of vestibular stimulation (see Fig. 14 in Chapter 10). We must therefore assume that vestibular stimulation modulated the neuronal response in these spared areas to a degree that, following stimulation, touch elicited conscious awareness. In this case we have a within subject design in which conditions with identical stimulus input differ solely with respect to the presence of phenomenological consciousness. Once again the location of activity relates to a specific content of consciousness.

We would also expect damage to the frontal component of the system to impair the ability to bring images to mind and maintain them. This might occur whatever the image modality. It is much more difficult to discover what the effects of such damage are like for the patient. The damage here is not affecting the content, but the system used for reporting that content (see Chapter 1). Thus the patient may not be able to tell us what his mental contents are like and we are left to infer them from his behaviour. We know that such patients have problems with carrying out actions across temporal discontinuities with the result that they have difficulty following through plans and are slaves to every passing irrelevance. However, the majority of cases in the literature display problems that extend well beyond simply holding things in mind. Their problem is much more obvious when it comes to manipulating things held in mind.

IV. MANIPULATING THINGS HELD IN MIND

Active memory enables a person to hold things in mind over an extended time period. Over and above simply holding something in mind humans have a highly developed facility to manipulate things held in mind. This ability to manipulate representations within an active memory system is captured by the concept of working memory [35]. Manipulating things in mind is critically important when we engage in cognitive acts such as conceptualising and planning. Planning involves complex cognitive operations that require a number of subprocesses [36]. First, to implement a plan it is necessary to have a goal. Second, it is necessary to prepare and implement responses aimed at achieving a series of subgoals while holding the end goal in mind. Finally, it is necessary to monitor and verify each response in relation both to the subgoals and the final goal. For effective planning these separate subcomponents must be integrated, a function often attributed to (and necessitating the concept of) a central monitor or central executive system [1]. Planning is one of those psychological functions that seems to be intimately associated with consciousness and conscious awareness has been identified with the phenomenal experience of the contents and regulatory operations of this central processor [37].

Plans can be thought of as prospective mental acts that free an individual from immediate environmental contingencies and enhance behavioural flexibility. Plans are also related to the concept of motivation or desire and are consequently bound up with the domain of emotion. In this regard a plan can be conceived of as a path from desire or motivation to an action. Deficits in planning are thus features of patients with psychomotor poverty as seen in depression and schizophrenia where the planning deficit may reflect the failure to initiate a plan or to carry through a plan once it has been initiated. Planning deficits are typically associated with anterior brain lesions, being a cardinal feature of patients with frontal lobe lesions [36]. This is well exemplified by the performance of frontal patients on the Wisconsin Card-Sorting test who show deficits in switching categories and marked perseverations [38]. Frontal lesion patients also have deficits in tasks involving self-ordered planning where they must impose their own structure on a task [39].

A. The Tower of London Task

One approach to the study of planning with functional imaging is to use a task that requires self-organised responding. The Tower of London provides a well validated example of such a task [40]. In essence, this task requires subjects to rearrange, in the minimum number of moves, a set of three coloured balls arranged on pegs or stacked on top of each other as in the task illustrated to attain a final configuration that matches a prespecified goal state (Fig. 7). To solve the problem the complete sequence of moves required must be planned and prepared in advance of making an actual response.

We used a computerised version of the task where subjects solved each problem using "mental" transformations of the initial position, before executing a single response to indicate the minimum number of moves needed to solve the problem. In the context of the study subjects were presented with a sequence of problems which took, in total, about 5 min to solve. Concealed within these sequences were runs of easy problems (two- and three-move

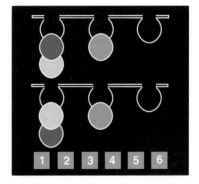

FIGURE 7. The Tower of London task. Given the starting position in the top row the task is to move one ball at a time (in the imagination) until the final position in the bottom row is achieved. The subject then indicates how many moves this will take by touching the appropriate number.

solutions) and difficult problems (four- and five-move solutions) presented during the 30-sec acquisition phase of a scan. Each subject was scanned six times during the task (three scans each with the easy and difficult conditions) and six times while performing a control condition in which the visual display and motor response were matched with the experimental task.

During this planning task activations were observed in the prefrontal, cingulate, premotor, parietal, and occipital cortices (Fig. 8). These activations bore striking correspondence to areas activated during our visuo-spatial working memory tasks. The one exception was an area of rostral prefrontal cortex that was uniquely activated in the planning task. Enhanced neural activity in this rostral prefrontal area, and in the visuo-spatial working memory system, was associated with increased task difficulty. This suggests that the rostral prefrontal area might be involved in the executive components of planning such as response selection and evaluation.

Manipulating something held in mind activates frontal regions and posterior brain regions. As planning involves holding in mind a representation of both the end goal and intermediate stages of the problem there must necessarily be engagement of an active memory system. From our study of active memory, and given the visuo-spatial nature of the Tower task, we interpret activations in the DLPFC, posterior parietal, and extrastriate visual cortices with this system. The activation of the rostral prefrontal cortex which was engaged to a greater extent in the more difficult problems, suggests that this region may implement executive processes concerned with the selection, monitoring, and evaluation of move sequences. Consistent with this suggestion are findings that rostrolateral frontal and DLPFC activations have been observed in "random" movement generation and motor sequence learning paradigms [41,42]. Activation of this rostral area has also been observed during retrieval of material from episodic memory [43–45]. An explanation for the commonality of activations is that they result from the need to evaluate and monitor responses. Anterior prefrontal lesions that characteristically lead to impaired performance in the Tower of London task almost invariably encompass this rostral area [40,46].

B. Failure to Manipulate Things Held in Mind

Deficits in planning are a feature of patients with psychomotor poverty as seen in depression and schizophrenia. In a series of studies Weinberger and his colleagues have shown that chronic schizophrenic patients show less prefrontal activation than normal controls when performing the Wisconsin card sorting task [47,48]. Andreasen and her colleagues have carried out a similar study using the Tower of London task [49]. In this study a similar difference between patients and controls was found, but in the anterior cingulate cortex. The reduced activation in this area was especially marked in patients with psychomotor poverty. A problem for the interpretation of all these studies concerns the performance of the patients which was worse than that of the controls. Since we might expect poor performance to be associated with reduced frontal activity, even in normal volunteers, it is not clear how to interpret these abnormal patterns of activity. We shall return to this problem in the next section (on response initiation) when we discuss studies of verbal fluency (another frontal task). We have concentrated in this section on the manipulation of things held in mind which is clearly a major component of executive tasks such as the Tower of London. However, another important component

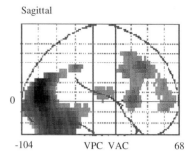

Sagittal

-104   VPC VAC   68

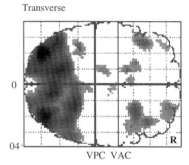

Transverse

04   **R**

VPC VAC

FIGURE 8. Brain activity associated withe Tower of London task. The brain regions active while volunteers are solving the Tower of London task are shown using the "glass brain" convention. All areas of activity are shown looking through the brain from two view points, from the side and from above. Bilateral activity can be seen in the parietal cortex and occipital cortex and in anterior cingulate and dorsolateral prefrontal cortex.

of executive tasks concerns the initiation of the search for a response or a plan of action and the inhibition of inappropriate responses or plans. Problems in this domain are particularly relevant to understanding psychosis. It is defects in initiation and maintenance (poverty of action) that are most characteristic of schizophrenic and depressed patients with negative features, while failure to suppress inappropriate actions are characteristic of schizophrenic patients with disorganised behaviour [50].

V. HOW DO WE CHOOSE WHAT TO DO?

A. Will, Action, and Planning

Planning has affiliations with the concept of action. The concept of action can encompass moving a limb, uttering a sentence, or performing a manipulation on a mental image. Action and planning are also closely tied to a concept of agency. However, not all actions involve a sense of agency. An example of this type of action occurs when we respond to an external cue telling us what to do and when to do it. Self-generated actions, on the other hand, are usually accompanied by a sense of agency and are determined principally by internal, as opposed to external, context [51]. William James suggested that this sense of agency arises when we are aware of choosing between several possible courses of action [17]. If one course of action dominates then we have little sense of choice (or agency) and action can be said to be stimulus or context driven. The necessity for choice is particularly likely to arise in novel situations where we have inadequate information for choosing one action rather than another, or situations in which different actions are roughly equal in the likelihood of achieving a desired outcome (the tyranny of choice). In line with the conceptual framework we have adopted for this chapter, we are concerned in this section with the ability to hold in mind several alternative actions in order to choose which one to initiate.

An important issue is whether there are common mechanisms for self-generated actions that are independent of modality. There is substantial neuroanatomical and electrophysiological evidence that the SMA plays a critical role in the generation of action [52,53]. For example, self-paced action in monkeys is strongly associated with increased activity in SMA. However, Neafsey in a trenchant criticism has suggested, on the basis of lesion studies, that SMA is concerned with the preparation of motor acts, rather than the intention to act [54]. The SMA is linked to the anterior cingulate portion of the limbic cortex, thus providing a pathway by which limbic outflow or evaluative signals could influence motor behaviour [51]. It may be the case that it is anterior cingulate cortex that has a special role in the intention to act.

Paus and colleagues contrasted novel and routine actions across three different modalities (manual, oculomotor, and speech), in experiments involving a contrast of routine and novel behavioural responses or the contrast of a prostimulus or antistimulus task [55]. For routine actions volunteers practiced extensively, for example, pressing one of three buttons in response to a cue in a manual task. For the novel action volunteers were informed of a new combination of stimuli–response associations just prior to scanning. Paus and colleagues contrasted novel and routine responses in three different modalities: finger movements, eye movements, and speech. In contrast to routine actions, novel actions activated anterior cingulate cortex with the precise location of the activity being dependent on modality.

We have carried out a series of studies in which volunteers were explicitly required to choose for themselves which of several responses to make. In one study subjects had to choose for themselves which of two fingers to move [56]. This was contrasted with a condition in which they simply moved whichever of two fingers was touched. During self-generated movement there was activity in DLPFC bilaterally and in anterior cingulate cortex. Similar results were obtained when volunteers had to choose between four possible joystick movements and this was compared with moving the stick in the same direction every time [41]. Once again activity was observed in DLPFC and anterior cingulate cortex when the movements were self-generated. In these studies volunteers chose which movement to make, but, because the tasks were paced, not when to make the movements. In another experiment, volunteers made the same movement every time, but chose for themselves when to make the movement [57]. Again, in this condition there was activity in DLPFC and anterior cingulate cortex.

The tasks discussed above are sometimes described as generation tasks, since volunteers have to generate a movement sequence for themselves. There have also been many studies of word generation. There are two basic forms of these tasks: generating many words in a particular category (*e.g.*, words beginning with F) and generating one word that goes with a cue word (*e.g.*, generating verbs for nouns, cake–eat) [58,59]. These tasks are rather different from the motor tasks we have already discussed. In the motor tasks volunteers consider all possible responses and choose one of them. In the verb generation task volunteers have, somehow, to summon into their minds a possible response from within a rather tightly specified category. Although the tasks have this different quality the pattern of activity associated with word generation is very similar to that seen in movement generation tasks. The main activity is again seen in DLPFC especially on the left and, in addition, there is activity in anterior cingulate cortex (Fig. 9).

A more complex situation in which people have to select between different actions occurs when they have to do two things at once (the dual task paradigm) [60]. Precisely how performance is achieved, whether both tasks are performed in parallel or in alternation, will depend upon the nature of the tasks. If the two tasks are routine and involve different modalities then they can probably be carried out in parallel without interference. However, if either or both tasks involve a degree of novelty and require focused attention, then there is likely to be interference. In this situation additional processes must be brought into play to "allocate resources" between the two tasks. We used a dual task paradigm in a study of memory where the primary task was to remember a series of word pairs [61] (see Chapter 15 for greater detail). This is achieved by processing the words at a semantic level, probably by searching for mediating concepts, and is associated with activation of left DLPFC. The secondary task was a paradigm in which subjects moved a cursor to one of four different target locations. In a routine version of this task the subject could predict the target location in advance because it appeared in an ordered sequence. This task had no effect on subsequent memory for the word pairs. When the sequence of targets was unpredictable the task required focused attention and caused impaired performance on the memory task. In the presence of this task the memory associated activation of DLPFC was eliminated, but activation of anterior cingulate was greatly enhanced (Fig. 10). This is an interesting result because, for once, activity in DLPFC and anterior cingulate was not positively coupled. The result confirms the idea

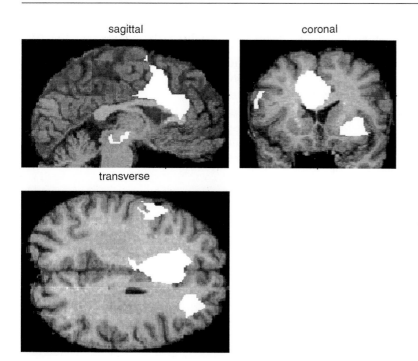

FIGURE 9. Brain activity associated with willed action. Areas of increased activity during the performance of a "willed action" task are shown superimposed on a structural image. Sagittal, coronal, and horizontal slices are shown. Activity can be seen in anterior cingulate cortex, and in left and right prefrontal cortex.

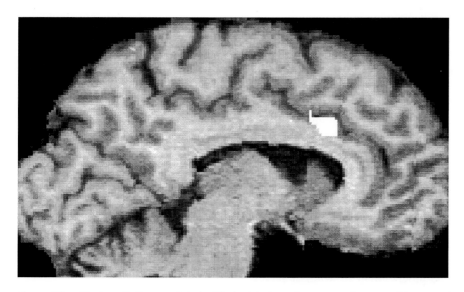

FIGURE 10. Brain activity associated with dual task performance. An area of increased activity in the anterior cingulate cortex is shown superimposed on a sagittal slice from a structural image. This was the area where increased activity occurred when volunteers had to perform two tasks at once.

that it is ACC and not DLPFC that is concerned with selection between different actions.

We have noted a striking difference in frontal activity associated with acquisition and retrieval of episodic memory (see Chapter 16). Acquisition tends to be associated with left frontal activity while retrieval is associated with right frontal activity. Presumably this difference reflects the different kinds of cognitive processes typically involved in acquisition and retrieval. Such processes are not necessarily unique to memory. On the basis of results discussed in this section we might speculate that left frontal activity is associated with the generation of items (bringing things into mind). In order to remember word pairs it is useful to generate "mediators", that is concepts that link two words. In contrast, right frontal activation might be associated with monitoring or checking items already held in mind.

B. Failures of Will

There are many neurological and psychiatric disorders that can best be characterised as manifestations of a specific problem with willed acts. In patients with SMA lesions there may be profound deficits of certain kinds of speech and motor acts. In these patients speech and motor action may occur in response to environmental cues but not as a result of the patient's own needs. For example, a patient may be perfectly able to respond to an outstretched hand and engage in a handshake but at the same time be unable to initiate a handshake [62,63] Nonvolitional integrated actions of the arm, the so-called alien hand sign, are reported in association with infarction of the SMA [64]. In these cases the arm contralateral to the lesion will "use" items (pencils, doorknobs, *etc.*) without the intention or knowledge of the patient.

A similar pattern of deficits has also been claimed in patients with Parkinson's disease. They can respond to cues, but have more difficulty with self-generated acts [51]. When they perform response generation tasks they are slower than controls, but produce sequences that are equally random. They also show significantly less activity in SMA than controls when performing these tasks [65]. The magnitude of this activity can be normalised by treatment with apomorphine [66]. These results are consistent with our earlier suggestion that SMA is concerned with the initiation of self-generated acts, but not with their selection.

Chronic schizophrenic patients with negative features (psychomotor poverty) have great difficulty with response generation tasks and often produce highly stereotyped sequences of responses [67,68]. There are, as yet, no data about the brain activity associated with this behaviour. Since the first study by Ingvar and Franzen it has been known that many schizophrenics show abnormally low resting blood flow in frontal cortex [69]. More recent studies show that this pattern is characteristic of patients with psychomotor poverty who show low blood flow specifically in DLPFC on the left [70]. However, this pattern is not unique to schizophrenia, but is also found in depressed patients with psychomotor retardation [71]. Furthermore, a symptom characteristic of poverty of will, namely poverty of speech, is strongly predictive of decreased perfusion of the left DLPFC independent of whether patients are diagnosed as depressed or schizophrenic [72]. Why should low frontal activity at rest be associated with symptoms of poverty of will? We suggest that when normal volunteers are at rest they are in fact actively engaged in generating thoughts and memories. Direct evidence for this notion comes from studies of "stimulus independent thoughts" and the sorts of activities which interfere with them [73]. Psychomotor poverty is (by definition) associated with poverty in the generation of all kinds of activity, including thoughts. This lack of activity is associated with a low resting flow in DLPFC.

We studied another aspect of response generation using a paced word fluency task in patients with schizophrenia. By using a paced task we could be sure that the patients produced the same number of words as the controls during the scan, even though their performance was probably worse in the sense that they took longer to generate each word. This approach avoids the problem of performance differences that makes interpretation of studies of abnormal groups so difficult. In a group of 18 chronic schizophrenic patients we found no differences from controls in the magnitude of the activations in DLPFC or anterior cingulate cortex [74]. However, in a group of 12 drug-free acute patients, while there was no difference in DLPFC there was significantly less activity in anterior cingulate cortex [75]. Treatment with apomorphine resulted in excessive activation of this area.

In summary, we might speculate that these results show that DLPFC is involved in generating potential responses, while anterior cingulate cortex is involved in selecting which one to produce. As we shall see in the next section, this response selection may depend upon the emotional state of the person or, perhaps, the emotional valence attached to the response options. In patients with schizophrenia, particularly those with psychomotor poverty, something has gone wrong with this system for generating and selecting responses. However, as we have already discussed in the section on active memory, engagement of frontal cortex alone is insufficient for making a response. There must be a dynamic interaction with posterior areas whose location depends upon the precise nature of the response being generated. At the end of this chapter we shall consider the nature of these interactions in more detail and present evidence that in schizophrenia a fundamental mechanism may be a breakdown of these interactions between frontal and posterior areas.

VI. EMOTION

A. What Is Emotion?

Influential theories suggest that there are a limited number of basic human emotions that include happiness, anger, fear, sadness, and disgust [76,77]. Understanding human emotion must ultimately involve specifying its neural basis and the mechanisms of its influence on cognition. As we have already implied, emotion has an important role in higher cognition, especially attention, will, and planning. We attend to what is relevant, we make decisions and plans on the basis of expected outcomes and the emotions they engender. What is termed emotion is often differentiated from mood though in many contexts, including the context of this chapter, the terms are used interchangeably. One theoretical differentiating feature is that emotions, as opposed to moods, are generally object directed. For example, emotions such as fear or disgust are invariably experienced towards an identifiable external object. Moods are generally objectless and are experienced without an obvious locus of attribution and provide a background hue to phenomenal experience. Moods are thus closely associated with self rather than object evaluation [78–80].

The acceptance of emotion as a pervasive component of human consciousness begs the question as to its function. Cognitive descriptions emphasise an evaluative function with emotional states reflecting the *"perceived propitiousness of current circumstances"* or the cue to an individual *"about the resources available to meet environmental demands"* [80,81]. These accounts describe an adaptive function arising out of the attribution of positive or negative value to current or future circumstances. A more extended cognitive account of emotion proposes a behavioural regulatory function invoked when individuals are confronted with incompatible goals in which rational choice cannot determine the desired outcome [82]. Emotions, in this context, prompt or bias behavioural choices in a manner that leads to outcomes that are better than random. In this respect emotions are an integral component of how to plan and enact plans. This theoretical account is supported by a neuropsychological literature on patients with acquired deficits of emotional experience who, critically, also have deficits in the regulation of behaviour. The most extended account of such a patient is that of EVR who, following resection of a prefrontal meningioma, not only had a profound inability to experience emotion, but also had a gross impairment of behavioural regulation [83,84].

B. The Neurophysiology of Emotion

The classical literature on emotion can be summarised as implying that fully formed emotions involve a complex of responses that incorporate motor, visceral/autonomic, and subjective feeling states. Evolutionary accounts equate emotion with different action tendencies such as approach or avoidance, each being associated with different emotional states [85–87]. The visceral/autonomic components of emotion are emphasised in the James–Lange theory where emotional experience is construed as the perception of peripheral physiological responses to events of value or significance [88,89]. The experiential component of emotion is emphasised in the anatomical and physiological accounts of Papez *et al.* [90–92].

Descriptions of the neural systems implicated in emotion derive principally from lesion studies in animals and observations in patients with focal brain pathology. It has long been known that damage to the amygdala results in marked emotional placidity (the Kluver–Bucy syndrome) highlighting the fact that regional brain damage can produce emotional change [93,94]. More recently it has been shown that damage to the amygdala in humans also affects the perception of emotion. In particular, patients with long-standing lesions of the amygdala have difficulty in recognising fear in the faces of others [95].

We examined the perception of emotion in normal volunteers by presenting a series of "morphed" faces, based on well validated prototypes, that represented two categories of facial emotion [96]. These faces also varied systematically in the degree of fear or happiness expressed which varied from 0% (neutral) to 125% (extreme fear or happiness) (Fig. 11). A comparison of the fearful with the happy expressions revealed a focal region of activation in the left amygdala. This neural response in the amygdala also displayed a sensitivity to the degree of expressed emotion as exemplified by an increasing response with increasing fearfulness and a decreasing response with increasing happiness (Fig. 12).

Although the data outlined provide compelling evidence for a role for the amygdala in processing fear it is the frontal lobes that are most intimately implicated in emotion. The landmark observations on Phineas Gage who,

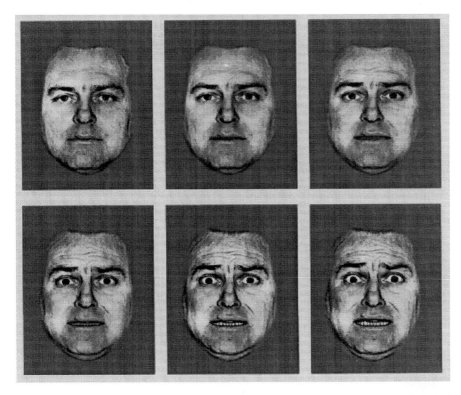

Figure 11. The expression of fear. Six faces are shown which vary systematically in the degree of fear expressed. The faces are derived from a neutral face (top left, 0%) and a standard fearful face (bottom middle, 100%) by morphing. The face on the bottom right expresses 125% fear.

following prefrontal damage, underwent a personality change best characterised as a lack of emotional regulation of behaviour, have not been bettered [97]. Subsequently, similar patients have been described in whom the common site of damage is orbital prefrontal cortex [98]. Another prefrontal region, anterior cingulate cortex, is also associated with emotion in that acquired lesions lead to indifference, amotivation, and akinetic mutism [99]. These observations have led to a suggestion that the anterior cingulate cortex initiates emotionally significant actions [51]. While lesion data suggest a dissociation between the role of the orbital frontal cortex mediating emotional experience and the regulation of cognition and the anterior cingulate mediating emotional expression *via* response selection, the precise contribution of different prefrontal regions to emotional regulation is unclear.

C. Pathological Emotion

Abnormalities of emotional regulation, particularly depression, represent common human psychopathological manifestations. The cardinal features of depression include low mood, loss of emotional reactivity, low self-esteem, guilty ruminations, and a pervasive sense of helplessness and hopelessness. Consistent with the proposal that mood is critical to cognition is the observation that pathological depression is invariably associated with alterations in memory, attention, intention, planning, and psychomotor function [100–104].

sagittal   coronal

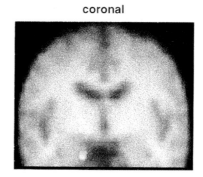

transverse

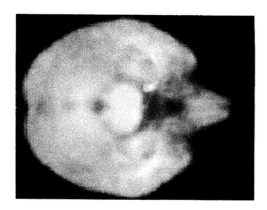

FIGURE 12.   Activity in the left amygdala associated with fear. When viewing fearful faces volunteers show increased activity in the left amygdala. This is shown as a yellow area superimposed on the average structural image for the six volunteers in sagittal, coronal, and transverse view.

Studying patients with affective disorders provides a potential means of addressing what brain regions are involved in emotional regulation and how emotion influences higher cognitive processes. We scanned a cohort of depressed patients in an "at rest" condition, when ill, and again on recovery and compared them to healthy controls matched for age and sex. The results enabled us to determine which brain regions were dysfunctional during a depressive episode and also to establish how function in these regions covaried with resolution of the depressed state. In the depressed state significant relative deactivations were evident in both supramodal and paralimbic brain regions that involved the anterior cingulate cortex, the left dorsolateral prefrontal cortex, and the left angular gyrus [105] (Fig. 13). When patients recovered, activity within these regions normalised implying state, rather than trait, abnormalities [106].

The simplest explanation for these findings in depression is that the identified pattern of hypoactivity represents an anatomical system involved in emotional regulation. The involvement of the anterior cingulate cortex is consistent with what might be predicted on the basis of human lesion studies and in particular with a proposal that the anterior cingulate is involved in emotional responses [5]. An alternative interpretation is that some or all

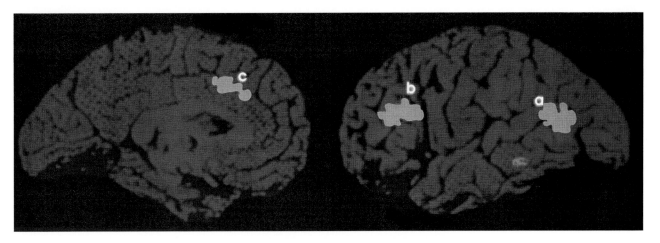

Figure 13. Reduced brain activity associated with the state of depression. The regions in the left dorso-lateral prefrontal cortex (b), anterior cingulate cortex (c), and angular gyrus (a) where there is decreased neural activity in resting state studies of depressed patients are displayed rendered onto an idealised brain.

of the identified brain regions contribute to systems that mediate cognitive processes other than mood, whose function has been modulated by inputs from some other region more critical to affective regulation.

The proposal that functional deficits in depression are manifestations of abnormally modulated brain systems predicts that the deficits should be associated with modes of symptom expression that reflect disruption of higher cognitive function. We found significant relationships between two symptom patterns and prefrontal activity [107]. An impairment of memory and attention was strongly associated with hypofunction in the medial prefrontal cortex, while another symptom constellation involving poverty of thought and action was associated with regional deficits seen in left DLPFC. We suggest that this latter syndrome represents a disorder of intentional behaviour. An abnormality in a system mediating intentional behaviour might be predicted to result in an absence of volition and a restriction of spontaneous or self generated motor and verbal behaviour. This in essence is a description of the syndrome of psychomotor retardation.

As already mentioned, precisely the same syndrome can be observed in chronic schizophrenic patients. Such patients show marked poverty of speech, thought and action, and also show reduced function in left DLPFC when at "rest." However, while flattening of affect is a feature of this syndrome, there is no evidence of depressed mood [108]. We believe that in schizophrenia the syndrome of psychomotor retardation is the consequence of a defect directly involving the physiological system underlying willed action. In contrast, in depression, the syndrome is a secondary consequence of the modulation of this "willed action" system by another region primarily concerned with mood.

This interpretation of functional deficits in depressed patients implies that the core system for mood regulation does not involve regions identified in our resting state study. This hypothesis begs the question as to the critical brain regions involved in a pure emotion. The human lesion and primate literature strongly implicates the orbital prefrontal cortex [83,109,110]. A manipulation of mood should consequently be associated with changed activity in regions such as orbital prefrontal cortex as well as with modulation of activity within circuitry concerned with cognition, particularly that involved in the regulation of volitional behaviour. These interpretations of the data from depressed patients can be subjected to empirical testing by scanning normal subjects in conjunction with mood induction procedures. Such an approach is particularly pertinent in that experimentally induced mood has been proposed as a model of mild retarded depression on the basis of the associated slowing of behavioural responses [111].

D. The Induction of Mood and Its Regulatory Effect on Cognition

An extensive psychological literature indicates that mood change can be induced in normal subjects and this experimental manipulation can impair cognition in a manner not dissimilar to that seen in depression [112,113]. A number of laboratories have reported findings based on studies of experimental mood induction. One such study scanned subjects while they recalled or imagined emotionally laden experiences, of an explicitly sad type, from their past lives [114]. In a contrast with a "rest" state this procedure showed a primary site of activation in the ventral prefrontal cortex. However, the design of the study meant that the experiment included a number of psychological processes that might in themselves account for the observed pattern of activation, such as the recall and maintenance of a representation in working memory. Another experiment studied normal subjects while they recalled affect-appropriate life events, including happy and sad events, and at the same time inspected sad or happy faces displayed on a screen [115]. In this study sadness was associated with activation of anterior cingulate, medial prefrontal, and mesial temporal cortex. However, the design of the study confounded two processes, recall of sad events and perceptual processing, which may themselves have interacted to influence the findings. A common feature of these studies is that they measured neural activity while mood was being actively induced.

For the purpose of our study we used a factorial design that involved the systematic manipulation of mood (to determine the functional anatomy of mood) while at the same time subjects performed psychological tasks (to establish how mood might modulate brain systems concerned with specific cognitive processes). In contrast to other studies the mood induction was performed between scans and involved a combination of the Velten technique, requiring repetition of negative or positive statements, in combination with a musical mood induction procedure that involved listening to sad, happy, or neutral music [116,117]. The subjects received 12 scans, 4 in each state. To determine the effect of mood on systems mediating cognition we had the subjects perform either a verbal fluency or a word repetition task in each of the mood states. We chose the verbal fluency task as we had already established that this task activated a network that included the DLPFC and anterior cingulate cortex, regions that are dysfunctional in clinical depression. More critically, verbal fluency engages a cognitive process that we hypothesise is dysfunctional in patients with the type of depression associated with psychomotor retardation. The design of the experiment therefore allowed us to determine which brain systems are activated when normal euthymic subjects undergo a change of mood and also to determine how these systems interact with those implicated in a specific higher cognitive process.

The induction of mood, happiness and sadness combined, resulted in significant changes of activity in a number of brain regions that included ventrolateral orbito-frontal cortex, DLPFC, and both medial and lateral premotor areas (Fig. 14). In the depressed mood condition alone, in addition to orbital frontal cortex, significant activations were observed in posterior cingulate and dorsal cingulate cortices, superior frontal gyrus, anterior SMA, right sensorimotor regions, and both insulae. As in previous studies the verbal fluency task activated left inferior and dorsolateral prefrontal cortices, cingulate cortex bilaterally, the rostral orbitofrontal cortex, and the left angular gyrus.

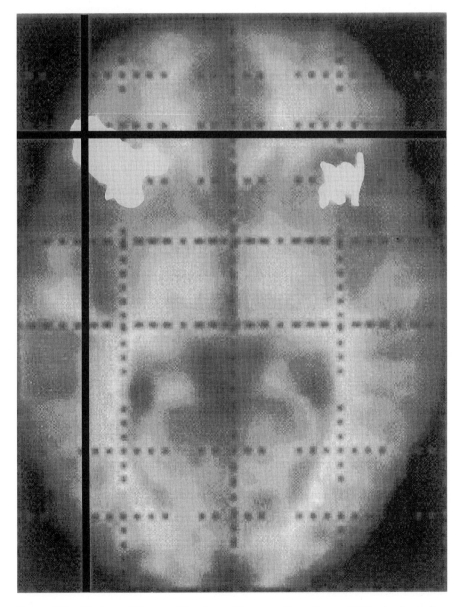

FIGURE 14. Brain activity resulting from the induction of mood. The brain regions which show the greatest change of activity in association with the induction of mood are shown superimposed onto a transverse MRI image at the level of the anterior and posterior commissures. The regions highlighted are in bilateral ventral prefrontal cortices.

The widespread pattern of activations associated with mood is in keeping with a concept of emotion as an integrated result of function in systems mediating subjective, visceral, and motor components of emotion. The common region activated in both sadness and happiness was the orbital frontal cortex. Although the study cannot fully disentangle the functional specificity of the various regional activations, it is tempting to suggest that orbital frontal activations represent the experiential components, insula and brain stem the visceral components, and SMA and cingulate the action components of emotion. The activation of orbital prefrontal cortex provides striking evidence that this region is central to the experience of emotions, consistent with reports that patients with lesions in this region lack sympathetically mediated skin conductance responses to emotionally arousing visual images and report an absence of the expected feelings to these stimuli [118]. This type of patient has also been described as suffering from an interoceptive agnosia—a lack of awareness of somatic bodily responses that function as critical cues to the meaning or value of situations and thoughts [84].

A critical additional finding was a significant attenuation of activation throughout the verbal fluency network under the condition of induced depression (Fig. 15). These attenuations subsume regions we had previously shown to be dysfunctional in depressed patients, namely the DLPFC and the anterior cingulate cortex. The profile of mood induced attenuations is also strikingly similar to the profile of brain areas that correlates with psychomotor retardation. This finding supports our contention that psychomotor retardation is a manifestation of modulated function in a system that mediates intrinsically based or self-motivated behaviour.

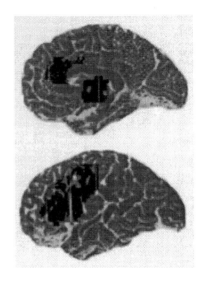

FIGURE 15. The effects of mood induction on cognitive activity. After the induction of a depressed mood there is an attenuation of the activation associated with the performance of the verbal fluency task. Brain regions affected include the anterior cingulate and dorsolateral prefrontal cortices. The regions of significant attenuation are displayed rendered on to an idealised brain.

VII. HOW DO WE KNOW WHAT IS IN THE MINDS OF OTHERS?

So far we have discussed brain systems underlying our ability to hold things in mind and the colouring that conscious experience gains from emotion. However, the most astonishing cognitive ability of all is that which enables us to infer what is in the minds of other people. We routinely explain and anticipate the behaviour of others on the basis of inferences about their current beliefs and intentions. This is sometimes referred to as "having a theory of mind" or "mentalising." This ability requires that we have in our brain a representation of the contents of the consciousness of other people that is independent of our own representation of the world. Deception is the acid test of this ability. Deception is a method of manipulating someone's behaviour by implanting a false belief in their mind. Deception comes naturally to us all, even in infancy, but there is evidence that it is not observed in monkeys [119]. Even in higher nonhuman primates such as chimpanzees, evidence for deception remains equivocal. In these circumstances we can have no data from animal studies directly relevant to the brain systems underlying mentalising abilities.

There have been speculations about a brain system underlying "social cognition" which involves temporal cortex (representing faces), amygdala (representing emotions), and orbital frontal cortex (concerned with social interactions) [120]. However, there is remarkably little knowledge about mentalising abilities from studies of patients with lesions. There is certainly evidence that frontal lesions, especially orbito-frontal lesions, lead to impairments

A 'Theory of Mind' story

A burglar who has just robbed a shop is making his getaway.
As he is running home, a policeman on his beat sees him
drop his glove. He doesn't know the man is a burglar, he just
wants to tell him he dropped his glove. But when the
policeman shouts out to the burglar, "Hey, you! Stop!", the
burglar turns round, sees the policeman, and gives himself
up. He puts his hands up and admits that he did the break-in
at the local shop.

Q: Why did the burglar do this?

A 'Physical' story

A burglar is about to break into a jewellers' shop. He
skillfully picks the lock on the shop door. Carefully he crawls
under the electronic detector beam. If he breaks this beam it
will set off the alarm. Quietly he opens the door of the store-
room and sees the gems glittering. As he reaches out,
however, he steps on something soft. He hears a screech and
something small and furry runs out past him towards the shop
door. Immediately the alarm sounds.

Q: Why did the alarm go off?

FIGURE 16. The 'theory of mind' story can only be understood on the basis of the
false belief of the burglar. The 'physical' story can be understood without considering
the mental states of the character.

of social behavior, but no formal investigations have ascertained the mentalising abilities of these patients using the various false belief tasks that have been
developed in other contexts. The study of autism provides strong evidence that
there is a dedicated brain system associated with mentalising ability [121].
The majority of people with this diagnosis show a very circumscribed disability
in mentalising while other abilities remain in the normal range.

Using tasks that have been developed and validated with autistic people
we looked for brain areas associated with mentalising abilities [122]. Volunteers read short stories while they were being scanned (Fig. 16). In one type
of story (theory of mind stories) the behaviour of the protagonists could only
be understood on the basis of their (false) beliefs. In a second type of story
the events could be understood on the basis of physical causality or general
knowledge. The beliefs and intentions of the characters were irrelevant. A
third condition consisted of unlinked sentences. One area of the brain was
uniquely activated while reading theory of mind stories in contrast to the
other two conditions. This was in left medial dorsal prefrontal cortex (Brodmann area 8/9; Fig. 17). The same area has been associated with mentalising
ability in a study in which volunteers listened to stories and in a study in
which volunteers made inferences about pictures [123]. We know very little
about the function of this area from other sources. Area 8 in the monkey is
often referred to as the frontal eye field, but in man imaging studies have
shown that the frontal eye field is more posterior and lateral and is in area 6
[124]. Area 8 has widespread cortical connections with parietal, temporal
polar, occipital, and anterior cingulate cortex. The only other brain imaging
study in which this area was activated involved a visual–visual conditional
task developed by Petrides [10]. There has been some speculation that men-

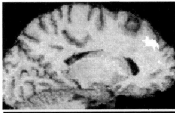
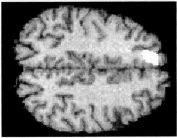

FIGURE 17. Brain activity associated with thinking about mental
states. When reading theory of
mind stories there was increased activity in the medial prefrontal cortex. This was not seen when reading
physical stories. The activity is
shown in white superimposed on
structural images in sagittal and horizontal view.

talising tasks are special cases of conditional tasks, but there is still considerable debate about the precise computational basis of such tasks. Our understanding of how the brain is able to mentalise will depend critically on further brain imaging studies in people.

VIII. THE NEUROPHYSIOLOGY OF CONSCIOUSNESS

A. An Extended System for Consciousness

One of our aims in this chapter has been to show that the content of consciousness is determined by the location of the associated brain activity and that this activity is in the same location during direct perception or action. For instance, when we hold the same perception or action "in mind" during imagery, recollection, or the mental manipulation of information. If this assumption is correct, it raises the question of how we distinguish between a direct perception, a memory or an act of imagination. If these states are to be distinguishable then they must be associated with different patterns of brain activity. We propose that this distinction critically depends upon frontal activity and, in particular, on the relationship between frontal activity and activity in the location that determines the contents of consciousness. The major difference between a direct perception and a mental image is that the nature of the direct perception is determined by events in the outside world. A mental image, by contrast, is determined from within and is the result of our own actions. Changes in perception have two sources. The first is caused by events and agents in the outside world that are outside our control. These changes are essentially unpredictable. The second results from our own actions (*e.g.*, moving our eyes across a scene). These changes are essentially predictable.

The well established mechanisms of corollary discharge and reafference copy provide one way in which the degree of predictability can be signaled [125,126]. The signals that lead to precisely determined movements of limbs or larynx can also be used to predict the sensory consequences of such actions (the forward model). Eye movements provide the most dramatic case. Each time we move our eyes, there is, in consequence, a rapid movement of our image of the world across the retina. It has been known for a long time that during rapid eye movements there is saccadic suppression. During the rapid movement of the eyes the image is effectively switched off. Paus and colleagues have performed an elegantly simple experiment to show the pattern of brain activity associated with this phenomenon [127]. Across a series of scans, volunteers lay in the dark and moved their eyes at different rates. Activity in the frontal eye fields was positively correlated with the rate of eye movements. However, in visual cortex and visual association areas the activity was negatively correlated with rate of eye movements. This result implies that each eye movement was accompanied by reduced activity in visual areas brought about by inhibitory corollary discharge and provides a physiological basis for saccadic suppression.

Similar observations have been made in the auditory system by recording neural activity from implanted electrodes. In the squirrel monkey cells have been found in the temporal cortex that respond to the vocalisations of other monkeys, but not when the monkey itself vocalises [128]. Creuzfeldt *et al.*, using implanted electrodes in patients undergoing neurosurgery, found areas of temporal cortex in which activity is reduced when patients vocalised [129]. The mechanism by which the sensory effects of our own actions can be predicted is likely to be intimately bound up with our sense of agency. In other words, we know we are in control of our actions because we can precisely predict their effects. We know almost nothing as yet about how we detect agency in the outside world, although this must be a very important ability in most mammals. It is likely that the mechanism for the detection of agency in others will be related to the mechanisms by which we are aware of our own agency. It should not be difficult to devise tasks in which volunteers have to detect that something is self-propelled or behaving in a goal directed manner [130].

Our proposal is that this modulation of perceptual areas by activity stemming from areas concerned with action generates differences in the overall patterns of activity that serve to identify the source of perceptions (internal or external). In principle, the same mechanism could be used to distinguish whether active representations derive from direct perception, memory or imagination. In these cases the critical interactions are likely to be with prefrontal rather than premotor areas. We have reviewed studies of active memory, of motor imagery, and of the manipulation of mental images. They all have shown activation in both prefrontal areas and sensory and/or motor association areas specific to the content of the mental image. However, there are other studies in which the relationship between frontal and posterior areas seems to be reciprocal since increased activity in one area is associated with decreased activity in the other.

B. Decreased Activity Associated with Willed Action

In the word generation task described in Section V.A volunteers had to summon into mind words beginning with a certain letter. In this task a representation of the word to be spoken becomes active in the absence of any presentation of that word to the senses. This task is associated with marked activation of left DLPFC and anterior cingulate. In the control task volunteers simply repeated the word that they heard. In this case there is an active representation of the word to be spoken which derives directly from the senses. In comparison with this control task there is reduced activity bilaterally in superior temporal cortex during word generation [56]. We have interpreted this result, which has been replicated many times, as evidence that the prefrontal cortex modulates temporal cortex during the intrinsic generation of words. We obtained a similar result with finger movements. When volunteers generated finger movements (contrasted with copying them) there was increased activity in prefrontal cortex and reduced activity in motor cortex and the region of the angular gyrus where lesions are associated with finger agnosia [56]. We have suggested a mechanism by which successful activation of a representation from sensory input (extrinsic, bottom–up) would require general activation of the network in which that representation was stored, while successful activation from an intrinsic source (top–down) would require a general reduction of activity in the same network [131]. However, the point we want to make here is that the difference in the level of activation also provides an indication of the source of the activation, *i.e.*, whether it was extrinsic or intrinsic. We suggest that, just as "corollary discharge" can label sensations as resulting from intrinsic actions, so the fronto-temporal interactions observed in word generation label inner representations as resulting from intrinsic actions. We anticipate that similar interactions will be identified that are associated with episodic memory and mental imagery.

A recurrent problem with the interpretation of brain imaging studies based on blood flow is that all measures are relative. We do not have a measure of absolute activity in any particular brain area, only a measure of activity relative to some other mental state. "Rest" is not associated with a lack of brain activity. We may be able to minimize sensory input and motor output in the "resting" state, but we cannot be sure about what kinds of mental activity are occurring. It may well be that at rest conscious, introspective processes predominate. Nevertheless, comparison with rest does provide some useful information on the word generation paradigm. We observed decreases of temporal lobe activity with word generation relative to word repetition. Word generation relative to rest is associated with increases of temporal lobe activity. However, these increases are not as large as those observed when we compare word repetition with rest [132]. Clearly delineation of the complex system level interactions within the brain that are a critical feature of conscious processes will require very careful choice of tasks and mental states for comparison.

C. Disconnections in the Extended System

In the major psychoses many of the key symptoms involve a loss of the feeling of agency or a false perception of agency in the outside world. For example patients with schizophrenia sometimes report that alien forces are controlling their actions (delusions of control) or that alien thoughts are being inserted in their minds (thought insertion). Auditory hallucinations are a particularly common feature of schizophrenia. There is increasing evidence that these experiences can be associated with patients' own subvocal speech or inner speech [133]. Functional imaging studies have shown that activity in Broca's area and left temporal cortex occurs during hallucinations [134]. All these observations suggest that schizophrenic patients are experiencing intrinsically generated activity as if it were extrinsically generated. A number of theories have been put forward essentially along the lines that patients with schizophrenia confuse memories and self-generated images with direct sensory perceptions (e.g., [135, Chap. 5]). We can now begin to think about how these descriptions at the psychological level can be translated into underlying physiology. On the basis of our discussion in the previous section we would predict that during the experience of schizophrenic symptoms something is going wrong with the interaction between prefrontal cortex and posterior brain areas concerned with the content of experience. The first direct evidence of such disconnections comes from studies of word generation in schizophrenia. We have already mentioned that when performing this task patients showed as much activation in DLPFC as controls. However, there was a striking failure to show the normal pattern of reduced activity in superior temporal cortex on the left (Fig. 18). This abnormality was observed both in chronic patients and in drug free patients in the acute phase of their illness [74,75].

We have yet to show whether this kind of disconnection can be directly related to the experience of symptoms such as auditory hallucinations and delusions of control. Preliminary studies of patients who are prone to hallucinate during remission suggest that they show abnormal patterns of brain activity when trying to imagine the sound of someone else's voice [136]. The location of this abnormal activity is in SMA and left superior temporal cortex. These areas are very likely to be part of the system involved in the generation and perception of speech.

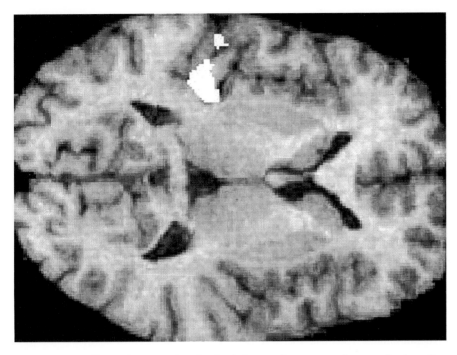

FIGURE 18. Failure of attenuation in the left superior temporal cortex in drug-free schizophrenic patients. In comparison to 6 normal controls, 12 drug-free schizophrenic patients show excess activity in the left superior temporal cortex during the performance of a word generation task.

IX. PERORATION

In this chapter we have discussed "higher order cognitive processes" as being various aspects of consciousness. We have taken a common sense and simplified view of consciousness as a state of "having things in mind". The content of consciousness (what it is we have in mind) is determined by the location of the associated brain activity in sensory and/or motor association cortex. Holding things in mind, manipulating things in mind, and getting ready to perceive or respond all require the additional function of prefrontal cortex. As yet there are few data to enable us to relate the location of frontal activity to different conscious functions, although a crude structure is beginning to emerge. Of course, none of these results tell us how consciousness emerges from brain activity, but through the technique of functional brain imaging we are beginning to get a very good idea of the locations and distributions of brain activity that are associated with consciousness.

References

1. T. Shallice. "From Neuropsychology to Mental Structure." Cambridge University Press, Cambridge, 1988.
2. J. A. Fodor. "Modularity of Mind." MIT Press, Cambridge, MA 1983.
3. S. Pinker. "The Language Instinct." Penguin Books, London, 1994.
4. N. Block. On a confusion about the function of consciousness. *Behav. Brain Sci.* **18,** 227–247 (1994).
5. A. Damasio. "Descartes Error." Grosset/Putnam, New York, 1994.
6. J. M. Fuster. "The Prefrontal Cortex." Raven Press, New York, 1989.

7. A. D. Baddeley. Working memory. *Science* **255,** 556–559 (1992).

8. P.S. Goldman-Rakic. Circuitry of primate prefrontal cortex and regulation of behaviour by representational knowledge. *In* "Handbook of Physiology—The Nervous System V" (V. B. Mountcastle, Ed.), pp. 373–417. Williams and Wilkins, Baltimore, 1987.

9. J. Jonides, E.E. Smith, R.A. Koeppe, E. Awh, S. Minoshima, and M. Mintum. Spatial working memory in humans as revealed by PET. *Nature* **36,** 623–625 (1993).

10. M. Petrides, B. Alivisatos, A. Evans, and E. Meyer. Dissociation of human mid-dorsolateral from posterior dorsolateral frontal cortex in memory processing. *Proc. Natl. Acad. Sci. USA,* **90,** 873–877(1993).

11. S. C. Baker, C. D. Frith, R. S. J. Frackowiak, and R. J. Dolan. The neural substrate of active memory for shape and spatial location in man. *Cereb. Cortex* **6,** 612–619 (1996)

12. H. R. Friedman and P. S. Goldman-Rakic. Coactivation of the prefrontal cortex and inferior parietal cortex in working memory revealed by 2DG functional mapping in the rhesus monkey. *J Neurosci.* **14,** 2775–2788 (1994).

13. K. M. Stephan, G. R. Fink, R. Passingham, D. Silbersweig, A. D. Ceballos Baumann, C. D. Frith and R. S. J. Frackowiak. Functional anatomy of the mental representation of upper extremity movements in healthy subjects. *J Neurophys.* **73,** 373–386 (1995).

14. C. Ceballos-Baumann, R. E. Passingham, C. D. Marsden, and D. J. Brooks. Motor reorganisation in acquired hemidystonia. *Ann. Neurol.,* **37,** 746–757 (1995).

15. H. Chertkov and D. Bubb. Functional activation and cognition: The ^{15}O PET subtraction method. *In* "Localization and Neuroimaging in Neuropsychology." Academic Press, San Diego, 1994.

16. D.H. Ingvar and L. Philipson. Distribution of cerebral blood flow in the dominant hemisphere during motor ideation and motor performance. *Ann. Neurol.* **2,** 230–237(1977).

17. W. James, "The Principles of Psychology." Holt, New York, 1890.

18. M. Corbetta, F. M. Miezin, G. L. Shulman, and S. E. Petersen. Selective attention modulates extrastriate visual regions in humans during visual feature descrimination and recognition. *In* "Exploring Brain Function with Positron Emission Tomography. CIBA Foundation Symposium" (D. J. Chadwick and J. Whelan, Eds.), pp 165–180. Wiley, Chichester, 1991.

19. M. Corbetta, F. M. Miezin, S. Dobmeyer, G. L. Shulman, and S. E. Petersen. Selective and divided attention during visual discriminations of shape, colour, and speed: Functional anatomy by positron emission tomography. *J. Neurosci.,* **11,** 2383–2402 (1991).

20. G. Fink, P. Halligan, J. Marshall, C. D. Frith, R. S. J. Frackowiak, and R. J. Dolan. Where does visual perception process the forest and trees? *Nature* **382,** 626–629 (1996).

21. M. Martin. Hemispheric specialization for local and global processing. *Neuropsychologia* **17,** 33–40 (1979).

22. L. C. Robertson, M. R. Lamb, and R. T. Knight. Effects of lesions of the temporal–parietal junction on perceptual and attentional processing in humans. *J. Neurosci.* **8,** 3757–3769 (1988).

23. G. Rees, R. S. J. Frackowiak, and C. D. Frith. Two modulatory effects of attention that mediate object categorization in human cortex. *Science* **275,** 835–838 (1997).

24. M. I. Posner and S. E. Petersen. The attention system of the human brain. *Annu. Rev. Neurosci.* **13,** 25–42 (1990).

25. F. Galton. "Inquiries into Human Faculty and Its Development." Macmillan, London, 1883.

26. R. E. Cytowic and F. B. Wood. Synesthesia. *Brain Cognit.* **1,** 23–35 (1982).

27. S. Baron-Cohen, J. Harrison, L. H. Goldstein, and M. Wyke. Coloured speech

perception: Is synaesthesia what happens when modularity breaks down? *Perception* **22,** 419–426 (1993).

28. E. Paulesu, J. Harrison, S. Baron-Cohen, J. D. G. Watson, L. H. Goldstein, J. Heather, R. S. J. Frackowiak, and C. D. Frith. The physiology of coloured hearing. A PET activation study of colour–word synaesthesia. *Brain* **118,** 661–676 (1995).

29. H. Komatsu, Y. Ideura, S. Kaji, and S. Yamane. Colour selectivity of neurons in the inferior temporal cortex of the awake macaque monkey. *J. Neurosci.* **12,** 408–424 (1992).

30. S. Zeki. Colour coding in the superior temporal sulcus of the rhesus monkey. *Proc. R. Soc. London B* **197,** 195–223 (1977).

31. L. Weiskrantz. "Blindsight. A Case Study and Implications." Oxford Univ. Press, Oxford, 1986.

32. J. L. Barbur, J. D. G. Watson, R. S. J. Frackowiak, and S. M. Zeki. Conscious visual perception without V1. *Brain* **116,** 1293–1302 (1993).

33. G. Bottini, E. Paulesu, R. Sterzi, E. Warburton, R. J. S. Wise, G. Vallar, R. S. J. Frackowiak, and C. D. Frith. Modulation of conscious experience by peripheral sensory stimuli. *Nature* **376,** 778–780 (1995).

34. G. Bottini, R. Sterzi, E. Paulesu, G. Vallar, S. F. Cappa, F. Erminio, R. E. Passingham, C. D. Frith, and R. S. J. Frackowiak. Identification of the central vestibular projections in man: A positron emission tomography activation study. *Exp. Brain Res.* **99,** 164–169 (1994).

35. A. D. Baddeley. "Working Memory." Oxford Univ. Press, Oxford, 1986.

36. A. R. Luria. "The Higher Cortical Functions in Man." Basic Books, New York, 1980.

37. C. Umilta. The control operations of consciousness. *In* "Consciousness in Contemporary Science" (A. J. Marcel and E. Bisiach, Eds.), pp 334–356. Oxford Univ. Press, Oxford, 1988.

38. B. Milner. Effects of different brain lesions on card sorting. *Arch. Neurol.* **9,** 90–100 (1963).

39. M. Petrides and B. Milner. Deficits in subject-ordered tasks after frontal- and temporal-lobe lesions in man. *Neuropsychologia* **20,** 249–262 (1982).

40. T. Shallice. Specific impairments of planning. *Phil. Trans. R. Soc. London* **298,** 199–209 (1982).

41. M. P. Deiber, R. E. Passingham, J. G. Colebatch, K. J. Friston, P. D. Nixon, and R. S. J. Frackowiak. Cortical areas and the selection of movement: A study with positron emission tomography. *Exp Brain Res.* **84,** 393–402 (1991).

42. I. H. Jenkins, D. J. Brooks, P. D. Nixon, R. S. J. Frackowiak, and R. E. Passingham. Motor sequence learning: A study with positron emission tomography. *J. Neurosci.* **14,** 3775–3790 (1994).

43. P. M. Grasby, C. D. Frith, K. J. Friston, C. Bench, R. S. J. Frackowiak, and R. J. Dolan. Functional mapping of brain areas implicated in auditory memory function. *Brain* **116,** 1–20 (1993).

44. E. Tulving, S. Kapur, H. J. Markovitsch, F. I. M. Craik, R. Habib, and S. Houle. Neuroanatomical correlates of retrieval in episodic memory: Auditory sentence recognition. *Proc. Natl. Acad. Sci. USA.* **91,** 2012–2015 (1994).

45. T. Shallice, P. C. Fletcher, C. D. Frith, P. Grasby, R. S. J. Frackowiak, and R. J. Dolan. Brain regions associated with acquisition and retrieval of verbal episodic memory. *Nature* **368,** 633–635 (1994).

46. A. M. Owen, J. J. Downes, B. J. Sahakian, C. E. Polkey, and T. W. Robbins. Planning and spatial working memory following frontal lobe lesions. *Neuropsychologia* **28,** 1021–1034 (1990).

47. D. R. Weinberger, K. F. Berman, and B. P. Illowsky. Physiological dysfunction of dorsolateral prefrontal cortex in schizophrenia III. A new cohort and evidence for a monoaminergic mechanism. *Arch. Gen. Psychol.* **45,** 609–615 (1988).

48. Berman, K. F., Illowsky, B. P., and Weinberger. D. R. Physiological dysfunction of dorsolateral prefrontal cortex in schizophrenia. IV. Further evidence for regional and behavioral specificity. *Arch. Gen. Psychol.* **45**, 616–622 (1988).

49. N. C. Andreasen, K. Rezali, R. Alliger, V. W. Swayze, M. Flaum, P. Kirchner, G. Cohen, and D. S. O'Leary. Hypofrontality in neuroleptic-naive patients and in patients with chronic schizophrenia: Assessment with xenon 133 single-photon emission computed tomography and the Tower of London. *Arch. Gen. Psychiatry* **49**, 943–958 (1992).

50. C. D. Frith, J. Leary, C. Cahill, and E. C. Johnstone. Disabilities and circumstances of schizophrenia patients—A follow-up study. IV. Performance on psychological tests: Demographic and clinical correlates of the results of these tests. *Br. J. Psychiatry.* **159** (Suppl. 13), 26–29 (1991).

51. G. Goldberg. Supplementary motor are a structure and function: Review and hypotheses. *Behav. Brain Sci.* **8**, 567–616 (1985).

52. E. A. Murray, and J. D. Coulter. Organisation of corticospinal neurons in the monkey. *J Comp Neurol.* **195**, 339–365 (1981).

53. J. Tanji and K. Kurata. Comparison of movement—Related activity in two cortical areas of primates. *J. Neurophysiol.* **48**, 633–653 (1982).

54. C. Brinkman and R. Porter. Supplementary motor area of the monkey: Activity of neurons during performance of a learned motor task. *J. Neurophysiol.* **42**, 681–709 (1979).

55. T. Paus, M. Petrides, A. Evans, and E. Meyer. Role of the human anterior cingulate cortex in the control of oculomotor, manual, and speech responses: A positron emission tomography study. *J. Neurophysiol.* **70**, 453–469 (1995).

56. C. D. Frith, K. J. Friston, P. F. Liddle, and R. S. J. Frackowiak. Willed action and the prefrontal cortex in man: a study with PET. *Proc. R. Soc. London B* **244**, 241–246 (1991).

57. M. Jahanshani, I. H. Jenkins, R. G. Brown, C. D. Marsden, R. E. Passingham, and D. J. Brooks. Self-initiated *versus* externally triggered movements. 1. An investigation using measurement of regional cerebral blood flow with PET and movement-related potentials in normal and Parkinson's disease subjects. *Brain* **118**, 913–934 (1995).

58. C. D. Frith, K. J. Friston, P. F. Liddle, and R. S. J. Frackowiak. A PET study of word finding. *Neuropsychologia.* **29**, 1137–1148 (1991).

59. M. I. Posner, S. E. Petersen, P. T. Fox, and Raichle. M. E. Localization of cognitive operations in the human brain. *Science* **240**, 1627–1631 (1988).

60. P. D. McLeod. A dual task response modality effect: Support for multiprocessor models of attention. *Q. J. Exp. Psychol.* **29**, 651–667 (1977).

61. P. C. Fletcher, C. D. Frith, P. M. Grasby, T. Shallice, R. S. J. Frackowiak, and R. J. Dolan. Brain systems for encoding and retrieval of auditory–verbal memory: An in vivo study in humans. *Brain* **118**, 401–416 (1995).

62. D. Laplane, J. Talaraich, V. Meininger, J. Banchaud, and J. M. Orgogozo. Clinical consequences of corticectomies involving the supplementary motor area in man. *J. Neurol. Sci.* **34**, 310–314 (1977).

63. A. R. Damasio and G. W. Van Hoesen. Structure and function of the supplementary motor area. *Neurology* **30**, 359 (1980).

64. G. Goldberg, N. H. Mayer, and J. U. Toglia. Medial frontal cortex infarction and the alien hand sign. *Arch. Neurol.* **38**, 683–688 (1981).

65. E. D. Playford, I. H. Jenkins, R. E. Passingham, M. D. Nutt, R. S. J. Frackowiak, and D. J. Brooks. Impaired mesial frontal and putamen activation in Parkinson's disease: A positron emission tomography study. *Ann. Neurol.* **32**, 151–161 (1992).

66. I. H. Jenkins, W. Fernandez, E. D. Playford, *et al.* Impaired activity of the supplementary motor area in Parkinson's disease is reversed when akinesia is treated with apomorphine. *Ann. Neurol.* **32**, 749–757 (1992).

67. C. D. Frith, and D. J. Done. Stereotyped responding by schizophrenic patients on a two-choice guessing task. *Psychol. Med.* **13**, 779–786 (1983).

68. N. Lyon, B. Mejsholm, and M. Lyon. Stereotyped responding by schizophrenic outpatients: cross-cultural confirmation of perseverative switching on a two-choice guessing task. *J. Psychol. Res.* **20,** 137–150 (1986).

69. D. H. Ingvar and G. Franzen. Abnormalities of cerebral blood flow distribution in patients with chronic schizophrenia. *Acta Psychiatr Scand.* **50,** 425–462 (1974).

70. P. Liddle, K. J. Friston, C. D. Frith, S. R. Hirsch, T. Jones, and R. S. J. Frackowiak. Patterns of cerebral blood flow in schizophrenia. *Br. J. Psychiatry* **160,** 179–186 (1992).

71. R. J. Dolan. Functional imaging in the neurobiology of the psychoses. *Sem. Neurosci.* **7,** 165–171 (1995).

72. R. J. Dolan, C. J. Bench, P. F. Liddle, K. J. Friston, C. D. Frith, P. M. Grasby, and R. S. J. Frackowiak. Dorsolateral prefrontal cortex dysfunction in the major psychoses: Symptom or disease specificity? *J. Neurol. Neurosurg. Psychol.* **56,** 1292–1298 (1993).

73. J. D. Teasdale, L. Proctor, and A. D. Baddeley. Working memory and stimulus-independent thought. *Eur. J. Cogn. Psychol.* **5,** 417–433 (1993).

74. C. D. Frith, K. J. Friston, S. Herold, D. Silbersweig, P. Fletcher, C. Cahill, R. J. Dolan, R. S. J. Frackowiak, and P. F. Liddle. Regional brain activity in chronic schizophrenic patients during the performance of a verbal fluency task. *Br J Psychiatry.* **167,** 343–349 (1995)

75. R. J. Dolan, P. Fletcher, C. D. Frith, K. J. Friston, R. S. J. Frackowiak, and P. J. Grasby. Dopaminergic modulation of an impaired cognitive activation in the anterior cingulate cortex in schizophrenia. *Nature* **378,** 180–182 (1995).

76. P. Ekman and W. V. Friesen. Felt, false and miserable smiles. *J Nonverb. Behav.* **6,** 238–252 (1982).

77. C. E. Izard. "Human Emotions." Plenum, New York, 1994.

78. C. Armon-Jones. "Varieties of Affect." Harvester Wheatsheaf, London, 1991.

79. N. H. Frijda. "The Emotions." Cambridge Univ. Press, Cambridge, 1994.

80. W. N. Morris. "Mood: The Frame of Mind." Springer-Verlag, New York, 1989.

81. R. M. Nesse. Evolutionary explanations of emotions. *Hum. Nature.* **1,** 261–289 (1990).

82. K. Oatley and P. N. Johnson-Laird. Towards a cognitive theory of emotion. *Cognit. Emotion* **1,** 29–50 (1987).

83. P. J. Eslinger and A.R. Damasio. Severe disturbance of higher cognition after bilateral frontal lobe ablation: Patient EVR. *Neurology* **35,** 1731–1741 (1985).

84. A. R. Damasio, D. Tranel, and H. Damasio. Individuals with sociopathic behavior caused by frontal damage fail to respond autonomically to social stimuli. *Behav. Brain Res.* **41,** 81–94 (1990).

85. M. B. Arnold. "Emotion and Personality." Columbia Univ. Press, New York, 1960.

86. R. Plutchik. Only four command systems for all emotions? *Behav. Brain Sci.* **5,** 442–443 (1982).

87. W. McDougall. "Outline of Psychology." Scribner, New York, 1994.

88. W. James. What is emotion? *Mind* **9,** 188–204 (1884).

89. C. G. Lange. "The Emotions." Williams and Wilkins, Baltimore, 1922.

90. J. W. Papez. A proposed mechanism of emotion. *Arch. Neurol. Psychiatry* **79,** 217–224 (1937).

91. P. D. MacLean. Some psychiatric implications of physiological studies on fronto-temporal portion of limbic system (visceral brain). *Electroencephalogr. Clin. Neurophysiol.* **4,** 407–418 (1952).

92. D. O. Hebb. "The Organisation of Behaviour." Wiley, New York, 1949.

93. L. Weiskrantz, Behavioural changes associated with ablation of the amygdaloid complex in monkeys. *J. Comp. Physiol. Psychol.* **49,** 381–391 (1956).

94. J. P. Aggleton and R. E. Passingham. Syndrome produced by lesions of the amygdala in monkeys. *J. Comp. Physiol. Psychol.* **95,** 961–977 (1981).

95. R. Adolphs, D. Tranel, H. Damasio and A. R. Damasio. Fear and the human amygdala. *J. Neurosci.* **15,** 5879–5891 (1995).

96. J. S. Morris, C. D. Frith, D. I. Perrett, D. Rowland, A. W. Young, A. J. Calder, and R. J. Dolan. A differential neural response in the human amygdala to fearful and happy facial expressions. *Nature* **383,** 812–815 (1996).

97. J. M. Harlow, Passage of an iron rod through the head. Boston Med. Surg. J **39,** 389–393(1848).

98. A. R. Damasio and G. W. Van Hoesen. Emotional disturbances associated with focal lesions of the frontal lobe. *In* "Neuropsychology of Human Emotion" (P. Satz, ed.), pp. 85–110 Guilford Press, New York, 1983.

99. B. Maxwell, D. A. Powell, and S. L. Buchanan. Multiple- and single-unit activity in area 32 (prelimbic region) of the medial prefrontal cortex during pavlovian heart rate conditioning in rabbits. *Cereb. Cortex* **4,** 230–246 (1994).

100. W. R. Miller. Psychological deficit in depression. *Psychol Bull.* **82,** 238–260 (1975).

101. H. Weingartner, R. Cohen, D. L. Murphy, J. Martello, and C. Gerdt. Cognitive processes in depression. *Arch. Gen. Psychol.* **38,** 42–47 (1981).

102. A. Calev, Y. Korin, B. Shapira, S. Kugelmass, and B. Lerer. Verbal and non-verbal recall by depressed and euthymic affective patients. *Psychol. Med.* **16,** 789–794 (1986).

103. R. G. Brown, L. C. Scott, C. J. Bench, and R. J. Dolan. Cognitive function in depression: Its relationship to the presence and severity of intellectual decline. *Psychol. Med.* **24,** 829–847 (1994).

104. R. Abrams and M. A. Taylor. Cognitive dysfunction in melancholia. *Psychol. Med.* **17,** 359–362 (1987).

105. C. J. Bench, K. J. Friston, R. G. Brown, L. Scott, R. S. J. Frackowiak, and R. J. Dolan. The anatomy of melancholia. Abnormalities of regional cerebral blood flow in major depression. *Psychol. Med.* **22,** 607–615 (1992).

106. C. J. Bench, R. S. J. Frackowiak, and R. J. Dolan. Changes in regional cerebral blood flow on recovery from depression. *Psychol. Med.* **25,** 247–262 (1995).

107. C. J. Bench, K. J. Friston, R. Brown, R. S. J. Frackowiak, and R. J. Dolan. Regional cerebral blood flow (rCBF) in depression measured by positron emission tomography (PET): The relationship with clinical dimensions. *Psychol. Med.* **23,** 579–590 (1993).

108. E. C. Johnstone and C. D. Frith. Validation of three dimensions of schizophrenic symptoms in a large unselected sample of patients. *Psychol. Med.* **26,** 669–679 (1996).

109. E. T. Rolls, J. Hornak, D. Wade, and J. McGrath. Emotion-related learning in patients with social and emotional changes associated with frontal lobe damage. *J. Neurol. Neurosurg. Psychiatry* **57,** 1518–1524 (1994).

110. E. T. Rolls. A theory of emotion and consciousness, and its application to understanding the neural basis of emotion. *In* "The Cognitive Neurosciences" (M. S. Gazzaniga, Ed.), pp. 1091–1106 MIT Press, Cambridge, MA, 1994.

111. J. D. Teasdale. Selective effects of emotion on information-processing. *In* "Attention: Selection, Awareness, and Control" (A. Baddeley and L. Weiskrantz, Eds.), pp. 374–389. Oxford Univ. Press, Oxford, 1993.

112. P. H. Blaney. Affect and memory. *Psychol. Bull.* **99,** 229–246 (1986).

113. H. C. Ellis and P. W. Ashbrook. The "state" of mood and memory research: A selective review. *In* "Mood and Memory" (D. Kuiken Ed), pp. 1–22. Sage, London, 1991.

114. J. V. Pardo, P. J. Pardo, and M. Raichle. Neural correlates of self-induced dysphoria. *Am. J. Psychiatry* **150,** 713–719 (1993).

115. M. S. George, T. A. Ketter, I. Parekh, B. Horwitz, P. Herscovitch, and R. Post. Brain activity during transient sadness and happiness in healthy women. *Am. J. Psychiatry.* **152,** 341–351 (1995).

116. E. Velten. A laboratory task for induction of mood states. *Behav. Res. Ther.* **6,** 473–482 (1968).

117. D. M. Clark, and J. D. Teasdale. Constraints on the effects of mood on memory. *J. Person Soc. Psychol.* **48,** 1595–1608 (1985).

118. W. J. H. Nauta. The problem of the frontal lobe: A reinterpretation. *J. Psychiatr. Res.* **8,** 167–187 (1971).

119. D. L. Cheney and R. M. Seyforth. "How Monkeys See the World." Chicago Univ. Press, Chicago, 1990.

120. L. Brothers. The social brain: A project for integrating primate behaviour and neurophysiology in a new domain. *Concepts Neurosci.*. **1,** 27–51 (1990).

121. U. Frith, J. Morton, and A. M. Leslie. The cognitive basis of a biological disorder: Autism. *Trends Neurosci.* **14,** 433–438 (1991).

122. P. Fletcher, F. Happe, U. Frith, S. C. Baker, R. J. Dolan, R. S. J. Frackowiak, and C. D. Frith. Other minds in the brain; a functional imaging study of "theory of mind" in story comprehension. *Cognition* **57,** 109–128 (1995).

123. B. M. Mazoyer, N. Tzourio, V. Frak, A. Syrota, N. Murayama, O. Levrier, G. Salamon, S. Dehaene, L. Cohen, and J. Mehler. The cortical representation of speech. *J. Cog. Neurosci.* **3,** 467–479 (1993).

124. T. J. Anderson, I. H. Jenkins, D. J. Brooks, M. Hawken, R. S. J. Frackowiak, and C. Kennard. Cortical control of saccades and fixation in man: A PET study. *Brain* **117,** 1073–1084 (1994).

125. W. Sperry. Neural basis of the spontaneous optokinetic response produced by visual inversion. *J Comp Physiol Psych.* **43,** 482–489 (1950).

126. E. von Holst and H. Mittelstaedt. Das Reafferenzprinzip (Wechselwirkungen zwischen Zentralnervensystem und Peripherie). *Naturwissenschaften.* **37,** 464–476 (1950).

127. T. Paus, S. Marrett, A. C. Evans, and K. Worsley. Imaging motor to sensory discharges in the human brain. *NeuroImage* **4,** 78–86 (1996).

128. P. Muller-Preuss and D. Ploog. Inhibition of auditory cortical neurons during phonation. *Brain Res.* **215,** 61–76 (1981).

129. O. Creutzfield, G. Ojeman, and E. Lettich. Neuronal activity in the human lateral temporal lobe. II. Responses to the subject's own voice. *Exp. Brain Res.* **77,** 476–489 (1989).

130. D. Premack and A. J. Premack. Origins of human social competence. *In* "The Cognitive Neurosciences" (M. S. Gazzaniga, Ed.). MIT Press, Cambridge, 1995.

131. K. J. Friston, C. D. Frith, P. Liddle, and R. S. J. Frackowiak. Investigating a network model of word generation with positron emission tomography. *Proc. R. Soc. London B* **244,** 101–106 (1991).

132. C. Weiller, C. Isensee, M. Rijntjes, W. Huber, S. Muller, D. Bier, K. Dutscheka, R. P. Woods, J. Noth, and H. C. Diener. Recovery from Wernicke's aphasia—A PET study. *Ann. Neurol.* **37,** 723–732 (1995).

133. C. D. Frith and P. C. Fletcher. Voices from nowhere. *Crit. Q.* **37,** 71–83 (1995).

134. P. K. McGuire, P. Shah, and R. M. Murray. Increased blood flow in Broca's area during auditory hallucinations in schizophrenia. *Lancet* **342,** 703–706 (1993).

135. C. D. Frith. "The Cognitive Neuropsychology of Schizophrenia." Erlbaum, Hove, 1992.

136. P. McGuire, D. A. Silbersweig, I. Wright, R. M. Murray, A. S. David, R. S. J. Frackowiak, and C. D. Frith. Abnormal inner speech: A physiological basis for auditory hallucinations. *Lancet* **346,** 596–600 (1995).

CHAPTER FIFTEEN

HUMAN MEMORY SYSTEMS

I. INTRODUCTION

Many aspects of cognition are uniquely human and it is ironic that memory, a faculty so central to personal human experience, is most shared across species. Memory is critical to the conduct of everyday life, providing a continuously updated working model and a unique personal record of the individual within an environment. Memory has a pivotal role in personal identity, a view first propounded by John Locke [1]. Memory is also integral to virtually all other cognitive functions and is expressed in the operation of other higher order psychological processes such as planning, reasoning, and problem solving. Its essential role in a wide range of psychological functions makes a powerful case that understanding the neurobiology of memory is critical to all domains of enquiry into the functional architecture of cognition. The isolated analysis of the functional anatomy of memory presented in this chapter might be interpreted as upholding the idea that brain function can be fractionated into discrete processes such as sensation, perception, attention, and memory. We adhere to this compartmentalisation only insofar as it provides a useful and conventionally recognised framework. The central aim of this chapter is to make explicit the contribution of functional imaging to understanding human memory function in terms of the conventional division into short- and long-term memory systems and to suggest that cognitive operations within memory are operations shared with other cognitive faculties.

II. THE STRUCTURE OF MEMORY

A. The Neurophysiology of Memory

At its simplest level memory embodies the notion of an information store and a persistence of this store over time. The most widely used concept that refers to this putative store is that of a memory engram defined as the *"state of a memory system before and after the encoding of an event"* [2]. William James speculating on the nature of this store inferred that it was *"a purely physical phenomenon, a morphological feature, the presence of these paths, namely in the finest recesses of the brain's tissue"* [3]. The medium for this long lasting memory storage remains uncertain although dynamic structural modification of synaptic circuitry remains the most plausible mechanism [4].

The neurophysiological basis of memory has important implications for the interpretation of functional imaging findings. Some forms of memory, such as short-term memory, are mediated by ongoing neural activity. Consequently functional imaging data must necessarily reflect the direct operations of this active memory system. Long-term memory, on the other hand, involves the establishment of stable patterns of neural connectivity. Data from functional imaging studies of long-term memory are thus less likely to reflect pure memory *per se*. This speaks to a distinction between the so-called memory trace or engram, which refers to the plastic component of memory, and sensory-motor elements from receptor to effector that are involved in the performance of a given memory task [5]. Tulving has made the point that the memory traces have no independent existence but only manifest themselves in combination with retrieval processes [2]. We suggest that it is these active processes or operations associated with long-term memory encoding or retrieval that are primarily reflected in patterns of neural activity obtained from functional imaging studies of long-term memory.

B. A Taxonomy of Memory

Memory is not a unitary construct. Cognitive psychology and neuropsychology have provided compelling evidence that memory can be dissociated into discrete processes. These processes can be distinguished from each other along a number of axes that include conscious access, functional role, capacity, temporal duration, and neural basis. The most fundamental and widely recognised distinction within memory is a dichotomy based upon temporal duration into short- and long-term components. These refer to a limited capacity store of brief duration and an high capacity system enduring over the lifetime of an individual [6]. An alternative description, based on functional role, is that of active and latent memory. These refer to memory that is currently guiding behaviour and a memory system that is largely functionally inactive but which can be activated in response to ongoing cues or behavioural contingencies. It is generally assumed that short-term memory (STM) and long-term memory (LTM) represent distinct or orthogonal systems. An issue that has direct bearing on this conjecture that can be addressed by functional imaging is the degree of anatomical overlap in the neuronal systems engaged by these psychologically distinct systems.

The concept of a short-term or active memory system has been extensively reformulated in terms of a working memory system that has provided a rich explanatory model for many of the behavioural observations on short-term memory [7]. Working memory enables the representation and selective attention to information not concurrently present in the sensory stream. Its functions are diffuse and include complex sentence comprehension, learning, mental arithmetic, reasoning, problem solving, and planning. In this sense its operations are unencapsulated and available to multiple cognitive domains. One structural account of working memory includes a core system, referred to as the central executive and "slave systems" that include a phonological loop and visuo-spatial sketch pad specialised for processing in the auditory–verbal and visual domains, respectively. However, these specified systems do not necessarily provide an exhaustive account of the modules or subsidiary systems available to working memory. A more extended analysis of the functioning of short-term memory systems is provided below.

From a functional perspective long-term memory can be described as latent in that it endures outside of conscious awareness but is available to conscious awareness in response to ongoing contingencies. The latent quality of long-term memory is consistent with an embodiment in the brain that involves enduring neural reorganisation. A widely accepted subdivision of long-term memory relates to the accessibility (declarative or explicit memory) or inaccessibility (procedural or implicit memory) of the retrieved elements to consciousness. Declarative memory is "unencapsulated" in the sense that its outputs are accessible to other cognitive systems, a feature shared with working memory. Within declarative memory, a division into semantic and episodic memory systems has been proposed [2]. Semantic memory is concerned with facts or knowledge about the world and is manifest in the process of knowing and, unlike episodic memory, has no necessary temporal or contextual landmarks. Only the cognitive referents but not the perceptual properties of input signals are registered in semantic memory. Episodic memory, on the other hand, deals with events that have a spatio-temporal dimension that provides an autobiographical context that we associate with the process of remembering [2]. Episodic memories are thus stored primarily in terms of their perceptual properties (Fig. 1).

The retrieval products of the memory systems described so far are all accessible to consciousness. A number of forms of memory reveal themselves solely in behaviour. In this sense they are unaccessible to consciousness and have no time or place event referents. These memory types fall under a general class referred to as nondeclarative memory. Examples include procedural memory and priming which manifest in skills, habits, or altered performance on indirect memory tests. Procedural memory and priming are, in contrast to declarative memory, prototypically modular and encapsulated. In other words, their functions are automatic, unconscious, and their outputs are generally unavailable to other cognitive operations. They represent forms of memory expressed solely in circumstances similar to those of initial learning. The dissociation from other systems of memory is exemplified by observations in amnesic patients who show intact procedural learning and priming [8]. Implicit memory processes are thought to be a function of the very modules engaged

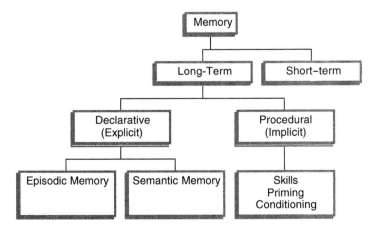

FIGURE 1 A taxonomy of memory.

in initial learning and may involve an adaptive tuning of neuronal groups within these processing modules [9,10]. Reactivation of these same neuronal configurations is a postulated mechanism for at least some forms of nondeclarative memory.

III. A FUNCTIONAL ANATOMY OF AUDITORY–VERBAL SHORT MEMORY

In the following sections we describe data that bear on the functional anatomy of human working memory. Working memory processes have been submitted to considerable modelling by cognitive psychologists. As a consequence the mapping of these processes is of broad theoretical interest and has direct bearing on the extent to which cognition may be mapped to physiology. The definition of working memory used here is the one originally proposed by Baddeley and Hitch [11] that refers to a limited-capacity, multicomponent cognitive system devoted to the temporary storage and active manipulation of information. Although alternative models of working memory have been described, based largely upon primate research, their implementation requires considerable pretraining and consequently are insufficient to describe the functional range of human working memory which includes executive, visuo-spatial, and verbal components. Human models of memory have the additional benefit that they are amenable to testing in the context of pathology. An illustration of this latter approach, based upon findings from developmental dyslexics, is presented below.

Early models of working memory, such as the "modal model" proposed by Atkinson and Shiffrin [12], postulated a unique short-term store where information has access from different sensory channels or from long-term memory for temporary manipulation and storage in long-term memory (for review, see Baddeley [13]). Such models could not easily accommodate the ability to carry out complex tasks such as reasoning or long-term learning with concurrent performance of tasks that, in theory, should have filled short-term memory capacities (*e.g.*, digit span tasks). The Baddeley and Hitch [11] model provided a more complex working memory model that could accommodate these observations. The central executive, the least specified component of the model, has been compared to the Norman and Shallice [14] Supervisory Attentional System and can account for observations that self-generated as opposed to routine acts interfere more powerfully with cognitive operations than simple span tasks.

In the Baddeley and Hitch model the central executive is supplemented by two slave systems specific for language and for visual material: a "phonological loop" and a visuo-spatial "sketch pad" (VSSP)[13]. Independence of verbal and visuo-spatial short-term storage has been demonstrated in psychological experiments in normal subjects [14–17]. Perhaps the most striking confirmation of this dichotomy comes from neuropsychological observations. Patients who fulfil the criteria of a classical double-dissociation have been described (see McCarthy and Warrington [18]). Patients affected by auditory verbal STM defects have diminished verbal span despite normal language function [19,20]. These same patients have an intact visuo-spatial short-term memory that contributes to the apparently paradoxical superior performance in verbal span tasks when stimuli are presented visually. The opposite dissociation is represented by patients with intact visuo-perceptive functions, defective visuo-spatial STM and intact auditory verbal STM [21,22].

A. Anatomical Studies of Working Memory

The component of human working memory known as the phonologial loop has received the greatest attention from cognitive psychologists. The phonological loop allows the maintenance through active rehearsal of verbal material, for example, when trying to remember a telephone number [23,24]. In the Salamè and Baddeley model, the phonological loop has two components: a subvocal rehearsal system, based on an articulatory code, and a short-term store, based on a phonological and acoustic code [25]. Independence of these components is indicated by observations of a differential interference of concurrent articulation (articulatory suppression) on the word length effect and on the phonological similarity effect. The word length effect refers to the fact that it is harder to keep words that take longer to articulate in short-term memory (*e.g.*, harpoon, Friday, coerce as opposed to bucket, wiggle, tipple). The phonological similarity effect accounts for the difficulty in remembering words that sound similar (can, mad, sat as opposed to bed, hall, frost) [26]. As articulatory suppression abolishes the word length effect but not the phonological similarity effect [23,24] this indicates that rehearsal processes based on an articulatory code are independent of short-term storage where auditory stimuli have privileged and direct access. However, when words are presented visually articulatory suppression also abolishes the phonological similarity effect, indicating that visual material needs rehearsal, or articulatory recoding, prior to access to a short-term store. These conclusions are supported by studies of the effect of unattended speech on verbal short-term memory performance for visually presented stimuli. Here, interference is maximal when unattended speech is phonologically similar to that being remembered. This is compelling evidence that the phonological loop is specialised for highly processed as opposed to early untransformed acoustic stimuli.

From the extensively specified cognitive psychology model, there are a number of predictions concerning the functional anatomy of the phonological loop. One prediction is that there should be a dissociation between areas concerned with rehearsal and storage. It can also be predicted that these anatomical sites have some degree of functional independence. Subvocal rehearsal in this model should involve areas concerned with language planning, while short-term storage should implicate areas involved in phonology but with functional independence from areas involved in early acoustic processing.

B. Functional Imaging Studies of Auditory Verbal Memory

We studied the neural correlates of verbal short-term memory with the explicit aim of dissecting the rehearsal from short-term storage components of the phonological loop [27]. The study involved four visually presented tasks, which were performed silently. Visual stimuli were either verbal (consonants of the Latin alphabet) or nonverbal (letters from the Korean alphabet presented to volunteers with no knowledge of Korean). In the verbal version subjects saw a sequence of six phonologically dissimilar consonants followed by a probe consonant. Subjects had to indicate whether or not the probe had been present in the preceding list. The task was considered to involve both the subvocal rehearsal system and phonological short-term storage. In the second verbal task subjects had to decide whether or not each consonant rhymed with a reference consonant (the consonant "B"). This task was considered to engage subvocalization exclusively. The results of this experiment are shown in Fig. 2.

Compared to its nonverbal equivalent, the memory task activated perisylvian areas primarily in the left hemisphere, including Broca's area, the superior temporal gyrus (Wernicke's area), the left insula (not directly visible in image renderings), and the inferior part of the supramarginal gyrus (BA 40). In addition there was also activation in supplementary motor area (SMA), left lingual gyrus, and cerebellum. Broca's and Wernicke's areas, insula, lingual gyrus, and SMA were also activated in the rhyming task, but the supramarginal area was not [27,28]. The findings fit well with the Baddeley and Hitch model of STM[11] and enabled us to conclude that the left temporoparietal junction at

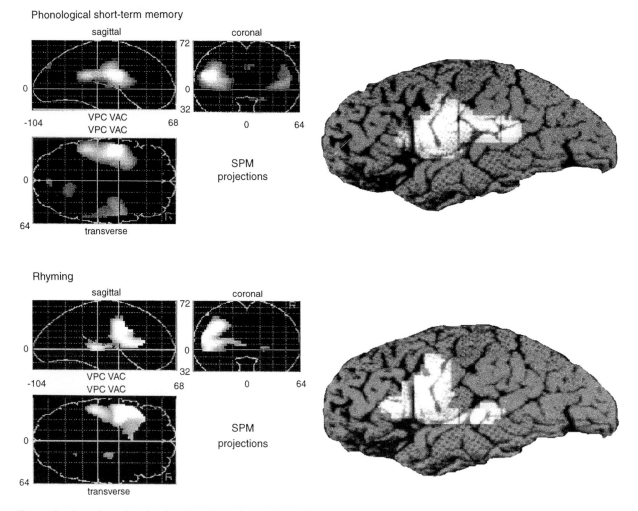

FIGURE 2 Location of activations during a phonological short-term memory tasks and a rhyming task for Latin letters in normal subjects. Left images show projections through sagittal, coronal, and transverse views of the brain. Right images aid interpretation of the areas of significant activation in the left hemisphere. Patterns of activation during phonological short-term memory and rhyming tasks are evident in the left temporo-parietal junction.

the supramarginal gyrus has a unique role in phonological short-term memory, operating as a short-term phonological buffer. Brain areas activated by the rhyming task we attributed to the functioning of the rehearsal system. This system notably involves Broca's area which, on the basis of the data, would appear to be specialised for rehearsal rather than short-term storage *per se*.

Converging evidence relating to the neural basis of verbal short-term memory is provided by phonology and language studies. Démonet *et al.* examined the neural systems engaged during either phonological or lexical–semantic processing [29]. The phonological task involved monitoring of sequences of phonemes in polysyllabic, consonant–vowel type, binaurally presented nonwords. Subjects had to respond whenever they detected the phoneme /b/ in a nonword if, and only if, the phoneme /d/ had been present in the preceding syllable. This phoneme detection task was compared with two other experimental conditions; a nonverbal task, in which subjects detected a rise of pitch in the third component of a triplet of pure tones, and a verbal task in which subjects detected words possessing two semantic criteria. In a comparison with the tones condition, the phoneme detection task activated both Broca's and Wernicke's areas. The activation of Broca's area was again interpreted as reflecting subvocal articulation used by subjects when performing the task. These results also conform to those published by Zatorre *et al.* [30]. Further analyses have shown that, in comparison to a word detection task, the phoneme detection task activated the same inferior part of the left supramarginal gyrus identified as the phonological short-term store by Paulesu *et al.* [27]. Such convergence is strong evidence that phoneme detection tasks engage phonological short-term memory. A lack of activation in a comparison of phoneme with pure-tone monitoring tasks can be interpreted as evidence that the left supramarginal region also possesses units that perform transformations other than phonological analysis (possibly with associative functions).

C. Early Acoustic Codes and Phonological Memory

We define early acoustic codes (EACs) as those cognitive abilities depending on explicit activity of primary auditory cortex (Heschl's gyrus). Prevalent views suggest that EACs should not contribute to verbal short-term memory [31]. On the other hand, nonverbal complex acoustic stimulation (orchestral music) has a small but significant interference effect on verbal span tasks. This suggests an alternative interpretation to a strict separation of EACs and verbal STM. Can data from brain physiology resolve these issues? Clearly, studies where stimuli are delivered auditorally are unsuitable. On the other hand, experiments involving inner speech mechanisms seem ideal. If the phonological codes subserving verbal working memory tasks also depend upon some form of mapping into EACs, then one might expect to see EAC activations due to reentrant activity even during inner speech based working memory tasks. This is perfectly plausible on anatomical grounds as there are feedback connections from associative to primary auditory cortex [32]. The spatial resolution of early PET activation experiments based on intersubject averaging could not exclude a contribution of EACs to phonological memory. However, we replicated our "inner speech" phonological short-term memory experiment using PET-MRI coregistration techniques both in single subjects and in group data [28]. Both analyses found no evidence that primary auditory cortex is activated during inner speech tasks indicating a functional independence of phonological STM and EACs.

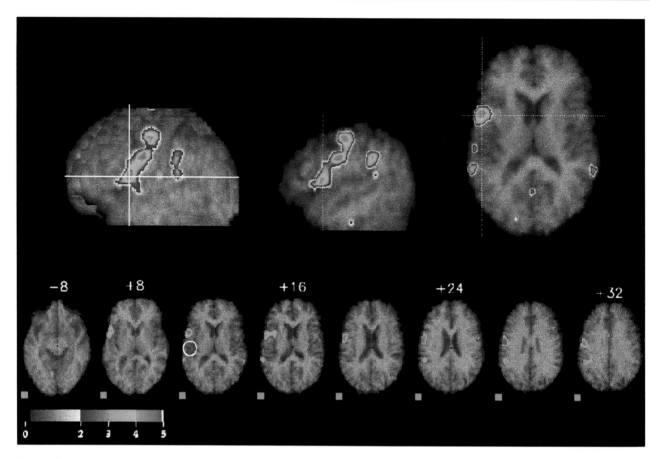

FIGURE 3 Phonological short-term memory seems independent from early acoustic codes. Data averaged from three subjects, performing the same inner-speech short-term memory task, are shown superimposed on averaged MRI images in stereotactic space. It can be readily seen that no activity is observed in this task within primary auditory cortex (Heschl's gyrus, inside the white circle).

The physiological basis of the interference of more complex patterns of nonverbal acoustic stimuli with verbal short-term memory remain to be explained. A recent study found that whilst monotonic series of noise bursts have no effect on verbal span, streams of changing tones (in time and/or in pitch) can be disruptive of serial recall of verbal stimuli [33]. Preliminary physiological evidence also indicates that nonmonotonic series of pure tones may compete for access to processing in the left supramarginal gyrus. Démonet *et al.* report that a nonverbal task in which subjects were instructed to detect a rise in pitch in the third component of a triplet of pure tones activates the lower bank of both supramarginal gyri (right much more than left) in comparison with an auditory lexical–semantic decision task [34]. Paulesu *et al.* asked subjects to listen to single words or to pure tones, both presented at varying intervals during PET scans (between 0.5 and 1.5 sec). Tones also varied in pitch within the frequencies of the human voice. Comparison of a pure tone task with a word listening task revealed bilateral (relative) activations in the supramarginal gyrus [28].

Taken together, these findings suggest that the lower bank of the left supramarginal gyrus is responsive to complex acoustic stimuli or to silent speech based phonological short-term memory tasks. Accordingly, a disruptive effect on verbal serial recall by complex acoustic patterns could be interpreted as competition between external stimulation and internal, short-term, phonological traces. This anatomical view of the interference effect is speculative and an explicit dual task experiment will be required to test the hypothesis formally.

To summarise, a number of predictions about the phonological loop have been verified in activation studies. The multicomponent nature of the loop is supported and specialisation of brain regions for short-term storage (the left temporo-parietal junction) and subvocalisation or articulatory rehearsal (Broca's area) have been demonstrated. Involvement of Broca's area in such processes meets predictions from cognitive psychology that rehearsal should be based on an articulatory (*i.e.*, speech planning) code. Finally, functional imaging also shows an independence between early acoustic codes and phonological memory. There remain large gaps in our knowledge of short-term memory that require further experimentation. The description of the anatomy of the rehearsal system is clearly underspecified such that a correspondence with cognitive psychological models is, at best, insufficient. Models and paradigms that can tease apart subcomponents of the rehearsal system are clearly needed. Classical paradigms used to refine the cognitive model of the phonological loop, as for example articulatory suppression, word length and phonological similarity effects, have not been widely used with functional imaging. An ideal cross-validation of cognitive and anatomical models of the phonological loop requires a correspondence between robust behavioural effects and regional brain physiology.

IV. THE FUNCTIONAL ANATOMY OF VISUO-SPATIAL SHORT-TERM MEMORY

A. The Anatomy of the VSSP

The VSSP is a convenient short-hand for Baddeley's account of visual short-term memory that incorporates processes of active visualisation used during mental imagery [13]. In this system, perceptual abilities are dissociable from STM in both humans [21] and primates [35]. The issue of a correspondence between visuo-perceptual codes and working memory codes and the extent of correspondence between human and primate visual working memory systems is the subject of this section.

The question to be asked is whether there are single or multiple visual working memory systems? A tenet of the physiology of visual perception is that attributes of the visual world (shape, colour, motion) are processed in segregated pathways with subsequent integration [36] (Chapter 9). A popular dichotomy also suggests that object and spatial knowledge are processed in ventral occipito-temporal and a dorsal occipito-parietal pathways, respectively [37]. This corresponds to the "what" and "where" pathways, a concept that has been criticised as an oversimplification [38].

The evidence for the existence of a seperate visual short-term storage system has been described by Posner and Keele [15]. Phillips has provided compelling evidence for a distinction between iconic visual memory (that covers span times of about 0.2–0.3 sec) and visual short-term memory (that covers span times as long as 8 sec) [39,40]. Phillips also performed a number of probe recognition experiments presenting, on a tachistoscope screen, matrices of squares of increasing complexity [40]. He studied the effect of increasing interstimulus intervals between stimulus and probe and the effects of shifting the position of the probes on performance. By shifting the position of the probe matrix on the screen, it is possible to interfere with performance when the interstimulus interval is very short (about 0.2 sec). For longer intervals, however, there is no effect of shifting the matrix which indicates that iconic memory relies on retinotopic coordinates and visual short-term memory on a more abstract coordinate system. An extension of this argument suggests that the memory component of the VSSP may be spatial rather than visual in nature [41]. Ellis and Allport (1985) have used the same argument to explain their finding of differential decay rates for viewer-centred coordinates and object-centred coordinates during a same–different matching task using photographs of common objects [42]. Why might a short-term visual memory store be spatial in nature? Marr (1982) provided a clue in his suggestion that object recognition *via* object-centred models would require a spatial model appended to a current model of the scene [43]. Thompson (1983) argues that this would be crucial for visual guidance of locomotion [44].

The distinction between visual and spatial codes in working memory has been proposed from a different perspective by neuropsychologists interested in mental imagery, which we consider here as part of the same VSSP [45]. Evidence of such a dissociation within mental imagery is provided by Levine *et al.* [46]. They reported a patient who, following occipito-parietal brain injury, was perfectly capable of describing and drawing objects from memory but unable to describe the relative spatial locations of well known things (*e.g.*, cities in the United States on a map, landmarks of his neighbourhood). We are not aware of the reverse dissociation (preserved imagery for spatial locations and impaired imagery for objects). The majority of mental imagery theorists hold that the visual buffer used for active visualisation is the same as that used for storage of visual information about the outside world [47].

In conclusion, the what and where dichotomy seems to hold explanatory power for the VSSP of working memory. However, the dichotomy is proposed in different ways by different authors; first, to distinguish between iconic and short-term memory; second, to distinguish between mental imagery codes for objects and for spatial locations. On this basis it is possible to predict that visual short-term memory tasks, combined with functional imaging, should reveal brain areas specialised for the "on-line" maintenance of information additional to that involved in simple perception. The simple "what and where" model offers the straightforward prediction that the elements of memory should be relatively segregated within each stream depending on the nature of the study material. On the other hand, the Humphreys and Bruce model suggests that memory for objects and memory for spatial locations should depend upon the activity of brain areas concerned with spatial coordinates as opposed to retinotopic coordinates [47].

B. The Functional Anatomy of Visuo-spatial Memory

To what extent do putative visual as opposed to spatial codes contribute to the VSSP in man? One study with bearing on this issue is that of Haxby *et al.* [48]. The authors asked the question whether the "what and where" dichotomy applies to the human brain. Subjects were required to perform a face matching, dot-location or sensorimotor control task. During each trial subjects were presented with three squares containing one picture each; one square appearing on the upper portion of a computer screen and two squares paired on the bottom of the screen. The subjects' task was to indicate which of the lower squares contained a picture of the same person shown in the upper square. In a spatial vision task subjects were challenged with a dot location matching task arranged identically to the face-matching task. Subjects indicated their responses (right or left) by pressing a key with the right or left thumb. The control sensorimotor task involved alternating right and left key press in response to visual presentation of empty squares. Compared to baseline, both tasks activated the lateral occipital cortex. Face discrimination alone activated a region of the occipito-temporal cortex, whereas the spatial location task activated a region of the lateral superior parietal cortex. The authors concluded that the data provided evidence for dissociable pathways subserving object and spatial visual processing. Given the amount of active exploration needed to deal with this complex matching to sample task (the spatial task, in particular, involved a degree of mental rotation) it can be argued that the data also provide evidence that these different codes may also contribute to working memory.

Jonides and colleagues directly addressed the issue of the anatomy of visuo-spatial working memory in an experiment involving two tasks [49]. In a memory condition subjects were briefly shown a pattern of dots for 200 msec on a computer screen. After a 3-sec delay they were required to indicate whether one of the dots would have fallen within a circle shown on the screen. A baseline task involved presentation of the dot pattern at the same time as the circle. A comparison of conditions revealed significant activation in the right hemisphere, in the parietal, occipital, premotor, and ventral prefrontal cortices. The authors interpret activation in BA 47 as the homologue of the principal sulcus in the macaque, a claim not supported by classical comparative anatomical studies [35], which suggest that the human homologue of the principal sulcus lies within BA 46.

We compared two tasks, one requiring shape similarity judgements on Korean letters and the other involving STM for strings of Korean letters (which cannot be coded phonologically by non-Korean speakers) to tasks where the stimuli were Latin letters [50]. These comparisons are the opposite of those in the experiment on the phonological loop [27]. The two systems challenged by the different material (Latin letters and the nonsymbolic line drawings of the Korean letters) we considered orthogonal rather than embedded and increased activation across both dimensions as analogous to a double anatomical dissociation between verbal and visual working memory systems. Immediate matching of the Korean letters, based on shape similarity, was dependent on bilateral dorsal occipital cortex activation with an additional small activation in the right ventral prefrontal cortex (Figure 4). Short-term memory for the same material, however, resulted in a much more extensive pattern of activation involving parietal cortex bilaterally (right more than left as in Jonides's experiment [49]) and also dorso-lateral prefrontal and ventral prefrontal cortices.

How do these data fit with the physiology of working memory described in primates? Experiments in macaques emphasise the role of dorso-lateral prefrontal cortex in visuo-spatial working memory. Lesion and cellular recording studies during delayed response or delayed-alternation tasks implicate the dorso-lateral prefrontal cortex near the principal sulcus (Walker's area 46). This area is massively connected with parietal cortex and diencephalic and limbic structures. Involvement of both DLPFC and parietal cortex during

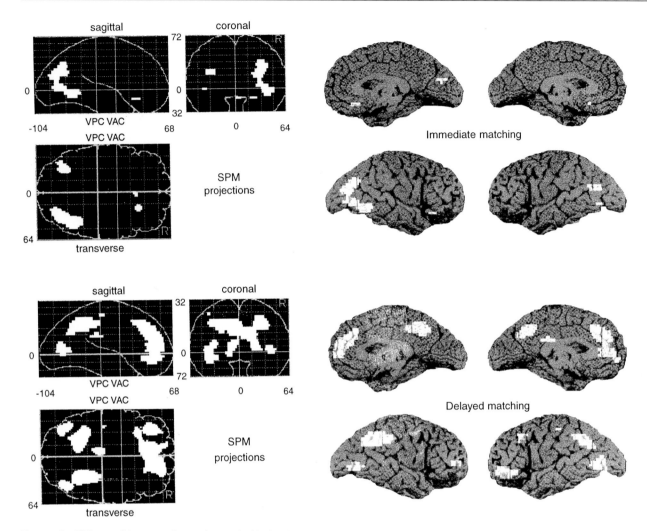

FIGURE 4   When subjects perform shape similarity judgements on nonsymbolic line drawings (visual immediate matching task) or perform a short-term memory task for strings of Korean letters (visual delayed matching task) distinct patterns of activation are observed. Strikingly greater activation is seen in anterior brain regions with delayed matching.

spatial delayed-response tasks is also suggested by imaging techniques using the 2DG autoradiographic method [51]. On the other hand, performance of matching-to-sample tasks, in which the remembered stimuli are objects rather than spatial locations, is sensitive to lesions of the inferior convexity of the frontal lobes (Walker's area 12) but insensitive to lesions near the principal sulcus. Further, the inferior convexity of the frontal lobes is massively connected to inferior temporal cortices where lesions selectively impair object matching [52]. Taken together, these data represent an anatomical double dissociation of "what and where" pathways within the frontal lobe.

Do the data fit those expected from cognitive psychology and neuropsychology? Jonides's experiment is straightforward and shows that brain areas involved in spatial processing are more activated when the tasks have a memory demand. Haxby's tasks, although not explicitly designed as working memory tasks, are likely to depend on active manipulation of stimuli and the results fit those predicted by Farah *et al.* [53]. Perception and visual working memory depend on different codes, either visual or spatial depending on the nature of material to be remembered. On the other hand, our data show that line drawings that can be considered as special instances of objects can be perceived and discriminated in a immediate-matching task by processes involving the occipital cortex alone [50]. Short-term memory for the same material, however, requires contributions from parietal and prefrontal cortices, including the dorso-lateral prefrontal convexity. This finding provides evidence for the model proposed by Humphreys and Bruce that visual short-term memory requires transformation of visual coordinates into viewer centred (spatial) coordinates [47]. Additional studies with a wider range of material are needed to assess whether these interpretations are indeed correct. In addition it is likely that a great deal of information on the physiology of the VSSP will emerge from experiments on mental imagery.

C. The Anatomy of the Central Executive System

The classical working memory theory is that the central executive represents the attentional component of working memory and that it allows integration of the activity of slave systems that are involved in strategy selection, planning, and retrieval during the performance of simple digit span tasks [13]. It is possible that the notion of a central executive is of *"a poorly specified and very powerful system that could be criticised as little more than an homunculus within the (working memory) model"* [54]. No functional imaging data are available that address this topic systematically. The conceptual similarities between the central executive and the supervisory attentional system of Norman and Shallice have already been mentioned [14].

If functional imaging was expected to give answers about the plausibility of the central executive concept, similarities would be expected between the anatomy that subserves performance across different memory tasks and that which combines these components. Whilst no convincing test of the central executive hypothesis has appeared in the functional imaging literature there are a number of experiments in which components of the executive functions have been investigated. These include attention, long-term episodic memory, willed action, random digit generation using above span lists of digits and dual task interference combined with episodic memory encoding tasks [55–59].

V. DYSFUNCTIONAL WORKING MEMORY

A. Neuropsychological Studies

Lesion studies on anatomical candidate sites for working memory have reported critical dissociations. The correspondence between findings from functional imaging studies in normal subjects and findings from patients is therefore critical. In this regard the phonological loop represents the most tractable problem. Pathological anatomical models of deficits of the rehearsal component of the phonological loop in patients have been described. Typically these patients have a limited verbal short-term memory buffer despite normal language understanding and production [31]. The same patients have preserved phonological skills that are necessary for performing a simple rhyme task. Metaanalysis of lesion sites in these patients led Shallice and Vallar to the conclusion that the core lesions is in the left inferior parietal cortex [31]. On the basis of their data a potential contribution of superior temporal cortex cannot be disregarded, as most lesions also involve the superior temporal cortex. Furthermore, it is the case that a lesion in a discrete brain area can have an impact on surrounding brain function. Thus, an isolated inferior parietal lesion may well cause reduced function in superior parietal cortex by disconnection. Shallice and Vallar's conclusion is complemented by observations identifying the temporo-parietal junction as the phonological store in normal subjects.

However, alternative interpretations of pathological data in the auditory verbal short-term memory syndrome suggest that acceptance of a correspondence between normal and patient anatomical data is premature. The properties of the phonological loop may arise from an interaction of the various anatomical components rather than from the cognitive contribution of a series of specialised brain areas. This idea predicts that lesions anywhere within the loop could lead to impaired verbal short-term memory. Alternatively, one could speculate that the residual behavioural skills observed in patients with a selective defect might arise from the activity of an intact right hemisphere. If this were so, modeling of the loop based on neuropsychological data should be reconsidered. There is evidence, however, to show that the first hypothesis is invalid. Indeed, the pathological literature offers preliminary evidence of a double anatomical dissociation within the phonological loop and has shown that patients with anterior perisylvian lesions involving Broca's area have significantly greater verbal spans than patients with posterior lesions [60]. This dissociation fits with one physiological model of the phonological loop, in which Broca's area is considered a relatively "memory independent" component concerned with rehearsal rather than with short-term storage. The acid test for this dissociation, however, would be activation studies that show that a spared component of the loop (that in normal subjects depends more heavily on the left hemisphere) can be activated during specific tasks. Independent activation of subcomponents of the loop would be a strong argument in favour of modularity of the system. In addition, such studies should allow a test of the right hemisphere hypothesis. We are not aware of any such activation studies in patients with acquired deficits.

However, there is an increasing wealth of functional imaging studies in developmental dyslexia that are addressing these issues. The basic deficit in dyslexia has been thought to involve a deficit of phonology [61,62]. Dyslexic children have difficulty mapping subsyllabic segments of speech (phonemes) onto graphemes. Early sensitivity to the phonological aspects of words determines how easily a child learns to map spoken words onto written words and so develop an alphabetic reading system [63,64]. Phonology plays a major role in verbal working memory as the short-term buffer is based on a phonological code. Not surprisingly, dyslexic patients show reduced verbal span and reduced abilities in manipulating verbal material on the basis of word sounds. Developmental dyslexia (and this may also apply to other developmental disorders) is therefore of particular interest for study by functional imaging because the behavioural abnormalities are not associated with macroscopic brain lesions. In such patients it is possible to circumvent many of the methodological problems associated with imaging studies of acquired disorders due to lesions.

B. Functional Imaging in Dyslexia

Since dyslexics seem to have a very circumscribed functional defect within the phonological loop, functional imaging studies of dyslexic people may inform the debate as to the precise role of the various brain areas implicated in normal phonological processing. One activation study has suggested that a component of the problem experienced by dyslexics may be due to a dysfunctional phonological loop [65]. In this study developmental dyslexics failed to activate their left planum temporale during a rhyming task, a result that complements pathological and structural imaging evidence of abnormal left planum temporale in dyslexia. Dyslexics also show difficulties in other phonologically based abilities (*e.g.*, verbal short-term memory) that depend on a more distributed neural system.

We examined whether alteration of planum temporale activity can explain phonological dysfunction [66]. We challenged five adult developmental dyslexics with established phonological loop tasks. The ease of the tasks was such that dyslexics were able to perform satisfactorily, despite psychological evidence of altered verbal short-term memory and word sound manipulation on more demanding tasks. Only a subset of the brain regions normally involved in phonological processing was activated, Broca's area during the rhyming task and the left parietal and temporal cortex during the short-term memory task. In contrast to normals, these areas were not activated in concert. Furthermore, the left insula was never activated in dyslexics (Fig. 4). One interpretation is that the defective phonological system in dyslexics results from a lack of connectivity between anterior and posterior areas involved in the articulatory loop. This may be due to a dysfunctional left insula which in normals could mediate functional integration between Broca's area and superior temporal and inferior parietal cortices.

The findings in dyslexics provide additional data about functional segregation within the anatomy of the loop. The isolated activation of Broca's area during a rhyming task supports the notion that this brain region is involved in both subvocalisation and probably also speech perception. The isolated activation of left temporo-parietal cortex during the memory task supports the suggestion of specialisation for functions consistent with a phonological buffer. Although similar conclusions could be drawn from normal subject studies, the results from dyslexics provide powerful confirmatory evidence. It is also evident from the results of this study that investigations of patients have a role in the grander enterprise of linking cognition to brain function.

VI. AUDITORY VERBAL EPISODIC LONG-TERM MEMORY

Long-term episodic memory has assumed increasing importance in the psychological literature on human memory with the recognition that this memory system is primarily impaired in amnesia. The classic amnesic syndrome results in a loss of episodic memory and can occur after a relatively circumscribed brain lesion. In this context it is surprising that functional imaging studies provide evidence for the involvement of widespread brain regions in episodic memory. The involvement of many of the identified regions does, however, find support in existing evidence from neuropsychology and animal experimentation. From the functional imaging and lesion literature the regions mutually shown to be of importance in episodic memory include the thalami [67–69], the medial temporal lobes [59,70–72], the prefrontal [58,67,73–75] and posterior cingulate cortices [58,59,68,76,77], cerebellum [59], and a medial parietal region called the precuneus [67,78]. These unexpected findings clearly require a functional explanation. For example, it has been suggested that the anterior cingulate cortex activations reflect the attentional demands of the memory tasks [67]. Similarly, the precuneus has been associated with visual imagery processes associated with episodic memory retrieval [78]. These issues of functional specialisation provide a focus for a discussion of functional imaging experiments of episodic long term memory.

A. Functional Maps of Episodic Auditory Verbal Long-Term Memory

In one of the first functional imaging experiments to explore the neural basis of episodic memory we studied subjects using a paradigm requiring the free recall of word lists [67]. Volunteer subjects were scanned under two separate conditions. In one condition the subjects were presented with 15-item word lists with prior instruction to immediately free recall as many items as possible. In order to subtract the auditory–verbal and the short-term memory components of this task the subjects were also scanned during the immediate free recall of 5-item word lists. This subtraction identifies a system primarily engaged by long-term episodic memory. The findings revealed widespread activations in the left and right prefrontal cortex, the posterior cingulate cortex, and the precuneus. In a between-group comparison with a neutral rest condition additional activations were seen in the thalamus, the anterior cingulate, and the lateral temporal cortices.

In a subsequent study we again addressed the issue of the functional anatomy of auditory–verbal memory using a different conceptual methodology involving a parametric approach [59]. The paradigm again involved word list learning but instead of a categorical comparison we used a graded task approach involving listening to, and repeating back, word lists that for each scan could vary in length from 2 to 13 items. The total word list length was, however, constant for each scan and consequently during any one scan subjects might hear a set of 3-item word lists, while in another the wordlists were, for example, 11 items in length. The adoption of a graded response type paradigm also necessitated a parametric approach to the data analysis. Using this design we were able to interrogate the data for significant correlations between brain activity and variation in independent variables that included word list length (memory load) and the degree of ongoing encoding. Thus, the graded task technique allowed a more intricate analysis of the data including a direct correlation of rCBF with components of memory performance measured as the proportion of each word list correctly recalled.

The primary patterns of activation revealed in this study were strikingly similar to those of the previous (cognitive subtraction) experiment. Overall, increasing list length was correlated with activations in bilateral prefrontal cortices, thalamus, anterior cingulate cortex, precuneus, and cerebellum. In an analysis of rCBF changes with performance we ignored scans for the shorter word lists, since performance was at ceiling and was assumed to reflect the predominant operation of short-term memory. Scans obtained during word lists 7 to 13 inclusive were weighted according to actual memory performance as this allowed optimal evaluation of brain systems engaged during successful learning. In this analysis there were again activations in the prefrontal, anterior cingulate and cerebellar cortices as well as in precuneus and thalamus. Most importantly we observed a significant bilateral hippocampal activation (left greater than right).

The interpretation of these early experiments is complicated by the fact that the rCBF changes due to the encoding, storage, and retrieval stages of memory are confounded. However, they define a complete system involved in overall memory function. The most fundamental components of memory processes are those associated with encoding and retrieval operations and it is therefore critical to consider experiments which dissociate these processes in order to define the related functional anatomy. Appropriate strategies, while conceptually simple, are not without important methodological difficulties, as will become apparent.

B. Encoding of Episodic Memory

Encoding is a simple term for a complex cognitive process that at its simplest refers to a process that converts an event into an enduring, and retrievable, memory. A degree of episodic encoding is an automatic part of any conscious experience in that learning can occur without conscious intent [80]. *Prima facie,* it seems unavoidable that the presentation of auditory verbal material will be associated with encoding and even simple tasks, designed to control for the auditory–verbal demands of a memory task, must necessarily involve a degree of encoding. This is an obstacle to studies of encoding based upon cognitive subtraction paradigms and two methodological approaches will be described that surmount this difficulty.

One approach employed a strategy that capitalised on the varying degrees of encoding that characterise different cognitive operations performed on auditory–verbal material [80]. The framework for this approach is derived from Levels of Processing Theory which states that deep, or more effective, encoding is a product of a greater degree of semantic processing [81]. A study of normal volunteers, using this approach, involved scanning subjects while they processed auditory–verbal material in one of two ways. The first task required a semantic decision which, within the theory, results in deep encoding, while the second task required an orthographic decision that results in shallow encoding. A comparison between the patterns of neural activation in the orthographic and the semantic decision tasks can be predicted to highlight areas engaged by effective encoding. The main finding from this study was that the primary area engaged during effective encoding was the left prefrontal cortex.

One potential drawback of this approach is that, although a semantic operation at encoding will improve subsequent recall if the cue is semantically based, it is also true that an orthographic/phonologic manipulation at encoding will result in a high degree of recall if the cue is orthographically/phonologically based [2]. We therefore adopted an alternative approach [58,68]. In our study brain activity was measured while subjects were presented with paired associate words (each pair consisting of a category and an appropriate exemplar, *e.g.,* Poet ... Browning). Subjects were given explicit prior instructions to facilitate remembering the associates. The control condition, designed to account for verbal input, involved passive listening to identically paced repetitions of the words "One thousand ... Two thousand." This control task also involves at least a degree of episodic encoding. However, this simple design does not control for priming/semantic processes that automatically occur in association with any encoding task. To overcome this pitfall we employed a dual task methodology. This has its basis in the finding that a distracting task interferes with episodic memory encoding but not with semantic/priming processes [82,83]. Subjects were therefore required to perform a distracting motor task (and also a nondistracting task to control for movement) simultaneously with the encoding task. A distracting secondary task interferes with episodic encoding and not with priming. We therefore reasoned that the areas involved in episodic encoding should be selectively attenuated by performance of the dual task.

The principal findings were that performance of the dual task resulted in an attenuation of activation in the left prefrontal cortex and in the posterior cingulate cortex (Fig. 5). Thus, our study indicated significant involvement of the left prefrontal cortex at encoding a finding also described by others [80]. The two foci comprise two of the four areas identified by more general tasks that encompassed both encoding and retrieval stages of episodic memory [59,67].

C. Retrieval of Episodic Memory

An early attempt to determine the neural basis of episodic memory retrieval used a word stem completion paradigm in which subjects had previously been presented with the entire words [70]. The neural associations of episodic retrieval were isolated by rCBF measurements taken during a baseline task in which subjects completed word stems that could not be used to form previously seen words and those obtained during a priming or implicit memory task. In this task subjects were unaware that word stems presented during the scanning period could be completed to form previously seen words. The main finding in association with the episodic memory retrieval tasks was activation of the right hippocampus and the right frontal lobe. A subsequently reported study measured rCBF in subjects engaged in recognition of sentences that had been presented 24 hr previously [84]. Here again there was a predominantly right-sided frontal activation together with a posterior medial parietal activation.

We examined episodic memory retrieval using identical verbal paired associates to those used in our encoding experiment [58,68]. This time, the initial presentation of the items occurred 5 min prior to scanning. Scans were

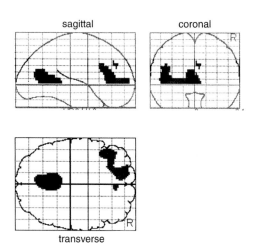

FIGURE 5   Regions activated in association with an episodic memory encoding task.

subsequently performed during the cued retrieval of word pairs while a control task employed word repetition. A comparison of the two tasks showed significant activation of the right frontal cortex, the anterior cingulate cortex, the left and right thalami, and the precuneus in association with episodic retrieval. This does not, however, represent a pure episodic memory paradigm since brain regions involved in retrieval from semantic memory will also be engaged. To identify these regions, subjects also underwent rCBF measurements while they performed a task specific to semantic memory. This task involved presentation of categories to which they had not previously been exposed with the prior instruction to provide a relevant exemplar, from semantic memory, to each category. Comparison of this condition with the control (repetition) task showed activation of the left and right thalamus and the anterior cingulate cortex. A direct comparison between the episodic and semantic retrieval conditions showed specific engagement of the right prefrontal cortex and precuneus. The importance of this dissociation is that it provided for the first time functional anatomical support for the taxonomic distinction between episodic and semantic memory (see Fig. 6).

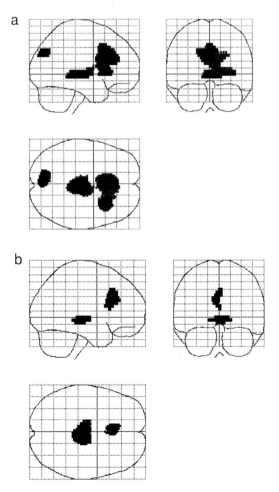

FIGURE 6 (a) Regions activated in association with an episodic memory retrieval task. (b) Regions activated in association with a semantic memory retrieval task. The differences, representing areas associated purely with episodic retrieval, are in the right prefrontal cortex and the precuneus (medial parietal region).

Functional imaging studies therefore indicate engagement of multiple brain regions during the performance of episodic memory tasks. Refinement of task design has indicated functional specialisation with the left prefrontal and posterior cingulate cortex for operations active during encoding and the right prefrontal cortex and precuneus for operations active at retrieval. These areas in combination encompass all of the regions we had previously identified in studies that confounded activations due to both encoding and retrieval operations. The findings clearly raise the issue of the contribution of individual brain regions to memory. To determine the predominant functional contribution of individual areas we took the approach of refining experimental tasks in order to manipulate the demands on cognitive subprocesses that we thought were critical to encoding and retrieval.

VII. FUNCTIONAL SPECIALISATION FOR MEMORY PROCESSES

A. Imagery in Retrieval

In all our studies involving episodic memory retrieval a medial parietal region, the precuneus, is consistently activated [58,59,67]. Common features of these studies were the use of concrete highly imageable words and the fact that subjects reported using imagery as a mnemonic strategy. Activation of the precuneus was confined to the retrieval process, which also suggested a possible relationship to visual imagery used as a mnemonic strategy during retrieval. To test this hypothesis of precuneus activation as a function of the engagement of visual imagery we compared patterns of activation during the retrieval of paired associates that differed in their visual imageability.

In this study we again used cued recall of previously learned paired associates [78]. In one condition subjects were scanned during the cued retrieval of strongly imageable paired associates (*e.g.*, River ... Stream). In another condition they retrieved weakly imageable word associates (*e.g.*, Justice ... Law). The prediction was that recall of imageable pairs alone would activate the precuneus. A potential confound of this approach is that the activations associated with recall of imageable pairs might be attributable to superior memory performance. This has its basis in empirical evidence for an advantage to recall of imageable over nonimageable material [85]. To overcome this confound we equalised performance across the 12 scans by variable prior rehearsal. This, in itself, is open to the criticism that changes of rCBF might be attributed to differing degrees of item novelty, a difficulty circumvented by a further methodological refinement. In both strongly and weakly imageable paired associates the strength of semantic association was varied systematically along a scale of 1 (strong association, *e.g.*, King ... Queen) to 6 (weak/no association, *e.g.*, Puppy ... Hurricane). This allowed us to vary the degree of novelty of the material within both groupings of scans (the six imageable conditions and the six nonimageable conditions) whilst maintaining a comparable degree of performance. In other words, within both the imageable and the nonimageable sets of scans, there was a variation in novelty that we were able to treat as a covariate whose effect could be statistically controlled. The experimental variation of semantic distance also provided an opportunity to address theories regarding the function of the prefrontal cortex at retrieval. We reasoned that differing degrees of relatedness between members of a pair should lead to differential engagement of processes subserved by the frontal lobes such as organisation, monitoring or verification.

The results of our study confirmed the main predictions. The precuneus was strongly activated in association with recall of visually imageable material (Fig. 7). This activation was unaffected by covarying out the effect of item novelty. Our hypothesis that precuneus activation reflects the use of imagery

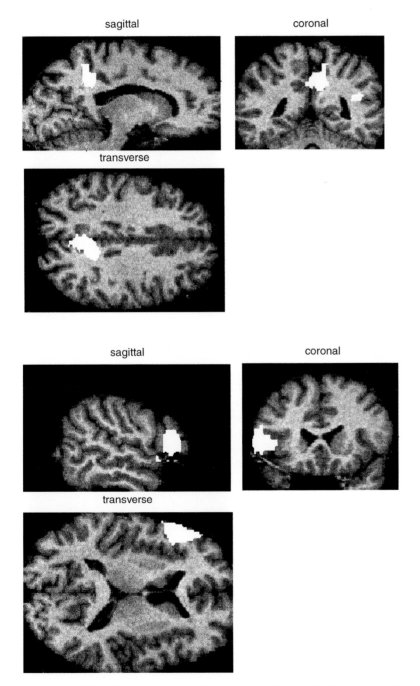

Figure 7   (a) Regions associated with retrieval of imageable/concrete verbal material. (b) Regions associated with retrieval of nonimageable/abstract verbal material. See text for description of regions.

as a mnemonic strategy at retrieval was therefore strongly supported. The opposite comparison, of nonimageable *versus* imageable recall, showed areas of significantly greater activity in the left inferior prefrontal cortex, anterior to Broca's area.

Our findings of activation of the precuneus, without activation of early visual processing areas in association with visual imagery implies that coherent image generation does not necessarily require activation of brain regions involved by perceptual processes. This is in accord with some, but not all, previous functional imaging studies of imagery where a consistent feature is activation of parieto-occipital and temporo-occipital areas. There are clear phenomenological differences in the quality of perceptual and imagined experience. The use of imagery in word pair recall necessitates only a degraded representation and it is possible that activation of early visual processing areas may be a feature of paradigms where there is selective attention to components of the generated images necessitating imagery of a more coherent nature than that required in paired associate recall [86]. Therefore, activation of the precuneus in the present study should not be taken to imply that it is the sole region involved in image generation. We would predict that attention to, for example, spatial or other components of a generated image would coactivate associated functionally specialised regions.

B. Nonimageable Retrieval

Words can be represented in memory according to orthographic, phonetic, semantic, and imageable attributes. Our study of episodic recall, involving concrete imageable nouns, was associated with preferential right prefrontal activation. The presence of predominant left prefrontal activation in nonimageable recall suggests that the pattern of prefrontal activation is a function of the nature of the recalled material (*i.e.*, imageable or nonimageable). It should be borne in mind that right sided activation is likely to be common to both types of retrieval. The imagery system is specialised for direct processing of signals concerning concrete objects and events that necessarily involves a spatial transformation. The verbal system is specialised for dealing with abstract linguistic units. Separate representational systems for attributes of words are supported by evidence that imageable and verbal components of stimuli are functionally independent in storage. One possibility, therefore, is that the differential left prefrontal activation for recall of nonimageable material may be linked to an independent access of word representations and images to language output systems [87]. A response in the imageable recall condition simply requires naming of an element in a composite image. In nonimageable recall prior reactivation of phonological or semantic links between the elements of a pair may be required prior to engagement of an output system. The prefrontal region in the recall of nonimageable material may thus be a final common pathway prior to activation of a word form in language output.

A parallel in the neuropsychological literature can be drawn with dynamic aphasia. Dynamic aphasia is associated with a lesion anterior to Broca's area in a region similar to that activated in the contrast of nonimageable with imageable word recall; it is characterised by a dissociation between normally generated speech and the ability to name, read, and repeat [18]. In the present context a composite image automatically accesses output in a manner akin to reading in dynamic aphasia; recall dependent on phonology or semantic association my require prior engagement of a prefrontal system.

C. The Effects of Practice and Semantic Relatedness

In examining the effects of varying semantic distance the results require careful interpretation. First, semantically distant paired associate lists were those associated with greater degrees of prior rehearsal and consequently these items were less novel. A change of activity associated with increasing semantic distance might equally reflect a changing degree of item novelty. We observed a significant negative correlation between activity in the left and right prefrontal cortex and the degree of prior rehearsal of test material. In the same regions, however, the most semantically distant paired associates (that had received the greatest amount of prior rehearsal) were associated with significant activations. Therefore, the simple explanation of increased activity in the prefrontal regions by the degree of prior rehearsal is not compelling. Bilateral prefrontal activations, associated with retrieval of word pairs that are unrelated (*e.g.,* puppy … hurricane) compared to those that are related (*e.g.,* car … truck) must reflect cognitive processes specifically required for the successful retrieval of semantically unrelated pairs (Fig. 8).

The cognitive processes involved in this type of retrieval are not immediately obvious. The recall of semantically unrelated associates is likely to involve processes such as monitoring putative responses and verification of their appropriateness. Such processes could conceivably account for prefrontal activation. The relative deactivations found in association with decreasing novelty might be interpreted as consistent with the

sagittal

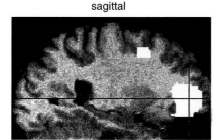

coronal

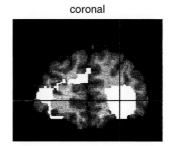

transverse

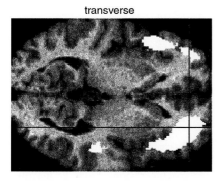

FIGURE 8 Brain regions associated with episodic memory retrieval when there is a systematic manipulation of semantic cueing. The regions shown are those which show maximal activity when the semantic cue is very closely related to the correct response and when the cue is semantically unrelated. Regions are described in the text.

suggestion that the prefrontal cortex is only engaged when novelty is a feature of task demand. However, alternative interpretations include an argument that cued recall of closely related pairs requires greater prefrontal activation because the almost obligatory response to a cue necessarily involves greater monitoring or verification of what might otherwise be an automatic response.

VIII. THE ROLE OF THE PREFRONTAL CORTEX IN EPSIODIC RETRIEVAL

A. Attempted *versus* Successful Retrieval

Right prefrontal activation has been a consistent feature of experiments involving retrieval of episodic memories [68,70,84,88,89]. The functional significance of this activation pattern is consequently of considerable theoretical interest. However, many experiments on episodic memory recall do not enable a distinction between attempted, or effortful, and successful retrieval. Two studies with bearing on this issue need to be considered. Tulving *et al.* compared the patterns of activation when subjects heard sentences that were either old or new [84]. A greater right prefrontal activation during recognition of old sentences was interpreted as consistent with retrieval success. Subsequently, Kapur *et al.* compared patterns of activation during a recognition memory task for words, previously encoded, in which the proportion of old and new words was either 15:85 or 85:15. The control was a semantic classification task. A similar degree of right prefrontal activation was seen in both memory tasks, leading the authors to conclude that this pattern of activation is a function of retrieval effort [90].

We examined the differential effect on brain activity of the actual retrieval of information compared to the attempted retrieval in an experiment involving a word recognition memory task [91]. Prior to scanning, subjects read a list of words and, to ensure effective encoding, were required to generate a short sentence using the target word. Subsequently, during scanning, they were presented with a longer list containing varying numbers of items seen at study. The varying density of old and new items (number of targets present being 0, 4, or 16) presented during the actual scan were embedded within longer lists that formed a run in to the scanning window. The actual task simply required subjects to identify whether or not each word had been previously seen. In the control tasks subjects were required to discriminate simple visual patterns (Xs or Os) presented with the same relative probability of occurrence as in the memory condition.

Compared to the "all new" condition, sequences containing old words were associated with activations in the right prefrontal and orbitofrontal cortices, the right anterior cingulate cortex, and the precuneus/cuneus. This result suggests that activity in all these regions is associated with retrieval success. A comparison of high *versus* low density target conditions indicated relative activation in a circumscribed region of the right prefrontal cortex that bordered area 46 and area 10, indicating these areas that are associated with successful retrieval (Fig. 9).

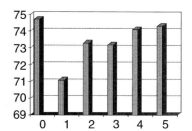

FIGURE 9 Graphic representation of cerebral blood flow in a right prefrontal region. Flow is maximal when the cue is strongly related to the required response (condition 5) and when it is unrelated (condition 0).

B. Incidental *versus* Intentional Retrieval

In a follow up to this study, we examined brain activations associated with attempting to retrieve as opposed to incidental retrieval. The study involved a manipulation of two factors. First, prescan, depth of processing was manipulated such that subjects encoded material in a deep or shallow way. Second, during scanning, subjects either performed an intentional memory task (recognition memory) or an incidental one in which they were required to make a non-memory-based semantic decision on test material containing a substantial proportion of items to which they had been exposed during the study phase. Thus, scanning occurred under four conditions, high and low levels of intentional and high and low levels of incidental retrieval. The findings revealed a dissociation between right frontal and left medial temporal function. When the recognition tasks were compared with semantic decision (incidental) tasks, right prefrontal cortex was active irrespective of whether the test phase had been preceeded by a deep or a shallow encoding operation. The medial temporal region, however, was sensitive to the prescan phase (being more active following deep encoding) irrespective of the nature of the task during scanning. Taken together, these results provide evidence that the retrieval-related right prefrontal activation hinges upon an intention to retrieve whereas the medial temporal activation possibly reflects a more automatic retrieval process [92] (see Fig. 10).

C. Post-retrieval Processes

The nature of post-retrieval-related activations was examined in a study in which subjects were required to perform two distinct episodic memory retrieval tasks. In one task optimal memory performance required an internal organising framework ("internally cued" retrieval) while in the other, that was balanced for auditory–verbal demands, subjects used external cues (provided by

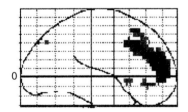
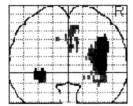
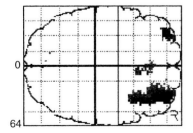

Figure 10 Regions showing increased activity in a verbal recognition memory task, when a higher proportion of words are correctly recognised compared to when no targets (previously seen words) are seen. See text for description of regions.

the experimenter) to guide retrieval ("externally cued" retrieval). Comparisons of the two memory tasks with their respective repetition control tasks, showed activation of the right, but not the left, prefrontal cortex in association with memory retrieval. Thus, even in a task that explicitly requires the need to organise material retrieval-associated frontal activity is predominantly right sided. The other striking finding was a double dissociation between the right dorsolateral and ventrolateral prefrontal regions. While both areas showed significant activity when each of the memory tasks was compared to its control conditions, internally cued memory retrieval activated right dorsolateral prefrontal cortex and the externally cued retrieval activated right venterolateral prefrontal cortex when the memory conditions were directly compared (Fig. 11). We suggest that the former task required, in addition to the setting up and maintenance of the organisational structure, a continual updating of recall plans in light of headings already covered and items already produced. Such processes must, necessarily, tax working memory and, in particular, monitoring of responses with respect to the overall structure to be reproduced (*i.e.*, organisational processes). The externally cued recall placed far fewer demands on these processes since, for each item recalled, subjects merely held in mind the cue provided by the experimenter without the need to refer to what had gone before or what was to come. This finding is consistent with the suggestion that ventral and dorsal parts of the lateral prefrontal cortex are differentially engaged depending on the demands of a task. In monkeys it has been suggested that the ventral prefrontal cortex acts directly upon the products of memory retrieval, particularly in relation to contextual operations (*e.g.*, salience, temporal sequence), while the dorsal prefrontal cortex is required for "complex, high-level planning" of intended acts [93,94]. Thus, lesions to DLPFC in monkeys lead to profound deficits in tasks that require animals to monitor their own responses or cues provided by the experimenter in order to guide the next response, whereas lesions to this region do not affect animals' performance on delayed response and delayed alternation tasks. Lesions specific to ventrolateral prefrontal cortex, on the other hand, do not lead to deficits on tasks requiring monitoring but do lead to a deficit in performance on spatial and nonspatial delayed alternation tasks. In the externally cued retrieval task, retrieval conditions (provided by a cue that provides the subject with a memory search "descriptor") change more frequently than in the internally cued task. The process of specifying the parameters that govern a search may be critical for right ventral prefrontal activation. A disorder of such a process would help to explain the confabulatory states found, at times, following anterior communicating artery aneurysms [74].

IX. RECONCILING FUNCTIONAL IMAGING AND NEUROPSYCHOLOGICAL DATA

Having considered functional imaging experiments of episodic memory it is necessary to address the significance of specific profiles of regional activation with respect to existing neuropsychological and psychological evidence. For simplicity individual brain areas will be discussed separately.

A. Frontal Lobes and Memory

Patients with frontal lobe damage perform normally on a wide range of intellectual tests [95]. Nevertheless, there is substantial evidence to indicate the

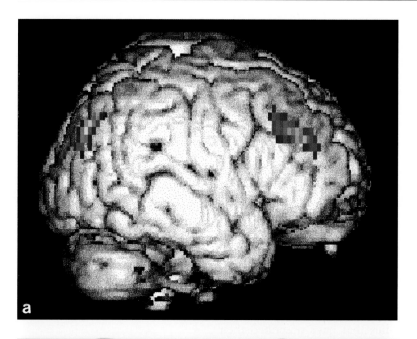

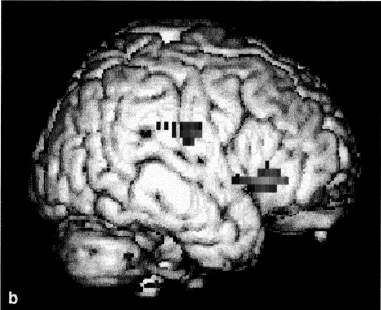

FIGURE 11 Regions activated during a verbal episodic memory retrieval task. (a) Regions active when external cueing is minimised and subjects are required to use a prelearnt organisational structure to optimise retrieval. The comparison is between this condition and an externally prompted retrieval. (b) Regions active when retrieval is prompted by externally provided semantic cues. This is the reverse of the comparison in (a). Regions described in text.

importance of the frontal lobes in selective cognitive functions. These operations include the organisation and planning of behavioural responses, strategy selection and implementation, monitoring of behavioural responses and behavioural flexibility [96]. Performance on memory tasks that do not engage these processes may conceivably be unimpaired in frontal lobe damaged patients. Conversely, impaired performance can be predicted in frontal patients for tasks that make demands on one or more such processes. Indeed, empirical evidence strongly supports this prediction. Deficits in frontal damaged patients include effects on memory for temporal sequence and for tasks that tax strategic organisational requirements [97–102]. This finding has led to the suggestion that there is a differential involvement of the frontal lobes depending upon whether an "associative/cue-dependent" search or a "strategic" search of memory is required [96].

From a theoretical perspective strategic memory search has elements in common with problem solving, requiring subsidiary processes of goal determination, response selection, monitoring, and verification. Like problem solving a strategic memory search is both volitional and effortful, functions traditionally ascribed to the frontal lobes. Shallice has suggested that the frontal lobes are vital to a process of "verifying that any candidate memories that have been retrieved are relevant" [96]. Our finding of increased right frontal activity in association with memory retrieval, and in particular during the identification of previously seen words compared with words not previously seen, provides support for this verification function.

The multiple specialisations of the frontal lobes are reflected in the number and range of functional imaging studies that have described their activation. Tasks involving internal generation of responses or "willed action" lead to marked activation of the left and, to a lesser extent, the right prefrontal cortex [56]. Merely listening to words or phonemes, when compared to listening to tones, results in left frontal activation [29]. Interpreting metaphorical sentences is associated with right frontal activity [103]. Additionally, motor learning, self-pacing, and working memory tasks have all been shown to engage the frontal lobes [104–106]. Virtually all functional imaging studies that have examined auditory–verbal long-term memory have shown either unilateral or bilateral frontal activation [107]. This finding implies that tasks that do not explicitly engage memory may share cognitive subprocesses with explicit memory tasks and an understanding of this common ground seems critical for an understanding of frontal function. We suggest that what these diverse tasks have in common is a need for planning and organisation together with outcome assessment that must also embody behavioural adaptation in response to unsatisfactory outcome or changing task demands.

The results of functional imaging studies are entirely concordant with neuropsychological evidence for the importance of the frontal lobes to memory function. Our earlier work showing bilateral frontal activations in combined encoding/retrieval tasks has been widely replicated. Subsequent experiments indicate that the left and right frontal lobes are predominantly activated at episodic encoding and retrieval, respectively. Reviewing studies that (intentionally or unintentionally) resulted in differing degrees of encoding and retrieval, Tulving suggested that lateralisation of function is an ubiquitous phenomenon encompassed by his so-called *HERA* (hemispheric encoding/retrieval assymmetry) hypothesis [88].

One critical question is whether left frontal activation at encoding reflects modality specific effects (*e.g.*, auditory–verbal demands) or more generic cognitive subprocesses. For example, it is possible that the left frontal activation at encoding is associated with organisational processes that are assumed to predominate at this stage. Conversely, right frontal activation may reflect greater engagement of monitoring and verification processes that predominate at retrieval. Evidence for the former assumption comes from our finding that a distracting task, when administered during episodic memory encoding, has a pronounced effect on left prefrontal activation [58]. This impaired activation is reflected, at a behavioural level, in impaired memory performance. It seems plausible to suggest that the organisational processes necessary for efficient encoding are disrupted by a distractor task and that this manifests as left prefrontal deactivation. Our demonstration that the retrieval of semantically unrelated word pair associates engages the frontal lobes to a greater degree than retrieval of semantically related pairs is evidence that they mediate the organisational and strategic aspects of memory encoding and retrieval. This conclusion is also supported by our finding of an association between right prefrontal activation and both retrieval success and the internal organisation of material at retrieval.

The finding of left frontal activity at retrieval of nonimageable material is at first sight puzzling. First, it reinforces the idea that the frontal activation in memory reflects subprocesses that may be present during both encoding and retrieval. In this respect the finding of relative lateralisation (left-encoding; right-retrieval) may be an oversimplification. The finding itself may indicate a specificity of function in this region for accessing either phonological representations of words or representations dependent upon semantic qualities.

B. Medial Temporal Lobes and Memory

The importance of the medial temporal lobes to episodic memory is well established [108]. The left medial temporal cortex and paleocortex are generally associated with verbal and the right side with visual aspects of memory. The specific importance of the hippocampus and surrounding areas (parahippocampal gyrus, amygdala, uncus) were first highlighted in the extensively reported descriptions of HM, who, following bilateral surgical ablation of these areas, developed a profound and permanent loss of episodic memory [69]. This finding has subsequently been widely replicated [109]. Since lesions of the monkey hippocampus impair recently acquired, but not more remotely acquired, memory, it has been suggested that the hippocampus plays a role in acquisition processes but not in the retrieval or consolidation of memory traces [72]. However, the exact role of the hippocampus in episodic memory remains speculative. It has been suggested that a hippocampal lesion is insufficient to produce amnesia and that more extensive lesions, that involve the entorhinal and perirhinal cortices, are necessary to produce the full range of deficits [110]. Whether the amnesic syndrome in patient HM was due to hippocampal damage or due to a disconnection of the temporal cortex from other neocortical regions has been questioned [111]. In this regard recent evidence suggests that lesions of the rhinal cortex may be more important in certain types of amnesia than lesions of the hippocampus [112].

Despite controversies concerning the effects of hippocampal lesions in animals and medial temporal lobe lesions in humans, the experimental data have had a major effect on concepts of the organisation of memory. Although initial observations on the patient HM indicated a dense amnesia following medial temporal lobe resection the perspective that such lesions led to a global amnesia has been modified by evidence that certain memory functions are retained. For example, on tests of implicit memory such patients perform comparably to normal subjects [113]. This neuropsychological evidence has given rise to an anatomical formulation of systems that are dependent and independent of the hippocampus. The hippocampus is considered important for declarative memory or knowledge acquired from specific encounters with the environment. The multimodal nature of declarative memories suggests that they must depend on the output of a range of cognitive modules or processing systems. The integration of these outputs in the form of coherent representations is one suggested function of the hippocampal system [114]. In other words, coactivations in different output modules converge on the hippocampus which registers their relational conjunctions. The hippocampus receives from, and feeds back to all sensory processing systems and together with its widespread connectivity with cortical association areas provides a unique anatomical arrangement to integrate function in distributed cortical regions that together form a coherent memory [115]. Furthermore, one means of reconciling animal evidence that the hippocampus codes for spatial context is an hypothesis that it is involved in registering conjunctions between stimuli. This formulation would be consistent with the view that the hippocampus is critical for memory that is dependant upon context, a key feature of episodic memory.

Despite an unquestionable importance in memory function, the medial temporal lobes have been activated in relatively few functional imaging studies of episodic memory [70,116]. One study that reported hippocampal activation used a cognitive subtraction approach with cued recall as the experimental paradigm [70]. Subjects were presented prior to scanning with word lists and during subsequent scans they were shown three-letter word stems with instructions to use them to make words which they had previously been shown. Activation of the right hippocampus was reported during episodic memory retrieval. In a subsequent report of the same study activation was reported only when the material presented was in the same sensory modality as during the learning phase and when it had the same visual characteristics (*i.e.*, when the same letter-case was used at retrieval as at encoding) [107].

In view of the large number of functional imaging experiments addressing episodic memory, it is surprising that activation of the hippocampus is relatively rare. It remains possible that hippocampal engagement during a memory task is reflected in altered patterns of activation without any net increase in overall activity (and, hence, without an increase of blood flow). Another possibility is that the hippocampus is continually active during both experimental and control tasks such that a cognitive subtraction technique will not demonstrate relative activation when one task is compared with another. Our graded task experiment, which demonstrated hippocampal activation, may indicate a need for experimental methodologies that differentially engage memory, making specific demands upon hippocampal function [70].

C. Diencephalon and Memory

Damage to diencephalic structures (thalami, mammilary bodies, mammilo-thalamic tract) from a wide range of aetiologies may result in amnesia [69]. The thalamus has widespread cortical and subcortical connections and evidence for its role in memory comes from both studies of amnesic patients and healthy volunteers [58,67,95,115]. In one study thalamic activation was found with memory retrieval from either episodic or semantic memory [58]. Thalamic activation has also been reported in verbal fluency tasks, which may reflect a memory retrieval component of such tasks [117]. It seems reasonable, however, to conclude that functional imaging studies have done little to clarify the role of diencephalic structures in memory.

D. Cingulate Cortex and Memory

Clinical studies have implicated the posterior cingulate cortex in episodic memory [76,77]. An important neural pathway connecting the prefrontal cortex with the hippocampus relays in this region [118]. Numerous functional imaging memory studies have reported activation in both anterior and posterior cingulate regions [58,67]. Involvement in encoding of episodic memory has been suggested by our experiment using a dual task methodology (see above). One interpretation is that cingulate activation reflects the attentional demands of a task, a suggestion borne out by the observation that in a dual task encoding paradigm the effect of a distractor task alone was to activate the anterior cingulate cortex. The anterior cingulate cortex appears to have a preeminent role in the maintenance of goal-directed behaviours, particularly those that require the suppression of external or internal interfering influences. Cingulate activations have been observed in studies that involve the internal generation of action, both motor and verbal, performance of the Stroop interference task, selective and divided attention during visual discrimination, auditory–verbal graded response memory tasks, and a verbal memory monitoring task requiring subjects to hold up to 10 numbers in mind [55–57,73,117,119–121]. The suggested role of the cingulate in the control of attention is lent credence by our finding that performance of a distracting task in the presence of memory encoding leads to significantly greater activation in anterior cingulate cortex than that found in memory encoding alone. One possibility is that activation of the cingulate cortex may result in modulatory influences on cortical regions that are not critical to immediate goal attainment, or tune the reponse of specific regions to enable more effective task related processing.

E. Precuneus and Memory

The precuneus is a medial parietal area, which incorporates Brodmann's areas 7 and 31 and which is structurally similar to the posterior cingulate cortex and has connections with prefrontal cortex, the temporal and occipital lobes, and the thalami [122–126]. Little is known about its specialised functions but activation of this area is a frequent accompaniment of functional imaging studies of memory [58,67,78,84,89]. The suggestion that activation in this region reflects the use of imagery in episodic memory is supported by our finding that it is significantly activated with the retrieval of imageable paired associates.

X. CONCLUSIONS

Neuropsychological divisions of memory have provided a framework for empirical research and the interpretation of deficits and dissociations in patients with discrete pathologies. In this regard there is strong psychological evidence for fundamental distinctions within memory such as between short- and long-term memory. Functional imaging techniques have provided a complementary approach to the study of memory that enables the establishment of correlations between large scale brain activity and specific memory processes as identified by psychological and neuropsychological studies.

At the broadest level, functional imaging experiments have vindicated neuropsychological models of both working memory and long-term memory. Anatomically dissociable brain systems have been shown to underpin visual and auditory verbal working memory. Within long-term memory functional imaging has provided evidence that the processes of encoding and retrieval are anatomically dissociable. The anatomical and physiological dissociation of brain systems involved in STM and LTM is less clear given the striking overlap of regions activated in experiments engaging these functions. This observation raises the question whether activations represent the engagement of processes common to both STM and LTM tasks. For example, both working memory and episodic memory necessitate the temporal organisation of events and tasks involving both types of memory have revealed common prefrontal activations. Another possibility is that the very tasks used to study LTM necessarily involve working memory. For example the common LTM paradigm of cued retrieval must involve maintenance of a cue within a working memory system during strategic memory search.

A long-standing issue in research is whether memory can be localised to a specific neural architecture or whether it represents a distributed property of the brain. Lesion studies, in animals and humans, implicate a number of brain areas as critical for memory function and have been interpreted as favouring a concept of local specialisation. However, the presence of memory deficits after discrete brain lesions does not necessarily imply that memory is a function of that specific region. It is equally plausible that a localised brain lesion may impair a psychological process related to the functioning of an anatomically distributed memory system. An alternative conceptualisation is that lesion studies address the importance of local networks in psychological processes related to memory function. The relative preservation of memory in the presence of extensive cerebral insults provides compelling evidence for memory as a distributed function of the brain. In this respect, functional imaging by studying the intact brain provides unique information about memory by describing memory processes at both a local network (the primary domain of lesion methodology) and a systems level. One clear impact of functional imaging studies is the emergence of a more dynamic view of memory that is now unambiguously seen as a process requiring the coordinated interaction of anatomically separate brain regions. A nexus of identifed regions with a high degree of regional specialisation for unitary processes that can be identifed with attributes of memory is an emerging view of the functional architecture of memory.

Is there convergence between findings from human functional imaging studies and studies in primates? This question can best be addressed by considering the role of prefrontal cortex in working memory. Primate studies have indicated a critical role for the sulcus principalis region of the left DLPFC in spatial working memory [35]. On the other hand, functional imaging experiments in humans suggest that the right DLPFC is more specialised for this type of memory [106]. Although differences in laterality might indicate important disjunctions between data from humans and primates they are overshadowed by a high degree of convergence in relation to other regions coactivated in conjunction with the prefrontal cortex. In the interpretation of similarities or differences it is important to bear in mind that psychological similarities across organisms may reflect convergent environmental selection rather than underlying physiological similarities.

An important distinction in memory studies is for memory with and without awareness. Memory with awareness is a critical feature of consciousness that can be distinguished from pure thought or perceptual awareness. Although consciousness is clearly a property of explicit memory the precise relationship still requires theoretical development. One viewpoint is that the hippocampal system is critical for conscious memory and during encoding binds together outputs of individual brain modules with those of a central system whose functioning contributes to the conscious experience of an event [127]. Because encoding was conscious, subsequent recollection also embodies the experience of consciousness. It is this recovered consciousness that may be a signal or marker that distinguishes memories from thoughts and percepts. While these issues await resolution it is clear that the study of memory is not only an end in itself but may provide critical evidence that speaks to the very nature of conscious experience.

References

1. J. Locke. Of identity and necessity from *Essay Concerning Human Understanding.* *In* "Personal Identity" (J. Perry, ed.), pp. 33–53. Univ. of California Press, Berkeley, 1994.
2. E. Tulving. "Elements of Episodic Memory." Oxford Univ. Press, Oxford, 1983.
3. W. James. "The Principles of Psychology." Holt, New York, 1890.
4. C. H. Vanderwolf and D. P. Cain. The behavioural neurobiology of learning and memory: A conceptual reorientation. *Brain Res. Rev.* **19,** 264–297 (1994).
5. J. M. Fuster. "The Prefrontal Cortex," 2nd ed. Raven Press, New York, 1989.
6. R. F. Thompson, T. W. Berger, and J. Madden. Cellular processes of learning and memory in the mammalian CNS. *Annu. Rev. Neurosci.* **6,** 447–491 (1983).
7. A. D. Baddeley. "Working Memory." Oxford Univ. Press, Oxford, 1986.
8. L. Squire and N. J. Cohen. Human memory and amnesia. *In* "The Neurobiology of Learning and Memory" (J. L. McGaugh, G. Lynch, and N. M. Weinberger, Eds.), pp. 3–64. Guilford Press, New York, 1984.
9. E. J. Furlong. "A Study in Memory." T. Nelson, London, 1951.
10. M. M. Merzenich, G. H. Recanzone, W. M. Jenkins, and K. A. Grajski. Adaptive mechanisms in cortical networks underlying cortical contributions to learning and nondeclarative memory. *In* "Cold Spring Harbor Symposia on Quantitative Biology," Vol. 55, The Brain. Cold Spring Harbor Laboratory, Cold Spring Harbor, NY, 1995.
11. A. D. Baddeley and G. J. Hitch. Working memory. *In* "Recent Advances in Learning and Motivation" (G. Bower, Ed.), 8th ed., pp. 47–90. Academic Press, New York, 1974.
12. R. C. Atkinson and R. M. Shiffrin. Human memory: A proposed system and its control processes. *In* "The Psychology of Learning and Motivation: Advances in Research and Theory" (K. W. Spence, Ed.), pp. 89–195. Academic Press, New York, 1968.
13. A. D. Baddeley. Working memory. **255,** 556–559 (1992).
14. D. A. Norman and T. Shallice. Attention to action: Willed and automatic control of behaviour. *In* "Consciousness and Self Regulation: Advances in Research" (R. J. Davidson, G. E. Schwartz, and D. Shapiro, Eds.), Vol. IV, pp. 1–18. Plenum, New York, 1986.
15. M. Posner and S. W. Keele. Decay of visual information from a single letter. *Science* **158,** 137–139 (1967).
16. A. D. Baddeley, N. Thomson, and M. Buchanan. Word length and the structure of short-term memory. *J. Verb. Learn. Verb. Behav.* **14,** 575–589 (1975).
17. A. D. Baddeley and K. Lieberman. Spatial working memory. *In* "Attention and Performance" (R. Nickerson, Ed.), Erlbaum, Hillsdale, NJ, 1980.
18. R. A. McCarthy and E. K. Warrington. "Cognitive Neuropsychology. A Clinical Introduction." Academic Press, Orlando, 1990.
19. T. Shallice and E. K. Warrington. The selective impairment of auditory verbal short-term memory. *Brain* **92,** 885–896 (1969).

20. A. Basso, H. Spinnler, G. Vallar, and E. Zanobio. Left hemisphere damage and selective impairment of auditory verbal short-term memory. A case study. *Neuropsychologia* **20,** 263–274 (1982).

21. E. K. Warrington and P. Rabin. Visual span and apprehension in patients with unilateral cerebral lesions. *Q. J. Exp. Psychol.* **23,** 423–431 (1971).

22. E. De Renzi and P. Nichelli. Verbal and non-verbal short-term memory impairment following hemispheric damage. *Cortex* **11,** 341–353 (1975).

23. D. J. Murray. Articulation and acoustic confusability in short-term memory. *J. Exp. Psychol.* **78,** 679–684 (1968).

24. B. A. Levy. Role of articulation in auditory and visual short-term memory. *J. Verb. Learn. Verb. Behav.* **10,** 123–132 (1971).

25. P. Salame and A. D. Baddeley. Disruption of short-term memory by an attended speech: Implications for structure of working memory. *J. Verb. Learn. Verb. Behav.* **21,** 150–184 (1982).

26. R. Conrad. Acoustic confusions in immediate memory. *Br. J. Psychol.* **55,** 75–84 (1964).

27. E. Paulesu, C. D. Frith, and R. S. J. Frackowiak. The neural correlates of the verbal component of working memory. *Nature* **362,** 342–344 (1993).

28. E. Paulesu, A. Connelly, C. D. Frith, K. J. Friston, J. Heather, R. Myers, D. G. Gadian and R. S. J. Frackowiak. Functional MR imaging correlations with positron emission tomography. *Neuroimaging Clin. North Am.* **5,** 207–225 (1995).

29. J-F. Demonet, F. Chollet, S. Ramsay, D. Cardebat, J-L. Nespoulous, R. Wise, A. Rascol and R. Frackowiak. The anatomy of phonological and semantic processing in normal subjects. *Brain* **115,** m1753–1768 (1992).

30. R. J. Zatorre, A. C. Evans, E. Meyer, and A. Gjedde. Lateralization of phonetic and pitch processing in speech perception. *Science* **256,** 846–849 (1992).

31. T. Shallice and G. Vallar. The impairment of auditory-verbal short-term storage. *In* "Neuropsychological Impairments of Short-Term Memory" (G. Vallar and T. Shallice, Eds.). Cambridge Univ. Press, New York, 1990.

32. K. Zilles. Cortex. *In* "The Human Nervous System" (G. Paxinos. Ed.). Academic Press, San Diego, 1990.

33. D. M. Jones, W. J. Macken, and A. C. Murray. Disruption of visual short-term memory by changing-state auditory stimuli: The role of segmentation. Mem. Cognit. **21,** 318–328 (1995).

34. J. F. Demonet, C. Price, R. J. S. Wise, and R. S. J. Frackowiak. Differential activations of right and left posterior sylvian regions by semantic and phonological tasks: A positron emission tomography study in normal human subjects. *Neurosci. Lett.* **182,** 25–28 (1994).

35. P. S. Goldman-Rakic. Circuitry of primate prefrontal cortex and regulation of behaviour by representational knowledge. *In* "Handbook of Physiology—The Nervous System" (V. B. Mountcastle, F. E. Bloom, and S. R. Geiger, Eds.), Vol. V, pp. 373–417. Williams and Wilkins, Baltimore, 1987.

36. S. Zeki and S. Shipp. The functional logic of cortical connections. *Nature* **335,** 311–317 (1988).

37. M. Mishkin, L. G. Ungerleider, and K. A. Macko. Object vision and spatial vision: two cortical pathways. *Trends Neurosci.* **6,** 414–417 (1983).

38. S. Zeki. "A Vision of the Brain." Blackwell Scientific, Oxford, 1993.

39. W. A. Phillips. On the distinction between sensory storage and short-term visual memory. *Percept. Psychophys.* **16,** 283–290 (1974).

40. W. A. Phillips. Short-term visual memory. *Phil. Trans. R. Soc. London* **302,** 295–309 (1983).

41. M. A. Brandimonte, G. J. Hitch, and D. V. M. Bishop. Influence of short-term memory codes on visual image processing. evidence from image transformation tasks. *J. Exp. Psychol.* (1992).

42. A. W. Ellis and D. A. Allport. "Multiple Representations for Visual Objects: A Behavioural Study." Paper presented at the Easter meeting of the Society for

the Study of Artificial Intelligence and Simulation of Behaviour, Warwick, April 10–12, 1985, unpublished.

43. D. Marr. "Vision." Freeman, San Francisco, 1982.

44. J. A. Thompson. Is continuous visual monitoring necessary in visually guided locomotion? *J. Exp. Psychol.* **9,** 427–443 (1983).

45. S. Kosslyn. The medium and the message in mental imagery: A theory. *Psychol. Rev.* **88,** 46–66 (1981).

46. D. N. Levine, J. Wallach, and M. Farah. Two visual systems in mental imagery: dissociation of "what" and "where" in imagery disorders due to bilateral posterior cerebral lesions. *Neurology* **35,** 1010–1018 (1985).

47. G. W. Humphreys and V. Bruce. "Visual Cognition: Computational, Experimental and Neuropsychological Perspectives." Erlbaum, Hove, 1989.

48. J. V. Haxby, C. L. Grady, B. Horowitz, L. G. Ungerleider, M. Mishkin, R. E. Carson, P. Herscovitch, M. B. Schapiro, I. Rapoport. Dissociation of object and spatial visual processing pathways in the human extrastriate cortex. *J. Neurosci.* **88,** 1621–1625 (1991).

49. J. Jonides, E. E. Smith, R. A. Koeppe, E. Awh, S. Minoshima, and M. Mintum. Spatial working memory in humans as revealed by PET. *Nature* **363,** 623–625 (1993).

50. E. Paulesu, C. D. Frith, C. J. Bench, G. Bottini, P. M. Grasby and R. S. J. Frackowiak. Functional anatomy of working memory: The visuospatial "sketchpad." *J. Cereb. Blood Flow Metab.* **13,** S551 (1993). [Abstract]

51. H. R. Friedman and P. S. Goldman-Rakic. Coactivation of the prefrontal cortex and inferior parietal cortex in working memory revealed by 2DG functiona mapping in the rhesus monkey. *J. Neurosci.* **14,** 2775–2788 (1994).

52. J. M. Fuster, R. H. Bauer, and J. P. Jervey. Functional interactions between inferotemporal and prefrontal cortex in a cognitive task. *Brain Res.* **330,** 299–307 (1985).

53. M. J. Farah. Is visual imagery really visual? Overlooked evidence from neuropsychology. *Psychol. Rev.* **95,** 307–317 (1988).

54. A. Baddeley. Exploring the central executive. *Q. J. Exp. Psychol.* **49,** 5–28 (1996).

55. J. V. Pardo, P. J. Pardo, K. W. Janer, and M. E. Raichle. The anterior cingulate cortex mediates processing selection in the Stroop attenentional conflict paradigm. *Proc. Natl. Acad. Sci. USA* **87,** 256–259 (1990).

56. C. D. Frith, K. J. Friston, P. F. Liddle, and R. S. J. Frackowiak. Willed action and the prefrontal cortex in man: a study with PET. *Proc. R Soc. London B* **244,** 241–246 (1991).

57. M. Corbetta, F. M. Miezin, S. Dobmeyer, G. L. Shulman, and S. E. Petersen. Selective and divided attention during visual discriminations of shape, colour, and speed: Functional anatomy by positron emission tomography. *J. Neurosci.* **11**(8), 2383–2402 (1991).

58. T. Shallice, P. Fletcher, C. D. Frith, P. Grasby, R. S. J. Frackowiak, and R. J. Dolan. Brian regions associated with acquisition and retrieval of verbal episodic memory. *Nature* **368,** 633–635 (1994).

59. P. M. Grasby, C. D. Frith, K. J. Friston *et al.* A graded task approach to the functional mapping of brain areas implicated in auditory–verbal memory function. *Brain* **117,** 1271–1282 (1994).

60. J. E. Metter. Neuroanatomy and physiology of aphasia. *Aphasiology* **1,** 3–33 (1987).

61. S. Brady and D. Shankweiler. "Phonological Processes in Literacy." Erlbaum, Hillsdale, NJ, 1991.

62. J. P. Rack, M. J. Snowling, and R. K. Olson. The nonword reading deficit in dyslexia: a review. *Reading Res. Q.* **27,** 29–53 (1992).

63. I. Y. Liberman, D. Shankweiler, F. W. Fischer, and B. Carter. Explicit syllable and phoneme segmentation in the young child. *J. Exp. Child Psychol.* **18,** 201–212 (1974).

64. U. Frith. Beneath the surface of developmental dyslexia. *In* "Surface Dyslexia"

(K. E. Patterson, J. C. Marshall, and M. Coltheart, Eds.). Routledge Kegan-Paul, London, 1985.

65. J. M. Rumsey, P. Andreason, A. J. Xametkin, T. Aquino, A. C. King, S. D. Hamburger, A. Pikus, J. L. Rapoport, R. M. Cohen. Failure to activate the left temporo-parietal cortex in dyslexia. An oxygen 15 positron emission tomography study. *Arch. Neurol.* **49**, 527–534 (1992).

66. E. Paulesu, U. Frith, M. Snowling, A. Gallagher, J. Morton, R. S. J. Frackowiak, and C. D. Frith. Is developmental dyslexia a disconnection syndrome? Evidence from PET scanning. *Brain* **119**, 143–157 (1996).

67. P. M. Grasby, C. D. Frith, K. J. Friston, C. Bench, R. S. J. Frackowiak, and R. J. Dolan. Functional mapping of brain areas implicated in auditory memory function. *Brain* **116**, 1–20 (1993).

68. P. C. Fletcher, C. D. Frith, P. M. Grasby, T. Shallice, R. S. J. Frackowiak, and R. J. Dolan. Brain systems for encoding and retrieval of auditory–verbal memory: An in vivo study in humans. *Brain* **118**, 401–416 (1995).

69. N. Butters and D. T. Stuss. Diencephalic amnesia. *In* "Handbook of Neuropsychology" (F. Boller and J. Grafman, Eds.), 3rd ed., pp. 107–148. Elsevier Science, Amsterdam, 1989.

70. L. R. Squire, J. G. Ojemann, F. M. Miezin, S. E. Petersen, T. O. Videen, and M. E. Raichle. Activation of the hippocampus in normal humans: A functional anatomical study of memory. *Proc. Natl. Acad. Sci. USA* **89** (1992).

71. W. B. Scoville and B. Milner. Loss of recent memory after bilateral hippocampal lesions. *J. Neurol. Neurosurg. Psychiatry* **20**, 11–21 (1957).

72. S. M. Zola-Morgan and L. R. Squire. The primate hippocampal formation: Evidence for a time-related role in memory storage. *Science* **250**, 288–290 (1990).

73. M. Petrides, B. Alivisatos, A. Evans, and E. Meyer. Dissociation of human mid-dorsolateral from posterior dorsolateral frontal cortex in memory processing. *Proc. Natl. Acad. Sci. USA* **90**, 873–877 (1993).

74. M. Moscovitch. Confabulation and the frontal system: Strategic *vs* associative retrieval in neuropsychological theories of memory. *In* "Varieties of Memory and Consciousness: Essays in Honor of Endel Tulving" (H. L. Roediger and F. I. M. Craik, Eds.), pp. 133–160. Hillsdale, NJ, 1989.

75. B. Milner, M. Petrides, and M. L. Smith. Frontal lobes and the temporal organisation of memory. *Hum. Neurobiol.* **4**, 137–142 (1985).

76. E. Valenstein, D. Bowers, M. Varfaellie, A. Day, and R. T. Watson. Retrosplenial amnesia. *Brain* **110**, 1631–1646 (1987).

77. P. Rudge and E. Warrington. Selective impairment of memory and visual perception in splenial tumours. *Brain* **114**, 349–360 (1993).

78. P. Fletcher, C. D. Frith, S. Baker, T. Shallice, R. S. J. Frackowiak and R. J. Dolan. The mind's eye—activation of the precuneus in memory related imagery. *Neuroimage* **2**, 196–200 (1995).

79. L. Hasher and R. T. Zacks. Automatic and effortful processes in memory. *J. Exp. Psychol.* **108**, 356–388 (1979).

80. S. Kapur, F. I. M. Craik, E. Tulving, A. A. Wilson, S. Houle and G. M. Brown. Neuroanatomical correlates of encoding in episodic memory: Levels of processing effect. *Proc. Natl. Acad. Sci. USA* **91**, 2008–2011 (1994).

81. F. I. Craik and R. S. Lockhart. Levels of processing: A framework for memory research. *J. Verb. Learn. Verb. Behav.* **11**, 671–684 (1972).

82. A. D. Baddeley, V. Lewis, M. Eldridge, and N. Thomson. Attention and retrieval from long-term memory. *J. Exp. Psychol.* **113**, 518–540 (1984).

83. L. J. Jacoby, D. Ste-Marie, and J. P. Toth. Redefining automaticity: Unconscious influences, awareness and control. *In* "Attention: Selection, Awareness and Control" (A. D. Baddeley and L. Weizkrantz, Eds.). Oxford Univ. Press, Oxford, 1993.

84. E. Tulving, S. Kapur, H. J. Markovitsch, F. I. M. Craik, R. Habib, and S. Houle. Neuroanatomical correlates of retrieval in episodic memory: Auditory sentence recognition. *Proc. Natl. Acad. Sci. USA* **91**, 2012–2015 (1994).

85. A. D. Baddeley. "Human Memory." Erlbaum, Hillsdale, NJ, 1991.

86. S. M. Kosslyn, N. M. Alpert, W. L. Thompson, V. Maljkovic, S. B. Weise, C. F. Chabris, S. E. Hamilton, S. L. Rauch, and F. S. Buonanno. Visual mental imagery activates topographically organized visual cortex: PET investigations. *J. Cognit. Neurosci.* **5,** 263–287 (1993).

87. A. Paivio. "Mental Representations." Oxford Univ. Press, Oxford, 1986.

88. E. Tulving, S. Kapur, F. I. M. Craik, M. Moscovitch, and S. Houle. Hemispheric encoding/retrieval asymmetry in episodic memory: Positron emission tomography findings. *Proc. Natl. Acad. Sci. USA* **91,** 2016–2020 (1994).

89. R. L. Buckner and E. Tulving. Neuroimaging studies of memory: Theory and recent PET results. *In* "Handbook of Neuropsychology" (J. Boller and J. Grafman, Eds.), 10th ed. Elsevier, Amsterdam, 1994.

90. S. Kapur, F. Craik, G. M. Brown, S. Houle and E. Tulving. Functional role of the prefrontal cortex in memory retrieval: A PET study. *Neuroreport* **6,** 1880–1884 (1995).

91. M. D. Rugg, P. C. Fletcher, C. D. Frith, R. S. J. Frackowiak, and R. J. Dolan. Differential activation of the prefrontal cortex in successful and unsuccessful memory retrieval. *Brain* **119,** 143–157 (1996).

92. M. Rugg, P. F. Fletcher, C. D. Frith, R. S. J. Frackowiak, and R. J. Dolan. Brain regions supporting intentional and incidental memory: A PET study. *Neuroreport* **8,** 1283–1287 (1997).

93. M. Petrides. Frontal lobes and memory. *In* "Handbook of Neuropsychology" (F. Boller and J. Grafman, Eds.), pp. 75–90. Elsevier Science, New York, 1989.

94. M. Petrides. Impairments on nonspatial self-ordered and externally ordered working memory tasks after lesions of the mid-dorsal part of the lateral frontal cortex. *J. Neurosci.* **15,** 359–375 (1995).

95. A. R. Mayes. "Human Organic Memory Disorders." Cambridge Univ. Press, Cambridge, 1988.

96. T. Shallice. "From Neuropsychology to Mental Structure." Cambridge Univ. Press, Cambridge, 1988.

97. W. Jetter, U. Poser, R. B. Freeman, and H. J. Markowitsch. A verbal long term memory deficit in frontal lobe damaged patients. *Cortex* **22,** 229–242 (1986).

98. A. P. Shimamura, J. S. Janowsky, and L. R. Squire. What is the role of frontal lobe damage in memory disorders? *In* pp. 173–198. Oxford Univ. Press, Oxford, 1991.

99. A. P. Shimamura, J. S. Janowsky, and L. R. Squire. Memory for the temporal order of events in patients with frontal lobe lesions and amnesic patients. *Neuropsychologia* **28**(8), 803–814 (1990).

100. F. W. Black. Cognitive deficits in patients with unilateral war related frontal lobe lesions. *J. Clin. Psychol.* **32,** 366–372 (1976).

101. D. L. Schachter. Memory, amnesia and frontal-lobe dysfunction. *Psychobiol.* **15,** 21–36 (1987).

102. J. S. Janowsky, A. P. Shimamura, M. Kritchevsky, and L. R. Squire. Cognitive impairment following frontal lobe damage and its relevance to human amnesia. *Behav. Neurosci.* **103,** 548–560 (1989).

103. G. Bottini, R. Corcoran, R. Sterzi, *et al.* The role of the right hemisphere in the interpretation of figurative aspects of language: A positron emission tomography activation study. *Brain* **117,** 1241–1254 (1994).

104. M-P. Deiber, R. E. Passingham, J. G. Colebatch, and R. S. J. Frackowiak. Cortical areas and the selection of movements: A study with positron emission tomography. *Exp. Brain Res.* **84,** 393–402 (1991).

105. I. H. Jenkins, D. J. Brooks, P. D. Nixon, R. S. J. Frackowiak, and R. E. Passingham. Motor sequence learning: A study with positron emission tomography. *J. Neurosci.* **14,** 3775–3790 (1994).

106. S. C. Baker, C. D. Frith, R. S. J. Frackowiak, and R. J. Dolan. The neural substrate of active memory for shape and spatial location in man. *Cereb. Cortex* **6,** 612–619 (1996).

107. R. L. Buckner, S. E. Petersen, J. G. Ojemann, F. M. Miezin, L. R. Squire, and M. E. Raichle. Functional anatomical studies of explicit and implicit memory retrieval tasks. *J. Neurosci.* **15**(1), 12–29 (1995).

108. M. L. Smith. Memory disorders associated with temporal-lobe lesions. *In* "Handbook of Neuropsychology" (F. Boller and J. Grafman, Eds.), pp. 91–106. Elsevier-Science, Amsterdam, 1989.

109. H. Dimsdale, V. Logue, and M. Piercy. A case of persisting impairment of recent memory following right temporal lobectomy. *Neuropsychologia* **1**, 287–298 (1964).

110. M. Mishkin. Memory in monkeys severely impaired by combined but not by separate removal of amygdala and hippocampus. *Nature* **273**, 297–298 (1978).

111. J. Horel. The neuroanatomy of amnesia: A critique of the hippocampal memory hypothesis. *Brain* **101**, 403–445 (1978).

112. M. Meunier, J. Bachevalier, M. Mishkin, and E. A. Murray. Effects on visual recognition of combined and seperate ablations of the entorhinal and perirhinal cortex in rhesus monkey. *J. Neurosci.* **13**, 5418–5432.

113. N. J. Cohen. Preserved learning capacity in amnesia: Evidence for multiple memory systems. *In* "Neuropsychology of Memory" (L. R. Squire and N. Butters, Eds.), pp. 83–103. Guilford Press, New York, 1984.

114. H. Eichenbaum and T. Otto. The hippocampus—What does it do? *Behav. Neurol. Biol.* **57**, 2–36 (1992).

115. D. G. Amaral. Memory: Anatomical organisation of candidate brain regions. *In* "Handbook of Physiology—The Nervous Systems" (V. B. Mountcastle, F. E. Bloom, and S. R. Geiger, Eds.), Vol. V, pp. 211–294. American Physiological Society, Bethesda, MD, 1987.

116. P. Grasby, C. Frith, K. J. Friston, R. S. J. Frackowiak, and R. J. Dolan. Activation of the human hippocampal formation during auditory–verbal long-term memory function. *Neurosci. Lett.* **163**, 185–188 (1993).

117. C. D. Frith, K. J. Friston, P. F. Liddle, and R. S. J. Frackowiak. A pet study of word finding. *Neuropsychologia* **29**, 1137–1148 (1991).

118. P. Goldman-Rakic, L. D. Selemon, and M. L. Schwartz. Dual pathways connecting the dorsolateral prefrontal cortex with the hippocampal formation and parahippocampal cortex in the rhesus monkey. *Neuroscience* **12**, 719–743 (1984).

119. E. C. Johnstone, T. J. Crow, C. D. Frith, and D. G. C. Owens. The Northwick Park "functional" psychosis study: Diagnosis and treatment response. *Lancet* **2**, 119–124 (1988).

120. C. J. Bench, C. D. Frith, P. M. Grasby, K. J. Friston, E. Paulesu, R. S. J. Frackowiak, and R. J. Dolan. Investigations of the functional anatomy of attention using the Stroop test. *Neuropsychologia* **31**, 907–922 (1993).

121. T. Paus, M. Petrides, A. Evans, and E. Meyer. Role of the human anterior cingulate cortex in the control of oculomotor, manual, and speech responses: A positron emission tomography study. *J. Neurophysiol.* **70**(2), 453–469 (1993).

122. B. A. Vogt, D. N. Pandya, and D. L. Rosene. Cingulate cortex of the rhesus monkey. I. Cytoarchitecture and thalamic afferents. *J. Comp. Neurol.* **262**, 256–270 (1987).

123. B. A. Vogt and D. N. Pandya. Cingulate cortex of the rhesus monkey. II. Cortical afferents. *J. Comp. Neurol.* **262**, 271–289 (1987).

124. J. S. Blum, K. L. Chow, and K. H. Pribram. A behavioural analysis of the organisation of the parieto-tempero-preoccipital cortex. *J. Comp. Neurol.* **93**, 53–100 (1950).

125. H. B. Pribram and J. Barry. Further behavioural analysis of parieto-temperopreoccipital cortex. *J. Neurophysiol.* **19**, 99–106 (1956).

126. C. von Economo. "The Cytoarchitectectonics of the Human Cerebral Cortex." Oxford Univ. Press, London, 1929.

127. M. Moscovitch. Models of consciousness and memory. *In* "Cognitive Neuroscience," pp. 1341–1355. MIT Press, Boston, 1995.

CHAPTER SIXTEEN

Measuring Neuromodulation with Functional Imaging

I. INTRODUCTION

Two principal modes of neurotransmitter action can be identified in the central nervous system. The predominant mode involves fast acting mechanisms of either an excitatory or an inhibitory nature, typically associated with neurotransmitters such as glutamate, aspartate, and GABA. A second type of neurotransmitter action, which operates on a slower time scale, has a primary mode of action that involves the alteration of target neuronal excitability and discharge patterns. These latter systems are further characterised by relatively low baseline firing rates and a prolonged duration of action following neurotransmitter release. Typical neurotransmitters in this class are noradrenaline (NA), dopamine (DA), and serotonin (5HT).

Fast and slow acting neurotransmitter systems have different functional roles in the central nervous system. Fast acting neurotransmitters are implicated primarily in signal or information transfer. By contrast slow acting neurotransmitters play a critical role in altering the excitability of cortical neurones to other extrinsic influences with relatively little effect on background resting potentials. The contingent nature and the long duration of action of this class of neurotransmitter are the basis for the ascription of the term neuromodulatory effects [1].

A pertinent example of neuromodulatory neurotransmitter influence comes from observations, based upon single cell recordings, in the nonhuman primate. In the nonhuman primate working memory is critically dependant on the functional integrity of the dorsolateral prefrontal cortex and its interactions with modality specific posterior brain regions [2]. Working memory in the primate is inextricably associated with sustained neural activity in prefrontal neurones as exemplified in delayed response tasks. As will be detailed later in this chapter task related neuronal activity, but not resting activity, is highly susceptible to the influence of pharmacological manipulations including the manipulation of dopaminergic inputs [3].

A critical issue and a major challenge in developing an understanding of human brain function is to establish how modulatory neurotransmitters influence human cortical function. Experimental protocols, using factorial designs, now enable these issues to be addressed in the intact human brain. The theoretical background and experimental basis to these approaches, with particular reference to dopamine neurotransmission, as well as an account of findings from neuroimaging studies of normal function and pathology provide the basis for this chapter.

II. NEUROMODULATION

A. The Cortical Anatomy of Dopamine

Monoaminergic inputs to the human cortex have, until recently, been considered diffuse and nonspecific. Evidence now suggests that these ascending projection systems display a high degree of anatomical specificity characterised by pronounced regional and laminar specialisation [4–7]. The ordered architecture of monoaminergic inputs to the cortex is compatible with an important regulatory role on cortical activity.

The high degree of organisation and functional role of monoaminergic systems is exemplified by a consideration of cortical dopamine projections. Dopamine inputs to the cortex have a bilaminar distribution, the highest levels being seen in upper cortical layers I to III and lower layers V and VI, with pyramidal neurons in particular being their principal target site [8]. In keeping with anatomical evidence of an ordered cortical dopamine input autoradiographic and immunoreactivity based studies in both the human and nonhuman primate have demonstrated dopamine receptors in the cortex [9]. Furthermore, consistent with anatomical data autoradiographic techniques also indicate a bilaminar cortical distribution of receptor labelling with the highest receptor labelling in cortical layers 1b and 11 and V and V1 [9]. The predominant cortical receptor is of the D1 type though D2 receptors are also present to a lesser degree [8,10].

Clues to the functional role of cortical dopaminergic inputs can be surmised from an ultrastructural analysis of the pattern of formed cortical synapses. The majority of cortical dopamine synapses form symmetric or triadic synapses, possibly with cortico-cortical glutaminergic inputs, onto the spines and dendrites of pyramidal cells [11]. The precision in the microanatomy of cortical dopaminergic inputs, with a localisation of D1 receptors to the very spines which receive glutaminergic inputs, provides an architectural arrangement through which dopamine can potentially modulate excitatory inputs [12,13].

B. Dopamine Regulation of Prefrontal Function

Modulatory effects of dopamine on glutaminergic inputs to pyramidal cells in the prefrontal cortex have now been repeatedly demonstrated [14–16]. These effects on prefrontal cortical function seem to be mediated via the D1 receptor [17]. Although the effects of dopamine on the firing of pyramidal cells are complex the net effect is inhibitory, an effect that can be elicited by direct iontophoretic application of dopamine or through stimulation of DA cell bodies [18,19]. However, the effects of dopamine perturbations on task related neuronal activity, rather than the spontaneous or baseline firing rate of target neurons, provides the most meaningful framework for an understanding of the role of dopamine on cortical processing. The term neuromodulation, as already described, is used to specify the situation whereby the main effects of a neurotransmitter are to modify the impact of other synaptic or nonsynaptic inputs on to common postsynaptic target cells [20]. This type of influence has been particularly well demonstrated in experiments that have examined the effects of iontophoretically applied noradrenaline to auditory cortical cells of unanesthetised squirrel monkeys, prior to, and following acoustic activation by species specific vocalisations. During exposure to auditory vocalisations the effect of applied noradrenaline was to enhance elicited activity in discrete neural ensembles relative to background spontaneous activity. This effect has been described as an enhancement of signal to noise characteristics of auditory cortical cells [21].

The most important postsynaptic effects of dopamine are evident in an alteration of the effectiveness of other excitatory or inhibitory synaptic inputs, particularly the modulation of target brain systems involved in cognitive operations [21–23]. Stimulation of dopamine cells in the ventral tegmentum blocks the excitatory effects on cortical neurons of thalamic stimulation [24]. Single cell recordings from the prefrontal cortex of monkeys, studied while performing delayed response tasks, have shown a differential cellular response to the microiontophoretic application of dopamine. A subpopulation of prefrontal cells, which increase their firing rate during a delay period, are further enhanced by dopamine manipulation while activity in cells not engaged by the task is unaltered or inhibited [25]. These effects can be conceived of as altering the state of a network subserving a specific psychological function by increasing task specific firing relative to background firing in specific populations of prefrontal cells [25]. The effects of neuroleptics on patterns of cellular activation has highlighted the receptor mediated mechanisms that underlie such a differential response. Haloperidol and fluphenazine both antagonised task related dopamine augmentation of cell firing but not the selective D_2 antagonist sulpiride. These observations suggest that a D_1 effect is responsible for dopamine mediated alteration of task related neuronal activity in prefrontal neurons [26]. A recent *ex situ* study on human cortex has demonstrated a dopamine facilitation of NMDA (*N*-methyl-D-aspartate) excitatory amino acid receptor action, an effect that seems to be mediated by the D1 receptor [27,28].

C. Dopamine Regulation of Working Memory

In terms of neurophysiological effects it seems that activation of dopamine D_1 receptors in particular may be related to the performance of delayed response tasks where the underlying processes involve the temporal organisation of behaviours guided by short-term memory [26]. Local injections of selective D_1 antagonists, such as SCH23390 and SCH39166, directly into the prefrontal cortex of rhesus monkeys induce errors and increased latencies on an oculomotor task that requires memory guided saccades [3]. The drugs had no effect on performance in a task that required visually guided saccades, indicating that sensory and motor functions were unaltered. Thus D1 receptors have a permissive role in the mnemonic or predictive functions of the primate prefrontal cortex [3].

Recent nonhuman primate experiments that combine iontophoretic analysis of dopamine receptors with single-cell recording during behaviour have produced a refined analysis of dopaminergic effects on prefrontal cortical neurones [29]. In an oculomotor delayed-response (ODR) paradigm, that requires the animal to remember the spatial position of a stimulus, the iontopheretic application of a low dosage of the selective dopamine antagonist SCH 39166 enhanced activity in neurones that showed maximal firing during the delay period between a cue and a motor response. This enhancement of neuronal response could be reversed by the iontophoretic application of the D1 partial agonist SKF 38393. These effects were specific to task dependant units and no effects were observed on the general excitability of cells studied. At higher dosages the same D1 antagonist inhibited prefrontal unit firing in a nonspecific fashion, as did the D2 antagonist raclopride, with an effect evident not only in the memory field cells but also in nonmemory task neurones [29]. The specificity of the D1 mediated effects implies that blockade disinhibits specific excitatory inputs to the same cell. The overall findings can be interpreted as consistent with a proposal that there is an optimal level of D1 receptor mediated activity for memory related neuronal function. A lack of dopamine inputs or an excess of dopamine can therefore have similar functional effects on task related cell firing.

D. Dopamine and Cognition in Humans

Dopamine inputs to the prefrontal cortex have an important function in the regulation of cognition in the nonhuman primate. Depletion of dopamine inputs impairs performance on tasks that are mediated by this brain region [30,31]. The role of monoaminergic cortical inputs in the regulation of neural systems mediating higher cognitive functions in humans is less well specified. Links between a specific neurotransmitter and a neuropsychological function can be made by relating drug-induced changes in neuropsychological performance with the neurotransmitter system targeted by the drug. Examples of this approach are the impairment of paired associate learning due to clonidine-induced alteration in noradrenergic neurotransmission [32]. Improved cognitive performance has also been reported in studies that augment central monoaminergic drive [33]. Increasing dopaminergic tone improves performance on selective and divided attention tasks while dopamine blockade impairs performance in normal subjects [34]. Increasing central dopaminergic tone with amphetamine in patients with schizophrenia has also been reported to improve performance on a cognitive task that involves a large working memory component [35].

A less direct approach has been to determine the neuropsychological deficits associated with neuropathologies that preferentially target a particular neurotransmitter system. An example of the latter approach is verbal fluency performance in patients with Parkinson's disease [36,37]. These approaches have inherent limitations, not least due to the fact that drug-induced changes in neuropsychological performance lack neuroanatomical specificity. Furthermore, the neuropsychological deficits in patients with specific diseases can rarely, if ever, implicate a specific neurotransmitter system.

III. FUNCTIONAL IMAGING OF NEUROTRANSMITTER EFFECTS

A. Direct Effects of Pharamacological Challenge

Cognitive activation studies in conjunction with functional imaging have shown robust changes in neuronal activity associated with discrete psychological processes. An obvious question is whether specific pharmacological challenges can be associated with reproducible neuronal responses. We used apomorphine (5 or 10 μg/kg), a nonselective dopamine agonist, as a pharmacological probe while carrying out repeated measurements of regional cerebral blood flow (rCBF) that extended over the course of action of the drug. Difference in the distribution of changes in rCBF, before and after drug, were used to identify areas activated by apomorphine. Compared to a placebo control experiment, both doses of apomorphine were associated with a remarkably similar profile of activation involving the anterior cingulate cortex. Apomorphine-induced increases of rCBF were also seen in the right prefrontal cortex at the 10 μg/kg dose and less significantly in the left prefrontal cortex. The similarity in the location of rCBF increases in the anterior cingulate with both doses of apomorphine is evidence for a significant biological effect and broadly in agreement with the reported stimulatory effects of dopamine agonists on cerebral blood flow (CBF) in animals and man. For example, in man the dopamine agonists apomorphine, piribedil, bromocriptine, and the dopamine precursor L-DOPA all increase CBF [38,39,39]. In the anaesthetized baboon apomorphine also increases CBF [40]. These results are also in line with some human studies in which a selective increase of prefrontal rCBF has been noted following dopaminergic challenge [35].

Apomorphine stimulates dopamine autoreceptors located on cell bodies or dendrites of dopaminergic neurones but also acts on dopaminergic receptors postsynaptic to dopamine neurones [41]. Either or both sites might be the pharmacological site of action of apomorphine by which the effects on rCBF are mediated. If a direct postsynaptic effect on dopamine receptors in the anterior cingulate is postulated then D_1 receptor stimulation would seem more likely as dopamine D_1 receptors are in higher concentration than dopamine D_2 receptors in cortical areas [42,43]. If a direct action on presynaptic dopamine autoreceptors is postulated then rCBF changes might be manifest in areas of dense dopaminergic terminal innervation. Unlike the restricted dopaminergic innervation of the rat cortex, in man, most cortical areas are innervated. However, innervation is most dense in the anterior cingulate and motor cortex where dopaminergic projections are to all cortical layers [44].

The demonstration of a regionally specific drug effect is open to the interpretation that what is being measured is local vascular effects. This possibility can be addressed in the context of a consideration of its neuromodulatory effects in that task specific effects cannot easily be accomodated by vascular explanations.

B. A Methodology for Measuring Modulatory Effects of Drugs

Understanding the regulatory role of dopamine and other modulatory neurotransmitters on cortical function in the human brain involves the specification of the neuroanatomical locus of interactions between modulatory neurotransmitter inputs and brain systems that mediate specific psychological processes [45]. The study of modulatory effects in humans requires a specific pharmaco-

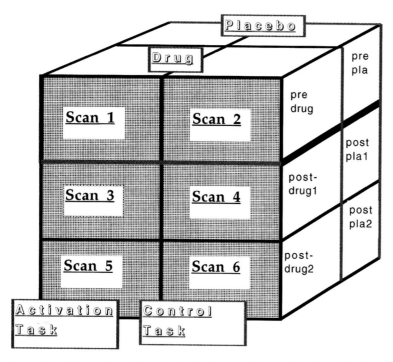

FIGURE 1 Schematic outline of the design used in combined psychopharmacological experiments. Scans 1, 3, and 5 correspond to the cognitive activation task while scans 2, 4, and 6 correspond to its reference control. Scans 1 and 2 refer to predrug scans while scans 3, 4, 5, and 6 represent postdrug or postplacebo scans. This design provides a means of assessing cognitive task and drug related activations as well as the interaction between drug and cognitive task.

logical manipulation and can be approached from the perspective of a factorial experimental design. At the level of an imaging experiment measurement of a neuromodulatory effect requires the stimulation of a large set of neurons (to be modulated) with the simultaneous activation of a neuromodulatory neurotransmitter system (the modulatory influence). This design involves combining two treatment effects within the same experiment with the effect of interest being that of the influence of the second treatment on the pattern of activity evoked by a first treatment. This neuromodulatory effect can be explicitly assessed from the interaction term (see Chapter 8).

In a combined psychological and pharmacological experiment the question being asked is what is the effect of a pharmacological manipulation on the pattern of activation induced by the psychological task. The interaction term in this case describes the subset of brain regions engaged by the psychological task in which there has been a significant modification of neuronal activity, either increases or decreases, brought about by the introduction of a drug. The basic design of a typical experiment is outlined in Fig. 1. The 2 by 3 layout of these experiments can be seen to enable the determination of three separate effects. These effects are that of the psychological task, that of the drug manipulation, and that of the effect of the drug on the pattern of cognitive task induced activation. It is this latter effect that is of primary interest in combined psychopharmacological studies.

C. Modulatory Effects of Dopamine in Normal Subjects

The question addressed in these experiments is what are the effects of dopamine manipulation on the pattern of psychological task induced neuronal activations in the prefrontal cortex? On the basis of an extensive primate literature we were in a position to predict that altering central dopaminergic drive would result in a significant modulation of cognitive task induced neuronal activation in the prefrontal cortex. We had previously shown that a task that involved the comparison of neuronal activity during the free recall of either sub (5 word)- or supraspan (15 word) lists elicited a robust and highly reproducible prefrontal activation [46]. On this basis the same psychological task was chosen while for the pharmacological challenge the requirement was for an agent that reliably altered central dopaminergic tone. Apomorphine was chosen because it is a widely used and potent D1 and D2 dopamine agonist.

In the cognitive task subjects were required to immediately free recall auditorily presented 5 (subspan)- and 15 (supraspan)-word lists while being scanned. Thus in the subspan condition subjects repeated a series of different groups of 5 words (45 words in all) while in the supraspan task the words were presented 15 at a time (45 in all). The essential difference between the supraspan and subspan task is the amount of auditory verbal material that has to be remembered. The subspan tasks was presented during three scans and likewise the supraspan task during three scans. A cognitive subtraction, *i.e.*, distribution of perfusion in the supraspan compared to that in subspan was used to identify the activation profile representing brain systems engaged by the increased auditory–verbal memory demand that necessarily involves encoding and retrieval [47]. Memory performance on the postdrug supraspan tasks was measured as the number of correctly recalled words in the three presentations of each 15 word list and this was then expressed as a percentage of the number correctly recalled in the predrug condition.

We studied the effects of apomorphine at two doses (5 and 10 μg/kg) to assess possible dose–response relationships. To control for possible nonspecific drug effects that might have independent effects on cortical neuronal activity we carried out a parallel experiment in a separate group of subjects under the same psychological activation conditions. However, for the drug challenge on this occasion we administered buspirone, a 5-HT$_{1A}$ partial agonist [48,49]. As buspirone has a distinct pharmacological profile to that of apomorphine we predicted that apomorphine and buspirone would have regionally distinct effects on memory-task induced increases in rCBF. To summarise, therefore, our first prediction was that apomorphine would modulate memory-induced activations in the prefrontal cortex. In contrast, as hippocampal activation is sensitive to 5-HT$_{1A}$ partial agonists [50,51], and 5-HT$_{1A}$ receptors are in high concentration in hippocampal and related brain structures [52,53], we predicted that buspirone would modulate memory-induced alterations of rCBF in the medial temporal cortex.

In all 24 normal, right handed, male subjects (age range 21–36) were studied. Each subject underwent six PET scans over a 75-min period. Two PET measurements were undertaken before ($t = -12$ min and -2 min) and four measurements after the administration of an active drug or placebo ($t = +15, +25, +45,$ and $+55$ min for apomorphine; $+25, +35, +55,$ and $+65$ min for buspirone; $+20, +30, +50,$ and $+60$ min for placebo). Scan times postdrug were chosen on the basis of the kinetics of buspirone and apomorphine, the time course of side effects and the induction of centrally mediated neuroendocrine responses [54,55]. Scan times for placebo were chosen so as to minimise the time difference between placebo scans and active drug scans (difference of 5 min only). Six subjects received placebo (saline sc), six apomorphine (5 μg/kg sc), six apomorphine (10 μg/kg sc), and six received buspirone 30 mg orally.

The profile of memory activation (supraspan minus subspan task) defined the brain system within which the modulatory effects of drug challenge were examined. The regions activated by the task included the prefrontal cortex and an area centred on the posterior cingulate cortex (Fig. 2). The prefrontal activations (Brodmann's areas (BA) 9/10/45,46) were bilateral and encompassed the middle and superior frontal gyri. The posterior activation was centred on the posterior cingulate cortex (BA 23) but also subsumed the posterior extent of the parahippocampal cortex (BA 27/30), the retrosplenial cortex (BA 29/30), and a medial parietal structure, the precuneus (BA 31), adjacent to the posterior cingulate.

Compared to placebo, and averaged across all postdrug scans, apomorphine 5 μg/kg attenuated memory-induced activations in the prefrontal

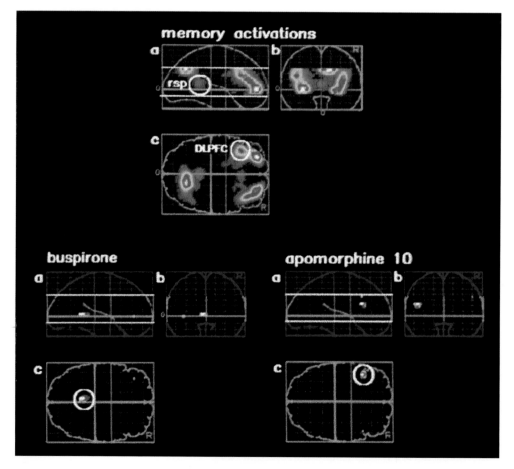

FIGURE 2 An example of a psychopharmacological interaction. (Top) The brain system activated during a long-term episodic memory task. (Bottom) The regions, within the memory system, where activation is attenuated by buspirone (left) and apomorphine, (right). These regions correspond to the retrosplenial and left dorsolateral prefrontal cortices.

cortex (BA 10/45/46). At the time of maximal drug induced impairment of memory function, derived from the percentage of words freely recalled, the maximal attenuation of activity was in the left dorsolateral prefrontal cortex (DLPFC). Compared to placebo, apomorphine 5 μg/kg augmented memory-induced activations in the precuneus (BA 31), posterior cingulate (BA 23), and retrosplenial cortex (BA 30). The effects of higher dose apomorphine were remarkably similar to those at the lower dosage. Averaged across all postdrug scans, and compared to placebo, apomorphine 10 μg/kg again attenuated memory-induced activations in the prefrontal region centred on BA 45/46. At the time of maximal impairment of memory function the maximal attenuation of activation was in the left dorsolateral prefrontal cortex. Compared to placebo, and similarly to the lower dose, apomorphine 10 μg/kg augmented memory-induced activations in the posterior cingulate cortex (BA 23), retrosplenial cortex (BA 30), and adjacent precuneus (BA 31).

The profile of interactions seen with buspirone and the same memory task was clearly distinct from that found with apomorphine. Compared to placebo, and averaged across all postdrug scans, buspirone attenuated memory-induced activations in the right prefrontal cortex (BA 10/46). In contrast to both doses of apomorphine, buspirone also attenuated memory-induced activations in the retrosplenial area (BA 30) and adjacent parahippocampal gyrus (BA 27/29/30). Areas of augmented activity were noted in the left DLPFC and in the posterior cingulate (BA 23) and adjacent precuneus (BA 31) The principle drug attenuations are illustrated in Fig. 2.

As the drugs had significant effects on cognitive task induced changes in neurophysiology an important question is whether they were manifest at the level of behaviour. Memory performance on the second and third supra-span tasks (relative to predrug performance) were examined. A significant effect of drug on memory performance was noted with performance increasing across presentations in the placebo group and decreasing in all active drug groups.

This series of studies demonstrates that distinct regional patterns of attenuations and augmentations of memory-induced activations can be distinguished following drug administration. Particularly striking was the observation that both doses of apomorphine resulted in a significant attenuation of activity in the left dorsolateral prefrontal cortex. In contrast, the effect of buspirone was a regionally distinct attenuation centred on the retrosplenial area. Furthermore, the maximal attenuation of memory-induced activation correlated in time with maximal impairment of memory function. In other words impaired neurophysiology was correlated in time with impaired performance on a behavioural measure. The specific interactions demonstrated are likely to result from differential effects on neurotransmitter systems targeted by these drugs and cannot easily be accounted for by nonspecific effects. The effects of both drugs on behaviour were associated with a differential effect on neurophysiology. One explanation is that the observed effects occur at the level of the vasculature. This seems most unlikely as the measured parameter is that of a differential effect on neuronal activations induced by a cognitive task. Furthermore, the effects are seen only under the condition of activation, whereas a direct effect on the vasculature should manifest under both control and activation conditions.

With apomorphine the attenuation of activation was limited to the prefrontal cortex. This confirms the hypothesis of a specific interaction between dopamine and memory function in this brain region. The finding is in agreement with animal data in terms of both regional effects and the impact on a task that engages a mnemonic function [31]. The findings are therefore entirely consistent with a neuromodulatory role for dopamine in the prefrontal cortex in man and closely parallel experiments in primates wherein spatial memory tasks, in particular, are significantly modulated by microiontophoretic application of dopamine [25]. The data from primates implicate a D1 mechanism and studies using selective dopaminergic agents are required to determine if similar explanations apply to humans.

The observation that the site of maximal memory attenuation of activity with buspirone was in the retrosplenial/parahippocampal region provides an indicator that the observed drug induced interactions are not a nonspecific effect of altered memory performance, that was similar under the conditions of both apomorphine and buspirone administration, but are specific to particular pharmacological manipulations.

In keeping with the regional attenuation of neurophysiological responses a decrease in memory performance was seen under all active drug conditions [56,57]. The experiment suggests that dopaminergic and serotonergic inputs, either directly or indirectly, are capable of modulating memory induced activations on a selective basis in different brain regions. The methodology and findings demonstrate that it is possible to link neurotransmission and neuropsychological functioning and, more importantly, to specify the neuroanatomical sites of such interactions.

IV. NEUROMODULATORY EFFECTS OF DOPAMINE IN SCHIZOPHRENIA

A. Theoretical Background

Dopaminergic dysregulation remains a theoretical cornerstone for research on the pathophysiology and treatment of schizophrenia. The most direct evidence for a dopaminergic dysfunction in schizophrenia is the psychotic inducing effects of dopaminergic agonists [58,59] and antipsychotic potency of dopaminergic antagonists [60,61]. The evidence linking dopamine dysfunction to schizophrenia is largely indirect and in terms of direct measurements of central dopamine the most robust finding has been that of elevated dopamine receptor numbers reported from postmortem investigations [62,63]. A difficulty with this latter type of evidence is the possible long lasting effect of prior exposure to neuroleptic medication. PET experiments that address the issue of dopamine receptor numbers in schizophrenia *in vivo* can overcome this deficiency by studying drug naive patients. Unfortunately, ligand based approaches have given rise to contradictory findings [64,65].

The mesolimbic–mesocortical dopamine system originates in the ventral tegmentum and a dysfunction of this system in particular is thought to be an important pathophysiological mechanism in schizophrenia [66,67]. It is noteworthy that there is substantial evidence that this system is highly susceptible to the influence of stress. Furthermore, the stress responsiveness of the mesolimbic component of this system is increased by pathology in the prefrontal cortex [68]. One of the most robust epidemiological findings in schizophrenia is that patients are highly susceptible to stressful environments which frequently lead to a reemergence of psychotic symptoms. An abnormality in dopamine function could therefore provide a bridge between clinical observation and biological mediating mechanisms.

Preliminary findings have suggested significant neuromodulatory effects of dopamine manipulation, with apomorphine or amphetamine, on the function of the dorsolateral prefrontal cortex in patients with schizophrenia [35]. To determine whether there are abnormal neuromodulatory effects of dopamine in schizophrenia we examined its regulatory role on cortical function in a placebo controlled experiment of normal and unmedicated acute schizophrenic subjects. Using a factorial experimental design the effect of a dopaminergic perturbation with apomorphine, on a cognitive task induced neuronal activation was directly compared across groups.

B. Modulatory Effects in Acute Unmedicated Schizophrenic Patients

The experiment involved 24 right-handed male subjects and comprised 12 unmedicated patients who met DSM III - R criteria for schizophrenia and 12 normal controls. Nine of the patients were neuroleptic and psychotropic medication naive while the remaining 3 were free of psychotropic medication for a minimum of 6 months. We scanned all subjects while they performed a paced verbal fluency task consisting of a paced orthographic verbal fluency (scans 1, 3, and 5), or a verbal word repetition control task (scans 2, 4, and 6). The tasks required a verbal response every 5 sec and by this means equality of response rate was ensured across experimental trials and subject groups. We had previously established that the cognitive activation, defined by the subtraction of the repetition control from the fluency conditions, activates a prefrontal network that includes the dorsolateral prefrontal cortex and the anterior cingulate cortex [69]. Under the same experimental conditions we scanned the subjects prior to (scans 1 and 2) or following (scans 3 to 6) an injection of either the nonselective dopaminergic agonist apomorphine, or placebo. The drug manipulation consisted of apomorphine, given subcutaneously in a dosage of 10 μg/kg, or placebo administered prior to scan 3. This dosage has a significant effect on neural activity in the prefrontal and anterior cingulate cortex [70]. Thus, control subjects and schizophrenic patients were studied under a condition of verbal fluency and verbal repetition prior to and following a subcutaneous injection of either apomorphine or placebo.

Six separate rCBF measurements, with an interscan interval of 10 min, were recorded from each subject. The factorial design enabled us to determine, from the interaction term, the effect of one treatment (the administration of the dopaminergic agonist apomorphine) on the effect of the other (the neuronal response to the cognitive activation). In this particular experiment the effect of interest is the differential effect across groups of dopamine perturbation on the pattern of neuronal activation induced by the cognitive challenge.

In normal subjects the cognitive activation, derived from a comparison of the neuronal response in the repetition condition from the fluency condition, showed the expected pattern of activation that included the left dorsolateral prefrontal cortex, thalamus, and anterior cingulate cortex. The same cognitive activation in schizophrenic patients, compared to normals, indicated a failure of activation localised to the anterior cingulate cortex (Fig. 3).

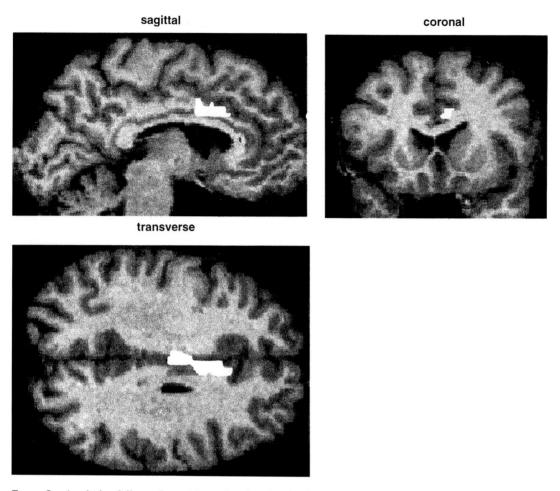

FIGURE 3   A relative failure of cognitive task-related activation in a group of untreated schizophrenic subjects when compared to healthy controls. PET results are superimposed onto an MRI scan rendered into standard stereotactic space. The region of significant difference is in the anterior cingulate cortex.

Following dopaminergic manipulation with apomorphine, this relative failure of task induced cingulate activation in schizophrenic patients was reversed. In the postapomorphine state schizophrenic patients displayed a significant augmentation of the neuronal response to cognitive activation in the anterior cingulate cortex relative to control subjects (Fig. 4). This effect was specific for verbal fluency induced activation as no differential effect of apomorphine on patterns of activation was evident under the repetition condition alone. The changes in rCBF at a selected pixel in the anterior cingulate cortex, pre- and postapomorphine, during cognitive activation for controls and schizophrenic patients are shown in Fig. 5.

The striking finding is that in patients with acute schizophrenia there was a significant effect of central dopaminergic manipulation on the pattern of neuronal response in the anterior cingulate cortex. The findings provide direct evidence of abnormal neuromodulatory effects of dopamine function on prefrontal function in schizophrenia and indicate that a critical anatomical locus of dysregulation is centred on the anterior cingulate cortex. One model of dopamine dysfunction in schizophrenia has suggested diminished tonic dopamine release, and upregulation of postsynaptic dopamine receptors with consequential increased postsynaptic responsiveness to phasic dopamine activation [71]. Increased postsynaptic sensitivity to phasic dopamine activation might also provide a mechanism for stress induced worsening of psychotic symptoms. Dopamine cells in the ventral tegmentum (VTA) are responsive to environmental cues and show an increase in discharge rate under stressful conditions [72,73]. Although the present findings are consistent with such a model they can equally well be interpreted in the context of a hyperdopaminergic state resulting in the modulation of extrinsic task induced activations in the cingulate cortex. In this model the effect of apomorphine is primarily presynaptic, resulting in a net decrease in dopminergic neurotransmission and consequently an enhanced excitatory response in the cingulate, which is now released from a tonic inhibitory dopamine input.

No treatment effects, either of task or drug, were observed in the dorsolateral prefrontal cortex of schizophrenic patients as has been reported by others [35,74,75]. The regional specificity of our finding is, however, consistent

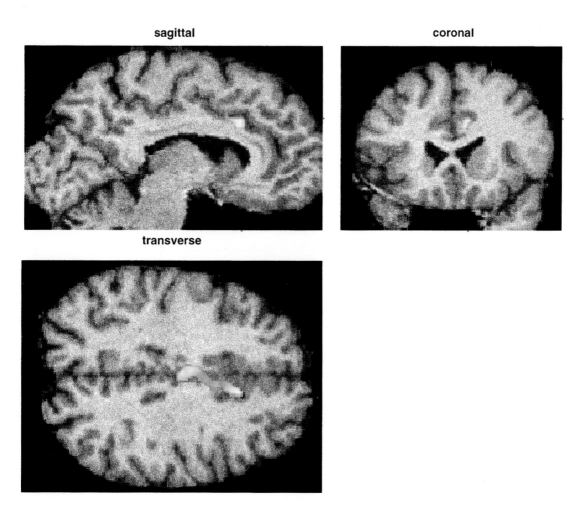

Figure 4 Relatively greater augmentaion of task-related anterior cingulate activity in schizophrenic subjects after the administration of apomorphine.

with evidence from other investigative modalities that indicate cingulate abnormality in schizophrenia. Core cingulate pathology has been described in neuropathological studies that report neuronal deficits, loss of interneurons and a decrease in GABA$_A$ receptors indicative of loss of GABAergic inhibitory cells [76–79]. Dopamine exerts an inhibitory effect on cortical activity and this effect is partially mediated via GABA release [80]. An alternative interpretation of our findings is that the loss of GABAergic inhibitory cells leads to a failure of dopaminergic inhibition of cortical activation.

C. Dopamine and Cortico-cortical Interactions in Schizophrenia

The findings of an abnormal neuromodulatory effect of dopamine in schizophrenia specifically implicate a dysfunction within the cingulate cortex. One perspective on this finding is that it points to a localised, or segregated, pathology in schizophrenia. However, an alternative view of higher brain function, complimentary to that of functional segregation, emphasises the integration of functionally specialised brain regions. Within this framework it has been proposed that the phenomenological features of schizophrenia can be conceptualised as representing abnormal interactions between different brain regions that mediate higher cognitive functions [81]. Empirical evidence bearing on this issue comes from a study of chronic medicated schizophrenic patients. In this study the patients were grouped into three categories on the basis of the expression of a classical symptom triad comprising psychomotor poverty, disorganisation, and reality distortion. A matched normal control group was also studied under the same experimental conditions. The study involved assessing the neural response to verbal fluency activation in a time series that was subsequently analysed in terms of functional connectivity. The principal observation, expressed across all schizophrenic groups, was of a task related failure of superior temporal deactivation in the presence of normal prefrontal activation. The findings were interpreted as suggesting a disruption of large-scale fronto-temporal interactions in schizophrenia [82,83].

In the context of our study of acute unmedicated patients, described above, we were able to replicate this finding of abnormal fronto-temporal interactions. During verbal fluency, relative to a repetition control condition, the schizophrenic patients again failed to show relative superior temporal deactivation. This striking replication indicated that the finding in chronic patients was not a function of neuroleptic medication or the stage of evolution of the illness but was present at its outset. As this study of unmedicated patients involved a manipulation of dopamine neurotransmission with apomorphine we were also able to ask the question whether this manipulation had any effect on prefrontal–temporal interactions. Consequently, we compared patterns of fronto-temporal interactions in the predrug and postdrug conditions. Following apomorphine administration there was a significant attenuation of the abnormal superior temporal activation, expressed in the nondrug state, in schizophrenic subjects. In other words, a manipulation of dopamine neurotransmission had a significant impact on abnormal patterns of cortico-cortical interactions in schizophrenia (Figs. 6 and 7).

Given that we have shown that the significant effect of apomorphine was on a task related activation of the cingulate cortex the observation of relative normalisation of fronto-temporal interactions in schizophrenia, post-apomorphine, suggests that the anterior cingulate cortex may be a source of abnormal cortical integration in schizophrenia. As already described the

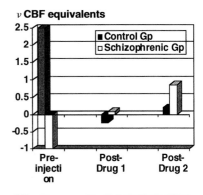

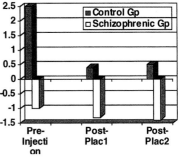

FIGURE 5 Graphic representation of the phenomena represented by Figs. 3 and 4. Activation from a region of the anterior cingulate cortex is shown both pre- and postapomorphine (top) and pre- and postplacebo (bottom).

sagittal   coronal

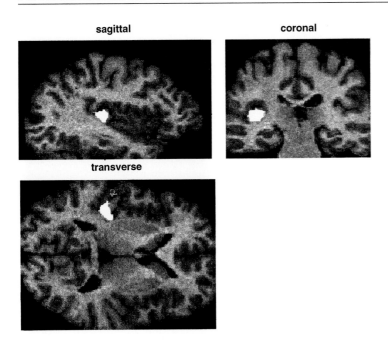

transverse

Figure 6 Failure of task-related deactivation in the left superior temporal cortex of a schizophrenic subjects when compared to healthy controls.

principal effects of dopamine on prefrontal function are mediated through the D1 receptor [17]. In the primate an enhancement of delay period activity via D1 receptor mechanisms suggests an influence on excitatory inputs responsible for the generation of delay period activity. That provides a mechanism through which dopamine can influence cognitive components of prefrontal function without affecting sensorimotor processing. The localisation of the D1 receptor to the spines of prefrontal cells that possess asymmetric synapses associated with glutaminergic inputs provides a mechanistic basis for the specific effects of D1 antagonists on cell firing. The enhancement of cingulate activity in schizophrenia following apomorphine could conceivably reflect a differential facilitation of excitatory inputs. The consequent enhancement of cingulate activity may enable it to exert an appropriate regulatory influence on more remote cortical regions that result in a normalisation of cortico-cortical interactions. Although the anterior cingulate cortex has multiple functional specialisations it has a critical role in attentional mechanisms that are core abnormalities in schizophrenia [84–86]. The predominant dopamine inputs to the cingulate are to layers II and III pyramidal cells that are the primary cortico-cortical output layers [87].

One possibility that emerges from these studies is that the anterior cingulate participates, directly or indirectly, in the pathogenesis of a dysfunctional neuronal integration in schizophrenia. A direct modulatory effect of cingulate activation on the temporal cortex has been demonstrated in primates [88]. A similar effect in humans is implied by a finding that cingulate activation is associated with modulation in a concurrent task-dependent cortical activation [89]. In the present study we have again observed abnormal fronto-temporal interactions that are modulated postdrug. This finding suggests that in schizophrenia there is a dysregulation in the dopaminergic modulation of cingulate neuronal activity with a consequent impairment in the functional

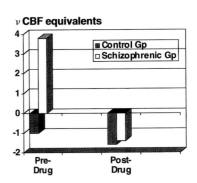

Figure 7 Graphic representation of the effect of apomorphine on the left superior temporal cortex of schizophrenic and control subjects. After the drug, there is a task-related deactivation in schizophrenic subjects akin to that seen in controls.

integration of more remote, but anatomically connected, cortical regions. A limitation of the present study that must caution against overinterpretation of the data is the restricted nature of the time series on which this inference is based.

V. CONCLUSIONS

Neuromodulatory neurotransmitters act not by directly affecting neuronal firing, but by modifying neuronal excitability such that responses to other neurotransmitters are altered [90]. Combined pharmacological and cognitive activation paradigms, in conjunction with functional imaging, now enable the *in vivo* specification of interactions between drugs and psychological functions in selective brain regions. Our observations of selective interactions between dopamine and memory function in the prefrontal cortex in normal volunteer subjects is consistent with a neuromodulatory effect. Similarly, the observation in schizophrenic patients point to abnormal neurmodulatory effects of dopamine in schizophrenia.

Cortical functions are the result of convergence of diverse afferent systems upon intrinsic neuronal elements. How these diverse synaptic inputs are integrated to produce a coherent output is a central question for the understanding of neuronal function [91]. Monoaminergic cortical afferent systems through their modulatory effects on cortical function may also act by influencing cortical integration. A dysregulation, due either to a functional increase or to a decrease in monoaminergic inputs, is likely to have profound effects on neuronal integration. In this respect the application of methodologies, similar to those described, that can examine these effects has powerful theoretical potential for the study of psychiatric disease.

Overall our studies provide direct evidence that monoaminergic projection systems have a high degree of regional functional specificity in their effects and provide a framework for linking neurotransmitter systems to specific psychological processes in humans. In schizophrenia our observation of an abnormal neuromodulatory effect of dopamine on the anterior cingulate cortex provides a basis for understanding how neurochemical abnormalities might result in abnormal cortico-cortical interactions and the consequent disintegration of mental function characteristic of this condition. Linking neurotransmitter systems to psychological processes provides a critical theoretical and mechanistic basis for the study of pathophysiological mechanisms in the major psychoses.

References

1. I. Kupfermann. Modulatory actions of neurotransmitters. *Annu. Rev. Neurosci.* **2,** 447–465 (1979).
2. P. S. Goldman-Rakic. Topography of cognition: Parallel distributed networks in primate association cortex. *Annu. Rev. Neurosci.* **11,** 137–156 (1988).
3. T. Sawaguchi and P. S. Goldman-Rakic. D1 dopamine receptors in prefrontal cortex: Involvement in working memory. *Science* **251,** 947–950 (1991).
4. R. M. Brown, A. M. Crane, and P. S. Goldman. Regional distribution of monoamines in the cerebral cortex and subcortical structures of the rhesus monkey: Concentrations and in vivo synthesis rates. *Brain Res.* **168,** 133–150 (1979).

5. P. Gaspar, B. Berger, A. Febvret, A.Vigny, and J. P. Henry. Cathecolamine innervation of the human cerebral cortex as revealed by comparative immunohistochemistry of tyrosine hydroxylase and dopamine-beta-hydroxylase. *J. Comp. Neurol.* **279,** 249–271 (1989).

6. R. D. Oades and G. M. Halliday. Ventral tegmental (A10) system: Neurobiology. 1. Anatomy and connectivity. *Brain Res. Rev.* **12,** 117–165 (1987).

7. G. C. Papadopoulos and J. G. Parnavelas. Monoamine systems in the cerebral cortex: Evidence for anatomical specificity. *Prog. Neurobiol.* **36,** 195–200 (1991).

8. J. F. Smiley, S. M. Williams, K. Szigeti, and P. S. Goldman-Rakic. Light and electron microscopic characterisation of dopamine-immunoreactive processes in human cerebral cortex. *J. Neurol. Neurosurg. Psychiatry* **321,** 325–335 (1992).

9. E. K. Richfield, A. B. Young, and J. B. Penney. Comparative distribution of dopamine D-1 and D-2 receptors in the cerebral cortex of rats, cats, and monkeys. *J. Comp. Neurol.* **28,** 409–426 (1989).

10. M. S. Lidow, P. S. Goldman-Rakic, D. W. Gallager, and P. Rakic. Distribution of dopaminergic receptors in the primate cerebral cortex: quantitative autoradiographic analysis using [^{3}H] raclopride, [^{3}H] spiperone and [^{3}H] SCH23390. *Neuroscience* **40,** 657–671 (1991).

11. P. S. Goldman-Rakic, C. Leranth, M. S. Williams, N. Mons, and M. Geffard. Dopamine synaptic complex with pyramidal neurons in primate cerebral cortex. *Proc. Natl. Acad. Sci. USA* **86,** 9015–9019 (1989).

12. J. Mantz, C. Milla, J. Glowinski, and A. M. Thierry. Differential effects of ascending neurons containing dopamine and noradrenaline in the control of spontaneous activity and of the evoked responses in the rat prefrontal cortex. *Prog. Neurobiol.* **36,** 195–200 (1991).

13. J. H. Morrison and S. L. Foote. Noradrenergic and serotonergic innervation of cortical and thalamic visual structures in old and new world monkeys. *J. Comp. Neurol.* **243,** 117–138 (1986).

14. L. A. Chiodo and T. Berger. Interactions between dopamine and amino acid-induced excitation and inhibition in the striatum. *Brain Res.* **375**(1), 198–203 (1986).

15. A. G. Knapp and J. E. Dowling. Dopamine enhances exciatatory amino acid-gated conductances in cultured retinal horizontal cells. *Nature* **325,** 437–439 (1987).

16. E. Pralong and R. S. G. Jones. Interactions of dopamine with glutamate- and GABA-mediated synaptic transmission in the rat entorhinal cortex in vitro. *Eur. J. Neurosci.* **5**(6), 760–767 (1993).

17. T. Sawaguchi and P. S. Goldman-Rakic. The role of D1-dopamine receptor in working memory: Local injections of dopamine antagonists into the prefrontal cortex of rhesus monkeys performing an oculomotor delayed-response task. *J. Neurophysiol.* **71,** 515–528 (1994).

18. B. S. Bunney and G. K. Aghajanian. Dopamine and noreinephrine innervated cells in the rat prefrontal cortex: Pharmacological differentiation using microiontophoretic techniques. *Life Sci.* **19,** 1783–1792 (1976).

19. A. M. Thierry, T. M. Jay, S. Pirot, J. Mantz, R. Godbout, and J. Glowinski. Influence of afferent systems on the activity of the rat prefrontal cortex: Electrophysiological and pharmacological characterization. *In* "Motor and Cognitive Functions of the Prefrontal Cortex" (A. M. Thierry, Ed.), pp 35–50. Springer-Verlag, Berlin Heidelberg, 1994.

20. R. K. Dismukes. New concepts of molecular communication among neurons. *Behav. Brain Sci.* **2,** 409–448 (1979).

21. S. L. Foote, R. Freedman, and A. P. Oliver. Effects of putative neurotransmitters on neuronal acitivity in monkey auditory cortex. *Brain Res.* **86,** 229–242 (1975).

22. T. J. Brozoski, R. M. Brown, H. E. Rosvold, and P. S. Goldman. Cognitive deficit caused by regional depletion of dopamine in prefrontal cortex of rhesus monkey. *Science* **205,** 929–932 (1979).

23. A. F. T. Arnsten and P. S. Goldman-Rakic. Alpha2-adrenergic mechanisms in the

prefrontal cortex associated with cognitive decline in aged nonhuman primates. *Science* **230,** 1273–1276 (1985).

24. J. H. Ferron, A. M. Thierry, C. LeDouarin, and J. Glowinski. Inhibitory influence of mesocortical dopaminergic system on spontaneous activity or excitatory response induced from the thalamic mediodorsal nucleus in the rat medial prefrontal cortex. *Brain Res.* **302,** 257–265 (1984).

25. T. Sawaguchi, M. Matsumura, and K. Kubota. Cathecolaminergic effects on neuronal activity related to a delayed response task in monkey prefrontal cortex. *J. Neurophysiol.* **63,** 1385–1399 (1990).

26. T. Sawaguchi, M. Matsumura, and K. Kubota. Effects of dopamine antagonists on neuronla activity related to a delayed response task in monkey prefrontal cortex. *J. Neurophysiol.* **63,** 1401–1411 (1990).

27. C. Cepeda, N. A. Buchwald, and M. S. Levine. Neuromodulatory actions of dopamine in the neostriatum are dependent upon the excitatory amino acid receptor subtypes activated. *Proc. Natl. Acad. Sci.* **90**(20), 9576–9580 (1993).

28. C. Cepeda, Z. Radisavljevic, W. Peacock, M. S. Levine, and N. A. Buchwald. Differential modulation by dopamine of responses evoked by excitatory amino acids in human cortex. *Synapse* **11**(4), 330–341 (1992).

29. G. V. Williams and P. S. Goldman-Rakic. Modulation of memory fields by dopamine D1 receptors in prefrontal cortex. *Nature* **376,** 572–575 (1995).

30. M. Le Moal and H. Simon. Mesocorticolimbic dopaminergic network: Functional and regulatory roles. *Pysiol. Rev.* **71,** 155–234 (1992).

31. T. J. Brozoski, R. M. Brown, H. E. Rosvold, and P. S. Golman. Cognitive deficit caused by regional depletion of dopamine in the prefrontal cortex of rhesus monkey. *Science* **205,** 929–932 (1979).

32. C. D. Frith, J. Dowdy, I. N. Ferrier, and T. J. Crow. Selective impairment of paired associate learning after administration of a centrally acting adrenergic agonist (clonidine). *Psychopharmacology* **87,** 490–493 (1985).

33. R. Klorman, L. O. Bauer, H. W. Coons, J. L. Lewis, J. Peloquin, R. A. Perlmutter, R. M. Ryan, L. F. Salzman, and J. Straus. Enhanced effects of methylphenidate on normal young adults cognitive processes. *Psychopharmacol. Bull.* **20,** 3–9 (1984).

34. C. R. Clark, G. M. Geffen, and L. B. Geffen. Role of monoamine pathways in the control of attention: Effects of droperidol and methylphenidate in normal adult humans. *Psychopharmacology* **90,** 28–34 (1986).

35. D. G. Daniel, D. R. Weinberger, D. W. Jones, J. R. Zigun, R. Coppola, S. Handel, L. B. Bigelow, T. E. Goldberg, K. F. Berman, and J. E. Kleinman. The effect of amphetamine on regional cerebral blood flow during cognitive activation in schizophrenia. *J. Neurosci.* **11,** 1907–1917 (1991).

36. J. M. Gurd and C. D. Ward. Retreival from semantic and letter-initial categories in patients with Parkinson's disease. *Neuropsychology* **27,** 743–746 (1989).

37. N. Wolfe, D. I. Katz, M. L. Albert, A. Almozlino, R. Durso, M. C. Smith, and L. Volicer. Neuropsychological profile linked to low dopamine: in Alzheimer's disease, major depression and Parkinson's disease. *J. Neurol. Neurosurg. Psychol.* **53,** 915–917 (1990).

38. U. Sabitini, O. Rascol, P. Celsis, G. Houin, A. Rascol, and J. P. Marc-Verges. Subcutaneous apomorphine increases regional cerebral blood flow in parkinsonian patients via peripheral mechanisms. *Brit. J. Clin. Pharmacol.* **32,** 229–234 (1991).

39. A. Guell, G. Geraud, Ph. Jauzac, G. Victor, and M. C. Arne-Bes. Effects of a dopaminergic agonist (pirbedil) on cerebral blood flow in man. *J. Cereb. Blood Flow Metab.* **2,** 255–257 (1982).

40. J. McCulloch and A. Murray-Harper. Cerebral circulation: Effects of stimulation and blockade of dopamine receptors. *Am. J. Physiol.* **233,** 222–227 (1977).

41. G. K. Aghajanian and B. S. Bunney. Doamine "autoreceptors." Pharmacological

characterisation by micro iontopheretic single cell recording studies. *Naunyn-Schmiedeberg's Arch Pharmacol.* **297,** 1–7 (1977).

42. R. Cortes, B. Gueye, A. Pazos, A. Probst, and J. M. Palacious. Dopamine receptors in human brain: autoradiographic distribution of D1 sites. *Neuroscience* **28,** 263–273 (1989).

43. M. Camps, R. Cortes, B. Gueye, A. Probst, and J. M. Palacios. Dopamine receptors in human brain: Autoradiographic distribution of D2 sites. *Neuroscience* **28,** 275–290 (1989).

44. B. Berger, P. Gaspar, and C. Verney. Dopaminergic innervation of the cerebral cortex: Unexpected differences between rodents and primates. *Trends Neurosci.* **14,** 21–27 (1991).

45. K. J. Friston, P. Grasby, C. D. Frith, C. Bench, R. J. Dolan, P. J. Cowen, P. F. Liddle, and R. S. J. Frackowiak. The neurotransmitter basis of cognition: psychopharmacological activation studies using PET. *In* "Exploring Brain Functional Anatomy with Positron Tomography," pp 76–92. Wiley, Chichester, 1991.

46. P. M. Grasby, C. D. Frith, K. J. Friston, C. Bench, R. S. J. Frackowiak, and R. J. Dolan. Functional mapping of brain areas implicated in auditory memory function. *Brain* **116,** 1–20 (1993).

47. S. E. Petersen, P. T. Fox, M. I. Posner, M. Mintun, and M. E. Raichle. Positron emission tomographic studies of the cortical anatomy of single-word processing. *Nature* **331,** 585–589 (1988).

48. S. J. Peroutka. Selective interaction of novel anxiolytics with 5-hydroxytryptamine1A receptors. *Biol. Psychiatry* **5**(20), 971–979 (1985).

49. J. Traber and T. Glazer. 5-HT1A receptor-related anxiolytics. *Trends Pharmacol. Sci.* **8,** 432–437 (1987).

50. A. Wree, J. Zilles, A. Schleicher, E. Horvath, and J. Traber. Effect of the 5-HT1A receptor agonist on the local cerebral glucose utilization of the rat hippocampus. *Brain Res.* **436,** 283–290 (1987).

51. P. A. T. Kelly, C. J. Davis, and G. M. Goodwin. Differential patterns of local glucose utilization in response to 5-hydroxytryptamine agonists. *Neuroscience* **25,** 907–915 (1988).

52. A. Pazos, D. Hoyer, M. M. Dietl, and J. M. Palacios. Autoradiography of serotonin receptors. *In* (N. N. Osborne and M. Hamon, Eds.), pp. 507–543. Wiley, New York, 1988.

53. A. Pazos, A. Probst, and J. M. Palacios. Serotonin receptors in the human brain. Autoradiographic mapping of serotonin-1 receptors. *Neuroscience* **21,** 97–122 (1987).

54. S. Gancher, W. Woodward, B. Boucher, and J. Nutt. Peripheral pharmacokinetics of apomorphine in humans. *Ann Neurol.* **26,** 232–238 (1989).

55. R. E. Gammans, R. F. Mayol, and J. A. Labudde. Metabolism and disposition of buspirone. *Am. J. Med.* **80**(Suppl. 3B), 41–51 (1986).

56. K. J. Friston, P. Grasby, C. J. Bench, C. D. Frith, P. F. Liddle, P. Cowen, and R. S. J. Frackowiak. Measuring the neuromodulatory effects of drugs in man with positron emission tomography. *Neurosci. Lett.* **141,** 106–110 (1992).

57. P. M. Grasby, K. J. Friston, C. J. Bench, C. D. Frith, F. Paulesu, P. S. Cowen, and P. F. Liddle. The effect of apomorphine and buspirone on regional cerebral blood flow during the performance of a cognitive task—measuring neuromodulatory effects of psychotropic drugs in man. *Eur. J. Neurosci.* **4,** 1203–1212 (1992).

58. M. Davidson, R. S. E. Keefe, R. C. Mohs, L. J. Siever, M. F. Losonczy, T. B. Horvath, and K. L. Davis. L-dopa challenge and relapse in schizophrenia. *Am. J. Psychiatry* **141,** 934–938 (1987).

59. J. A. Lieberman, J. M. Kane, D. Gadaleta, R. Brenner, M. S. Lesser, and B. Kinon. Methylphenidate challenge as a predictor of relapse in schizophrenia. *Am. J. Psychiatry* **141,** 633–638 (1984).

60. P. Seeman, T. Lee, M. Chau-Wong, and K. Wong. Antipsychotic drug doses and neuroleptic/dopamine receptors. *Nature* **261,** 717–719 (1976).

61. I. Creese, D. R. Burt, and S. H. Snyder. Dopamine receptor binding predicts clinical and pharmacological potencies of antischizophrenic dugs. *Science* **192,** 481–483 (1976).

62. A. J. Cross, T. J. Crow, and F. Owen. 3H-Flupenthixol binding in postmortem brains of schizophrenics: Evidence for a selective increase in dopamine D2 receptors. *Psychopharmacology* **74,** 122–124 (1981).

63. P. Seeman, N. H. Bzowej, H. C. Guan, C. Bergeron, G. P. Reynolds, E. D. Bird, P. Riederer, K. Jellinger, and W. W. Tourtellote. Human brain D1 and D2 dopamine receptors in schizophrenia, Alzheimer's, Parkinson's and Huntington's diseases. *Neuropsychopharmacol.* **1,** 5–15 (1987).

64. L. Farde, F. A. Wiesel, S. Stone-Elander, C. Halldin, A.-L. Nordstrom, H. Hall, and G. Sedrall. D2 Dopamine receptors in neuroleptic-naive schizophrenic patients. *Arch. Gen. Psychiatry* **47,** 213–219 (1990).

65. D. F. Wong, H. N. Wagner, Jr., L. E. Tune, R. F. Dannals, G. D. Pearlson, J. M. Links, and C. A. Tamminga. Positron emission tomography reveals elevated D2 dopamine receptors in drug-naive schizophrenics. *Science* **234,** 1558–1563 (1986).

66. S. H. Snyder. Amphetamine psychosis: A model schizpohrenia mediated by cathecolamines. *Am. J. Psychiatry* **130,** 61–67 (1973).

67. J. R. Stevens. An anatomy of schizophrenia? *Arch. Gen. Psychiatry* **29,** 177–189 (1973).

68. A. Y. Deutch, W. A. Clark, and H. R. Roth. Prefrontal cortical depletion enhances the responsiveness of mesolimbic dopamine neurons to stress. *Brain Res.* **521,** 311–315 (1990).

69. C. D. Frith, K. J. Friston, P. F. Liddle, and R. S. J. Frackowiak. Willed action and the prefrontal cortex in man: A study with PET. *Proc. R. Soc. London B* **244,** 241–246 (1991).

70. P. Grasby, K. J. Friston, C. J. Bench, *et al.* The effect of apomorphine on regional cerebral blood flow in normal volunteers. *Schiz. Res.* **6**(2), 149 (1992).

71. A. A. Grace. Phasic *versus* tonic dopamine release and the modulation of dopamine system responsivity: A hypothesis for the etiology of schizophrenia. *Neuroscience* **41,** 1–24 (1991).

72. M. Fabre, E. T. Rolls, J. P. Ashton, and G. Williams. Activity of neurons in the ventral tegmental region of the behaving monkey. *Behav. Br. Res.* **9,** 213–235 (1983).

73. M. E. Trulson, and D. W. Preussler. Dopamine-containing ventral tegmental area in freely moving cats: Activity during the sleep–wake cycle and effects of stress. *Exp. Neurol.* **83,** 367–377 (1984).

74. D. R. Weinberger, K. F. Berman, and B. P. Illowsky. Physiological dysfunction of dorsolateral prefrontal cortex in schizophrenia. III. A new cohort and evidence for a monoaminergic mechanism. *Arch. Gen. Psychiatry* **45,** 609–615 (1988).

75. K. F. Berman, B. P. Illowsky, and D. R. Weinberger. Physiological dysfunction of dorsolateral prefrontal cortex in schizophrenia. IV. Further evidence for regional and behavioral specificity. *Arch. Gen. Psychiatry* **45,** 616–622 (1988).

76. F. M. Benes, J. Davidson, and J. E. Bird. Quantitative cytoarchitectural studies of schizophrenic cortex. *Arch. Gen. Psychiatry* **43,** 31–35 (1986).

77. F. M. Benes, J. McSparren, E. D. Bird, J. P. SanGiovanni, and S. I. Vincent, Deficits in small interneurons in prefrontal and cingulate cortex of schizophrenic and schizoaffective patients. *Arch. of Gen. Psychiatry* **48,** 996–1001 (1991).

78. F. M. Benes, S. I. Vincent, G. Alsterberg, E. D. Bird, and J. P. SanGiovanni. Increased GABAa receptor binding in superficial layers of schizophrenic cingulate cortex. *J. Neurosci.* **12,** 924–929 (1992).

79. S. Akbarian, W. E. Bunney, Jr., S. G. Potkin, S. B. Wigal, J. O. Hagman, C. A. Sandman, and E. G. Jones. Altered distribution of nicotinamide—Adenine dinucleotide phosphate-dia-phorase cells in frontal lobe of schizophrenics implies disturbances in cortical development. *Archives of Gen. Psychiatry* **50,** 169–177 (1993).

80. S. Retaux, M. J. Besson, and J. Penit-Soria. Opposing effects of dopamine D2 receptor stimulation on the spontaneous and the electrically evoked release of [^{3}H] GABA on rat prefrontal cortical slices. *Neuroscience* **42**, 61–71 (1991).

81. K. J. Friston and C. D. Frith. Schizophrenia: A disconnection syndrome? *Clin. Neurosci.* **3**, 89–97 (1995).

82. K. J. Friston, C. D. Frith, P. Fletcher, D. Silbersweig, P. Liddle, R. J. Dolan, and R. S. J. Frackowiak. Abnormal fronto-temporal interactions in schizophrenia. *In* "Biology of Schizophrenia and Affective Disorders" (S. J. Watson, Ed.). Raven Press, New York, 1994.

83. C. D. Frith, K. J. Friston, S. Herold, D. Silbersweig, P. C. Fletcher, C. Cahill, and R. J. Dolan. Regional brain activity in chronic schizophrenic patients during the performance of a verbal fluency task. *Br. J. Psychiatry* **167**, 343–349 (in press).

84. E. Bleuler. "Dementia Praecox or the Group of Schizophrenias." Int Press, New York, 1950.

85. A. McGhie and J. Chapman. Disorders of attention and perception in early schizophrenia. *Br. J. Med. Psychol.* **34**, 103–116 (1961).

86. P. Liddle, K. J. Friston, C. D. Frith, S. R. Hirsch, T. Jones, and R. S. J. Frackowiak. Patterns of cerebral blood flow in schizophrenia. *Br. J. Psychiatry* **160**, 179–186 (1992).

87. J. H. Fallon and S. E. Loughlin. Monoamine innervation of cerebral cortex and a theory of the role of monoamines in cerebral cortex and basal ganglia. *In* "Cerebral Cortex: Further Aspects of Cortical Function, Including Hippocampus" (E. G. Jones & A. Peters, Eds.), Vol. 6, pp. 41–128. Plenum, New York, 1987.

88. P. Muller-Preuss and D. Ploog. Inhibition of auditory cortical neurons during phonation. *Brain Res.* **215**, 61–76 (1981).

89. P. C. Fletcher, C. D. Frith, P. M. Grasby, T. Shallice, R. S. J. Frackowiak, and R. J. Dolan. Brain systems for encoding and retrieval of auditory–verbal memory: An in vivo study in humans. *Brain* **118**, 401–416 (1995).

90. C. Kaczmarek and K. Levitan. What is neuromodulation? *In* "Neuromodulation" (C. Kaczmarek and K. Levitan, Eds.), pp. 3–17, New York, Oxford University Press, 1987.

91. K. J. Friston, C. D. Frith, R. E. Passingham, R. J. Dolan, P. F. Liddle, and R. S. J. Frackowiak. Entropy and cortical activity: Information theory and PET findings. *Cereb. Cortex* **2**(3), 259–267, (1992).

PART THREE

FUTURE PERSPECTIVES

CHAPTER SEVENTEEN

BRAIN MAPS: LINKING THE PRESENT TO THE FUTURE

I. ATLASES, MAPS, AND THEIR APPLICATION TO HUMAN NEUROSCIENCE

The nervous system is fertile ground for map making. Ever since the earliest investigators of nervous system function, physical as well as theoretical depictions of brain function have been visualised using some form of mapping methods. If one focuses on the structural aspects of brain anatomy, an important difference between geographical maps of the Earth and neuroanatomical maps of the brain is quickly realised. That is, that while there is one single unique physical reality to the geographical organisation of Earth, neuroanatomy must represent a variable physical reality that differs from individual to individual. Thus, human brain map atlases of structure and function require a representation that accounts for variance between individuals. Further, neuroscientists have yet to agree definitively on a standard reference system and nomenclature to define brain location. This again differs from geographical maps where the conventions of longitude, latitude, and altitude represent a universal standard.

Despite these differences between geographical and neuroanatomical maps, there are many similarities. Both Earth and brain maps can represent a seemingly infinite number of variables. For Earth maps these may take the form of population density, crime rate, transportation systems, temperature, environmental pollutants, *etc.* [1,2]. Similarly, brain maps can describe regional blood flow, metabolism, receptor density, fibre connections, *etc.* Both Earth and brain maps can be depicted at different scales. For the Earth maps this can range from global depictions to local neighbourhoods. In the brain, maps can be equally global, regional, nuclear, cellular, or ultrastructural. Both Earth and brain maps change over a wide time scale. The continental drifts that occur over hundreds of millions of years can be contrasted with meteorological maps that vary from minute to minute. Evolutionary changes in brain anatomy can similarly be contrasted with electrophysiological fluctuations that occur in the millisecond time range.

Atlases are abstract representations of physical realities. While we are most familiar with geographical maps, they are, in fact, an aspect of almost all disciplines. Their utility is in the organisation and visualisation of information so as to provide better insights about the subject matter and as a tool for data exploration. This may be as simple as plotting a route from city A to city B or as complex as examining celestial movement based on composite space and Earth sensors. Maps need not represent simply physical realities but can also be used to depict abstract concepts, temporal patterns, or theoretical constructs [1,2].

One can conclude this analogy by examining the types of data depiction schemes that have been used for Earth and are now, with ever increasing regularity, being applied to the brain. Three-dimensional spherical models of Earth, such as globes, are commonly found in most elementary school classrooms. Flattening of this true representation of the earth induces aberrations that have led to many schemes for the projection and flattening of the three-dimensional surface onto a flat sheet. All of these approaches result in either errors or discontinuities in the representation. The complex gyral patterns of the human brain represent a similarly difficult task [3–5]. The heterogeneous internal structure of Earth is rarely depicted in anything more complex than cross-sectional slices. The same can be said of brain maps. The challenge of producing a flattened brain map that depicts both cortical surface and internal nuclei is a formidable task indeed.

The advent of digital representation provides a meaningful and highly flexible new tool to aid in the map making process. With a true three-dimensional representation, the observer can select, scale, and view any orientation at will provided that the appropriate data set is available for survey. Quantifiable information can then be retrieved by pointing to the appropriate location in space and opening a file that produces tabular data about a given region or a selected view of detailed structure at a higher degree of magnification.

This concept raises yet another problem. Tools are available for analysing brain structure at a macroscopic level, particularly with the advent of *in vivo* imaging techniques such as X-ray computed tomography (CT) and magnetic resonance imaging (MRI). Microscopic anatomy has been of interest to investigators for more than a century. The same can be said, although for a shorter time frame, of ultrastructural anatomy of the brain. Critical, though largely missing components of these methods, are the appropriate bridging technologies that can span the gamut from macroscopic to microscopic and microscopic to ultrastructural scales. Yet, in order to have a continuous, smooth scaling from the ultrastructural level to the macroscopic level such methods must be established.

In this chapter, we will explore the types of maps that can be produced of the nervous system and the opportunities as well as constraints that currently exist for their development and ultimate use. It should be realised, however, that the creation of formal digital and standardised approaches to mapping of the brain are less of a luxury and more of a requirement in the current neuroscientific era as the explosion in neuroscientific information demands an organised approach to communication between neuroscientists that will increase both the efficiency and the quality of data analysis [6–12].

Collaborating on these efforts and in the ideas expressed in this chapter are my colleagues in the International Consortium for Brain Mapping (ICBM), including Arthur Toga, Ph.D., from UCLA, Alan C. Evans, Ph.D., from the Montreal Neurological Institute, and Peter Fox, M.D., and Jack Lancaster,

Ph.D., from the University of Texas Health Sciences Center for San Antonio. Support for this work was provided by the Human Brain Project in the United States through the National Institutes of Mental Health and the National Institute for Drug Addiction. We are grateful for the support of the Pierson–Lovelace Foundation, the Brain Mapping Medical Research Organization and The Ahmanson Foundation.

II. ATLAS DESIGNS

A. Current Approaches

Most atlases of the human brain and, for that matter, the brains of other species [13], are derived from one, or at best a few, individual specimens [14–18]. Such atlases may take the form of anatomical references or they may represent a particular feature of the brain [19], such as a specific neurochemical distribution [20] or cerebral cortical cytoarchitecture [14]. In existing atlases, proportional scaling systems are typically employed to reference a given brain to the atlas brain. The commonly used human atlases include those of Talairach and Tournoux [18] and Schaltenbrand and Wahren [16]. In the former, provisions were created to attempt to make individuals comparable by subdividing the brain into 12 volumes referenced to the anterior and posterior commissures. Linear scaling is used to stretch or constrict the 12 volumes so as to approximate the shape and position of a given brain to the atlas brain. The Talairach atlas was derived from the brain of a 60-year-old French woman. It depicts one hemisphere assuming interhemispheric symmetry. With the exception of the upper midbrain, the atlas excludes the brain stem and cerebellum.

Atlases such as that of Talairach and Tournoux [18] have proven very useful for anatomical normalisation required for surgical procedures, particularly those at brain sites close to the origins of the reference system (*i.e.*, the anterior and posterior commissures), such as the thalami and basal ganglia. It is predictable that such an atlas would be successful for areas of the brain that have low intersubject variability and for sites close to the landmarks of the reference system. Such atlases will be progressively less accurate in more highly variable portions of the brain such as the cerebral cortex (particularly neocortical and perisylvian regions) and in brain regions known to be highly asymmetric between the two cerebral hemispheres (*e.g.*, planum temporale) [21–26].

While these atlases were used to develop reference systems primarily for use in intraoperative planning, detailed atlases of brain cytoarchitecture [14,27], fibre tract connections [28], chemoarchitecture [20], and myeloarchitecture [29] were developed and frequently referenced, particularly to identify regions of the cerebral cortex.

B. Limitations of Current Atlas Tools

The anatomical variability between individual human brains is well known. Given the still undefined relationship between neuronal structure and function, an atlas based on an unvarying anatomy cannot succeed fully. One need only look at the functional and structural specialisation of the hemispheres to recognise the depth of this problem [21–26,30]. Single modality atlases are also of limited value, as the mapping from, for example, a neurochemical atlas to a functional assay, can lose accuracy only when transformed through a third (*i.e.*, anatomical) reference space.

Perhaps equally important is the fact that conventional atlases are typically published rather than maintained in a digital, electronic form. While printed atlases represent essentially an understanding frozen in time, a digital atlas grows and evolves. It can be resampled, annotated, and manipulated in a wide variety of ways. By its very nature, atlases that can be updated by new data improve in accuracy with time, achieving better statistics as more information is added. Further, digital atlases can be readily segmented into subpopulations by, for example, age, gender, race, behavioural abilities, handedness, or chemical composition.

Since no common reference space has been defined for the human brain, past atlases, including all of those referenced above, were never cross-referenced to allow a realistic and defensible means of comparing information relevant to the topic of one atlas with another. As mapping the human brain in all its complexity becomes a reality, comparing and correlating brain maps across modalities and subjects will improve our understanding of normal and pathologic variability [31,32]. Past atlases, because they were based on single specimen, or at best a few specimens, did not take into account the full range of anatomical variability between individuals. Correlations that result in multimodality brain maps will enable a more complete understanding of the complex and integrative responses that typically must still be studied one variable at a time. Digital atlases that use a common coordinate system allow comparisons between data sets acquired with different modalities. In addition, they allow comparisons with previously published atlas templates.

Previous brain atlases, based on single subjects, describe structural human brain neuroanatomy in a rigid and intolerant system that does not retain information about variability of structure, much less function. As noted above, the commonly used Talairach atlas [18] provides little information below the diencephalon and specifically omits the cerebellum entirely. While these approaches work reasonably well for structures near the origin of the coordinate system (anterior–posterior commissures), their accuracy diminishes as the distance from the origin increases. The errors are particularly large for the cerebral cortex of the human brain where it can reach magnitudes of 1–1.5 cm. This is undoubtedly due both to the limitations of affine transformations used in these atlases as well as the significant amount of variation in human cortical morphometry. Unlike animal stereotaxy, in human neurosurgical atlases it is not possible to base coordinate systems entirely on external bony landmarks because of the high degree of human intersubject variation for these structures [33]. Thus, issues pertaining to the generalisability of such atlases, variability within a population or accuracy of anatomic delineations (when performed) have largely been ignored. Similarly, issues pertaining to correlations across modalities in subjects have remained unexplored until recent times [34,35].

The ability to correlate any volume or model within a common coordinate system not only enables one to generate new anatomical models but also allows a comparison of current data with previously published atlas templates. Such a system could form the basis for mapping the brain of other species, typically with less variability in morphometrics, and may ultimately enable computational models of phylogenetic [36–39] and ontogenetic development.

Developing atlases of the human brain provides the greatest challenge, due to both practical and ethical limitations on experimentation and to the great morphometric variability of the human brain. Variance between human brains is becoming better understood. As was noted above, this occurs not only for gyral patterns but also for interhemispheric differences [25]. Microscopic variation in the human brain also exists as does the boundaries of microscopic (*i.e.*, cytoarchitectural) [24,40] and macroscopic (gyral/sulcal) [41] landmarks. Since variations between brains, both micro- and macroscopic in nature, exist and yet past published atlases represent one or, at best, a few brains, it is impossible to make generalisations about these varying anatomies for the entire species.

As in all anatomical atlases, past approaches in human brain atlasing have included systematic experimental error induced by postmortem changes in tissue, sectioning or imaging artefacts, and unpredictable size distortions resulting from chemical processing of the tissue. While some attempts have been made to minimise these changes, by attention to chemical, photographic, and radiological techniques, they nevertheless exist. Further, since the observations were largely qualitative and based on visual information of a single observer, rigorous comparisons between techniques, observers, or laboratories has been lacking.

Attempts at developing atlases and deformation tools from populations of subjects have been reported [33,42–50], typically derived from a single modality and have demonstrated the utility of such an approach (Fig. 1).

III. INPUT SOURCES FOR BRAIN MAPPING ATLASES

A wide variety of techniques are available for providing information about the structure and function of the human brain [10]. They differ in a variety of key characteristics including spatial and temporal resolution, the volume and frequency of data sampling, the interval of measurement repetition, their requirements for sedation or anaesthesia, and their degree of invasiveness. Highly invasive techniques, primarily those that require direct access to brain tissue, can be applied only postmortem or intraoperatively and, thus, by their very nature, are applied only in subjects that have cerebral abnormalities. As such, data from these sources can be compared only with, but should not be considered typical of, normal brain structure and function.

Macroscopic techniques that can be used to evaluate human brain structure include X-ray CT, MRI, and MRA, as well as digital postmortem cryosectioning [51] (Fig. 2). Functional techniques applicable to the human brain on a macroscopic scale include positron emission tomography (PET), single photon emission computed tomography (SPECT), functional MRI, magnetic resonance spectroscopy, stable xenon enhanced CT, transcranial magnetic stimulation [52–54], EEG, MEG, as well as intraoperative direct cortical stimulation and recording in the awake patient. Microscopic techniques that can be applied to the human brain include a wide variety of electrophysiological surface and depth recordings, optical intrinsic signal imaging, and postmortem tissue analyses that span the gamut from structural anatomy to cyto-, chemo-, and myeloarchitecture. A clear understanding of the types of data that these different input sources provide is important in understanding their applicability for human brain atlasing as well as the resultant data types that would result from a modality-specific atlas using any particular methodology. In addition,

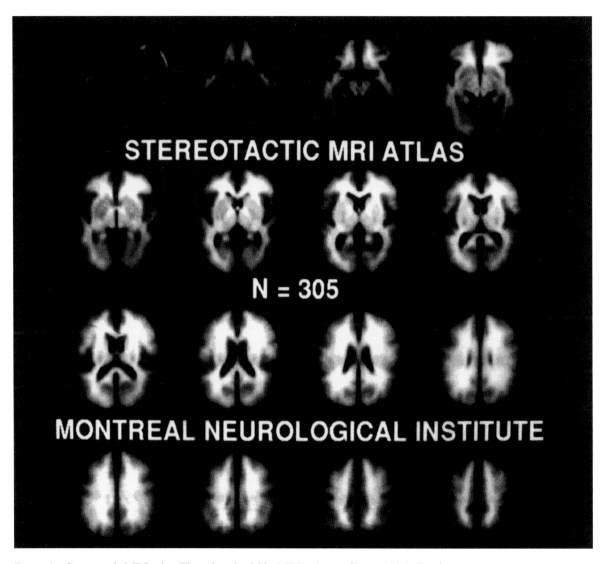

FIGURE 1   Stereotaxic MRI atlas. Three hundred fifty MRI volumes (2-mm-thick slices) were mapped by linear transformation into stereotaxic space, intensity normalised, and averaged [45].

differences between techniques with regard to key variables and methodology are important in the valid cross-referencing of data obtained using specific techniques, both within and between subjects.

A. Critical Variables in Brain Mapping Techniques

While an infinite number of variables can be represented in maps, the two most obvious and immediately important are those of spatial organisation and temporal pattern. The resolution, both temporal and spatial, of measurements made with most brain mapping techniques is one factor that defines their applications. Spatial resolution determines the scale and, hence, the types of measurements that are attainable with the method. By convention, high

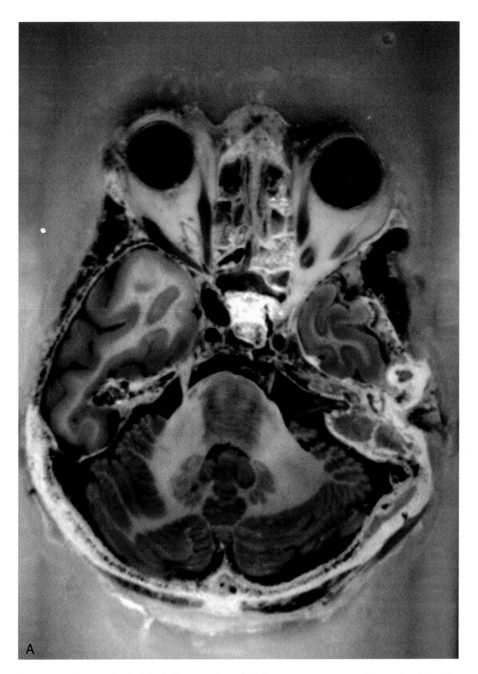

FIGURE 2 Human brain block face sectioned with a cryomacrotome. These horizontal images are at the level of the orbits and hippocampus and illustrate the detail that can be seen. Grey and white matter differences are easy to appreciate. The inner and outer mantles of the bony skull are clearly visible. The full 1024-pixel resolution of the primary image is not represented in this reproduction. (A) Note the fact that the specimen is not symmetrical. The blocking and positioning of the head in the cryomacrotome is not exact, but since the volumes are reconstructed and subsequently resampled this does not affect the final result. (B) High-resolution primary imagery of selected human brain subregions. Here the hippocampus, alveus, taenia fibria, lateral geniculate body, and posterior cerebral artery in the ambient cistern are visible in one section of a complete cryotomy series. This approach is useful for architecturally complex regions such as hippocampus, brain stem, and cerebellum, where it yields detail far higher than *in vivo* imaging modalities such as MRI (data courtesy of A. Toga [51]).

435

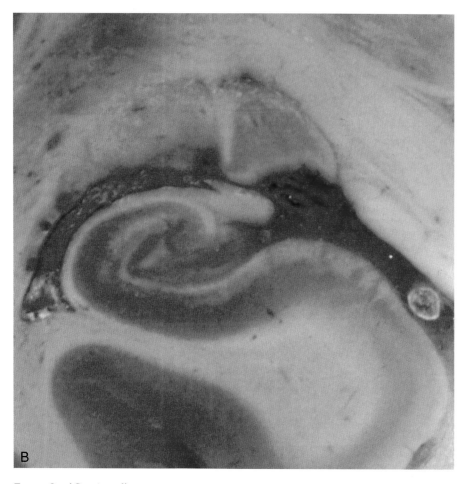

FIGURE 2   *(Continued)*

resolution devices are capable of accurately defining smaller structures. With increasing spatial resolution one moves up the scale from macroscopic (*e.g.*, CT, MRI, PET, SPECT), to microscopic (*e.g.*, light microscopy, confocal microscopy, optical intrinsic signal imaging), to ultrastructural measurements (*e.g.*, electron microscopy).

Similarly, temporal resolution is an important determining factor in the types of data that can be acquired with a given method and hence its applications in neuroscience research. On the temporal resolution spectrum one could begin with the lowest forms of temporal resolution. Examples in this category would include the ability to examine fossilised remains and cranial casts, both within and between species, in order to evaluate the evolution of the macroscopic aspects of the nervous system in a time frame of thousands to millions of years [37]. Structural *in vivo* imaging over years with serial studies performed longitudinally in the same individual can provide insights into maturation, development, aging, and the structural impact of the natural course of diseases. Techniques that provide temporal resolution in the time frame of hours provide the opportunities for examining other types of events. For example, ligands labeled with radionuclides can be injected into subjects and these individuals can then be studied with PET or SPECT, with kinetic data being collected for many hours. Positron emitting isotopes with half-lives of approximately 2 hr (*e.g.*, fluorine-18) are ideally suited to this type of experiment. The 2-hr half-life of fluorine-18, when incorporated into an appropriate molecule, can provide insights into the uptake of the compound in the brain, the selective binding to specific receptor subtypes as well as the clearance of unbound compound from nonspecific sites in the brain.

Techniques that allow for measurements in the time frame of minutes include PET measurements of cerebral blood flow, volume, glucose, and oxygen metabolism. Techniques that provide accurate data in the time frame of seconds to hundreds of milliseconds include fMRI, optical intrinsic signal imaging and tracer dye techniques. Finally, electrophysiological (*e.g.*, EEG) and magnetoencephalographic (MEG) techniques would be those chosen to examine events in the millisecond time frame.

In addition to evaluating time and space factors in the domain of brain mapping, there are numerous other variables that are important to consider and which help to define the applicability of a given technique to a neurobiological question. Sampling volume is the critical variable of this type. The *in vivo* brain imaging methods such as PET, MRI, CT, and SPECT provide global macroscopic views of the entire intracranial contents. At the other end of the spectrum would be depth electrodes used for intracellular recording that provide data from individual or small clusters of neurons. In general, sampling volume is inversely related to spatial resolution. This rule does not, however, hold for the relationship of sampling volume to temporal resolution. For example, fMRI, when used with echo planar techniques, can sample the entire intracranial contents but still maintains a relatively high temporal resolution.

Sampling frequency is another key variable to assess. Some methods allow for only a single examination, a situation typical of postmortem or autoradiographic experiments. Other methods have a sampling frequency dictated by the need for clearance of an indicator substance (*e.g.*, PET or SPECT radiopharmaceuticals, intravascular dyes, *etc.*), a factor that may also determine the upper limit of measurement that can be performed based on radiation or toxin exposure levels. Techniques that are entirely noninvasive are the most frequently repeatable. Included in this category would be fMRI, EEG, and MEG. Human experiments can be performed in animal models if brain size is adequate (*e.g.*, PET studies in primates). Animal experiments can often not be performed in humans because of logistic or ethical issues.

The degree of invasiveness is an important factor in evaluating methods for brain mapping applications. As was noted above, completely noninvasive methods most minimally perturb normal brain function and, from the point of view of safety, have the widest range of applications because the risks of their use are so low. Measurements that involve the administration of substances that can produce toxic or allergic reactions as well as those that contain radioisotopes have added risk and more limited use because of exposure factors. Measurements that require direct access to brain tissue, such as optical intrinsic signal imaging, depth or surface electrophysiology, are reserved for clinical situations where human subjects require surgery for specific neuropathological disorders or for animal models. These approaches, by their very nature, require physical manipulation of the brain tissue or its surrounding structures and, as such, have an inherently higher propensity to alter functional integrity. Human subjects evaluated with these techniques are, by definition, patients with cerebral abnormalities and, as such, are not examples of normal brain function.

Other factors that should be kept in mind when evaluating brain mapping methods include whether there are any requirements for anaesthesia or other medications that may alter brain function. For studies of postmortem tissue one should consider whether a given method examines this tissue *in situ* or in excised specimens. Finally, the costs and complexity of establishing a given method for use in one's laboratory are additional considerations in defining the applications of specific techniques. In fact, these factors can often be the driving force in determining whether a specific laboratory can make use of a particular method.

IV. TOOLS FOR BUILDING HUMAN BRAIN ATLASES

A. Spatial Normalisation

Spatial normalisation of data sets between modalities and individuals is required for successful human brain mapping techniques. Such methods must include not only the three spatial dimensions and time (*i.e.*, serial studies of the same subject or kinetic studies in the same session) but also the incorporation of several different mapping technologies derived from separate methods. The most straightforward case is the spatial normalisation of data sets obtained from the same individual using the same modality. This within-subject, within-modality alignment and registration amounts to a linear transformation that includes a rigid component (*i.e.*, no change in size or shape) amounting to rotation and translation of the data set. The nonrigid component of scaling allows for the adjustment of size while maintaining shape as invariant. The result is a nine-parameter fit (rotation, translation, and scaling along each of the three spatial axes). A variety of techniques exist for this kind of spatial normalisation, including landmark matching [18,47,48,55,56], surface contouring [57–59], and densitometric [35,60] approaches. Comparisons of the efficiency and accuracy of these methods have been made and indicate that the densitometric approach has been most successful to date [34] (Table 1).

TABLE 1

Specific Approaches to Spatial Normalisation

Approach	References
Principal axes	
Extrinsic fiducials	35, 141–143
Talairach-like approaches	18, 47, 48
Intrinsic landmarks	56, 144
Contours	59, 145
Cross-correlations	60, 83
Deformations	
a. Point-based warping	144, 146, 147
b. Density-based warping	35, 55, 60
c. Global matching	83
d. Local matching	55, 148

The problem of within-subject, between-modality spatial normalisation is more difficult and requires a thorough knowledge of the behaviour of the instrument collecting the data and distortions that it may induce in its multidimensional representation. For the simple case of comparisons between tomographic techniques, geometric distortions can be defined using standardised phantoms and adjustments made for differing voxel sizes as part of the scaling procedure. When methods involve surface (*e.g.*, scalp EEG) or subsampled volumes of the entire brain (optical intrinsic signal imaging, depth electrode recordings) far greater difficulties exist in accurately localising these measurements in a true three-dimensional map of the individual's structural neuroanatomy.

By far the most difficult issue is transformation between different individuals. The central problem of such transformations, as a mechanism for comparing structural or functional neuroanatomy across individuals, is the residual nonlinear variability in human neuroanatomy persisting after linear transformation. A single linear transformation that corrects for rotational and scale differences between brains will lead to a misregistration of corresponding cortical landmarks by as much as 1–2 cm [18,61,62]. Using linear stereotactic mapping, three-dimensional image data are linearly mapped into a standardised brain-based coordinate space such that all brains have the same extent in three orthogonal directions and each plane of the resliced volume can be directly compared with an anatomical atlas. The most commonly employed space is that of Talairach [18]. This method is central to brain mapping studies for localisation of activation foci [47,48]. It is based on the identification of the anterior–posterior commissural (AC–PC) line, extending to the cortical edge in the AP direction and a set of perpendiculars to this line from the AC and PC points to the cortical edge. Strict application of the method [63] requires the proportional scaling to be partitioned into three piece-wise linear components in the AP direction (pre-AC, AC-PC, post-PC), two in the CC direction (above/below AC–PC), and to be independent for each hemisphere. This scheme is intended to overcome problems introduced by nonlinear variability between individuals. Most centers have either retained a single scale along each dimension or have applied full nonlinear warping techniques to address the nonlinearity issue directly. In one approach, the Talairach space is used both for anatomical analysis with MRI data and for functional activation studies with PET, using preregistered MRI images for defining the required transformation. A series of five well separated midline landmarks are selected that yield a least square fit approximation to the AC–PC line [64]. Validation studies in 37 young normal individuals indicate an angular discrepancy of -0.24 ± 2.9 mm and a vertical translational error of 1.2 ± 1.0 mm. A recently implemented automated method, which uses a general multiscale feature matching technique, has also been developed [65,66].

After brain data are transformed with stereotactic resampling using linear algorithms, residual anatomical variability remains. Major sulci can vary in position by 1–2 cm within a normal population [18,61,62]. Thin-plate spline procedures [56] for nonlinear, three-dimensional image deformation, based on continuous coordinate transformations which map one set of landmarks onto an equivalent set of homologous points, decompose the overall deformation into a series of principal warps of decreasing geometric scale [67]. A set of 26 anatomical landmarks in each of 16 separate MRI data sets have been matched to corresponding structures in a master MRI data set. The three-dimensional warping algorithm can then be applied to each of the MRI volumes to bring them into registration with the master volume, using all deformation terms or just the first three which define the affine component of the overall transformation. Nonlinear transformations exhibit a sharper appearance in more detail than linear versions reflecting superiority of the nonlinear approach for bringing homologous structures in the neighbourhood of individual landmarks into precise alignment. An estimate of nonlinear variability has been measured and averages 6.25 mm over 60 structures [67].

A problem with interactive landmark-based approaches is the subjectivity of landmark choice, that is, the dependence of the resultant transformation on the number and distribution of landmarks selected and the behaviour of the algorithm in regions distant from any landmark. An alternate approach is that of image feature matching [55]. One approach has been to apply three-dimensional feature matching procedures that use recursive evaluation of feature cross-correlation functions between two image sets [65,66,68]. The algorithm operates in a multiscale loop, beginning with heavily smoothed versions of the images and successively sharpening the images at each iteration. This reduces the likelihood of encountering local minima during the search and is approximately four times faster than the single stage high resolution optimisation. To measure intersubject registration accuracy, 20 random linear transformations have been applied to each MRI volume of the head from 17 young normal volunteers and the algorithm applied to recover the transformation. For each trial two measures of registration are calculated: the root mean square (RMS) difference between input and recovered parameters and the RMS registration error between 48 landmarks, manually identified in each volume. Over the 340 trials, the RMS error for rotation, translation, and landmark distance were less than or equal to 0.1°, 0.1 mm, and 0.2 mm, respectively. For intersubject registration, each data set in turn was identified as the target and the other 16 volumes coregistered to it. Over 272 trials, the linear transformation recovered by multiresolution registration yielded an RMS distance of 6.65 mm. This measure is dominated by nonlinear anatomic variability rather than landmark homology error. It is also in good agreement with the mean measure of anatomical variability of 6.25 mm obtained using the thin-plate spline technique discussed above [56].

1. General Methods

The development of algorithms for positioning of multiple three-dimensional digital volumes is essential for the development of any atlas or brain reference system as well as for extending single subject analysis to group evaluations. These algorithms are required to transform three-dimensional images into a stereotactic coordinate system [48,65,66,68]. Numerous approaches to cross-modality alignment and registration have been proposed. These include surface matching [57,59], homologous landmark matching [56,64,69], density feature matching [35,60] or geometric based (*e.g.*, principal axes) strategies [70]. Each approach has its advantages and limitations depending on the data type and inherent defects such as incomplete coverage, intensity distortions, geometric distortions, lack of contrast, and modality-specific inconsistencies. In addition, different approaches are more or less complex to implement and execute.

The most common application of cross-modality alignments and registration is between MRI and PET to enable quantitative assessment of structure and function relationships [71]. In order to provide better anatomic localisation, several methods for incorporating MRI data with PET images have been developed. Surface fitting techniques match the inner table of the skull from MRI data with the inner table surface observed in PET transmission scans [59]. Evans *et al.* [44] employed multiple landmarks and transformations including translation, rotation, and scaling to minimize the root mean square among corresponding points. Fox *et al.* [72] utilized the stereotactic method to equate data from MRI and PET. Woods *et al.* [35,60] employed a method that divided the two images voxel by voxel and iteratively adjusted rotation and translation parameters to minimise the standard deviation of the voxel ratios. SPM96 can be used to solve the between-modality problem by matching both images to two templates of the same modality. Because the relative positions of the templates are known, the between-modality mapping can, therefore, be derived (see Chapter 3).

2. Deformations

Warping is a subspecialty of image processing that deals with geometric transformation techniques [73]. Already these approaches have been applied to warp one brain on to another [74,75]. These transformations redefine the spatial relationship between points in image sets. For the purposes of multimodality and multisubject brain comparisons, warping is defined as those geometric transformations that alter brain shape. They do not include simple repositioning. The implementation, whether density or spatially based, of the warping is dependent on the type of data and their resolution. For example, if anatomic landmarks are easily obtained, spatially based algorithms may be employed. The location and number of landmarks are crucial to the goodness of fit. In other cases, density based warping algorithms can maximise the cross-correlation coefficients between data sets without the identification of landmarks. Initial work was based on the success of two-dimensional deformations [48] to produce a three-dimensional plastic deformation for the removal of nonlinear variability in brain shape. If one allows elastic deformations in any plane a three-dimensional approach is required [76].

3. Brain to Atlas

Neuroanatomic labels are used to communicate between investigators while digital atlases use coordinate space to quantitate location. Equating the relationship between neuroanatomic labels and a Cartesian (or polar) coordinate systems is one of the by-products of warping to a digital atlas. In addition, segmentation of neuroanatomic structures within three-dimensional data sets using anatomic templates such as the Talairach and Tournoux [18] stereotactic atlas of the human brain helps make functional measurements between subjects comparable. Fitting anatomic templates to data will greatly increase the number of structures that can be identified. It also provides a common reference system [77,78] for multisubject comparison and, ultimately, the development of a data base with normative data [31,44]. Clinical usefulness has also been tested. Clark *et al.* [79] presented initially encouraging results for a statistical model that assessed the probability of whether a patient was normal or had Huntington's disease using PET data and these methods.

Warping a brain to an atlas can be accomplished by sequentially mapping two-dimensional sections through the data set on to an atlas template, assuming the sections are oriented identically. Alternately, the reconstructed three-dimensional volume can be repositioned, warped, and resampled to correspond with atlas templates [80]. Typically, the spatial resolution of the atlas is significantly less than that of the experimental data so that loss of accuracy due to resampling is not a problem. Warping can be performed to any degree and can be either spatially [81,82] or density based [42].

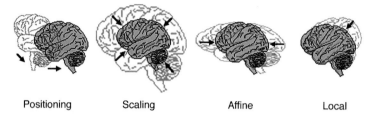

FIGURE 3　Deforming and warping techniques can be either density based or spatially based. Points and contours, when available, provide spatial information for deforming. Deformations across modalities may have to rely upon spatially based methods because the density patterns may not correlate. This figure illustrates a continuum of deformations, from pure positioning to local deformations that regionally alter the shape and form of the data set.

4. Brain to Brain

In order to remove the morphometric variability between data sets one can impose density based local deformations on the three-dimensional volume data set of high resolution postmortem digital anatomy. First, the data sets are histogram equalised and filtered to eliminate high frequency or artefactual contamination of the warpings. Then the volume to be warped is subjected to principal axes and centre of mass repositioning. Overall scaling and affine transformations are then applied. If a three-dimensional grid is placed on the volume, then the elastic forces can be computed at each point when derived using the cross-correlation function between the two volume data sets. An image similarity function can be computed as a least square polynomial approximation of the image correlation in the spherical region around the grid point. Results of this procedure demonstrate the forces required for the elastic deformation as shown in Fig. 3.

5. Atlas to Brain

Segmentation of data sets may be aided by the mapping of anatomic descriptions such as atlas contours to the data itself. To date, experiments have been limited to the deformation of the Talairach atlas [83] and the Paxinos and Watson rat brain atlas [82].

B. Reference Spaces

The most commonly used reference space for the human brain is the one defined in the atlas of Talairach and Tournoux [18]. This uses a simple x,y,z Cartesian coordinate system to organise data with a template-based approach that these authors defined. Despite the limitations in this approach that have been previously discussed, it remains the most widely used reference space, currently.

1. Probabilistic Reference Space

As will be discussed in more detail below, it is possible to organise data in a probabilistic reference system that describes variance throughout a population. When focused on neuroanatomy, structure probabilities result. A given voxel might, therefore, have an 80% likelihood of belonging to structure A, 10% to structure B, and so on. Functional and other data can also be referenced to the anatomy but the probability is modality specific; that is, local cerebral blood flow at locale X and rate Y are in the 80th percentile. The very nature of the brain data correlations includes the notion that probabilities are constantly being refined as data are added to such a system. The evolution of a probabilistic reference space will, of course, require recalculation of transforms in an iterative fashion. Transformations to map an individual into a probabilistic space will accumulate and help to redefine that space. Variance, trends, or extremes cause changes of the probability which in turn require recomputation of the transformations.

2. Morphing and Minimum Distance Fields

The explicit geometry of surface methods complement volume-based approaches. Morphing refers to the process of changing the shape and form of an object to take on the characteristics of another. Surface model manipulations can achieve this for neuroanatomical structures. The approach applies to three-dimensional models of function as well and may provide insight into the recruitment of additional systems during the evolution of a response or a reduction in involved systems as a response becomes more efficient. Surfaces can come from interactive techniques such as outlining [84] or automatic ones like isosurface creation [85]. However, manipulating surfaces using either direct or implicit methods presents a number of problems. To address such problems, one may use distance fields; the scaler fields derived from a synthesised triangle base surface model of either anatomic or physiologic data sets [86]. By interpolating at successive intervals, it is possible to animate a continuously deforming surface. It is also possible to use this approach to smooth and filtre (*i.e.*, a low pass Gaussian filter) a model that may contain high frequency noise or artefacts. Other applications include computing a model at a fixed distance larger or smaller than the source and blending several substructures into a single joined unit. To apply these implicit surface methods to a given surface model one must first represent the models by scaler fields. The distance field represents the distance from a surface at an assigned magnitude. Surface model distance fields have been used to remove surfaces [58] and interpolate between the upper and lower boundaries of a structure [82]. Published atlas descriptions of anatomic boundaries can be morphed to take on the shape and form of data contained in a probabilistic reference space.

C. Segmentation

Image segmentation is based on the existence of characteristics of the image, features such as intensity, intensity gradient, or texture (*i.e.*, variance) that can be used to group two-dimensional pixels or three-dimensional voxels into labeled anatomical regions [87]. For brain MRI, intensity thresholding in one image gives inadequate separation between tissue types and multiple echoes or pulse sequences are employed in multispectral classification algorithms [88–96]. Region growing, edge detection, and morphological operators can be used with single or multiple image segmentation to impose connectivity among segmented voxels and hence correct from this classification [97–102]. Even so, the image information is rarely adequate to distinguish more than three tissue types that need not be contiguous. Therefore, a priori knowledge in the form of production rules for hierarchical classification, spatial relationships or geographical likelihoods must be used to label structures at the local level [55,103–114]. The relative rigidity of the normal brain compared with,

Table 2

Segmentation Utilities

1. *Manual delineation of contours on successive two-dimensional slices:* Used for definition of polygonal volumes-of-interest (VOIs) in existing brain atlases and for obtaining convex hulls around the cortex.
2. *Region growing, edge detection, erosion, dilation, morphological operators:* To impose connectivity constraints on three-dimensional regions obtained tissue classification process.
3. *Interactive three-dimensional voxel-painting:* Used for labeling or editing three-dimensional volumes or surfaces.
4. *Surface extraction, volume, and surface rendering:* Marching cubes algorithm [85], surface shading, volume-rendering [139].
5. *Multiaxial triangulation, texture mapping:* Generates three-dimensional surfaces from orthogonal two-dimensional contours; superimposes views from one volume on cut-planes through another volume [74,140].
6. *Interactive analysis of extracted cortical topology:* Including tools for tracing sulci, delimiting gyri, and labeling all enclosed surface voxels [119].

for instance, the thorax and abdomen, means brain image segmentation is especially well suited to the use of prior models for local structure. Evans *et al.* [44,115] have made fundamental and explicit use of stereotactic image transformations to produce spatial constraints on three-dimensional neuroanatomic segmentation.

1. Low Level Tools for Region Definition

Prerequisites for neuroanatomical segmentation are low level tools for regional definition, manual labeling of voxels, editing of images, and other aspects of the process as defined in Table 2.

2. Tissue Classification

Multi-spectral tissue classification of MRI volumes into gray/white/CSF yields a three-dimensional map of the likelihood of membership in a given tissue class. The classification algorithm employs the ID3 decision tree classifier [116] operating on $3 \times 3 \times 3$ voxel neighbourhoods and T1- and T2-weighted intensity and/or variance features for each voxel. This algorithm represents tissue classification rules in the form of a binary decision tree where each tree node represents a test on a feature and each leaf represents a tissue class. A top–down divide-and-conquer strategy is used to grow the tree by recursively partitioning user-provided tissue training samples into progressively smaller subsets that eventually correspond to tissue classes [109]. ID3 uses an entropy function that examines the feature values of each training sample to determine which continuous intensity feature best partitions the samples into two classes at every node until a minimum-entropy stopping criterion is reached. An error-cost complexity pruning algorithm is then applied to reduce the total number of branches such that the cost of pruning, in terms of misclassified samples, is minimised. The pruned tree selected is the smallest tree with a misclassification rate within one standard error of the minimum. This classification procedure has been applied to 12 three-dimensional single gradient-echo MRI data sets previously transformed into stereotactic space [109], using intensity and variance as features. The proportion of all data sets for which a voxel was assigned to a given tissue class represents a likelihood function for membership in that class. The data can be used as a constraint on subsequent classifications by rejecting a particular voxel classification that has a probability lower than some preset threshold (*e.g.*, periorbital fat should not be classified as cerebral white matter). Alternatively, statistical search strategies for identifying significant activation foci in a brain mapping experiment can be confined to particular tissue classes (*e.g.*, grey matter) by use of the appropriate probability mask.

3. Model-Based Regional Parcelation

Tissue classification algorithms do not specifically label individual brain structures, such as caudate nucleus, automatically. For such parcelation, *a priori* information is needed to augment the intensity/gradient/texture features of the image, in the form of explicit geometric models or rules constraining the spatial relation of labeled structures. A three-dimensional volume-of-interest (VOI) atlas has been constructed by manual outlining of individual brain regions on 64 2-mm-thick adjacent MRI slices [44]. Sixty structures in each hemisphere were identified including deep grey matter structures, major gyri, ventricles, and white matter zones. The data exist as a tesselated geometrical model that can be resliced along any two-dimensional plane or warped in three dimensions to fit an image volume. Usually a template is matched to MRI before being applied to a correlated PET image for functional measurement [115]. This three-dimensional model has been employed in two ways for regional parcelation of individual MRI data sets.

a. Manual Deformation of Atlas to Image Here the VOI atlas is deformed to match the individual image volume by manual identification of corresponding three-dimensional landmarks in the VOI atlas and image, using the thin-plate spline algorithm [56]. The algorithm was applied in three dimensions to fit the VOI atlas to each of the 16 three-dimensional MRI data sets [67]. The 26 landmarks used for warping individual volumes to fit a master MRI data set were employed to warp the VOI atlas to fit each individual MRI volume. The VOI atlas has also been used to quantify nonlinearities in anatomical correspondence among the 16 brain data sets when using a simple linear stereotactic transformation [67]. A three-dimensional warped atlas fitted to each brain in its original coordinate space can be considered a labeled version of that brain. Hence, application of normal linear stereotactic transformation, defined on the MRI volume, without knowledge of the atlas locations results in a spread of equivalent points from different brains arising from the morphometric nonlinearities across the individual brains. RMS deviations in individual atlas locations then characterise the locations that characterise the local nonlinear variability. Results indicate a 6- to 7-mm variability in the location of the three-dimensional center of gravity of 60 brain regions.

b. Automatic Matching of Image to VOI Atlas It is possible to use automatic identification of individual brain regions by combining multiscale image feature-matching, the concept of stereotactic space and the VOI atlas. The VOI atlas and the MRI volume upon which the VOI atlas was originally defined are first mapped into stereotactic space. Hence, mapping an individual MRI volume into this space by feature matching against the resident MRI also fits it to the VOI atlas. An inverse transformation fits the VOI atlas to the new MRI in its original space. The multiscale nature of the feature matching algorithm facilitates the recursive application of the linear cross-correlation optimisation to individual neighborhoods defined on a three-dimensional grid with a dimension equal to the current scale. Hence, an overall nonlinear transformation is obtained by successive local linear transformations [65,66,68].

4. *Cortical Surface Labelling*

The study of variability in cortical anatomy across the normal population merits special consideration. Many methods already exist for visualising the cerebral cortex by extraction of isovalued surfaces, with or without subsequent polygonalisation. These techniques are susceptible to artefacts introduced by noise or signal inhomogeneities and do not enforce topological continuity (*i.e.*, there can be holes in the surface). Moreover, the unstructured representation of the cortex as 105–107 cuberilles or polygons is ill-suited for point-to-point comparison of equivalent surfaces across a population. This goal has motivated attempts to use analytic representations to replace the isosurface. Such parametric representations are continuous, relatively compact, and can often be expressed at different scales (*i.e.*, resolutions) in a hierarchical fashion. The problem of quantifying, as opposed to visualising, the cortical surface and measuring its variability across subjects is defined. Moreover, many secondary gyri have a highly variable manifestation or may be absent altogether. Even major sulci may have variable branching patterns. Van Essen and Maunsell [116a] suggested mapping the cortex to a flattened surface space, with examples in macaque and cat brains. Since then, various approaches have been made to apply such techniques with MRI data from the human brain. Jouandet *et al.* [117] outline the cortex manually on successive cortical slices while Carman *et al.* [118] and Sereno and Dale [4] have employed similar surface tension models to define the cortical anatomy.

MacDonald and colleagues [119] have developed a procedure that combines the advantages of polygonal, parametric, and hierarchical representations with a fast converging elastic deformation model. The vertices of a starting parametric surface, defined by a polygonal mesh, are moved towards a boundary surface, defined by a set of discrete boundary points, along a direction normal to the current parametric surface and for a distance controlled by a weighting factor for each boundary point. The weighting is linear such that zero weighting leaves the point unmoved and unit weighting moves it directly to the boundary surface. The algorithm proceeds iteratively, adjusting all mesh points at each iteration, until equilibrium is obtained with all mesh edges of almost equal length. The model allows a simple control of the surface resolution, by subsampling of the boundary points, and hence the degree of sulcal detail apparent in the fitted surface. The boundary points are usually isosurface voxels obtained by intensity or gradient thresholding but can also include additional manually defined boundary points reflecting specific surface targets with increased weighting. The mesh form of the parametric surface guarantees a continuous single surface topology and also allows a direct one-to-one mapping from a three-dimensional cortical manifold to a spherical projection. Corresponding sulci and gyri are evident and can be identified by cartographic lines of latitude and longitude.

D. Visualisation

Visualising the mapping of one modality to another, once they have been warped to coincidence, can be accomplished in a variety of ways. Surface based methods include direct mapping of function using false colouring without shading [120]. Flattening surfaces [3–5,116,121,122] can aid in the visualisation of multimodality maps. Employing colour space (hue, saturation, and value) in specific ways permits the mapping of function on structure while preserving shading cues [123]. Texture mapping function on anatomically defined polygonal surfaces can utilise shading and colour to indicate depth and magnitude [58]. We [115,124] visualised multiple modalities by assigning function to a colour scale and structure to grey scale in a voxel rendered model.

E. Data Base

A brain atlas is, in essence, a data base. While it can be visualised as a pictorial representation, the more common map-based approach, it is, nevertheless, a data base that is ideally maintained in a digital format. Since the most common language of neuroscience is that of neuroanatomy, a data base that is referenced by neuroanatomical terms or graphic representations of neuroanatomy is the most sensible. Using this type of format, one can input as a query, a neuroanatomical term or, alternately, click on a given voxel in a three-dimensional representation of the brain in order to reference information about that brain region [31] (Fig. 4).

Brain atlas/data bases can be modality-specific, population-specific, or composite data bases that allow linkage across many forms of data organisation. The latter approach produces the most comprehensive information system. This metadata base, allows access through the common neuroanatomy to individual data bases that may be functional, behavioural, bibliographical, or any of an infinite number of other groupings. By clicking on a given voxel or inputting a specific term, one would then be able to reference a table of modality- or population-specific attributes about that voxel. In essence, the reference space for the atlas becomes the framework structure of a system upon which modalities, functions, bibliographies, or other organisational approaches are attributes. One can ask for a specific attribute based on an anatomical location or one can ask for the set of locations that fulfil a certain criterion list of attributes.

Such metadata bases also allow for metaanalysis. For example, if one identified a specific function for a collection of voxels in neuroanatomical space, one could see whether these boundaries coincided with any other attribute boundaries. For example, Watson and colleagues [125] identified a region on the dorsolateral surface of the temporal–occipital junction of the human brain that increased its blood flow during the perception of visual motion. Through traditional (*i.e.*, published references) approaches, rather than digital data base searches, it was identified that this same region had a consistent relationship to early myelinisation [29]. We also noted that this cortical activation site had a consistent relationship to the gyral and sulcal anatomy of the region. Had there been a metadata base from which the separate attributes of functional activation, behaviour, myelinisation, and cortical anatomy could have been referenced, the identification of these coincident relationships for the human visual motion centre would have been trivial to identify. In the traditional approach, the identification of such relationships was difficult and is often not even attempted. This difficulty, in turn, leads to a loss of insight and potential value as new data are acquired. Having all neuroscientific data of this sort organised through atlases in a data base format, not only would such observations become simplified and in some cases made feasible, but new observations could be obtained solely from the metadata

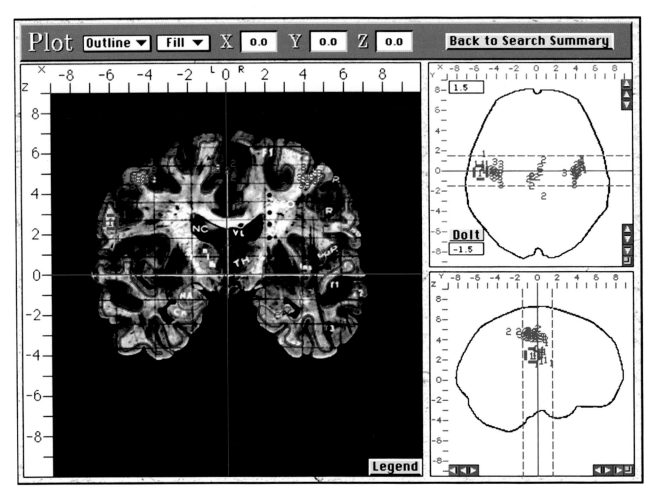

FIGURE 4 This is an example of one coronal section from the Talairach atlas used with the BrainMap data base system [32]. The views from above the head and from the right side of the head indicate the location (solid line) and extent for data plotting (dotted lines) of the coronal slice. Overlayed onto the grey scale atlas image are outlines of the cortical grey matter, white matter, and a ventricle.

base without a need for the addition of any new experimental information. A number of such data bases are already under development and are being continuously updated [32,126].

While neuroscience databasing and atlasing is currently still at an early stage, the field can look to a number of examples and insights provided from data bases developed for other disciplines, such as meteorology. In neuroscience, as in other fields requiring data base management, semantic compatibility is the greatest challenge [31]. Consistency of nomenclature is a critical aspect of any data base organisation. This does not necessarily mean that a single unique nomenclature system must be used. It does, however, require that for any nomenclature system, the appropriate translators are provided to reference it with a nomenclature system used for the data base–atlas system. Failure to successfully achieve this criterion leads to confusion and lack of utility of the resulting product. This has been a problem for the Human Genome Project.

A second factor is the sociology of sharing data. At present, a considerable amount of data go unpublished and, therefore, unreported. This is due to the overwhelming volume of data collected in laboratories worldwide about the human brain, its digital incompatibilities, and the proprietary wishes of the investigators who collect them. For human brain atlases and data bases to be ever growing and evolving, investigators must be willing to provide data, even in raw and uninterpreted forms, to the data base system. This notion could be developed as a prerequisite for traditional publication or simply an entry criterion for the data base project itself. A third key factor for such a data base is the quality of the entered data. Entries in the data base could be ranked with a figure of merit representing the confidence one had in the entered material. Rather than establishing a rigid system for judging such quality, they could simply be rated as to whether they were raw data, interpreted data, peer-reviewed data, or peer-reviewed and independently validated data. As such, the data base user could select from among these confidence attributes expanding or restricting the scope of data sets accessed based on the reliability criterion selected with a query.

V. ATLAS LINKAGES

As was discussed in the section on data bases, linking data sets is a critical aspect of any atlas project. This idea has already been addressed with regard to individual data sets where cross-correlations between modalities and techniques are the most fundamental type of linkage. This problem was further addressed in the section on data bases where comparisons between data sets organised by input modality or population could be linked through a common reference system of nomenclature. More difficult is the linkage of atlases across different scales, in either the spatial or the temporal domains. This difficulty is a problem because few techniques have the ability to span many orders of magnitude in either of these domains. Critical bridging technologies that link scales are lacking. One exception is postmortem digital cryomacrotome neuroanatomy.

High resolution postmortem cross-sectional cryomacrotome digital data from the entire human head is a unique technique that has the ability to span spatial resolution domains from the macroscopic world achieved with human *in vivo* imaging devices such as MRI, PET, SPECT, and CT to the microscopic world of light microscopy [51,127–130]. Existing devices have the capacity to section the human head at 20-μm intervals with an in-plane spatial resolution of approximately 200 μm in the x and y directions. The resultant data sets are 2–3 gigabytes in size. Spatial resolution can be increased in the plane of section by digitising smaller regions of each plane in raster fashion and reassembling them in a tesselated fashion, much like a quilt. Alternately, higher resolution digitising devices may increase spatial resolution by a factor of four in the plane of section, leading to an overall increase in spatial resolution of a factor of 16 in x and y. The resultant data base would be on the order of 32–48 gigabytes in size. These improvements would result in a spatial resolution of approximately 20 μm in each dimension.

The following approach could be used to incorporate microscopic data from small sections of the brain into an existing macroscopic atlas framework. Consider the following. A series of postmortem cryomacrotome human brains are stained with a series of conventional and commonly used neuroanatomical "landmark" stains (*e.g.*, Nissl, acetylcholinesterase, *etc.*). Using a state-of-the-art imaging device, these sections would be digitised and sampled at the 20-μm resolution specified above. The resultant data sets would be warped and entered into an atlas as an additional attribute feature. Then consider an investigator who studies GABA receptors in a surgically removed human hippocampus. This investigator would like to determine where the receptors from the hippocampi of a given specimen population fall with regard to other data in the atlas system. In preparing tissue, the investigator would process every Nth section using one of the "landmark" stains that are part of the atlas. The investigator would then digitise the information from both the GABA receptor sections and the landmark stained sections. Using alignment, registration, and warping tools that are part of the atlas system, the investigator would register the landmark stained sections with the atlas and then use the same mathematical transformations to enter the GABA receptor information into the hippocampal region of the atlas. Once referenced, data base queries and visualisation of these new data could be performed in the atlas system and shared with other investigators. A similar approach allows for referencing between newly acquired *in vivo* data and stored postmortem specimens that should aid in relating functional localisation with macroscopic and microscopic anatomy [33].

VI. PROBABILISTIC ATLAS APPROACH

A digital, probabilistic atlas based on a large population will rectify many of the current atlas problems discussed above. Its development from a large population provides, most importantly, retention of spatial and densitometric variance (Fig. 5). Such a system should be thought of as an ever evolving process rather than a single solution. The evolutionary aspect of such a system recognises the fact that as additional data are progressively added to it, its accuracy improves and the number and content of the subpopulations it depicts is increased. Landmarks are derived from the intersubject stability of structures rather than by simple assignment based on the anatomical features of a single brain. Since such an atlas can be fully three-dimensional and include the entire intracranial contents, as well as bony landmarks and surface features, morphometric calculations can be performed rigorously and efficiently. Its digital, electronic structure provides efficient statistical and computational comparisons between individuals or groups. The application of informatic principles, statistical methods, and mathematical approaches makes such an atlas a source of new information about the brain rather than simply a tool for localisation during procedures.

Because the probabilistic atlas approach is tolerant of differences between subjects and modalities, past or current systems can be incorporated into it easily by digitising the published atlases and transforming them into the newly defined probabilistic reference space. Thus, one could interrogate the probabilistic atlas for information using its own coordinates or those from any other reference system that had been entered into the data set (*e.g.*, the atlases of Talairach, Brodmann, *etc.*). In addition, information about physiology, neurochemistry, and an infinite number of relevant maps can be layered onto the anatomic atlas as additional features or attributes that can be referenced using such a system (Fig. 6). Interestingly, the probabilistic atlas auto-

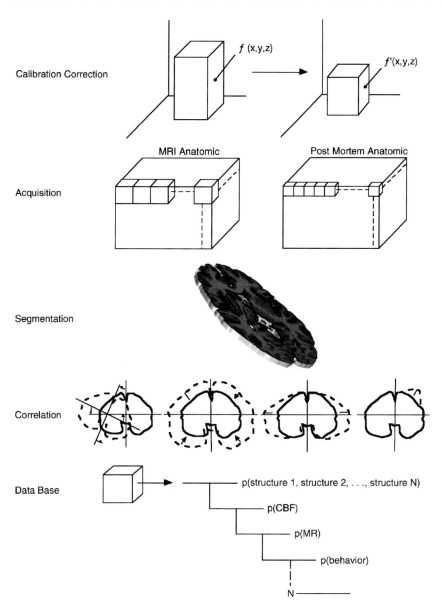

FIGURE 5 The steps required to achieve the goal of developing a probabilistic reference system for the human brain. Row 1 demonstrates the requirement of calibrating acquisition instruments and correcting data for acquisition-induced errors. Row 2 corresponds to the data set acquisition at different spatial resolutions. Row 3 indicates manual, semiautomated, and automatic image segmentation. This step is critical to identifying neuroanatomical structure boundaries in high resolution postmortem human cryomacrotome data sets as well as in lower resolution *in vivo* MRI data sets. Row 4 demonstrates alignment and registration of images using a combination of scaling, affine, linear, and nonlinear transformations and includes local deformations required to optimise the correlation between brain data volumes, a critical component of between-subject image correlation. The bottom row depicts the data base in which all of this information will be organised into a probabilistic reference system with search and query capabilities that will allow access to any aspect of the stored data and link this data base to other existing data bases.

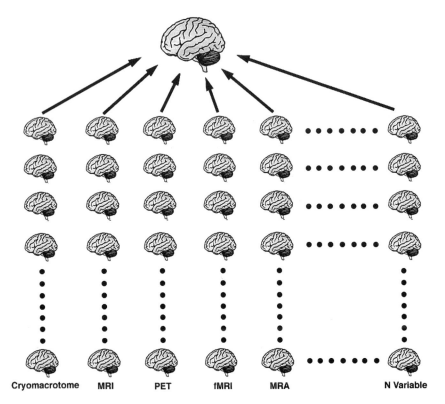

Cryomacrotome   MRI   PET   fMRI   MRA   N Variable

FIGURE 6 Data sets incorporated in the development of a probabilistic reference system. By acquiring sets of data from subjects by a variety of input modalities we can establish the mean and variance for each feature in a probabilistic fashion and store them in the ultimate data base that would be referenced to the voxel field established for the probabilistic reference system. Data sets that include postmortem cryomacrotome human brains and structural MRI images of human subjects. Other variables that could be added might include PET, functional MRI (fMRI), MR angiography (MRA), cerebral blood volume, receptor density, electrophysiological data, and behavioural variables.

matically provides variability information for data referenced by current, standard atlases.

The resulting system becomes an important source of data for testing models of structure, physiology, phylogeny, ontogeny, and disease states. The addition of bibliographic references and text enhance its utility. Knowledge of variability between ages in a population provide important insights about development and maturation of the brain, while information about evolutionarily older *versus* newer brain structures should provide clues to the phylogenetic history of the human brain and factors that have influenced it. Last, such a system would provide for the valid comparison of data collected by different investigators at different laboratories through the use of a common reference system.

Early efforts at averaging data sets with an eye towards probabilistic approaches to brain atlasing have proven useful. The current stereotaxic atlas of Talairach and Tournoux [18] was derived from the postmortem sectioning of the brain of a single 60-year-old female. Slice separation is variable, typically 3–4 mm, and the atlas data from orthogonal planes are inconsistent. Given (i) the known variability in human cortical anatomy, (ii) the prevailing differences between local implementation of the stereotaxic transformation at individual centers and the original piecewise linear Talairach framework, and (iii) that most brain mapping studies are performed on young normal subjects, the precise anatomical localisation of focal activation derived from PET using the Talairach atlas alone is problematic and can lead to overinterpretation of results [131]. These uncertainties prompted work at the Montreal Neurologic Institute towards a three-dimensional probabilistic atlas of normal gross neuro-anatomy, defined within stereotaxic space. Figure 1 shows a composite MRI data set from 305 young right-handed normals (239 males, 66 females; mean age 23.4 ± 4.1) after transformation of each MRI volume into Talairach space and intensity normalisation. Each MRI volume was acquired as 64 contiguous 2-mm-thick images [44,46,115]. The transformed atlas is $256 \times 256 \times 160$ in size, with voxel dimensions of $0.67 \times 0.86 \times 0.75$ mm. The average normalised intensity MRI data set illustrates the effect of anatomical variability in different brain areas and serves as a low resolution, large sample atlas of gross neuro-anatomy in Talairach space. This data set has been distributed to 35 centres for use with the Talairach atlas.

The data set contains striking features not normally apparent on individual MRI images. In the central regions, the noise reduction consequent upon image averaging outweighs the resolution loss caused by anatomical variability and allows for the discrimination of subtle intensity differences. For example, the dorsomedial nucleus of the thalamus is visible and the contrast between cingulum bundles and adjacent grey matter is enhanced. Other white matter structures, such as the internal capsule are distinguishable in coronal sections. In the mesencephalon, the substantia nigra, red nucleus, and adjacent white matter tracts and CSF spaces are markedly evident. At the cortex, anatomical variability leads to a loss of contrast for secondary sulci but major sulci are well defined. The ascending arm of the cingulate sulcus appears highly conserved. Comparison of left and right hemispheres, performed by reflecting one hemisphere around the midline of stereotaxic space and subtracting the images, reveals features consistent with previous findings [21,22,132–135]. There is clear evidence of left occipital petalia and right frontal petalia [23]. Heschl's gyrus is seen to be differently represented with the appearance of a second sulcus on the left, although this may be a consequence of the well known asymmetry in the planum temporale with left being considerably larger than right.

While useful as a qualitative indicator of local anatomical variability, the composite MRI intensity atlas is insufficient as a quantitative tool. For this purpose, the MRI intensity for each voxel in each MRI volume must be replaced by an anatomical label, (e.g., caudate, or precentral gyrus) and a probability assigned for each voxel having a particular label (Fig. 7). This requires a precise segmentation of each MRI volume into component structures, surface features and tissue types. Manual labelling of 305 brain volumes is prohibitively time consuming but completely automatic and accurate image parcelation at the regional level is, as was discussed above, a yet unsolved problem.

In conceptualizing the probabilities that would be used in such a system, one must keep in mind that localisation probability is not completely independent for all structures. That is, while the size, shape and position of the head of the caudate can vary from subject to subject, it is invariably anterior to the putamen within the context of the striatum. While both putamen and caudate

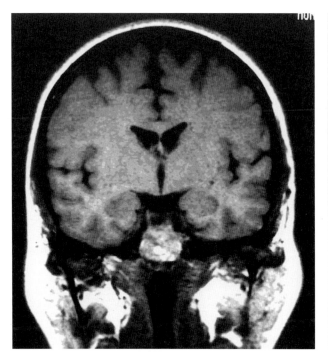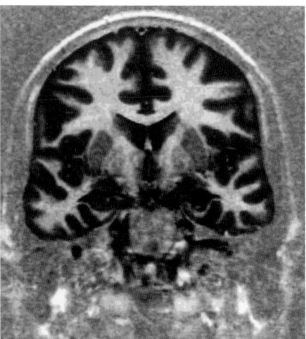

FIGURE 7   Demonstration of good grey/white contrast with inversion recovery pulse sequence (right). On the left a standard T_1-weighted sequence, on the right one of a 64-slice inversion recovery acquisition (TR=5700, TE=21 msec, TI=478 msec, acquisition time 24 min), demonstrating good brain–CSF separation.

may vary in size, shape, and orientation, they are always in the same relative position to one another. As such, one can express their localisation as a conditional probability keeping their anatomical order in mind. In fact, the relationship of all brain structures maintains a conditional probability to one another. This fact helps constrain the probabilistic aspects of building an atlas of this type.

One might question why one would begin by developing a probabilistic human brain atlas rather than using a species that is smaller and has presumably a more consistent neuroanatomy. Most neuroscientific information is derived from rodents, specifically rats. Cortical studies have focused on the macaque monkey [136]. Recent advances in imaging techniques, however, have led to a rapid expansion in the amount of functional and structural information currently available about the human brain [6,7,137]. Thus, human neuroscience is undergoing a rapid growth of experimental data. The human brain is particularly challenging because its presumed variance is greatest, with regard to structure and function, relative to other species.

Unlike other species, such as the rat, there are not vast amounts of human neuroscientific data already collected using methods and systems not easily compatible with a digital, electronic atlas. Thus, newly acquired information about the human brain will be relatively easy to incorporate into the appropriate reference standards to allow the use of newly developed probabilistic atlas approaches.

Perhaps most obvious is the fact that the study of the human brain is most relevant to understanding behavioural properties unique to humans and few other species (*e.g.*, language). Equally important is the fact that information about the human brain will lead to a better understanding of disorders that affect it and the means by which to rigorously analyse and compare data relevant to the treatment of neurological, neurosurgical, and psychiatric disorders.

A consortium of institutions (the International Consortium for Brain Mapping (ICBM)) has joined forces to develop a digital probabilistic atlas through funding provided by the Human Brain Project in the United States. The first step in developing a probabilistic atlas is to describe the geography of the brain. This fact leads to the natural conclusion that one must begin with structural anatomy. Ideally, this anatomy would be described *in vivo*. Fortunately, modern structural imaging techniques, such as MRI, have the ability to provide three-dimensional image sets of the entire anatomy of the human head at a resolution of approximately 1 mm in all dimensions (Fig. 7). Thus, the bulk input to the development of the probabilistic atlas and reference system will be from the study of normal human subjects, obtained in large numbers, who have been carefully characterised in terms of their demographic features and their general medical, neurological, and psychiatric health. Such a data set will be macroscopic, scalable, extensible, and, presumably, manageable as a first step in the atlas building process. Importantly, it will serve as a framework for higher resolution and, ultimately, microscopic approaches that will follow.

In order to achieve accurate neuroanatomical identification and to obtain data sets with a spatial resolution that exceeds that of MRI, high resolution postmortem cross-sectional cryomacrotome data from the entire human head will also be an important part of the feasibility study of this project (Fig. 2) [51,127–130]. As described earlier in this chapter, existing devices can produce spatial resolutions as high as 20 μm in all dimensions. In addition, sections that include neural elements as well as bone and soft tissue can be saved for future analysis. By obtaining and comparing MRI and postmortem high resolution cryomacrotome images of nonhuman primates, the relationship between *in vivo* and postmortem anatomy can be rigorously defined.

The development of a probabilistic atlas and reference system from these data sets will require an iterative approach (Fig. 5). This approach will be necessary on all fronts. For example, segmentation of the images into neuroanatomical structures will be hierarchical, beginning on a manual basis and, as progressively more automated approaches are developed, these will be employed. Initial segmentation will proceed from tissue characterisation (*e.g.*, grey matter, white matter, other matter) to the boundary identification of large cortical and subcortical structures and, ultimately, to nuclear and subnuclear groups. Initial data analysis will employ the macroscopic MRI data sets that progress to the use of high resolution cryomacrotome data as the tools for managing this degree of detail are developed. Computational models and methods used to deform and warp data between subjects will progress in simple linear approaches to more complex nonlinear local deformations (Fig. 5). The reference space and coordinate system itself will iteratively evolve from an initial starting point that uses Talairach space [18] to a newly developed three-dimensional volume.

In the course of establishing the data bases and reference system, initial estimates for the range and correlation of morphological variance will be derived [31]. Further, the acquisition of large data sets and their management will test the capacities for data storage, compression, visualisation and communication. Thus, this project will also serve as a test bed for neuroscientific transfer, visualisation schemes, mathematical methods, and statistical approaches.

The probabilistic reference system can be thought of in two forms. First, there will be a visualisable aspect of the atlas that allows one to see representative and neuroanatomically identifiable images of the human brain. Interrogation of this three-dimensional image will require a number of display formats including three-dimensionally rendered surface features, arbitrarily oriented planes of section, and, possibly, flattening approaches such as those applied in geographical cartography [3–5,118]. Second, highlighting a segment of this visualisable atlas will open a data base of information about the regions in question. Most responses for a given brain region query will be probabilistic in nature. For example, location probability would give estimates of the site in the nervous system that has been identified (*e.g.*, 92% head of caudate, 6% anterior limb of internal capsule, 1% anterior horn of lateral ventricle, less than 1% other regions). Average values and their variance for other features would also, ultimately, be available (*e.g.*, blood flow ± SD, glucose metabolism ± SD, *etc.*). Based on anatomical site, nonprobabilistic information could also be provided. This might include a bibliography of references pertaining to that brain region.

Thus, the ultimate atlas and reference system would have both visualisable (Fig. 8) and data base formats (Fig. 4). Such an approach provides for both visually intuitive and efficient means of interacting with the final product as well as statistical and modeling capabilities that a data base format provides [31]. Access to the atlas and reference system is envisioned to come through workstations. It is predictable that the rapidly increasing speed and storage capacity of computers matched with their progressively declining cost per unit storage, should result in very efficient, high capacity and low cost workstations that are commensurate with the types of data sets envisioned for such a project.

A surprising number of misconceptions exists with regard to probabilistic systems and average brain approaches. For example, there are those that consider an average brain system as one that would not allow for the study of individual subjects. This surprising common misconception disregards the fact that spatial transformations conserve original data and do not destroy them. A population-based probability atlas allows an investigator to take data from one individual subject and place it into a reference system for a population that defines the anatomical uncertainty for structure and function. In our implementation, transformations are bidirectional. That is, an individual subject's brain can be deformed or warped into the reference system and then, using the same mathematical methods, be dewarped or backtransformed into its original state. In an ideal system, no data loss or distortion should occur in this process. As a result, individuals within a given experiment can be more easily and effectively studied and compared. Further, individuals or subpopulations can be compared to other populations that have been previously entered into the data base by different investigators, thereby facilitating the determination of interexperiment or interlaboratory reproducibility.

While it is easy to conceive how such a system might work for tomographically obtained data sets, those working with nontomographic data sets (*e.g.*, electrophysiological, EEG, optical intrinsic signal data) may consider it irrelevant for their purposes. The proposed atlas is based on neuroanatomy. This is the most fundamental language of communication in neuroscience. As such, it allows appropriate reference and localisation to any structure in the brain

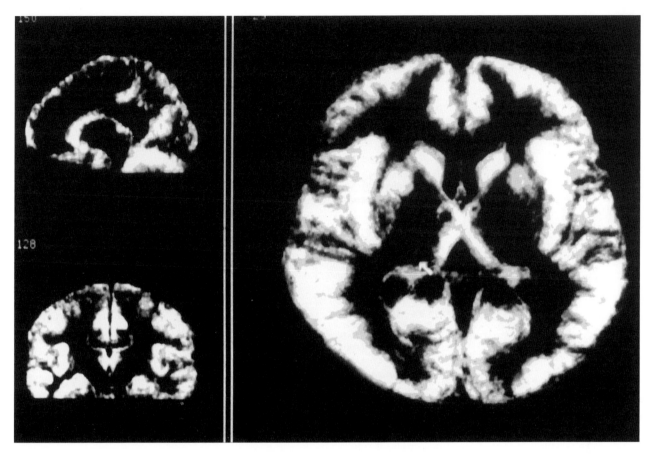

FIGURE 8 Grey matter probability map in stereotaxic space. Twelve MRI volumes (3 mm slice thickness) from normal subjects were classified, using intensity and variance as features, into grey/white/CSF classes. A group probability map for each tissue type constructed by determining the proportion of subjects assigned a given tissue label at each voxel (data courtesy of A. Evans [46]).

from any signal source. In the development of the reference system, cross-sectional and tomographic data will serve as the initial data sets. Once established, however, appropriate vehicles for entering nontomographic data will be developed. For EEG data, for example, systems already exist to localise scalp electrode placement three-dimensionally either through the use of paired tomographic image sets or by nontomographic localisation methods [138].

The more difficult problem is that of entering microscopic data from brain sites that were analysed on a regional basis (*e.g.*, the study of an isolated hippocampus). Nevertheless, such data can also be incorporated into a probabilistic reference system and atlas as was described above in the section on atlas linkages and landmark stains.

Last, it should be kept in mind that the creation of a probabilistic atlas of the human brain is not an exercise in library science. The atlas results from a series of fundamental, hypothesis-driven experiments (Fig. 9) and from merging mathematical statistical approaches with morphological and physiological problems posed with regard to the nervous system. The atlas will create new data and insights into the organisation of the human nervous system in health and disease, its development and its evolution.

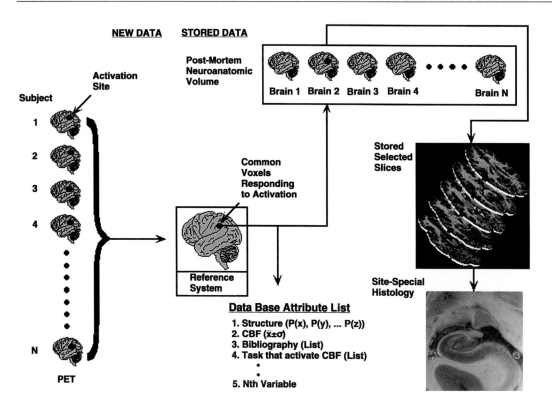

FIGURE 9 Use of the probabilistic reference system. This figure demonstrates inverse use of the reference system once developed. In the center is a representation of the probabilistic reference system. On the left, labeled "NEW DATA," one might envision a series of behavioural tasks performed in a group of subjects by measuring cerebral blood flow changes during the performance of a behavioural task with PET. When these new data sets are aligned, registered, and warped into the reference system, a site of common blood flow activation is identified. At this site we can query the data base for a biological feature attribute list that would tell us, as a function of probability, the location in neuroanatomical terms of this site, its average blood flow and variance, a bibliography related to the information known about this site, and other tasks that have activated this site in terms of functional imaging. In addition, using the inversion component of the reference system, one could dewarp from the probabilistic reference system to an individual cryosectioned human brain. Using boundary coordinates obtained from the reference system one would identify the specific sections that contain this activation site and then perform detailed microscopic histology or neurochemical evaluations of that site. As such, hypothesis and data driven experiments would emerge to evaluate the site-specific microscopic structure that sustains particular functional tasks in the human brain. The concept of processing large numbers of entire human brains at a microscopic and cytoarchitectural level is a massive undertaking that, without a framework or hypothesis driven question, will be less rewarding. Finally, since the microscopic information is rigorously linked to a specific constellation of voxels in the probabilistic data base, that information can automatically be added to the feature attribute list for those voxels.

VII. CONCLUSION

A wide range of brain mapping techniques currently exists for use in human subjects and animal models. Each has its own unique advantages and disadvantages and all vary on a continuum with regard to spatial and temporal resolution as well as sampling frequency and volume. Special issues with regard to the sites that these methods can access, their degree of invasiveness, requirement for anaesthesia, and repeatability all contribute to the selection of the appropriate approach for a given neurobiological situation. As has been stressed throughout this chapter, it is important to understand the limitations and constraints for each method so as to interpret the results appropriately and to use the resultant data to build reliable hypotheses that can be rigorously tested with further experimentation. The ideal brain mapping technique would have extremely high spatial and temporal resolution with the capacity to sample a large volume of the brain continuously. Its costs would be low as would its invasiveness, making it applicable in many settings, in human subjects as well as animal models. At present, no such method exists. Nevertheless, the combination of data sets acquired from many different techniques synthesised into an ever growing atlas of brain structure and function provides the most unifying means by which to span the spectrum of all these variables. Current and developing tools as well as the increasing power and decreasing cost of digital approaches to the management of such data sets make this goal appear to be not just a possibility in the near future but an actual requirement as the volume of information and the need to standardise it across laboratories, experiments, and species continues to grow.

Developing tools and mapping the brain are important challenges for neuroscience as we enter the twenty-first century. The rapid increases in the quality and variety of techniques that provide input for brain mapping experiments are overwhelming. Simultaneously, the speed and memory capacity of computing devices is advancing at an ever accelerating pace while cost is dropping, making powerful desktop manipulations of brain mapping data not only feasible but a reality in most laboratories. The appropriate mathematical and statistical models are being developed to develop advanced population-based probability atlases of the human brain and the data bases to use them.

Once a proper framework for the organisation and storage of neuroscientific data across spatial scales and temporal domains is available the results of every experiment and clinical examination involving the nervous system could ultimately have an appropriate place for future reference. This program depends on the ingenuity and farsightedness of the creators of the reference system to provide an approach that is flexible, compatible with existing as well as future technologies and one that is presented in a manner that is acceptable, in both the technical and the sociological sense, to the neuroscience community at large. Such a system will be neither easy to create nor inexpensive. Nevertheless, when one examines the amount of data, collected in both clinical and research settings today, that becomes inaccessible soon after acquisition, one quickly realises the economy of developing a system for storage and reference of these untapped and yet very costly data. Time and funds spent to organise and store these data that reflect the convenience of the investigators as well as the confidence and credibility ratings for the quality of each data set will provide a usable system that will stand the test of time.

Finally, one should return to the concept of using these systems not simply as libraries or data bases but rather as rich sources of neuroscientific information upon which one can base hypothesis generation. Such hypotheses could then be tested against actual data that need not be collected personally. Similarly, the ability to correlate rigorously *in vivo* human data acquired tomographically or by other methods with postmortem tissue that is available for the myriad of immuno-, histo-, and biochemical stains provides a two-way system for developing a more thorough understanding of the microscopic anatomy of the brain that is driven by hypotheses generated from human *in vivo* experiments (Fig. 9). Given the rapid growth and the amount of neuroscientific information and the pace with which it increases, such organisational, storage, and conceptual systems should no longer be considered a luxury but rather a necessity for the twenty-first century.

References

1. E. R. Tufte. "The Visual Display of Quantitative Information." Graphics Press, Cheshire, 1983.
2. E. R. Tufte. "Envisioning Information." Graphics Press, Cheshire, 1990.
3. D. Felleman and D. Van Essen. Distributed hierarchical processing in the primate cerebral cortex. *Cereb. Cortex* **1,** 1–47 (1991).
4. M. I. Sereno and A. M. Dale. A technique for reconstructing and flattening the cortical surface using MRI images. *Soc. Neurosci. Abstr.* **18**(1), 585 (1992).
5. M. I. Sereno, C. T. McDonald, and J. M. Allman. Analysis of retinotopic maps in extrastriate cortex. *Cereb Cortex* **4**(6), 601–620 (1994).
6. M. Barinaga. Neuroscientists reach a critical mass in Washington. *Science* **262,** 1210–1211 (1993).
7. M. Huerta, S. Koslow, and A. Leshner. The Human Brain Project: An international resource. *Trends Neurosci.* **16,** 436–438 (1993).
8. D. Koshland. The dimensions of the brain. *Science* **258,** 199 (1992).
9. J. C. Mazziotta. Physiologic neuroanatomy: New brain imaging methods present a challenge to an old discipline. *J. Cereb. Blood. Flow. Metab.* **4,** 481 (1984).
10. J. C. Mazziotta and S. Gilman. "Clinical Brain Imaging: Principles and Applications." Davis, Philadelphia, 1992.
11. J. C. Mazziotta and S. H. Koslow. Assessment of goals and obstacles in data acquisition and analysis for emission tomography: Report of a series of international workshops. *J. Cereb. Blood Flow Metab.* **7,** S1–S31 (1987).
12. C. M. Pechura and J. B. Martin. "Mapping the Brain and Its Function." National Academy Press, Washington DC, 1991.
13. G. Paxinos and C. Watson. "The Rat Brain in Stereotaxic Coordinates." Academic Press, Sydney, 1986.
14. K. Brodmann. Beitrage zur histologischen lokalisation der grosshirnrinde. Dritte mitteilung: Die rindenfelder der niederen affen. *J. Psychol. Neurol. Lpz.* **4,** 177–226 (1905).
15. T. Matsui and A. Hirano. "An Atlas of the Human Brain for Computerized Tomography." Igako-Shoin, New York, 1978.
16. G. Schaltenbrand and W. Wahren. "Atlas for Stereotaxy of the Human Brain." Yearbook Medical Publishers, Chicago, 1977.
17. J. Talairach, M. David, P. Tournoux, H. Corredor, and T. Kvasina. "Atlas d'anatomie stereotaxique; reperage radiologique indirect des noyaux gris centraux des regions mesecephalo-sous-optique et hypothalamique de l'homme [Atlas of stereotaxic anatomy: Indirect radiologic regions in humans]." Masson, Paris, 1957.
18. J. Talairach, and P. Tournoux. "Co-planar Stereotaxic Atlas of the Human Brain." Thieme, New York, 1988.
19. J. Van Buren and D. Maccubbin. An outline atlas of the human basal ganglia with estimation of anatomical variants. *J. Neurosurg.* **19,** 811–839 (1962).
20. A. Mansour, C. A. Fox, H. Akil, and S. J. Watson. Opioid-receptor mRNA expression in the rat CNS: Anatomical and functional implications. *Trends Neurosci.* **18,** 22–29 (1995).
21. A. Galaburda, M. Le May, T. Kemper, and N. Geshwind. Right–left asymmetries in the brain: Structural differences between the hemispheres may underlie cerebral dominance. *Science* **199,** 852–856 (1978).

22. N. Geshwind and W. Levitsky. Human brain: Left–right asymmetries in the temporal speech areas. *Science* **161,** 186–187 (1968).

23. M. Le May and D. Kido. Asymmetries of the cerebral hemispheres on computed tomograms. *J. Comput. Assist. Tomgr.* **2,** 471–476 (1978).

24. J. Rademacher, A. Galaburda, D. Kennedy, P. Filipek, and V. Caviness. Human cerebral cortex: Localization, parcellation, and morphometry with magnetic resonance imaging. *J. Cognit. Neurosci.* **4,** 352–374 (1992).

25. G. Schlaug, L. Jancke, Y. Huang, and H. Steinmetz. In vivo evidence of structural brain asymmetry in musicians. *Science* **267,** 699–701 (1995).

26. J. Wada, R. Clarke, and A. Hamm. Cerebral hemispheric asymmetry in humans. *Arch. Neurol.* **32,** 239–246 (1975).

27. C. Von Economo. "The Cytoarchitectonics of the Human Cortex." Oxford Univ. Press, New York, London, 1929.

28. W. J. S. Krieg. Connections of the cerebral cortex. I. The albino rat. A topography of cortical areas. *J. Comp. Neurol.* **84,** 221–275 (1946).

29. P. Flechsig. Developmental (myelogenetic) localisation of the cerebral cortex in the human subject. *Lancet* **2,** 1027–1029 (1901).

30. H. Steinmetz, J. Volkman, L. Jancke, and H. Freund. Anatomical left–right asymmetry of language-related temporal cortex is different in left and right handers. *Ann. Neurol.* **29,** 315–319 (1991).

31. P. T. Fox and J. L. Lancaster. Neuroscience on the net. *Science* **266,** 1793 (1994).

32. P. T. Fox, S. Mikiten, G. Davis, and J. Lancaster. Brain map: A database of human functional brain mapping. *In* "Functional Neuroimaging: Technical Foundations" (R. Thatcher, M. Hallett, T. Zeffero, E. John, and M. Huerta, Eds.), pp. 95–105. Academic Press, San Diego, 1994.

33. J. K. Vries, S. McLinden, and L. Banks. Computerized three-dimensional stereotactic atlases. *In* "Modern Stereotactic Neurosurgery." Little Brown, Boston, 1988.

34. S. C. Strother, J. R. Anderson, X. L. Xu, J. S. Liow, D. C. Bonar, and D. A. Rottenberg. Quantitative comparisons of image registration techniques based on high-resolution MRI of the brain. *J. Comput. Assist. Tomogr.* **18,** 954–962 (1994).

35. R. P. Woods, J. C. Mazziotta, and S. R. Cherry. MRI-PET registration with automated algorithm. *J. Comput. Assist. Tomogr.* **17**(4), 536–546 (1993).

36. P. Harvey and J. Krebs. Comparing brains. *Science* **249,** 140–146 (1990).

37. H. Jerison. Brain size and the evolution of mind. *In* "Fifty-Ninth James Arthur Lecture on the Evolution of the Human Brain," pp. 1–90. American Museum of Natural History, New York, 1989.

38. I. Divac. Monotremunculi and brain evolution. *Trends Neurosci.* **18,** 2–4 (1995).

39. S. Rapoport. Integrated phylogeny of the primate brain, with special reference to humans and their diseases. *Brain Res. Rev.* **15,** 267–294 (1990).

40. P. E. Roland and K. Zilles. Brain atlases-a new research tool. *Trends Neurosci.* **17**(11), 458–467 (1994).

41. E. Armstrong, A. Schleider, H. Omran, M. Curtis, and K. Zilles. The ontogeny of human gyrification. *Cerebral Cortex* **1,** 56–63 (1995).

42. R. Bajcsy, R. Lieberson, and M. Reivich. A computerized system for the elastic matching of deformed radiographic images to idealized atlas images. *J. Comput. Assist. Tomogr.* **7**(4), 618–625 (1983).

43. C. Bohm, T. Greitz, D. Kingsley, B. Berggren, and L. Ollson. Adjustable computerized stereotaxic brain atlas for transmission and emission tomography. *Am. J. Neuroradiol.* **4,** 731–733 (1983).

44. A. C. Evans, S. Marrett, J. Torrescorzo, S. Ku, and L. Collins. MRI-PET correlation in three dimensions using a volume of interest (VOI) atlas. *J. Cereb. Blood Flow Metab.* **11,** A69–A78 (1991).

45. A. C. Evans, D. L. Collins, and B. Milner. "An MRI-Based Stereotactic Brain Atlas from 300 Young Normal Subjects." Proceedings 22nd Annual Symposium of the Society of Neuroscientists, Anaheim, 1992.

46. A. C. Evans, M. Kamber, D. L. Collins, and D. MacDonald. An MRI-based probabilistic atlas of neuroanatomy. *In* "Magnetic Resonance Scanning and Epilepsy" (S. Shorvon, Ed.), pp. 263–274. Plenum, New York, 1994.

47. P. T. Fox, J. Perlmutter, and M. Raichle. A stereostatic method of anatomical localization for positron emission tomography. *J. Comput. Assist. Tomogr.* **9**(1), 141–153 (1985).

48. K. J. Friston, C. D. Frith, P. F. Liddle, and R. S. Frackowiak. Plastic transformation of PET images. *J. Comput. Assist. Tomogr.* **15**(4), 634–639 (1991).

49. H. Steinmetz, G. Furst, and H. J. Freund. Cerebral cortical localization: Application and validation of the proportional grid system in magnetic resonance imaging. *J. Comput. Assist. Tomogr.* **13**, 10–19 (1989).

50. A. W. Toga, M. Samaie, and B. Payne. Digital rat brain: A computerized atlas. *Brain Res. Bull.* **22**, 323–333 (1989).

51. A. W. Toga, K. Ambach, B. Quinn, M. Hutchin, and J. S. Burton. Postmortem anatomy from cryosectioned whole human brain. *J. Neurosci. Methods* **54**(2), 239–252 (1994b).

52. R. Michelucci, F. Valzania, D. Passarelli, M. Santangelo, R. Rizzi, A. M. Buzzi, A. Tempestini, and C. A. Tassinari. Rapid-rate transcranial magnetic stimulation and hemispheric language dominance: Usefulness and safety in epilepsy. *Neurology* **44**, 1697–700 (1994).

53. A. Pascual-Leone, J. Valls-Solé, E. M. Wassermann, and M. Hallett. Responses to rapid-rate transcranial magnetic stimulation of the human motor cortex. *Brain* **117**, 847–858 (1994).

54. E. M. Wassermann, A. Pascual-Leone, and M. Hallett. Cortical motor representation of the ipsilateral hand and arm. *Exp. Brain Res.* **100**, 121–132 (1994).

55. R. Bajcsy and S. Kovacic. Multiresolution elastic matching. *Comput. Vis. Graph. Imag. Process.* **46**, 1–21 (1989).

56. F. L. Bookstein. Thin-plate splines and the atlas problem for biomedical images. *In* "Lecture Notes in Computer Science 511: Information Processing in Medical Imaging" (A. Colchester and D. Hawkes, Eds.), pp. 326–342. Springer-Verlag, Heidelberg, 1991.

57. D. Levin, C. Pelizzari, G. Chen, and M. Cooper. Retrospective geometric correlation of MR, CT, and PET images. *Radiology* **169**, 817–823 (1988).

58. B. A. Payne and A. W. Toga. Surface mapping brain function on 3D models. *IEEE Comput. Graph. Appl.* **10**, 33–41 (1990).

59. C. Pelizzari, G. Chen, D. Sperling, R. Weichselbaum, and C. Chen. Accurate three-dimensional registration of CT, PET, and/or MRI images of the brain. *J. Comput. Assist. Tomogr.* **13**, 20–26 (1989).

60. R. P. Woods, S. R. Cherry, and J. C. Mazziotta. Rapid automated algorithm for aligning and reslicing PET images. *J. Comput. Assist. Tomogr.* **16**(4) 620–633 (1992).

61. H. Steinmetz and R. J. Seitz. Functional anatomy of language processing: Neuroimaging and the problem of individual variability. *Neuropsychologia* **29**(12), 1149–1161 (1991).

62. D. BvK. Keyserlingk, K. Niemann, and J. Wasel. A quantitative approach to spatial variation of human cerebral sulci. *Acta Anatomica* **131**, 127–131 (1988).

63. D. Lemoine, C. Barillot, B. Gibaud, and E. Pasqualini. *In* "Lecture Notes in Computer Science 511: Information Processing in Medical Imaging" (A. Colchester and D. Hawkes, Eds.), pp. 154–164. Springer-Verlag, Heidelberg, 1991.

64. A. C. Evans, S. Marrett, P. Neelin, L. Collins, K. Worsley, D. Weiqian, S. Milot, M. Ernst, and D. Bub. Anatomical mapping of functional activation in stereotactic coordinate space. *NeuroImage* **1**(1), 43–53 (1992).

65. D. L. Collins, T. M. Peters, and A. C. Evans. *Proc. IEEE Symp. Adv. Med. Image Processing Med.* **80**, 105–110 (1992).

66. D. L. Collins, W. Dai, T. M. Peters, and A. C. Evans. Visualization in biomedical computing. *Proc. SPIE* **1808**, 10–23 (1992).

67. A. C. Evans, W. Dai, L. Collins, P. Neelin, and S. Marrett. Warping of a com-

puterized 3-D atlas to match brain image volumes for quantitative neuro-anatomical and functional analysis. *Proc. SPIE Image Processing* **1445,** 235–246 (1991).

68. D. L. Collins, P. Neelin, T. M. Peter, and A. C. Evans. Automatic three-dimensional intersubject registration of MR volumetric data in standardized Talairach space. *J. Comput. Assist. Tomogr.* **18**(2), 192–205 (1994).

69. D. Hill, D. Hawkes, J. Crossman, M. Gleeson, T. Cox, E. Bracey, A. Strong, and P. Graves. Registration of MR and CT images for skull base surgery using point-like anatomical features. *Br. J. Radiol.* **64,** 1030–1035 (1991).

70. N. Alpert, J. Bradshaw, D. Kennedy, and J. Correia. The principle axis transformation: A method for image registration. *J. Nuclear Med.* **31**(10), 1717–1722 (1990).

71. N. C. Andreasen, G. Cohen, G. Harris, T. Cizadlo, J. Parkkinen, K. Rezai, and V. W. Swayze. Image processing for the study of brain structure and function: Problems and programs. *J. Neuropsychol. Clin. Neurosci.* **4**(2), 125–133 (1992).

72. P. T. Fox, M. Mintun, E. Reiman, and M. Raichle. Enhanced detection of focal brain responses using intersubject averaging and change-distribution analysis of subtracted PET images. *J. Cereb. Blood Flow Metab.* **8,** 642–653 (1988).

73. G. Wolberg. "Digital Image Warping." IEEE Computer Society Press, Los Alamitos, 1990.

74. A. W. Toga. "Three-Dimensional Neuroimaging." Raven Press, New York, 1991.

75. A. W. Toga. A digital three dimensional atlas of structure/function relationships. *J. Chem. Neuroanat.* **43,** 313–318 (1991).

76. S. Keibel, J. Asburner, J. B. Poline, and K. Friston. "MRI and PET Co-registration—A Cross Validation of SPM and AIR." *NeuroImage,* in press.

77. C. Bohm, T. Greitz, R. Seitz, and L. Eriksson. Specification and selection of regions of interest (ROIs) in a computerized brain atlas. *J. Cereb. Blood Flow Metab.* **11,** A64–A68 (1991).

78. M. W. Wilson and J. M. Mountz. A reference system for neuroanatomic localization on functional reconstructed cerebral images. *J. Comput. Assist. Tomogr.* **13**(1), 174–178 (1989).

79. C. M. Clark, C. Ammann, W. R. Martin, P. Ty, and M. R. Hayden. The FDG/PET methodology for early detection of disease onset: A statistical model. *J. Cereb. Blood Flow Metab.* **11**(2), A96–A102 (1991).

80. A. W. Toga. Visualization and warping of multimodality brain imagery. *In* "Functional Neuroimaging: Technical Foundations" (R. Thatcher *et al.* Eds.), pp. 171–180. Academic Press, San Diego, 1994.

81. A. W. Toga, P. K. Banerjee, and E. M. Santori. Warping 3D models for interbrain comparisons. *Neuroscience* **16,** 247 (1990). [Abstract]

82. A. W. Toga, B. A. Payne, and E. M. Santori. Leminar analysis of a 3D reconstruction of the superior colliculus. *Soc. Neurosci. Abstr.* **15,** 1792 (1989).

83. A. W. Toga and P. Banerjee. Registration revisited. *Neurosci. Methods* **48,** 1–13 (1993).

84. C. Leventhal and R. Ware. Three-dimensional reconstruction from serial sections *Nature* **236**(5344), 207–210 (1972).

85. W. E. Lorensen and H. E. Cline. Marching cubes: A high resolution 3D surface construct algorithm. *Comput. Graph.* (*Proc. Siggraph*) **8**(6), 163–169 (1987).

86. B. A. Payne and A. W. Toga. Distance field manipulation of surface models. *Comput. Graph. Appl.* **12**(1), 65–71 (1992).

87. R. O. Duda and P. E. Hart. "Pattern Classification and Scene Analysis." Wiley, New York, 1973.

88. D. Y. Amamoto, R. Kasturi, and A. Mamourain. *In* "Proceedings of the Xth International Conference on Pattern Recognition," pp. 603–607. IEEE Computer Society Press, Los Alamitos, 1990.

89. H. S. Choi, D. R. Haynor, and Y. Kim. Partial volume tissue classification of multichannel magnetic resonance images—a mixel model. *IEEE Trans. Med. Imag.* **10,** 395–407 (1991).

90. G. Gerig, J. Martin, and R. Kikinis. *In* "Lecture Notes in Computer Science 511:

Information Processing in Medical Imaging" (A. Colchester and D. Hawkes, Eds.), pp. 175–187. Springer-Verlag, Heidelberg, 1991.

91. A. Herrmann, D. N. Levin, X. Hu, K. K. Tan, and S. Galhotra. "Segmentation and 3D Display of MR Images of Brain Lesions." Proc. 7th SMRM Meeting, 1988.

92. G. R. Hillman, T. A. Kent, and A. Kaye. Measurement of brain compartment volumes in MR using voxel composition calculations. *J. Comput. Assist. Tomogr.* **15**(4), 640–646 (1991).

93. I. Kapouleas and C. A. Kulikowski. A model based system for the interpretation of MR human brain scans. *Proc. SPIE–Int. Soc. Optic. Eng. Med. Imag. II* **914,** 429–437 (1988).

94. R. Kikinis, F. A. Jolesz, and G. Gerig. 3-D Imaging in medicine: Algorithms, systems, applications. *NATO ASI Series F* **60,** 441–454 (1990).

95. M. I. Kohn, N. K. Tanna, G. T. Herman, S. M. Resnick, P. D. Mozley, R. E. Gur, A. Alavi, R. A. Zimmerman, and R. C. Gur. Analysis of brain and cerebrospinal fluid volumes with MR images: Methods, reliability and validation. *Radiology* **178,** 115–122 (1991).

96. K. O. Kim and A. Pfefferbaum. Segmentation of MR brain images into cerebrospinal fluid spaces, white and gray matter. *J. Comput. Assist. Tomogr.* **13**(4), 588–593 (1989).

97. H. E. Cline, W. E. Lorensen, R. Kikinis, and F. Jolesz. Three-dimensional segmentation of MR images of the head using probability and connectivity. *J. Comput. Assist. Tomogr.* **14**(6), 1037–1045 (1990).

98. H. E. Cline, C. L. Domoulin, and H. R. Hart. Three-dimensional reconstruction of the brain from magnetic resonance images using a connectivity algorithm. *Magn. Reson. Imaging* **5,** 345–352 (1987).

99. R. T. Fan, S. S. Trivedi, L. L. Fellingham, and A. Gamboa-Aldeco. Soft tissue segmentation and 3D display from computerized tomography and magnetic resonance imaging. *Proc. SPIE Med. Imag. Int. Soc. Optic. Eng.* **767,** 494–504 (1987).

100. K. H. Hoehne and W. A. Hanson. Interactive 3D segmentation of MRI and CT volumes using morphological operations. *J. Comput. Assist. Tomogr.* **16**(2), 285–294 (1992).

101. D. Marr and E. Hildreth. Theory of edge detection. *Proc. R. Soc. London Biol.* **207**(1167), 187–217 (1980).

102. A. Rosenfeld and A. C. Kak. "Digital Picture Processing," 2nd ed. Academic Press, New York, 1982.

103. M. Bomans, K. H. Hoehne, U. Tiede, and M. Riemer. 3-D segmentation of MR images of the head for 3-D display. *IEEE Trans. Med. Imag.* **2,** 177–183 (1990).

104. S.-Y. Chen, W.-C. Lin, and C.-T. Chen. Sensor integration for tomographic image segmentation. *Proc SPIE Med. Imag. III* **3,** 1387–1388 (1988).

105. B. L. Dalton and G. du Boulay. *Proc. SPIE Med. Imag. II* **914,** 456–464 (1988).

106. R. Dann, J. Hoford, S. Kovacic, M. Reivich, and R. Bajcsy. Evaluation of elastic matching system for anatomic (CT, MR) and functional (PET) cerebral images. *J. Comput. Assist. Tomogr.* **13**(4), 603–611 (1989).

107. R. Dann, J. Hoford, S. Kovacic, M. Reivich, and R. Bajcsy. Three-dimensional computerized brain atlas for elastic matching: Creation and initial evaluation. *Med. Imag. II 1988: SPIE Proc.* **914,** 600–612 (1988).

108. A. P. Dhawan and S. Juvvadi. *Proc. SPIE Med. Imag. II* **914,** 422–428 (1988).

109. M. Kamber, D. L. Collins, and G. S. Francis. Model-based 3D segmentation of multiple sclerosis lesions in dual-echo MRI data. *Proc. Second Conf. Visualiz. Biomed. Comp. Chapel Hill, NC* **1808,** 590–600 (1992).

110. D. N. Kennedy, P. A. Filipek, and V. S. Caviness. Anatomic segmentation and volumetric analysis in nuclear magnetic resonance imaging. *IEEE Trans. Med. Imag.* **7,** 1–7 (1989).

111. S. B. Serpico, F. Sturaro, G. Vernazza, and S. Dellepiane. Fuzzy-reasoning ap-

proach to understanding of 2D NMR images. *Proc. 9th Annu. Conf. IEEE Eng. Med. Biol. Soc.* **4,** 1980–1981 (1987).

112. E. Sokolowska and J. A. Newell. Multi-layered image representation: Structure and application in recognition of parts of brain anatomy. *Pattern Recognit. Lett.* **4,** 223–230 (1986).

113. M. W. Vannier, R. L. Butterfield, D. Jordan, W. A. Murphy, R. G. Levitt, and M. Gadd. Multispectral analysis of magnetic resonance images. *Radiology* **154,** 221–224 (1985).

114. G. Vernazza, S. B. Serpico, and S. G. Dellepiane. *IEEE Trans. Circ. Syst. CAS* **34**(11), 1399–1416 (1987).

115. A. Evans, S. Marrett, P. Neelin, L. Collins, K. Worsley, W. Dai, S. Milot, E. Meyer, and D. Bub. Anatomical mapping of functional activation in stereotactic coordinate space. *NeuroImage* **1**(1), 43–63 (1992).

116. J. R. Quinlan. Induction of decision trees. *Machine Learning* **1,** 81–106 (1986).

116a. D. C. Van Essen, and J. H. R. Maunsell. Two-dimensional maps of the cerebral cortex. *J. Compar. Neurol.* **191,** 255–281 (1980).

117. M. L. Jouandet, M. J. Tramo, D. M. Herron, A. Hermann, W. C. Loftus, J. Bazell, and M. S. Gazzaniga. Brainprints: Computer-generated two-dimensional maps of the human cerebral cortex in vivo. *J. Cognit. Neurosci.* **1**(1), 88–117 (1989).

118. G. J. Carman. (1990). "Mapping of the Cerebral Cortex," Unpublished doctoral dissertation, Caltech, Pasadena, CA.

119. D. MacDonald, D. Avis, and A. C. Evans. Multiple surface indentification and matching in magnetic resonance imaging: Visualization in biomedical computing 1994. *Proc. SPIE* **2359,** 160–169 (1994).

120. N. Kehtarnavaz, E. A. Philippe, and R. J. P. DeFigueirado. A novel surface reconstruction and display method for cardiac PET imaging. *IEEE Trans. Med. Imag.* **3**(3), 108–115 (1984).

121. E. L. Schwartz, B. Merker, E. Wolfson, and A. Schaw. Applications of computer graphics and image processing to 2D and 3D modeling of the functional architecture of visual cortex. *Comput. Graph. Appl.* **8,** 13–23 (1988).

122. E. L. Schwartz, A. Schaw, and E. Wolfson. A numerical solution to the generalized mapmaker's problem: Flattening nonconvex polyhedral surfaces. *IEEE Trans. Pattern Recognit. Mach. Intelligence* **11**(9), 1005–1008 (1989).

123. P. B. Heffernan and R. A. Robb. A new procedure for combined display of 3-D cardiac anatomic surfaces and regional functions. "Proceedings IEEE Computer Cardiology," pp. 111–114. IEEE Computer Society Press, Silver Spring, MD, 1984.

124. J. C. Mazziotta, D. Valentino, S. Grafton, F. Bookstein, C. Pelizzari, G. Chen, and A. W. Toga. Relating structure to function in vivo with tomographic imaging. *In* "Exploring Brain Functional Anatomy with Positron Tomography," pp. 93–112. Wiley, Chichester, 1991.

125. J. D. G. Watson, R. Myers, R. S. J. Frackowiak, R. P. Woods, J. C. Mazziotta, S. Shipp, and S. Zeki. Area V5 of the human brain: Evidence from a combined study using positron emission tomography and magnetic resonance imaging. *Cereb. Cortex* **3**(2), 79–94 (1993).

126. P. E. Roland, C. J. Graufelds, J. Wahlin, L. Engelman, M. Andersson, A. Ledberg, J. Pedersen, S. Ackerman, A. Dabringhaus, and K. Zilles. Human brain atlas: For high-resolution functional and anatomical mapping. *Hum. Brain Mapping* **1**(3), 173–184 (1994).

127. B. Quinn, K. A. Ambach, and A. W. Toga. Three-dimensional cryomacrotomy with integrated computer-based technology in neuropathology. *Lab. Invest.* **68,** 121A (1993).

128. W. Rauschning. Serial cryosectioning of human knee joint specimens for a study of functional anatomy. *Sci. Tools* **26,** 47–50 (1979).

129. A. W. Toga, K. L. Ambach, and S. Schluender. High-resolution anatomy from *in situ* human brain. *NeuroImage* **1**(4), 334–344 (1994).

130. M. B. M. Van Leeuwen, A. J. H. Deddens, P. O. Cerrits, and B. Hillen. A modified

mallory-cason staining procedure for large cryosections. *Stain Technol.* **65,** 37–42 (1990).

131. W. Drevets, T. Videen, A. MacLeod, J. Haller, and M. Raichle. PET images of blood flow during anxiety: Correction. *Science* **256,** 1696 (1992).

132. Chang, H. C. Chui, and A. R. Damasio. Human cerebral asymmeries evaluated by computed tomography. *J. Neurol. Neurosurg. Psychiatry* **43**(10), 873–878 (1980).

133. A. B. Rubens, U. W. Mahowald, and J. T. Hutton. Asymmetry of the lateral (sylvian) fissures in man. *Neurology* **26**(7), 620–624 (1976).

134. D. R. Weinberger, P. Luchins, J. Morihisa, and R. J. Wyatt. Asymmetry volumes of the right and left frontal and occipital regions of the human brain. *Ann. Neurol.* **11,** 97–102 (1982).

135. S. F. Witelson. Anatomic asymmetry in the temporal lobes: Its documentation, phylogenesis, and relationship to functional asymmetry. *Ann. NY Acad. Sci.* **299,** 328–354 (1977).

136. F. Crick and E. Jones. Backwardness of human neuroanatomy. *Nature* **361,** 109–110 (1993).

137. C. M. Pechura and J. B. Martin. "Institute of Medicine (US) Committee on a National Neural Circuitry Database." National Academy Press, Washington, DC, 1991.

138. G. H. Barnett, D. W. Kormos, C. P. Steiner, and H. Morris. Registration of EEG electrodes with three-dimensional neuroimaging using a frameless, armless stereotactic wand. *Stereotact. Funct. Neurosurg.* **61,** 32–38 (1993).

139. M. Levoy. Volume rendering: Display of surfaces from volume data. *IEEE Comput. Graph. Appl.* **8**(3), 29–37 (1988).

140. A. W. Toga and T. L. Arnicar. Image analysis of brain physiology. *Comput. Graph. Appl.* **5**(12), 20–25 (1985).

141. J. Zhang, M. Levesque, C. Wilson, R. Harper, J. Engel, R. Lufkin, and E. Benkhe. Multimodality imaging of brain structures for stereotactic surgery. *Radiology* **175,** 435–441 (1990).

142. G. Golub and C. Van Loan. "Matrix Computations." Johns Hopkins Univ. Press, Baltimore, 1983.

143. A. C. Evans, D. L. Collins, P. Neelin, D. MacDonald, M. Kamber, and T. S. Marrett. Three-dimensional correlative imaging: Applications in human brain mapping. *In* "Functional Neuroimaging and Technical Foundations" (R. Thatcher, M. Hallett, T. Zeffero, E. John, and E. Huerta, Eds.), pp. 145–161. Academic Press, San Diego, 1994.

144. F. L. Bookstein, B. Chernoff, R. L. Elder, J. M. Humphries, G. R. Smith, and R. E. Strauss. "Morphometrics In Evolutionary Biology." The Academy of Natural Sciences of Philadelphia, 1985.

145. D. Levin, X. Hu, K. Tan, S. Galhotra, C. Pelizzari, G. Chen, R. Beck, C. Chen, M. Cooper, J. Mullan, J. Hekmatpanah, and J. Spire. The brain: Integrated three-dimensional display of MR and PET images. *Radiology* **172,** 783–789 (1989).

146. J. C. Olivio, E. Kahn, S. Halpern, and P. Fragu. Image registration and distortion correction in ion microscopy. *J. Microsc.* **164,** 263–272 (1991).

147. P. A. Kenny, D. J. Dowsett, D. Vernon, and J. T. Ennis. A technique for digital image registration used prior to subtraction of lung images in nuclear medicine. *Phys. Med. Biol.* **35**(5), 679–685 (1990).

148. C. Broit. (1981). "Computer and Information Science," Unpublished doctoral dissertation, Univ of Pennsylvania.

CHAPTER EIGHTEEN

FUNCTIONAL IMAGING WITH MAGNETIC RESONANCE

I. INTRODUCTION

In the spring of 1991 the first of a group of new methods for mapping human brain function was successfully tested at the MRI Center of the Massachusetts General Hospital (MGH) in Boston. These methods use the supremely noninvasive technique of magnetic resonance imaging to create images of the brain that are sensitive to local changes in blood flow. In identification of cortical areas active for a particular brain task, they promise a spatial resolution of 2 mm, a temporal resolution of 1 sec, and the opportunity to rescan a single subject as often as desired. As might have been expected, legions of brain researchers have since leapt upon magnetic resonance functional neuroimaging, or functional MRI (fMRI) as it is more frequently called, attempting to apply it to various studies in cognitive neuroscience. Whilst the underlying phenomenon is simple, in the sense that many MRI scanners were found to have the capability of performing fMRI studies once the technique had been discovered, quantification of the effect in relation to cortical electrical activity has been elusive, and for those unversed in MRI the origins of the functional signal require some explanation.

II. PRINCIPLES OF fMRI

A. Sources of Contrast in MRI

The MRI signal in normal clinical use comes almost entirely from the protons of tissue water. The image intensity depends primarily on the density of these protons, of course, but can be profoundly affected by the local environment of the water molecules. After excitation with a pulse of radiofrequency magnetic field (RF pulse), which changes the alignment of the proton magnetic moments from being parallel to the large static field produced by the MRI magnet, the protons recover their original alignment quite slowly, in several tenths of a second to seconds. During this time the magnetisation which has thus been created in the direction transverse to the steady magnetic field induces a signal voltage in an antenna surrounding the object or body being scanned. If the water protons are excited again before full recovery, a smaller signal is obtained. The rate of recovery, described by a "longitudinal relaxation time," T1, depends on the type of tissue containing the relevant water molecules. For instance, in cerebrospinal fluid, which is close to pure water, protons relax in about 3 sec, while in brain white matter, where water molecules interact strongly with lipid membranes and intracellular organelles, the recovery time is reduced to about 0.5 sec.

Clearly, by varying the repeat time between RF pulses, the contrast between tissue regions of long and short T1 can be changed dramatically. However, another type of relaxation also offers a means of distinguishing tissue types. As we have seen, in order to observe an MRI signal the proton magnetisation must be tipped away from the main field direction to create a component of magnetisation precessing about this axis in the transverse plane. To produce maximum signal, the phase angle which the magnetisation vector makes in the transverse plane must remain constant across the object, allowing the magnetisation to add up constructively from each proton. However, small differences in the magnetic environment of each spin will cause them to precess at slightly different frequencies, resulting in a dispersion of phase angles and hence a signal which decreases with time. The decay of signal is generally roughly exponential, and can be characterised by a time constant T2, the "transverse relaxation time." In addition, if there are magnetic field variations across the object, which may be caused by the presence within the object of paramagnetic particles, such as an MRI contrast agent containing gadolinium, or simply by the spatial inhomogeneity of the object, there is a further phase dispersion causing a more rapid decay of the signal. This additional relaxation is denoted by T2′. Together the two effects result in a signal decaying with a time constant T2*, where $1/T2* = 1/T2 + 1/T2'$.

Until the late 1980s the decay of signal associated with local magnetic field inhomogeneities, called T2* relaxation, was considered a nuisance and represented a limitation upon MR imaging. To mitigate this, either the so-called "spin-echo" technique was used, in which a second "refocussing" RF pulse following the initial excitation pulse removed the effects of dephasing, or the time between the RF excitation pulse and the acquisition of signal was reduced as much as possible, as in FLASH (Fast Low-Angle Shot imaging) [1].

It was only when it was realized that the presence of a paramagnetic substance in the bloodstream could act as a vascular marker, giving useful contrast, that sequences without a refocussing pulse, with a relatively long time between the excitation pulse and data acquisition (20–80 msec), began to be used. Initially the paramagnetic contrast agent was exogenous, a nontoxic compound of gadolinium introduced into the bloodstream via a leg vein. A fraction of a millimole of contrast agent per kilogram of body weight is sufficient to give a loss of signal from tissue surrounding cerebral blood vessels of perhaps 40% as a bolus of contrast agent passes through. The group at MGH pioneered the application of this approach to brain perfusion, using the Central Volume Theorem [2] to obtain local cerebral blood flow as the ratio of blood volume to mean transit time. Early studies [3,4] examined the passage of contrast agent through the brains of rats and later dogs, making increasing use of an ultrafast MRI imaging technique known as echo-planar imaging (EPI), invented by Sir Peter Mansfield in 1977 [5], which acquires a complete image in less than 100 msec, and thus allows "snapshots" of the contrast agent distribution as it passes rapidly through the brain.

In a landmark paper published in 1991, Belliveau and collaborators finally applied the technique to functional activation studies in humans [6]. The subjects were given visual ("photic") stimulation while a bolus of contrast agent was injected into a leg vein, and single slice images of the brain in the plane of the calcarine fissure were obtained at 0.75-sec intervals to monitor the bolus passage. By integrating the time course of image intensity, estimates of relative blood volume were obtained and compared (by image subtraction) with those obtained when the subjects were at rest in darkness. Consistent increases (up to 30%) of blood volume in primary V1 visual cortex were observed.

Subsequent developments rapidly overtook this pioneering work. Ogawa [7] and Turner [8], working independently, had shown in laboratory animals that similar changes of MRI image contrast extending around the blood vessels could be obtained simply by changing the oxygenation state of the blood. This observation arose from the fact (noted by Faraday, and measured by Pauling and Coryell [9]) that deoxyhaemoglobin is more paramagnetic than oxyhemoglobin, which itself has almost exactly the same magnetic susceptibility as tissue. Thus deoxyhaemoglobin can be seen as nature's own contrast agent. Interventions to the state of the brain that create an imbalance between oxygen uptake and blood flow will thus inevitably cause a change of MRI signal around the cortical vessels, if MR imaging sequences are used that are sensitive to magnetic field inhomogeneity.

This development culminated in the work of Kwong *et al.* [10] and Ogawa *et al.* [11], who succeeded in showing that the change in deoxyhaemoglobin in human visual cortex, while the subject viewed a bright light, was sufficient to cause measurable changes in gradient-echo MRI images of a slice passing through the calcarine fissure. The technique was dubbed "blood oxygenation level dependent contrast" (BOLD). Thus the way was opened to functional mapping studies of the human brain without use of contrast agent, with no radiation dose, and with the high spatial resolution of MRI.

Meanwhile, another MRI method for noninvasive monitoring of blood flow was under development. This approach, begun at Pittsburgh in 1990 [12], uses a blood labeling technique akin to diffusible tracer studies. In this case, the label is applied using a preparatory radiofrequency pulse, before the MRI data acquisition sequence, which tags the spins of protons in arterial blood flowing into the brain region of interest. The label is evanescent, disappearing with the relaxation time constant T1(typically 1–2 sec), so that it is not possible to build up a large concentration of labelled spins in brain tissue. However, the label, which consists of inverting the nuclear spins, freely diffuses through the capillary walls into the tissue and reduces the MR signal there by up to 2%, sufficient to be measured with reasonable accuracy if care is taken [12]. Variations on this approach, now known as arterial spin tagging (AST) have been developed, in which the spins in the slice to be imaged are labelled, while unlabelled arterial spins move into the slice and change the image intensity proportionally to local CBF. Potentially AST methods can be quantified to give absolute values for local cerebral perfusion, although a number of important correction terms need to be evaluated.

AST has more recently been combined with EPI to measure relative changes in blood flow during activation. EPISTAR (echo-planar MR imaging and signal targeting with alternating radio frequency) [13] involves inversion of the MR spins in a thick slab of the brain/head which is physically close to the section of interest. The effect of labelled spins, carried by the blood into the imaging slice, is observed as a signal change within the slice, and blood flow changes can be monitored by comparing images with and without activation. This method enables haemodynamics to be investigated by varying the delay between inversion and detection. The change of signal related to brain activity observable with this technique depends on the relaxation time T1, both directly [13] and indirectly, since the magnetic labeling of the blood decays with the T1 of blood. T1 increases with magnetic field, and thus the sensitivity of EPISTAR should also increase with field strength.

B. Imaging Techniques

For human brain activation studies it is highly desirable to obtain image data quickly. There are several reasons for this, apart from the obvious need to avoid experiments lasting many hours. The first is that many perceptual and cognitive tasks of interest can be continued only for a few minutes without habituation, fatigue, or boredom. Second, the spatial resolution is generally on the order of 1–2 mm, which means that effective head immobilisation is essential. The longer a subject is lying in an uncomfortable position inside the MRI magnet, the greater the chance of large movement. Third, it is important to sample the activation state of the whole brain as synchronously as possible. Since MRI usually obtains image data one slice at a time, and 20–30 slices are necessary to cover the entire brain, this implies acquisition of a slice in a time very short compared with the haemodynamic response time of the cerebral vasculature of 6–8 sec. The only successful MRI technique capable of this speed with reasonable spatial resolution and good signal : noise ratio is EPI [14], as previously mentioned.

It has to be acknowledged that compared with slower MRI techniques, the spatial resolution of EPI is somewhat impaired (to about 2 mm), while the temporal resolution is improved to about 100 msec. Furthermore, the rate of information capture, that is, the signal to noise per unit time, is highest for EPI and its variants (such as single-shot GRASE [15] and single-shot spiral EPI [16]). However, EPI images (especially the gradient-echo version of EPI) suffer more than the other techniques from distortion and signal loss arising from magnetic field inhomogeneities in the brain, which often derive from the natural susceptibility differences between brain and air and are thus not amenable to correction by improved shimming (adjustment of the static field homogeneity with a set of correction coils).

C. Characteristics of BOLD and AST fMRI

The difference in susceptibility between fully oxygenated and deoxygenated blood is small (about 0.02×10^{-6} cgs units), and thus image intensity changes in BOLD contrast studies are generally small, less than 15% at a magnetic field of 2 T even when the haemoglobin oxygen saturation is reduced to 20% in acute hypoxia [17]. In brain activation studies at 1.5 T [10] the signal change is no more than 2–4%. Experiments [18] and model calculations [19–21] have shown that the change in T2* relaxation rate associated with this signal loss increases with the static magnetic field of the MRI scanner, so that the change of signal is typically about three times larger at 4 T than at the more commonly used field strength of 1.5 T for the same echo time and sequence type. Given the improved signal : noise ratio at higher field (roughly proportional to field strength) there is a strong case for the use of high magnetic fields for this type of functional MRI. At 4 T, signal changes of up to 30% have been observed for visual stimulation, with typical single-shot background noise of 0.5% or less, giving z values of 60 or more for some pixels. Of course, for more subtle brain activations in association cortex, intensity changes are generally much smaller, from 2 to 8% at this field strength, and proportionately lower at the more commonly used field of 1.5 T. At the lower field strength it is often necessary to perform averaging over images to obtain significant results, although single-subject studies remain eminently feasible.

By contrast with BOLD, AST methods characteristically have a poorer contrast to noise ratio. Here the change in signal depends on the relaxation time T1, which increases only weakly with field strength. At 1.5 T the contrast : noise is about one-third of that obtainable with BOLD, and signal averaging is always required. One benefit of the EPISTAR method is that the signal from static tissue in each slice is nulled in the absence of perfusion [13], so that the large background "anatomical" signal plays no part in functional studies. This means that the large subtraction errors in functional maps resulting from head movement and consequent image misregistration, which bedevil BOLD studies, are not found.

A major disadvantage of AST methods in general, however, is the considerable difficulty in obtaining multislice data. This problem arises from the fact that the nuclear spins of the water protons carry the label in the blood, and that once these spins have moved into a slice to be imaged, they are disturbed by the RF pulse needed in image acquisition, so that the blood must be relabelled for each image. Since it takes 1–2 sec for the label to move into the capillary bed, during which time no other RF pulse can be allowed to affect it, it is not feasible to obtain volume data at the rate of 10 slices per second, as is feasible with BOLD EPI methods.

Comparing areas in BOLD and AST functional images apparently activated by a simple brain stimulus, there is a very large measure of agreement. It can be shown that AST images (when obtained correctly) selectively show areas of increased capillary flow, and changes in arterial and venous flow are not represented. BOLD images show primarily oxygenation changes in small venules overlying neurally active cortical tissue, since these contain the majority of the blood experiencing local changes in oxygenation [22,23]. On the scale of the spatial resolution of EPI, the activated areas seen on BOLD and AST images overlap, with residual differences ascribable to the lower sensitivity of AST, as discussed earlier. Higher resolution BOLD images, at high magnetic field that selectively enhances contributions from smaller cortical vessels, may show yet more local oxygenation changes such as those associated with differential oxygen demand from adjacent cortical columns. AST is unlikely to be able to provide such fine discrimination, since it appears that the arteriolar control of blood flow lacks sufficient precision to selectively supply such small structures, except in specialised cortex such as rat whisker barrels [24].

D. Comparisons with PET Scanning

A number of groups have compared results obtained with fMRI and PET methods, for the same subjects performing the same tasks. When the poorer spatial resolution of PET is taken into account, the spatial localisation of the two methods is in good agreement [25] and a parametric study, in which finger pressure was varied, showed that changes in fMRI signal, averaged over a group of six volunteers, are proportional to changes in PET measurements of rCBF [26].

E. Typical fMRI Experimental Parameters

In a typical fMRI experiment, a subject lies on the bed of an MRI scanner while viewing a screen illuminated by an LCD video projector, or listens to auditory input via headphones, or performs some other form of cognitive task, while a sequence of images is obtained. When EPI is used, commonly 3–10 images per second are acquired, for a period of 5–10 min. The subject's head is kept still using foam pads or one of a number of proprietary methods for head immobilisation. Ideally, multislice images are obtained, giving upwards of 50 consecutive images of the entire brain during the experimental run. In-plane resolution is typically 2–3 mm, with a field of view of 16–24 cm, and slice thickness is between 3 and 10 mm. With a repeat time of 3 sec for any particular slice, effects on the image caused by cardiac and respiratory pulsations are relatively small compared with functionally related changes and are mostly confined to large vessels and CSF [27,28]. However, head movement of even as little as 0.5 mm can cause an apparent change of signal in a given voxel of as much as 40%.

III. SPECIAL ISSUES RELEVANT TO FUNCTIONAL BRAIN MAPPING

Functional neuroimaging with magnetic resonance imaging is therefore a technique that can provide information additional and complementary to that available with PET. The study of brain activity using fMRI poses a set of problems beyond those that have been addressed for PET. We can group these into three broad categories. (i) The fMRI signal depends on the effects that changes in cerebral physiology, consequent on changes in neural activity, have on MRI physics. There are therefore many aspects of fMRI imaging techniques that need to be refined to facilitate optimal data acquisition. (ii) The design of fMRI experiments reflects the temporal resolution of fMRI and the large number of measurements that will typically be made. At the same time the design needs to take account of the fact that unlike PET, fMRI is not measuring absolute blood flow changes but a relative change in the oxygenation of venous blood. These design issues also have implications for data processing; *i.e.*, the normalisation and statistical methods used to find significant activations need to address the particular characteristics of fMRI data. (iii) The high magnetic field, restricted space, and noise of the scanner make special demands on the methods of stimulus presentation and subject accommodation within the system.

A. MRI Physics

A T_2^* dependent effect is the dominant source of activation in BOLD-contrast fMRI images. It is not the only source, and two issues need to be considered in data analysis. The first can be paraphrased by the question "Brain or vein—oxygenation or flow?" [29] and the second relates to the question of the spatial accuracy of the T_2^* signal in locating neuronal activity.

NMR-sensitive spins in flowing blood do not obey the same simple T_1 relaxation effects as in stationary tissue; as fresh blood moves into the imaging slice it has higher signal intensity than blood that has been repeatedly excited by the slice selection radiofrequency pulses. Blood flow changes correlated with a stimulus can therefore lead to increased MRI signal levels in large vessels. Incorrect interpretation of these signals as BOLD effects can be avoided by anatomical inspection and minimised by the choice of MRI technique. Single slice imaging methods are very susceptible to these in-flow effects; multiple slice EPI provides a more uniform state of signal saturation.

BOLD signals can originate within and surrounding the smallest capillaries and the largest venous vessels. Optical imaging techniques [23] have shown that blood vessels during stimulation become more highly oxygenated over an area, a few millimetres in diameter, around the site of neuronal activity. This may impose an intrinsic resolution limit for fMRI. An additional constraint is that oxygenation changes can be detected several millimetres downstream in the venous system from the site of neuronal activity. Mapping of the macrovasculature may be required to remove these BOLD signals and optimise the spatial accuracy of fMRI [30].

Functional MRI techniques are deliberately sensitised to differences in T_2^* so that the magnetic properties of deoxyhaemoglobin can manifest themselves as image contrast. An unfortunate consequence of this fact is that the images are also sensitised to other sources of magnetic field inhomogeneity, most significantly macroscopic effects. These are detrimental to image quality. The magnetic susceptibility differences between air, bone, and different tissue types cause large scale inhomogeneity, particularly at the high field strengths typically used for fMRI. Components of inhomogeneity within the imaging plane cause geometric distortion and those collinear with the slice selection direction cause a loss of intensity [31]. This signal loss effect is particularly severe at the anterior frontal pole near to the sinuses, and near the ears. Geometric distortions are a serious problem with EPI because of the very low frequency per point in the phase encoding direction. This distortion needs to be minimised by selection of the imaging parameters; otherwise serious misregistration in relation to anatomical images can result. "Unwarping" schemes have been proposed to correct for these effects in postprocessing [32]. A delicate trade-off is required to improve the image homogeneity sufficiently so that more difficult areas of the brain, such as the medial ventral frontal cortex and the brain stem, may be investigated without sacrificing too much sensitivity in BOLD contrast. A number of MRI techniques, for instance using a combination of spin and gradient echoes, have been put forward to tackle this problem.

B. Experimental Design

This section addresses the key issues which inform the design of fMRI experiments. First we introduce the rationale for designing experiments with alternating periods of rest and activation. Second, we discuss some of the physical constraints imposed by the fMRI environment. Finally the important differences in the processing of fMRI data are highlighted.

1. fMRI Time Series Signal and Noise

Experimental design for fMRI is distinct from experimental design for PET in many respects. Data from an fMRI experiment forms a time series containing perhaps many hundreds of measurements at each voxel. If the data are acquired sufficiently fast (*e.g.*, every 6 sec or less) this time series can show temporal autocorrelations or temporal smoothness due to the effect of the slow haemodynamic response function, and other physiological variations. The haemodynamic response function effectively convolves an underlying neural time series with the response function to give the observed fMRI time course [33]. In this context, time-dependent changes in the BOLD signal may be represented, in frequency space, as the sum of several frequency components (where the spectral density is the Fourier transform of the autoco-variance function). Each frequency component has a different source; heuristi-cally these sources can be thought of as either signal, related to functionally activated brain areas (*i.e.*, neuronal activity convolved with the hemodynamic response function), or systematic noise arising from aliased physiological bio-rhythms or slow movement artifacts. The successful experimental design will therefore be one in which signal and noise in the fMRI time series are not confounded. Much of the noise appears as a low frequency component of the fMRI time series and is largely due to cardiac and respiratory aliasing. For example, if scans were acquired every 6 sec and the subject's respiratory cycle was 6.1 sec, then each scan would be 0.1 sec out of phase. Over a prolonged period of scanning, this asynchrony would create an artefactual signal of low frequency (0.1 Hz). Other low frequency components relate to Meyer's waves and related phenomena that are caused by slow periodic haemodynamic changes (probably due to intrinsic autoregulatory feedback of cerebrovascular tone). In what follows we present a characterisation of noise, dealing first with periodic noise and then with nonperiodic noise components.

2. Periodic Noise Sources

Two important sources of periodic physiological noise in brain fMRI are the cardiac and respiratory cycles. The heart cycle causes both periodic blood flow and pulsatile bulk motion due to induced pressure variation. The blood flow effects are confined mainly to vessels but the pulsatile motion can extend throughout the entire brain. Respiration causes both a generalised variation in blood oxygenation and bulk displacement of the head in reaction to breathing. Both oxygenation changes and small tissue displacements can cause image voxel intensity changes. The blood oxygenation level contributes directly through the BOLD contrast mechanism. Motion, which is small com-pared to the image voxel size, can be considered to operate on a given voxel at a certain time according to a Taylor expansion in image spatial derivatives about the voxel [34].

The expected time course of measured physiological noise depends not only on the sources but also on the imaging TR (repetition time). If the TR is short compared to both cardiac and respiratory cycles (*i.e.*, TR $\ll$ 1 sec) then both will be seen as straightforward periodic functions. In a frequency spectrum (neglecting harmonics) each will appear as a peak with a central "mean" frequency and with widths representing departure from strict periodic-ity. A schematic spectrum is shown in Fig. 1.

A very short TR is achievable with single slice EPI imaging (TR ~ 100 msec). For such short TR measurements simple notch filters can be applied,

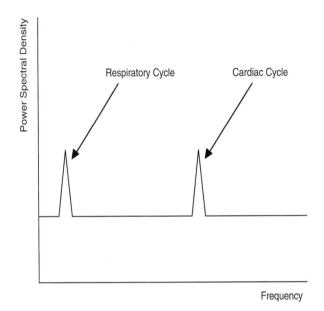

Figure 1 Schematic physiological noise spectrum.

centred on the mean cardiac and respiratory frequencies. Clearly any activation frequency component within the notch filter stop bands will be discarded along with the noise. If whole brain multislice EPI or other slow single slice techniques are used, the TR is typically several seconds. This is above the Nyquist limit for both the cardiac and respiratory noise and so aliasing will occur. In general, for a sampling frequency F_R and a noise of frequency F_N the measured frequency F_M is as shown in Fig. 2.

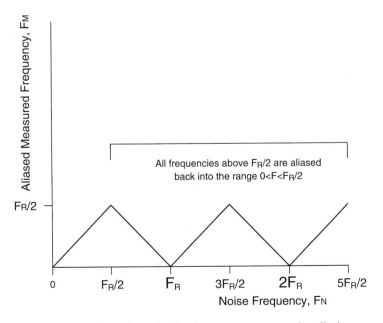

Figure 2 Transformation of noise frequency spectrum by aliasing.

The graph in Fig. 2 demonstrates that the aliased spectral density function depends primarily on the spectral width of the noise. If the noise is centred at an arbitrary frequency but extends over a width of $\Delta F_N > F_R$ then its aliased contribution will extend across the entire measurement frequency spectrum. In this situation (*i.e.*, nonmonochromatic noise and TR long compared with noise period) a simple notch filter would not be appropriate.

3. Nonperiodic Noise Sources

In addition to respiratory and cardiac related noise, low frequency noise components—typically manifesting as "drifts and shifts"—are evident in fMRI time courses. These can arise because of long-term physiological shifts, movement related noise remaining after realignment and adjustment, or from instrumental instability. The spectrum of this noise typically has a "1/f" characteristic, so-called because the spectral power density falls linearly with increasing frequency. In addition both the subject and scanner will contribute thermally generated white noise. These two generic types of noise combine to generate the form of spectrum seen in Fig. 3. In summary the noise spectrum of the fMRI signal comprises a low-frequency and wideband component. Periodic physiological noise sources can appear as focal peaks in the spectrum (short TR) or increased wideband noise (long TR).

4. Dealing with Low-Frequency Noise

Two techniques can be used (often, in combination) to counter noise. First, noise processes can be modelled and their estimated contribution removed from a measured signal. This technique is used, for example, to remove movement-related signal variation mediated by differential spin excitation histories [34]. Second, an experiment can be designed to take account of the characteristic features of the measurement system, for example the noise and sensitivity frequency spectra. An appropriate example in the present context is the method of "chopping." Chopping involves alternating between stimulus or task conditions to generate a time-dependent activation with a fundamental frequency sufficiently high to minimise contributions from 1/f noise without

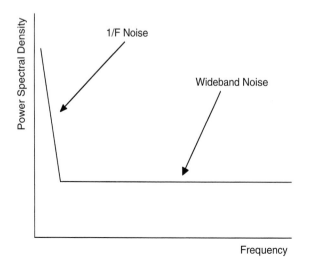

FIGURE 3 Schematic nonperiodic noise frequency spectrum.

being so high as to be attenuated by the sluggish haemodynamic response. Chopping utilises the high temporal resolution of fMRI to compensate for its poorer low-frequency noise performance. This leads to a choice of chopping frequencies between ~1 cycle/few minutes (a typical low-frequency noise cut-off point) and 1 cycle/10 sec (above which the signal would be attenuated by the haemodynamic response function). These effects are summarised in both the time and frequency domains in Fig. 4.

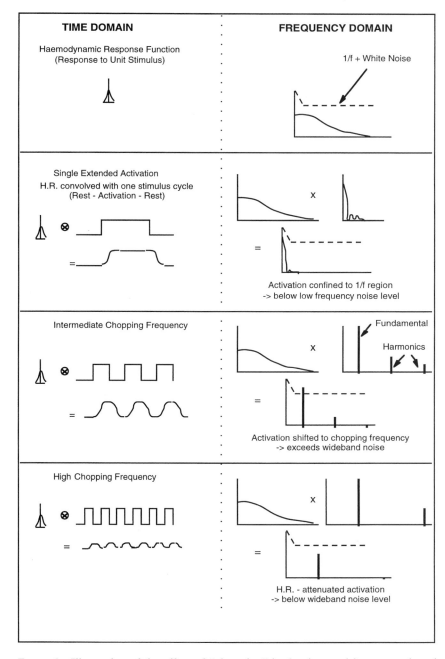

Figure 4 Illustration of the effect of "chopping" in the time and frequency domains.

5. Practical Implications

In practise many find that it is convenient to design experiments with control and activation periods alternating every 30 or 40 sec. In the context of the theoretical analysis presented above, this ensures that activations of interest and physiological noise are confounded as little as possible. The recurring control periods provide a constant baseline that can be used to assess low-frequency baseline drift caused by physiological noise. Low frequency effects may be assessed explicitly by comparing control periods at the beginning and end of the experiment or modelling time effects in the control periods explicitly. However, it is simpler and more practical to apply a high pass filter to the data to isolate the high frequency effects of interest and remove most of the (low frequency) physiological noise. It is important to set the filter periodicity appropriately with regard to the experimental design in order not to remove signals of interest. For example, a signal of interest of periodicity 60 sec can be achieved by alternating periods of 30-sec activation (five whole brain acquisitions with a TR of 6 sec) with 30 sec rest. Subsequently applying a high-pass filter of periodicity 120 sec will remove noise but leave the signal of interest intact. This is illustrated in Fig. 5.

6. Measuring Sustained Effects

Although it is desirable to alternate epochs of a control state and activation during an fMRI experiment, it is apparent that certain phenomena such as motor learning or sustained attention do not lend themselves to this approach. In these cases the neural phenomenon of interest is elicited only during a sustained period of activity. These types of experiment are therefore extremely vulnerable to confounding with the low frequency effects of physiological noise. It may not be possible unambiguously to attribute any changes in BOLD signal to a process of interest rather than to unrelated physiological states. It is therefore helpful to compare activation states with adjacent reference baseline states wherever possible. In short, this means that the assessment of enduring cognitive or sensorimotor states must be framed in terms of condition by time interactions. In relation to this problem it should be noted that the approach outlined here of alternating epochs of a reference condition and an activated condition does not require that the reference condition is necessarily rest. The constraint is merely that reference conditions are repeated through the course of the experiment at a frequency that is high relative to low-frequency sources of noise. We reemphasise here the need for alternating task conditions. All BOLD contrast fMRI experimental designs should embody the concept of a contrast between two experimentally specified states; there may be no such thing as "steady state" BOLD contrast fMRI.

7. Length of Epoch and the Evoked Haemodynamic Response

It is not clear how long the alternating periods of rest and activation should be. MRI data are fundamentally different from those acquired with PET, not only in the source of the detected signals but also in the duration of data acquisition. Whole brain volumes can be acquired in 5–10 sec, a duration that corresponds roughly to the time constant of the haemodynamic response function. The fMRI signal response reflects the time dependent changes in the relative quantities of oxyhaemoglobin and deoxyhaemoglobin. In primary sensory cortex a peak in the fMRI BOLD signal is reached between 5 and 8 sec after the onset of stimulus [35]. The haemodynamic response

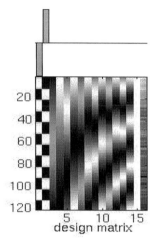

FIGURE 5 The use of the high-pass filter in a data set which involved alternating cycles of rest and finger opposition. The first two columns in the design matrix indicate that there is activation for 10 scans (60 sec) and then rest for 10 scans (60 sec); *i.e.*, the rest–activation cycle is 120 sec. The high-pass filter is set at 240 sec to remove noise but leave the signal intact. The next 12 columns of the design matrix denote the high-pass filter. Each column represents a sine wave of gradually increasing frequency. It can be seen from the third from right column that the highest frequency column of the design matrix has three complete cycles over 120 scans (720 sec), *i.e.*, 240 sec. Thus the signal of interest, which has a periodicity of 120 sec, is left intact.

function for such data has been fitted to a Poisson distribution [33]. In data analysis, the sensory input waveform is often convolved with the haemodynamic response function and tested for correlation with the fMRI time series. Significant correlations between brain activity and sensory input may otherwise be missed and a loss of statistical power can result. It should be noted, however, that the haemodynamic response function may be time dependent and may vary across brain regions. These are important considerations when developing strategies for processing fMRI data.

Most fMRI studies to date have been performed using a boxcar design with alternating epochs of rest and a single activation task of about 30 sec. These studies usually assume that sustained activation occurs during each cycle. For primary sensory cortex the time course of activation shows that this is generally the case. However, it may not be safe to assume that this feature applies to all areas of the brain, for different tasks, or that activation is sustained at a constant level for the duration of an experiment.

In primary visual cortex an activated state of venous oxygenation has been shown to persist throughout a 15-min stimulus [36,37]. Other researchers have found contradictory evidence, suggesting that the elevated signal has returned to baseline within 2–3 min of stimulus onset [38]. In a cognitive motor task we [39] demonstrated biphasic temporal responses in the anterior cingulate over a 30-sec period. This is an important observation because these significant responses cannot be classified as "activations" when averaged over the entire epoch. We have explored the form of the haemodynamic transients evoked during this task using a multivariate analysis [40]. Having identified a significant evoked response using MANCOVA, its form was then characterised with canonical variates analysis. This approach has the advantage that it makes no prior assumptions about the form of the evoked haemodynamic response. The study investigated two motor sequencing conditions, differing only in that in one the subject made a predetermined movement (cued visually) and in the other a random direction was specified by a visual cue. The evoked fMRI responses for the two conditions were significantly different. The message to take from this work is that the evoked haemodynamic response to different types of task may differ, not only in the degree to which they are expressed but also in their form and shape.

8. Intersubject Averaging

In many fMRI experiments it is likely that several subjects will be studied, and this raises the question of how best to proceed with data analysis. As there are no limits on the volume of data that can be acquired in a single subject, it is possible to perform an experiment as a series of single case studies. The resultant statistical parametric maps can be displayed directly as an anatomical rendering of that subject's brain. Localisation of function is therefore undertaken by referring directly to the surface anatomy. Such a solution characterises the data most fully in terms of both the similarities and differences between the functional anatomy of each subject. Reporting of such data poses problems; a qualitative description of areas activated in common across subjects is necessary rather than a quantitative comparison between subjects. The comparison of results between different groups becomes more difficult as results are not reported in a standard anatomical space.

The ability to normalise fMRI data into a common stereotactic space, such as that of Talairach and Tournoux allows the reporting of significant activations in a common reference space. However, the deformations introduced by single subject normalisation may compromise anatomical resolution. Spatial normalisation also allows intersubject averaging of data. However, the intersubject variability of gyral anatomy is significantly greater than the anatomical resolution of fMRI and so it is likely that a significant degree of spatial smoothing will be required to detect areas activated in common across subjects. This inevitably compromises the spatial resolution of fMRI, one of its most attractive features, but facilitates comparison with PET work where similar smoothing is employed for group studies.

It is likely that the use of these related approaches will depend on the nature of the question being studied.

C. Data Analysis

The analysis of fMRI data differs in some important ways from that of PET data. The time needed to analyse fMRI data is not trivial; statistical analysis alone, for 1200 16-slice images on an 8-CPU Sun SparcServer, can take approximately 72 hr. Here we highlight some of the special issues in fMRI data processing.

1. Movement-Related Effects

Imaging the human brain with functional MRI relies on detecting small signal changes in the presence of very large baseline signals. However, changes of signal intensity can also arise from head motion; this represents one of the most serious confounds in fMRI studies. Despite restraints on head movement, willing and cooperative subjects still show displacements of up to 1 mm or so. With very young, old, ill, or disturbed subjects head restraints may not be appropriate. In such circumstances head movements of several millimetres are not uncommon. Movement-related components in fMRI time series can arise from the following:

a. Differences in the Position of the Object in the Scanner   Spatial variation in sensitivity will render the signal a function of the object's position at the time of scanning. This spatial variability can include large scale field inhomogeneity or can be expressed at a much finer scale. An important example of the latter is found in slice-selective irradiation, used for example in multislice acquisition. The degree to which spins are excited in any small volume of the object will depend on an interaction between the local magnetic field and the Fourier transform of the slice-selective pulse. For example, the excitation of spins in a small region on the edge of a slice will be exquisitely sensitive to small displacements in and out of that slice. In other words, signal intensity will be a strong function of position relative to the volume excited or the scanner's frame of reference.

b. Differences Due to the History of the Position of the Object   If the number of excited spins is a function of position in the scanner it follows that the number of excited spins (and implicitly the signal) will also be a function of position in previous scans. This dependency is due to changes in saturation of spin magnetisation that is a function of the number of spins excited in the previous scan. This excitation will in turn be a function of position and so, by induction, a function of all previous positions. In summary, the current signal is a function of current position and the spin excitation history. The spin excitation history is in turn determined by the history of past movements. This effect will manifest if the recovery of magnetisation in the z direction is incomplete by the time the next slice-selective pulse arrives (*i.e.*, if TR is comparable to T_1 which is certainly the case for many fMRI studies). Generally speaking, movement within the plane of a slice will not change the set of spins excited and should not contribute to this effect.

In summary, movement-related effects can be divided into those that are some function of position of the object in the frame of reference of the scanner and a component that is due to movement in previous scans. This second component depends on the history of excitation experienced by spins in a small volume and consequent differences in local saturation. The spin excitation history will itself be a function of previous positions. This characteristic feature of MRI suggests an autoregression-moving average (ARMA) model for the effects of previous displacements on the current signal [34]. The spin excitation history is important because it suggests that realignment alone is not sufficient to deal with all movement-related effects. This approach [34] to image realignment and adjustment entails: (i) estimating the movement parameters by comparing each scan in the time series to a reference scan, as described in the section on spatial transformation, (ii) realigning the time series using these parameter estimates and, (iii) adjusting the values of each voxel by removing any component that is correlated with a function of movement estimates, obtained at the time of the current scan and the previous scan. This function is based on a first order ARMA model of movement-related effects.

It has been shown [34] that in an extreme case as much as 90% of the variance in an fMRI time series can be accounted for by the effects of movement after realignment and that this component can successfully be removed. A danger with this approach arises if there is stimulus-correlated motion, where some image intensity changes caused by neuronal activity, and not by motion, will be removed from the time series.

2. Temporal Autocorrelations and Statistical Modeling

Analysis of an fMRI time series involves fitting a model to the observed data; the model is composed of several different components specified in the design matrix. However, the general linear model used for PET data analysis assumes that each scan represents an independent observation. The presence of temporal autocorrelation in fMRI time series is a violation of this assumption. The approach we have adopted is to extend the general linear model to accommodate these temporal autocorrelations. The variance estimators are recalculated under the assumption that the data represent an uncorrelated set of observations that have been convolved with some smoothing kernel. The resulting statistics are then distributed with the t distribution whose effective degrees of freedom are a function of the smoothing kernel. The effective degrees of freedom are less than the number of scans and correspond roughly to the number of scans divided by the width of the smoothing kernel. This approach assumes the temporal autocorrelation function is known or can be estimated. In many instances it can be deduced from the temporal smoothing kernel applied to the time series to increase signal to noise. This temporal smoothing is considered in the next section.

3. Smoothing in Space and Time

Smoothing in space enhances the signal to noise ratio of the data and allows intersubject averaging by blurring differences in gyral anatomy between subjects. The validity of statistical inferences also depends on the data being sufficiently smooth to allow use of the theory of random Gaussian fields. On the other hand, fMRI has high anatomical resolution and so there is a trade-off between the degree of smoothing and the spatial resolution to be considered. Our approach has been to use the least degree of smoothing that is compatible with the smoothness being large enough to ensure the validity of the statistical inferences (*i.e.*, a smoothness of at least 2 voxels).

As noted in previous sections fMRI time series contain a number of signals; these include uncorrelated noise (*e.g.*, quantum noise and thermal noise), correlated noise (*e.g.*, physiological noise from cardiac and respiratory cycles), and correlated signal that conforms approximately to changes in neural activity convolved with a haemodynamic response function [33]. Correlated noise can arise directly from cardiac and respiratory cycles, their physiological modulation (*e.g.*, the heart rate variability signal), or aliasing of these effects due to an interaction with the repeat time.

Smoothing in time or convolution of the fMRI time series with the haemodynamic response function will, in principle, enhance signal relative to noise, particularly thermal and other noise with high frequency components. This denoising device is predicated on the "matched filter theorem" and is based on the conjecture that "interesting" haemodynamics are the result of convolving an underlying neuronal process with a haemodynamic response function. As such the signal is always at least as smooth as the response function. Clearly the optimum smoothing kernel is related to the haemodynamic response function. "Optimum" refers to the kernel that maximizes variance in the signal frequencies relative to other frequencies. It is generally accepted that the haemodynamic response function has an associated delay and dispersion of about 6–8 sec. This corresponds to a Gaussian kernel of width $\sqrt{6} = 2.45$ to $\sqrt{8} = 2.83$ sec and it is this sort of kernel that is usually applied to time series with short (<6 sec) TR.

D. fMRI Hardware and Environment

1. Hardware

The design of commercially available fMRI scanners can constrain experimental design. The Siemens Vision system can acquire up to 1024 measurements during a single run before pausing for data processing. A measurement can be any number of axial slices (48 slices representing whole brain acquisition) at variable repeat times; nevertheless data acquisition is likely to be discontinuous within an experiment. This may be significant for paradigms studying sustained physiological or psychological phenomena.

At short TR, T_1 relaxation effects become prominent in the early measurements of a time series. If TR is chosen such that significant saturation occurs during the time series (likely for any TR less than 10 sec) then a number of dummy scans (typically two to eight) should be acquired prior to those in the experiment. This will establish an equilibrium magnetisation by the time the experiment begins and will improve the realignment and statistical analysis.

2. The Scanning Environment

In contrast to PET, the fMRI environment embodies physical constraints that may restrict the stimulus presentation and subject's response. In addition to the limitations discussed below, it should be noted that access of the experimenter to the subject during the experiment is limited, as the subject needs to be placed completely inside the bore of the magnet.

The bore of the magnet is just wide enough to enclose a subject. The subject's head is surrounded by a radiofrequency transmit/receive head coil and immobilised with foam padding. A mirror mounted above the subject allows viewing of projected visual stimuli. Although the bore is restricted, it is possible to produce a wide field of view by placing a projection screen close to the subject (an apparent distance of 40 cm). This allows a field of view of greater than 50°. Arm movement at the shoulder is possible but restricted and can result in head motion.

Customised apparatus is required for the recording of responses within a magnetic environment. Recording of EEG and EMG presents special technical problems, which have been surmounted in several laboratories.

The gradient switching required by echoplanar imaging can create high levels of auditory noise. By means of careful acoustic engineering, this noise can be very substantially reduced, but this is not normally found in commercial

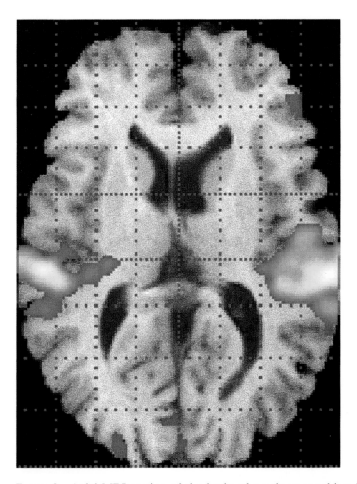

FIGURE 6 Axial MRI section of the brain of a volunteer subject listening to words presented at the rate of 1 per second. Superimposed in colour are the areas showing significant change of BOLD signal during the task, as compared with rest periods in which the subject heard only the noise of the scanner. A time series of 120 whole-brain echo-planar images, with 3 mm isotropic resolution, was obtained using a Siemens Vision MRI scanner working at 2 T field strength. The analysis was performed using statistical parametric mapping. The maximum z score was 14 (G. Rees, unreported data).

MRI equipment. Despite the use of shielded gradient coils, the ambient noise levels within the bore of an MRI magnet during imaging may exceed 90 dB. Nevertheless, stimulus delivery through appropriately isolated earpieces make presentation of auditory stimuli such as words feasible. It has proved possible to detect activation in both primary auditory cortex and auditory association areas using these techniques. However, acoustic noise may still present a limitation to certain types of experiment. The noisy environment also makes communication with the subject difficult whilst imaging is in progress.

IV. APPLICATIONS OF fMRI

Since fMRI methods are entirely noninvasive, multiple, indeed longitudinal, studies on single subjects may be performed, and large representative groups of volunteers may be recruited so that population studies can be performed. Furthermore, by comparison with other functional brain mapping techniques, such as PET, EEG, magnetic source imaging, and near-infrared spectroscopic imaging, fMRI has excellent spatial resolution and quite good temporal resolution. These features have lent themselves to a variety of novel experiments with human subjects (*e.g.*, [41]) and suggest others which may have considerable clinical benefit in cases of brain pathology.

Figure 6 shows an axial MRI section of the brain of a subject listening to words presented at the rate of 1 per second. Superimposed in colour are the areas showing significant change of BOLD signal during the task, as compared with rest periods in which the subject heard only the noise of the scanner. The analysis included accurate image realignment, temporal and spatial smoothing, high-pass filtering to remove aliased physiological noise, and statistical evaluation using the General Linear Model. What is strikingly noticeable is the exquisite definition of the primary auditory areas A1, bilaterally in the superior temporal lobes, corresponding to the visible anatomy of Heschel's gyri.

References

1. A. Haase, J. Frahm, D. Matthaei, W. Hänicke and K-D. Merboldt. FLASH imaging: Rapid NMR imaging using low flip angle pulses. *Magn. Reson.* **67**, 258–266 (1986).
2. G. N Stewart. Researches on the circulation time in organs and on the influences which affect it. *J. Physiol.* **15**, 1 (1894).
3. A. Villringer, B. R. Rosen, J. W. Belliveau, J. L. Ackerman, R. B. Lauffer, R. B. Buxton, Y. S. Chao, V. J. Wedeen and T. J. Brady. Dynamic imaging with lanthanide chelates in normal brain—contrast due to magnetic-susceptibility effects. *Magn. Reson. Med.* **6**, 164–174 (1988).
4. J. W. Belliveau, H. L. Kantor, I. L. Pykett, R. R. Rzedzian, E. Berliner, P. Beaulieu, F. S Buonanno, T. J. Brady and B. R. Rosen, Real-time proton susceptibility-contrast imaging of cerebral physiology. *Proc. Soc. Magn. Reson. Medicine*, **1**, 222 (1988).
5. P. Mansfield. Multiplanar image formation using NMR spin echoes. *J. Phys. C* **10**, L55-L58 (1977).
6. J. W. Belliveau, D. N. Kennedy, R. C. McKinstry, B. R. Buchbinder, R. M. Weisskoff, M. S. Cohen, J. M. Vevea, T. J. Brady and B. R. Rosen. Functional mapping of the human visual-cortex by magnetic-resonance-imaging. *Science* **254**, 716–719 (1991).
7. S. Ogawa, T. M. Lee, A. S. Nayak and P. Glynn. Oxygenation-sensitive contrast

in magnetic-resonance image of rodent brain at high magnetic-fields. *Magn. Reson. Med.* **14**, 68–78 (1990).

8. R. Turner, D. Le Bihan, C. T. W. Moonen, D. Despres and J. Frank. Echo-planar time course MRI of cat brain deoxygenation changes. *Magn. Reson. Med.* **22**, 159–166 (1991).

9. L. Pauling and C. D. Coryell. The magnetic properties and structure of hemoglobin, oxyhemoglobin and carbonmonoxyhemoglobin. *Proc. Natl. Acad. Sci. USA*, **22**, 210–216 (1936).

10. K. K. Kwong, J. W. Belliveau, D. A. Chesler, I. E. Goldberg, R. M. Weisskoff, B. P. Poncelet, D. N. Kennedy, B. E. Hoppel, M. S. Cohen, R. Turner, H-M. Cheng, T. J. Brady and B. R. Rosen. Dynamic magnetic resonance imaging of human brain activity during primary sensory stimulation. *Proc Natl Acad USA* **89**, 5675–5679 (1992).

11. S. Ogawa, T. M. Lee, A. R. Kay and D. W. Tank. Brain magnetic-resonance-imaging with contrast dependent on blood oxygenation. *Proc. Natl. Acad. Sci. USA* **87**, 9868–9872 (1990).

12. D. S. Williams, J. A. Detre, J. S. Leigh and A. P. Koretsky. Magnetic-resonance-imaging of perfusion using spin inversion of arterial water. *Proc Natl Acad Sci USA* **89**, 212–216 (1992).

13. R. R. Edelman, B. Siewert, D. G. Darby, V. Thangaraj, A. C. Nobre, M. M. Mesulam and C. Warach. Qualitative mapping of cerebral blood-flow and functional localization with echo-planar MR-imaging and signal targeting with alternating radio-frequency. *Radiology* **192**, 513–520 (1994).

14. M. K. Stehling, R. Turner and P. Mansfield. Echo-planar imaging–magnetic-resonance-imaging in a fraction of a second. *Science* **254**, 43–50 (1991).

15. D. A. Feinberg and K. Oshio. GRASE (gradient-echo and spin-echo) MR imaging—a new fast clinical imaging technique. *Radiology* **181**, 597–602 (1991).

16. C. B. Ahn, J. H. Kim and Z. H. Cho. High-speed spiral-scan echo planar NMR imaging. *IEEE Trans. Med. Imag.* **5**, 2–7 (1986).

17. P. Jezzard, F. Heineman, J. Taylor, D. Despres, H. Wen, R. S. Balaban and R. Turner. Comparison of EPI gradient-echo contrast changes in cat brain caused by respiratory challenges with direct simultaneous evaluation of cerebral oxygenation via a cranial window. *NMR Biomed.* **7**, 35–44 (1994).

18. R. Turner, P. Jezzard, H. Wen, K. K. Kwong, D. LeBihan, T. Zeffiro and R. S. Balaban. Functional mapping of the human visual-cortex at 4 and 1.5 Tesla using deoxygenation contrast EPI. *Magn. Reson. Med.* **29**, 277–279 (1993).

19. S. Ogawa, R. S. Menon, D. W. Tank, S. G. Kim, H. Merkle, J. M. Ellermann and K. Ugurbil. Functional brain mapping by blood oxygenation level-dependent contrast magnetic-resonance-imaging—A comparison of signal characteristics with a biophysical model. *Biophys. J.* **64**, 803–812 (1993).

20. R. M. Weisskoff, C. S. Zuo, J. L. Boxerman and B. R. Rosen. Microscopic susceptibility variation and transverse relaxation—Theory and experiment. *Magn. Reson. Med* **31**, 601–610 (1994).

21. R. P. Kennan, J. H. Zhon, and J. C. Gore. Intravascular susceptibility contrast mechanisms in tissues. *Magn. Reson. Med.* **31**, 9–21 (1994).

22. R. Turner and A. Grinvald. Direct visualization of patterns of deoxygenation and reoxygenation in monkey cortical vasculature during functional brain activation. *Proc. Soc. Magn. Reson.* **1**, 430 (1994).

23. D. Malonek and A. Grinvald. Interactions between electrical-activity and cortical microcirculation revealed by imaging spectroscopy—Implications for functional brain mapping. *Science* **272**, 551–554 (1996).

24. S. B. Cox, T. A. Woolsey and C. M. Rovainen. Localized dynamic changes in cortical blood-flow with whisker stimulation corresponds to matched vascular and neuronal architecture of rat barrels. *J. Cereb. Blood Flow Metabol.* **13**, 899–913 (1993).

25. E. Paulesu, A. Connelly, C. D. Frith, K. J. Friston, J. Heather, R. Myers, D. G.

Gadian and R. S. J. Frackowiak. Functional MR imaging correlations with positron emission tomography. Initial experience using a cognitive activation paradigm on verbal working memory. *Neuroim. Clin. N. Am.* **5**, 207–225 (1995).

26. C. Dettmers, A. Connelly, K-M. Stephan, R. Turner, K. J. Friston, R. S. J. Frackowiak and D. G. Gadian. Quantitative comparison of functional magnetic resonance imaging with positron emission tomography using a force-related paradigm. *NeuroImage* **4**, 194–200 (1996).

27. D. C. Noll, W. Schneider and J. D. Cohen. Artifacts in functional MRI using conventional scanning. *Proc. Soc. Magn. Reson. Med.* **3**, 1407 (1993).

28. T. H. Le and X. Hu. Retrospective estimation and correction of physiological artifacts in fMRI by direct extraction of physiological activity from MR data. *Magn. Reson. Med.* **35**, 290–298 (1996).

29. J. Frahm, K-D. Merboldt, W. Hanicke, A. Kleinschmidt, and H. Boecker. Brain or vein—oxygenation or flow? On signal physiology in functional MRI of human brain. *NMR Biomed.* **7,** 45–53 (1994).

30. R. S. Menon, S. Ogawa, D. W. Tank, and K. Ugurbil. 4 Tesla gradient recalled echo characteristics of photic stimulation induced signal changes in the human primary visual cortex. *MRM* **30,** 380–386 (1993).

31. J. Frahm, K-D. Merboldt, and W. Hanicke. Direct FLASH MR imaging of magnetic field inhomogeneities by gradient compensation. *MRM* **6,** 474–480 (1988).

32. P. Jezzard and R. S. Balaban. Correction for geometric distortion in echo-planar images from B_0 field variations. *MRM* **34**, 65–73 (1995).

33. K. J. Friston, P. Jezzard, and R. Turner Analysis of functional MRI time series. *Hum. Brain Mapping* **1**, 153–171 (1994).

34. K. J. Friston, S. Williams, R. Howard, R. S. J. Frackowiak, and R. Turner. Movement related effects in fMRI time series. *MRM* **35**, 346–355 (1996).

35. P. A. Bandettini. MRI studies of brain activation: Temporal characteristics. *In* "Functional MRI of the Brain (Workshop Syllabus)," pp. 143–151. Society of Magnetic Resonance in Medicine, Berkeley, CA, 143–151 1993.

36. P. A. Bandettini, T. L. Davis, K. K. Kwong, P. T. Fox, A. Jiang, J. R. Baker, J. W. Belliveau, R. M. Weisskoff and B. R. Rosen. FMRI and PET demonstrate sustained blood oxygenation and flow enhancement during extended visual stimulation dutations. *Proc. Soc. Magn. Reson* **1**, 453 (1995).

37. A. M. Howseman, O. Josephs, D. Porter, E. Mueller, R. S. J. Frackowiak, and R. Turner. Sustained activation in visual cortex using EPI and FLASH fMRI. *NeuroImage* **3**, S8 (1996).

38. G. Kruger, A. Kleinschmidt and J. Frahm. Dynamic MRI sensitized to cerebral blood oxygenation and flow during sustained activation of human visual cortex. *Magn. Reson. Med.* **35**, 797–800 (1996).

39. K. J. Friston, C. D. FrithD, R. Turner, and R. S. J. Frackowiak. Characterising evoked hemodynamics with fMRI. *NeuroImage* **2**, 157–165 (1995).

40. K. J. Friston, C. D. Frith, R. Turner, and R. S. J. Frackowiak. Characterising dynamic brain responses with fMRI: A multivariate approach. *NeuroImage* **2**, 166–172 (1995).

41. A. Karni, G. Meyer, P. Jezzard, M. M. Adams, R. Turner and L.G. Ungerleider. Functional MRI evidence for adult motor cortex plasticity during motor skill learning. *Nature* **377**, 155–158 (1995).

CHAPTER NINETEEN

IMAGES OF THE FUTURE: A PHILOSOPHICAL CODA

I. INTRODUCTION

This is the final chapter. In this chapter we look to the future. This is not a prospectus or even a manifesto for future research, but a critical consideration of influences that might shape imaging neuroscience in the years to come. These influences include the collective ambitions and perspectives of scientists involved in the field and the methods available to them. In this chapter we will try to provide an organisational framework for various approaches to imaging neuroscience and to relate them to the biological sciences in general. We start at a rather general level and then provide some more concrete illustrative examples in the context of our proposed framework. By design, a number of themes have recurred in this book, for example, the dialectic between functional segregation and functional integration in the brain. Clearly, we think that these themes are important. We shall return to them to clarify why we consider them crucial in dictating the important research questions that imaging neuroscience must address in the future.

One of the main distinctions we make is that between principles and maps. This distinction is meant to highlight the difference between mapping the brain and discerning the principles that underlie the organisation of these maps. Although some people treat the "mapping" component of "human brain mapping" with some disdain, we do not use that term here in any trivial sense. Mapping requires a careful and exhaustive delineation of functional anatomy in terms of both spatial, or anatomical, organization and the temporal dynamics that uniquely define functional specificity. The first section addresses the distinction between maps and principles with a comparison to developments in other biological sciences. The subsequent sections then consider a variety of issues that we think will have an impact on neuroimaging research in the near future. These issues relate both to how functional and cognitive anatomy are defined and to the sorts of principles that underlie functional organisation in the brain. We start by considering what we are measuring and how these measurements relate to the dynamics of interactions or transactions among neuronal populations in different cortical areas and subareas. We then examine how models of brain activity currently employed to analyse imaging data will continue to evolve to the extent that they can be used independently to simulate brain responses and inform our understanding of these responses. We then return to the relationship between functional segregation and integration and look at future developments in the analysis of effective connectivity and how one might integrate the empiricism of neuroimaging with theoretical neurobiology. In the penultimate section we consider some of the different classes of brain phenomena that are open to investigation using neuroimaging and provide some specific examples of new approaches. This section is a prelude to the final section which reviews the distinction between principles and maps in the light of what we are looking for, what we are measuring, and how we are measuring it.

II. PRINCIPLES AND MAPS

The problem facing imaging neuroscientists is clearly not a trivial one. Indeed, it is worth reflecting on what the problem is. What are the objectives of imaging neuroscience? To help define the answer to this question imagine a conversation between an imaging neuroscientist, a neuropsychologist, a neurophysiologist, and a molecular biologist. The molecular biologist asks, somewhat provocatively, "*So why are you doing all this brain mapping?*" This question has an edge to it because he secretly considers the imager to be a source of competition for research funding. "*Well I want to know how the brain works,*" replies the imager, impressed with his own simple honesty. "*That's a little ambitious isn't it?*" responds the neuropsychologist kindly (the neuropsychologist is more warmly disposed to neuroimaging than he might admit—he is currently in the middle of an fMRI experiment on his favourite patient). "*Indeed. Perhaps I should qualify that by saying I am interested in how the brain works at a systems level,*" responds the imager with a wary eye on the molecular biologist and the neurophysiologist. The neurophysiologist stirs, he is thinking many things and is trying to be constructive. (This is not as easy for him as it might be. He has spent many years using multiunit recordings to study phase locking and synchronisation in extrastriate cortex, has just reviewed yet another neuroimaging submission to *Nature*, obviously based on less than a week's data acquisition. Finally, his most promising postdoc has just elected to leave neurophysiology to learn about fMRI.) "*Do you really believe that you can make any sensible inference, even at a systems level, with your current spatial and temporal resolution?*" he asks politely. "*Yes I think I can,*" replies the imager. "*Clearly, I have to accept that I am measuring population dynamics at a fairly gross level but, assuming that the pool activity means something, I think we can learn a lot about the brain from imaging data. Perhaps I should qualify my previous answer by saying that I am interested in how the brain works at a systems level, in terms of large scale population dynamics.*" The neurophysiologist, warming to the argument, asks "*But surely you would admit that most of the fundamental organisational principles of the brain, for example, functional specialisation, were discovered through electrophysiological and anatomical studies?*" The imager responds, "*That is true but the first demonstration of functional specialisation in normal humans used neuroimaging. Furthermore, I can image the entire brain simultaneously and I think that this is important, especially in relation to looking at how different areas interact.*" The neurophysiologist: "*That may be the case but what happens if most important interactions are embodied in terms of phase relationships and timing at a temporal scale you cannot see?"* The imager replies, *"I acknowledge that this is a potential problem but there are two observations I would ask you to consider: First, neuroimaging works remarkably well, suggesting that at least one component of the possibly many types of neuronal interaction is expressed at the level of aggregated activity."* The neurophysiologist smiles to himself; we will never know why! The imager continues: *"The second thing is that fast dynamic interactions involving mechanisms like synchronisation may be coupled in an obligatory way to changes in mean activity, although I do not know this."* *"Well, perhaps you should find out,"* suggests the neurophysiologist. The neuropsychologist interrupts, earnestly but gently: *"Certainly, looking at the history of neuropsychology I think that we have gained much understanding about functional anatomy without necessarily understanding the fine scale mechanisms that underpin it. In fact,"* he continues, enthused by his own theme, *"I would have thought that the lesion deficit model has proved a most robust way of implicating a cortical area in a particular cognitive function. I mean how do you know,"* to the electrophysiologist, *"that your synchronisation is not merely an epiphenomenon, or,"* smiling at the imager, *"your activations are not purely incidental and that the critical processing is going on only in a small part of the system that you activate?"* The imager, irked by the word "incidental" replies, *"Well how do you know that your circumscribed lesion is not simply disrupting the integration of a distributed system?"* The molecular biologist, in an attempt to restore a feeling of bonhomie, restates his question: *"So, in the light of this debate, what is the question that you are trying to answer? I mean, are you going to tell us anything really useful about the mechanisms of brain function?"* The imager thinks for a while. *"Yes, I think we can. Indeed from your perspective we have a number of facts to offer. First, we can identify which regions and systems are involved in learning, memory, and plasticity for you to study at a molecular level. Second, we can give people drugs during neuroimaging experiments and can therefore lend our interpretations a neurochemical specificity. However, in answer to your more general question, I want to understand the principles behind the anatomical and dynamic organisation of the brain, at a systems level, in terms of large scale neural populations and I want to relate these principles, insofar as they can be related, to an understanding of the brain at a cognitive, neurophysiological, and molecular level. There, will that do?"* At that point a fifth person joins the party—a neuroanatomist. They summarise their discussion for him and he comments happily: *"Of course, the basis of all understanding of brain function is anatomy."* They all agree wholeheartedly—after all he is paying for dinner!

A. How Does a Forest Work?

If the imaging neuroscientist wants to understand organisational principles then he is faced with a great challenge. Imagine that we take you to an edge of a great English or even Central European forest. We then ask you *"Tell us how this forest works."* You may reply *"What do you mean? What does a forest do?"* We might reply, smugly, *"If you can answer that, you have answered a greater question than we have posed to you. There are lots of people interested in this forest and they study it using a variety of techniques. Some are interested in a particular species of flora or fauna, some more in its geography. You won't have time to talk to them, but you can read what they write in specialist journals. We should warn you, however, that many of them have very specific interests and tend to study those parts of the forest that are easily accessible.*" You accept the challenge and just to make things interesting, we place two restrictions on your investigations. First, you can measure only one thing. Second, although you can take measurements wherever you want, you can only take them at weekly intervals. You would then be confronted with a problem not unlike that facing neuroimaging. Of all the diverse aspects of neuronal dynamics, imaging is sensitive only to haemodynamic responses, which themselves are a very derived metric of underlying neuronal activity. Third, haemodynamic responses, and hence their measurement, have rather poor spatial and temporal characteristics and therefore resolvability. Although we can measure things everywhere, they can be measured only very sparsely in time. Clearly things are not quite so bad for brain mapping in the sense that different stimuli and tasks can be presented to subjects or different measures of their behavioural responses can be made. Furthermore, we can investigate subjects with specific lesions or defined psychological impairments in a way that facilitates a greater understanding than if we were given just one forest to observe. However, there are similarities between the two tasks. Faced with the forest problem we would simply acquire data generating map after map after map of the measured variable. We would try to make inferences, try to understand principles underlying the changes measured, initially at any one point and then collectively, looking at influences of the variable in one part of the forest on changes in another part. We might try and relate these measures to meteorological changes, look for seasonal variations and so on. In short, we would make maps and then try to characterise the dynamic behaviour of these maps. What, however, is the primary objective of such mapping in the first instance? Is it the careful construction of detailed maps or is it the interpretation of their dynamics and the discovery of simple rules or principles that govern them. We propose that both components are crucial to a more complete understanding. We now develop this argument further in relation to the development of evolutionary thinking [1] and other [neuro]biological fields.

III. THE NEURAL BOTANIST

Imaging neuroscience has often been referred to, sometimes in a disparaging way, as neophrenology or mental cartography. Cartography or map making is a corner stone of neuroimaging. Consider the development of evolutionary theory from Lamarckian ideas to a Darwinian perspective and the theory of natural selection [1]. The latter was predicated on a detailed map or taxonomy of different species and phenotypic variations among members of the same species. The idea was preceded by a "botanical" enterprise that was as fundamental as the idea itself. Without this painstaking observation and classification of animals and plants the notion of natural selection would not have arisen. The Darwinian synthesis, embracing Mendelian genetics as its mechanism, was similarly dependent on the earlier work of taxonomists. Without a Darwinian synthesis it is difficult to imagine how modern day molecular genetics would have become such a powerful tool for understanding our own structural and functional ontology. Similar examples of the importance of map making and observation can be found in many fields, not the least of those being anatomy. For example, our understanding of the pathophysiology of schizophrenia dates back to the careful observations of symptom profiles in patients suffering from dementia praecox [2]. Kraepelin's early subdivision of the different types of schizophrenia, variously revised over the decades, and refined using modern day statistics (*e.g.*, factor analysis) is now operationally crucial to schizophrenia research [3]. As in evolutionary theory there is a drive in schizophrenia research to elucidate mechanisms and pathophysiology that is deeply rooted in the initial taxonomies, classifications and maps. The point we are making is that a detailed cartography is a prerequisite to subsequent theorising and any integration of imaging neurosciences with neuroanatomy, molecular biology, neurophysiology, and other neuroscience disciplines.

In imaging neuroscience the cartographic component is very explicit and concrete. We find out which brain areas activate in response to the various aspects of cognitive and sensorimotor processing. As illustrations of how such maps will become successively refined and more detailed, consider two examples. First, maps will become more detailed with the increasing resolution of imaging techniques. We are already at a point where it is possible to imagine that the thick, thin, and interstripe organization of V2 can be directly observed with fMRI. Temporal resolution is already in the order of seconds and could be supplemented with magneto- or electrophysiological information with a resolution of milliseconds. Second, at a slightly more abstract level, one might think explicitly about a successive refinement of the taxonomy of regionally specific effects. Neuroimaging, to date, has largely focussed on "activations." In this book we have shown that regionally specific effects not only conform to an anatomical taxonomy (*i.e.*, which anatomical area is implicated) but also to a taxonomy based on the type of experimental design that generated the imaging data. A clear cut example is found in the distinction between regionally specific activations and regionally specific "interactions." The interpretation of these two "species" of regional effects is very different and one might anticipate that simply acknowledging such differences will improve the characterisation of functional anatomy. We will return to this point later. In our view, neophrenology should not be a demeaning term. Indeed, the essence of the proposals in Chapter 17 on multimodal and probabilistic brain atlases is a challenging attempt to recapitulate the essential and enabling observations of anatomists, natural historians, taxonomists, and neurologists in the 19th century. This challenge is not simply a question of collating data but also involves spotting important distinctions (*e.g.*, activations and interactions) in the nature of the things we observe.

On the other hand, map making *per se* is not the only aspiration of imaging neuroscience. Understanding the principles or invariant features of such maps, and the mechanisms associated with these features, is an ultimate aim. Returning to the analogy with evolution and molecular biology, one exciting development in genetics over the past decades has been the study of gene–gene interactions, how the discourse, at a molecular level, among various parts of the genome and cell infrastructure comes to shape ontology and neurodevelopment and how these interactions are subject to various epigenetic influences. A simple analogy can be made between mapping the human brain and mapping the human genome and between the mechanistic understanding of gene–gene and epigenetic interactions and functional integration between specialised areas in the cortex. We refer, of course, to analyses of population level neuronal interactions between different cortical areas, what mediates them, and how they contribute to cognitive or sensorimotor processing. A distinction needs to be made between identifying an interaction, either at a genetic level or in terms of, say, interactions between two extrastriate areas, and the principles that govern all such interactions. A concrete example of this idea is the difference between demonstrating a modulatory influence of posterior parietal cortex on prestriate cortical area V5 (the human homologue of macaque V5 and owl monkey area MT) and the general principle that reverse projections from higher order to lower order areas are more modulatory than their forward projecting counterparts. Note, however, that this principle depends upon a complete characterisation of all parietal interactions with extrastriate areas, if only to demonstrate that there are no, or few, exceptions. This fact simply reiterates the importance of adequate, dependable cartographic data, in this instance, a cartography of parieto-occipital connections and their nature.

Another example of principles that derive from empirical observations can be taken from the work of complexity theorists who postulate that certain degrees of "connectivity" at the level of gene–gene interactions give rise to complex dynamics [4]. This principle, termed sparse connectivity, has also emerged in relation to the complexity of neuronal interactions [5]. In both instances the mathematical models used to demonstrate the principle are predicated on an empirical mapping of the systems being modelled. What then are the categories of principle that are likely to emerge from imaging neuroscience? We already have a few examples. The principle of functional segregation is now very well established and fully endorsed by the results of human neuroimaging studies. We often refer in this volume to the principle of functional integration and yet it is not entirely clear what that principle really is. If we define functional specialisation in terms of regionally or anatomically specific responses that are sensitive to the context in which they are evoked, then, by analogy, functional integration can be thought of as anatomically specific interactions between neuronal populations that are elicited in a stereotyped fashion by a particular processing demand and are similarly context-sensitive. Functional integration is a phenomenon and in a sense a principle, but not a terribly useful one. Examples of more useful principles would include a principle of sparse connectivity which might state that functional integration is mediated by sparse extrinsic connections in the brain that preserve specialisation within systems that have dense intrinsic connections. A second example, referred to above, might be that relative to forward connections, backward connections are modulatory.

Our point is that detailed empiricism is a necessary prerequisite for the emergence of organisational principles. For some neuroimaging scientists definition of principles is the ultimate goal but such principles can and will only be derived from maps of the brain. For others, relating activation maps to cognitive architectures and psychological models of cognitive processing is the ultimate aim but even this more limited program requires a principled approach to map building in the first place. In subsequent sections we will return to the distinction between principles and maps using some specific examples from our recent work.

IV. Neuronal Dynamics and Haemodynamics

In this section we consider some issues that need to be resolved in the future that concern (i) the relationship between neuronal dynamics and what we actually measure and (ii) what aspects of neuronal dynamics are important. The brain is a connected dynamic system whose interactions are mediated by regular or irregular volleys of spikes communicated down axons of intrinsic and extrinsic connections. In neuroimaging we measure a consequence of changes in the chemical and electrical activity at both pre- and postsynaptic membranes which themselves may generate new spike discharges. The exact relationship between neuronal activity and the associated haemodynamic response remains incompletely understood. The problem, however, is not only to relate measurable changes in neurophysiology to underlying neuronal activity, but also, given the choice, to consider what aspect of neuronal activity we would measure if we had the opportunity to do so directly. These problems will probably be resolved by using different techniques. The relationship between unit activity in neurons and the ensuing changes in neuronal and glial metabolism, haemodynamics and measurable signals in fMRI and PET have been greatly informed by autoradiographic studies in animal models and steady-state measures of blood flow, oxygen, and glucose metabolism with PET. This issue has become salient again with the development of fMRI, but now the issues pertain more to the phasic nature of changes in oxygenation and the dynamics of haemodynamic transients elicited by neuronal activation. The mechanisms operating at these different physiological levels will probably be best understood using biophysical models and a combination of neurophysiology and imaging using optical techniques [6]. The second problem, namely, which aspect of neuronal dynamics it is important to measure, is somewhat more fundamental. If we want to base our characterisation of functional anatomy on a meaningful neuronal metric, then we have to be sure that the metric or measure is a proper one. In short, one would like to be confident that whatever aspect of neuronal interactions are measured, they relate in some systematic way to a neuronal code.

A. The Neuronal Code and Why It Is Important for Neuroimaging

It is not easy to construct a comprehensive and simple taxonomy of neuronal codes because there are many possible perspectives when considering what might constitute a code or metric for neuronal interactions. Furthermore, many aspects of putative codes are related to each other and must be disentangled. However, it is possible to identify some important distinctions. One of the more important distinctions relates to whether the exact timing of neuronal discharges is crucial for mediating interactions. An alternative view is that spike trains can be considered as stochastic processes, so that it is not the exact time of arrival of a spike but the density, or rate of firing at a particular time that is important [7]. These views have implications for the way that neuronal discharges are modelled. If the important measures are embedded in a temporal patterning of discharges then we should consider spike trains as point processes. Conversely, a "rate code" perspective would allow us to treat activity in neurons as stochastic processes. The phrase "temporal coding" has been used variously to emphasise the importance of the timing of spike events. In one usage it confers importance on the timing of individual spikes [7]. It is also used to refer to codes that have an explicit time domain, usually in the context of population dynamics [8]. The second use of the term "temporal code" subsumes synchronisation models of interactions between neuronal populations [9]. These synchronisations may be oscillatory, but they do not have to be [10]. From the perspective of neuroimaging the distinction between temporal coding and rate coding is important because it is conceivable that changes in the temporal patterning of impulses can change without any necessary change in the rate of firing. In the sense that neuronal and glial metabolism and the ensuing haemodynamic responses will be largely functions of the rate of firing, neuroimaging may be very insensitive to temporal codes. Is this a fundamental problem?

Potentially, it is! We use "neuronal code" to denote an aspect of neuronal dynamics that has to be measured before the influences that one neuronal system exerts over another become apparent. One can consider this to be a necessary condition for any code (whether it codes for anything in the sense of "meaning" or not). This operational definition of a neuronal code has important implications for imaging neuroscience where the challenge is to measure the right thing. Imagine that you are given a tape recording of a series of clicks and asked *"Is there anything going on here?"* You could either measure changes in the rate of clicks, using some suitable time window, or look at the distribution of interclick intervals. If you had been given a recording of a Geiger counter moving in the vicinity of a radioactive source, then measuring the interclick intervals would tell you nothing (you would conclude that it was a random point process). If, however, you measured the density of clicks you would discern a modulation of its Poisson rate. On the other hand, if you received a recording of some Morse code, any temporal structuring or repeating patterns would be completely overlooked by a metric based purely on rate. This example is analogous to the problem presented to imaging neuroscience. Is then the neuronal code a rate code or a temporal code? Even if, in most brain areas, the exact timing of a single impulse may not be important clearly the temporal patterning is. The overwhelming empirical evidence in support of fast dynamic synchronised interactions among neuronal populations suggests that the phase relationship (*i.e.*, timing) of neural discharges is an important aspect of interactions. Our own work in this area, using MEG data, suggests that synchronisation *per se* may only be one aspect of neuronal interactions that rely on stereotyped temporal patterns of activity. This work indicates that not only are coherent interactions important, as evidenced by the comodulation of a specific frequency in two brain areas, but that there is a high degree of mutual information among different frequencies. In short, our observations suggest that neuronal transients in one part of the brain can be statistically associated with transients in another part of the brain with different frequency structures [11]. The implication of these observations is that the brain does, in fact, use a temporal code.

What then are the implications of this conclusion for neuroimaging? If our measurements are sensitive only to discharge rate, they are potentially blind to a whole temporal dimension of neuronal discourse. In short, we could be measuring the wrong thing. However, as pointed out above, changes in integrated activity of large neuronal populations can be used to demonstrate regionally specific responses, and, as shown elsewhere in this book, to make meaningful inferences about interactions between different areas. One explanation for the arresting efficacy of neuroimaging is that temporal coding and rate coding are two perspectives on the same underlying neuronal dynamics. In other words, a change in the temporal patterning of interactions necessarily implies a change in rate, rendering neuroimaging vicariously sensitive to the temporal component of neural codes. A useful heuristic is to consider that mean discharge rates will increase monotonically with the degree of synchronisation; *i.e.*, a mutual entrainment of interacting populations is facilitatory, in terms of overall activity, for all the populations engaged in the synchronous exchange of signals. In previous chapters we have cited both empirical and theoretical evidence for this suggestion.

In terms of future research, computational neurobiology will probably find an important role in addressing the issue of neural codes and their relationship to neuroimaging data. One of the themes of this chapter is that theoretical neurobiology has a key part to play in imaging neuroscience, both as a constraint on empirical inferences that are made on the basis of imaging data and as a generator of models that inform the interpretation of those data. Our question about the relationship between temporal and rate aspects of neuronal codes provides a good example of this view. The relationship between integrated discharge rates in two connected populations, as a function of the degree of synchronisation between them, is clearly open to numerical analysis using computational methods. One could simply simulate two neurobiologically realistic populations, using appropriate electrophysiological time constants and anatomical constraints on modelled extrinsic and intrinsic connectivity, to examine their behaviour. Already such large scale synthetic neuronal models are providing insights into transactions between different cortical areas that could not be obtained from simply observing the living brain [12]. The importance of a computational approach is that very specific "lesions," or perturbations, can be applied to physiological or anatomical components of the model in a way that would not be possible in a living system. We will return to the relationship between computational or mathematical models of neuronal systems and the mathematical characterisation of real data in the next section.

V. MODELS OR TOOLS?

In this section we consider the status of various models that are used to analyse or characterise brain function and how they are likely to develop over the next few years. Three broad types of model are used in neuroscience. First, there are biologically plausible mathematical neural network models or synthetic neural models. Second, there are the mathematical models employed in linear and nonlinear system identification, and third, the statistical models we are all familiar with for characterising empirical data. One of the main points of this section is to suggest that as time goes on the increasing sophistication of statistical models makes them indistinguishable from those used to identify an underlying system. An example of this idea will be provided below. Similarly, synthetic neural models that are currently used to emulate brain systems and study their emergent properties will lend themselves to reformulation in terms of those required for system identification. The importance of this notion is that (i) the parameters of synthetic neural models, for example the connection parameters and time constants, can be estimated directly from empirical observations and (ii) the validity of statistical models, in relation to what is being modelled, will increase. Another way of looking at the distinctions between the various models (and how these distinctions might be eroded) is to realise that we use models either to emulate a system or to define the nature or form of an observed system. When used in the latter context empirical data are used to determine the exact parameters of a specified model, and in statistical models inferences can be made about the parameter estimates. In what follows we will review statistical models and how they may develop in the future and then turn to an example of how one can derive a statistical model from one normally associated with nonlinear systems identification. The importance of this example is that it shows how a model can be used not only as a statistical tool but also as a device for emulating brain behaviour under a variety of different circumstances.

A. Linear Models

The most prevalent model in this book is the general linear model. The linear model simply expresses the response variable (*e.g.*, haemodynamic response) in terms of a linear sum of explanatory variables or effects in a design matrix. Inferences about the contribution of explanatory variables are made in terms of parameter estimates. There are a number of ways in which the general linear model might be developed in neuroimaging as the nature of research questions and inferences become more sophisticated. We will consider three examples: First, nearly every experiment described in this book, and indeed in the imaging neuroscience literature, is based upon a "fixed-effects model." The alternatives are "random-effects models" and "mixed (random and fixed)-effects models." The distinction between these models relates to the sources of variability in the measurements that are included in the model, and through this feature, the scope or sphere over which the inferences can be made. In fixed-effects models we assume that, for example, subject-specific effects are "as measured" and are fixed. In a mixed-effects model we would allow for the fact that subjects come from a larger population and the observed subject effects have some inherent variability, by virtue of the fact that we have selected only a small sample of subjects from the population. This distinction can be seen from two points of view. In the first the degrees of freedom that allow us to make, say, inferences about differential activations in two populations, are limited by the number of scans. In the second the degrees of freedom are much smaller and are dictated by the number of subjects. This has the implication that the inferences that we make in a fixed-effects model apply to, and only to, the subjects studied. In other words, we are making an inference about what would happen if we scanned the same subjects again and again. In a random, or mixed-effects model, although the degrees of freedom are much smaller, the inference obtained is applicable to the population from which the sample was taken. This is a fundamental distinction and has special relevance to studies that purport to show effects such as sex differences. Most analyses, hitherto, have used fixed-effects models and can be interpreted only in relation to the actual groups of men and women studied. To make more wide-ranging comments on sexual dimorphism or differential activations one should employ a random or mixed-effects model. The development of such models is currently under consideration and represents one important future trend, namely a refinement of existing techniques.

A second refinement, that we anticipate will find an increasing role in imaging statistics, is that of model selection. Generally, when using simple statistical models, one has to choose from among a hierarchy of increasingly comprehensive models that embody more and more effects. Some of these effects may or may not be present in the data and the question is: "*Which is the most appropriate model*?" One way to address this question is to see if successively adding extra effects significantly reduces the error variance. At the point at which a fit is not significantly improved one can cease elaborating the model. This principled approach to model selection is well established in other fields and will probably be very useful in neuroimaging. One important application of model selection is in the context of parametric designs and the characterisation of evoked haemodynamic responses with fMRI. In parametric designs it is often the case that some high order polynomial expansion of an interesting variable (*e.g.*, the rate or duration of stimulus presentation) is used to characterize a nonlinear relationship between it and the evoked haemodynamic response. Similarly, in modeling evoked haemodynamic responses in fMRI data the use of expansions in terms of temporal basis functions has proved to be very useful. These two examples have a common feature. They both have an "order" that has to be specified. The order of the polynomial regression approach is simply the number of higher order terms employed and the order of the temporal basis function expansion is simply the number of basis functions used. Both of these approaches are potentially very powerful and are likely to enjoy increasing use. Model selection has a use in determining the most appropriate or best order for a model. Both nonlinear parametric models and models based on temporal basis functions bring us to a third and final example of new trends using the general linear model.

Recall that, in general, the contribution of experimentally designed effects is reflected in the parameter estimates relating to these effects. In the case of polynomial expansions, or temporal basis functions, these are sets of coefficients of the high order terms or basis functions. Unlike simple activations (or effects corresponding to a particular linear combination of parameter estimates), inferences based upon such high order models inevitably are a collective inference about all coefficients together. This inference is made with the F ratio and speaks to the usefulness of the SPM{F} in more advanced characterisations of imaging data. We anticipate that, with increasing sophistication of multiple regression analyses and other instances of the general linear model that use expansions, the SPM{F} will become more important as an inferential tool than equivalent maps of the t statistic (SPM{t}). We have already seen the SPM{F} used in the context of nonlinear regression in Chapter 6. We now present a second example that takes us to models used in nonlinear systems identification and possibly beyond.

B. Nonlinear Models

The problem we started with was "*How can we best characterise the relationship between a stimulus waveform and an evoked haemodynamic response recorded by fMRI?*" Hitherto, the normal approach to this problem has been to use a stimulus waveform that conforms to the presence or absence of a particular stimulus, convolve (*i.e.*, smooth) this with an estimate of the haemodynamic response function, and see if the result can predict what is actually observed. Using an estimate of the haemodynamic response function assumes knowledge of the nature or form of this response and furthermore, by using a first order convolution, precludes any contribution of nonlinear effects. A much more comprehensive approach would be to use nonlinear systems identification, and to identify a stimulus with the input and an observed haemodynamic response with the output. This approach posits a very general form, or model, for the relationship between stimulus and response and uses the observed inputs and outputs to determine the parameters of the model employed to optimise the match between observed and predicted outputs, in this instance, haemodynamic responses. The approach that we have adopted is to use a mathematical device called a Volterra series expansion. This expansion can be thought of as a nonlinear convolution. It is, in fact, a more general model and can be shown to emulate the behaviour of any nonlinear, time invariant, dynamic system. The results of such an analysis is a series of Volterra

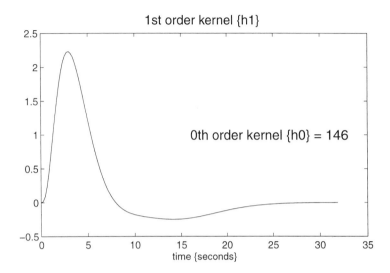

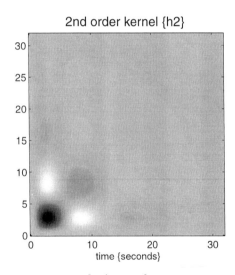

FIGURE 1   Volterra kernels h^0, h^1, and h^2 based on parameter estimates from a voxel in the left superior temporal gyrus at -56, -28, 12 mm. These kernels can be thought of as a characterisation of the second order haemodynamic response function. The first order kernel (top) represents the (first order) component usually presented in linear analyses. The second order kernel (bottom) is presented in image format. The colour scale is arbitrary; white is positive and black is negative.

kernels of increasing order. The zero order kernel is simply a constant, the first order kernel corresponds to the haemodynamic response function usually arrived at in linear analyses and the second and higher order kernels embody nonlinear dependencies of response on stimulus input. By using a series of mathematical devices (second order approximations and expansions of coefficients in terms of temporal basis functions) we have been able to reformulate the Volterra series model in terms of the general linear model and to use our standard techniques to estimate and make statistical inferences about such kernels. An example of the kernel estimates for a voxel in periauditory cortex is shown in Fig. 1. This estimate is based on a parametric study of evoked fMRI responses to words presented at varying frequencies

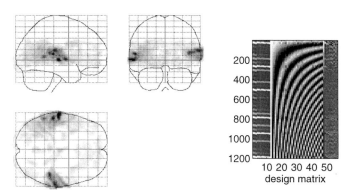

Figure 2 (Left) SPM{F} testing for the significance of the first and second order kernel coefficients (h^1 and h^2) in a word presentation rate single-subject fMRI experiment. This is a maximum intensity projection of a statistical process of the F ratio, following a multiple regression analysis at each voxel. The format is standard and provides three orthogonal projections in the standard space conforming to that described in Talairach and Tournoux [13]. The grey scale is arbitrary and the SPM{F} has been thresholded ($P < 0.001$ uncorrected). (Right) The design matrix used in the analysis. The design matrix comprises the explanatory variables in the general linear model. It has one row for each of the 1200 scans and one column for each explanatory variable or effect modeled. The left-hand columns contain the explanatory variables of interest $x_i(t)$ and $x_i(t)$, $x_j(t)$, where $x_i(t)$ is word presentation rate convolved with the ith basis function used in the expansion of the kernels. The remaining columns contain covariates or effects of no interest designated as confounds. These include (left to right) a constant term (h^0), periodic (discrete cosine set) functions of time, to remove low frequency artefacts and drifts, global or whole brain activity $G(t)$, and interactions between global effects and those of interest $G(t) \cdot x_i(t)$ and $G(t) \cdot x_i(t)$, $x_j(t)$. The latter confounds remove effects that have no regional specificity.

and is fairly typical of a nonlinear haemodynamic response function. The associated SPM{F}, shown in standard anatomical space [13], testing the significance of the Volterra kernels is shown in Fig. 2 along with the design matrix used.

At this point we could stop and conclude that the evoked fMRI responses are very significantly nonlinear and characterise them in terms of the kernel coefficients (Fig. 1). However, we can go further and use the parameter estimates to specify a model that can be used to emulate responses to a whole range of auditory inputs. As an example of using a model in this way consider the fMRI response to a pair of words that are presented close together in time, as distinct from when they are presented in isolation. Figure 3 demonstrates the results of this simulation and shows that the presence of a prior stimulus attenuates the response to a second word, when it is close in time. The key feature is that we are now performing a "virtual" experiment on the model, presenting it with stimuli that were never actually used. Indeed, we can go further and determine the model's response to a single word. The results of this analysis are shown in Fig. 4 along with the empirically determined fMRI responses from a real experiment where single words were presented in isolation. The latter experiment is an example of event-related fMRI which we will return to below.

In conclusion, the distinction between analytical and predictive models may, in the future, become sufficiently unconstrained and general to provide

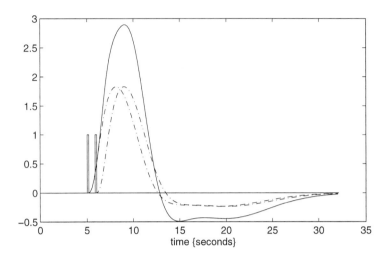

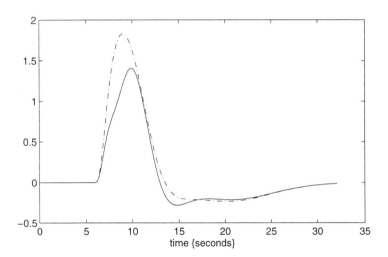

FIGURE 3 (Top) The simulated responses to a pair of words (bars) (one second apart) presented together (solid line) and in isolation (broken line) based on the second order haemodynamic response function in Fig. 1. (Bottom) The response to the second word when preceded by the first (broken line), obtained by subtracting the response to the first word from the response to both, and when presented alone (broken). The difference reflects the impact of the first word on the response to the second.

a basis for simulated experiments to predict results that can then be empirically tested.

VI. BRIDGES IN THE BRAIN

A. Recursion—A Principle of Principles?

Of the many recurrent themes in neuroscience two turn up again and again, namely "recursion" and "connectivity." Recursion seems fundamental to neurobiology and is expressed at many different levels. At a cognitive science

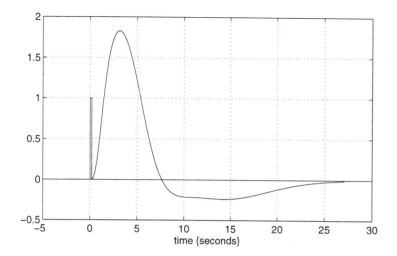

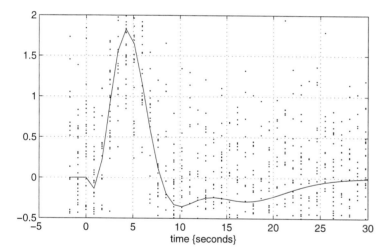

FIGURE 4 (Top) Haemodynamic response to a single word (bar at 0 sec) modeled using the Volterra kernel estimates of Fig. 1. (Bottom) The empirical event-related response in the same region based on an independent event-related single-subject fMRI experiment. The solid line is the fitted response using only first order kernel estimates and the dots represent the adjusted responses.

level, metarepresentations are an example of the recursive application of the notion of a representation to itself. Metarepresentations (probably better termed *m*-representations or second order representations) are mentalistic representations of one's own or another's mental representation. *M*-representations are crucial to "Theory of Mind" and for tasks where, in order to attribute meaning to the behaviour of others, one has to have a representation of the beliefs and intentions of the other person. In short, in some circumstances, the representation of a representation is a more important construct than the representation itself.

The same recursive theme can be found at the level of global brain theories. Neural Darwinism, the theory of selection of neuronal groups [14] or their dynamics, is predicated on evolutionary selection of selective mechanisms at a neuronal level, mediated by the evolutionary value of adaptive "neuronal value systems" in the brain (*i.e.*, the value of value) [15]. Again, the power of the idea is not simply due to natural selection itself but to the embedding of one selective process in another. The extension of this idea to even lower levels (*e.g.*, the selective consolidation of an individual presynaptic configuration in the context of neuronal selection) is appealing and eschews the awkward question often put to these sorts of theories: "*What is the unit of selection?*" A neuroanatomical example of recursion is the columns of columns (*e.g.*, minicolumns and macrocolumns) that characterise the microanatomical infrastructure of cerebral cortex. This final example brings us to the relationship between recursion and functional segregation. At what scale is function segregated in the brain? In terms of colour opponent cells, can functional specialisation be expressed in the lateral geniculate nuclei at the level of individual neurons, or is it expressed at a level of 100 μm (*i.e.*, the size of ocular dominance columns in primary visual cortex) or, perhaps, at the level of a millimetre or two in the thick stripe structures of V2 participating in the processing of visual motion. Or, is functional segregation expressed in terms of a centimetre or two as indicated by the extensive activations of V5 in humans exposed to moving stimuli. The question is obviously facile. Functional segregation is expressed at many different levels, or spatio-temporal scales, with functional segregation within functionally segregated areas. Is this a problem for neuroimaging, with intrinsic lower limits on spatial resolution? Obviously, from one perspective it is, in the sense that neuroimaging is denied access to fine microscopic aspects of specialisation and selective responses. However, it may be the case that the principles of functional segregation are similar over all levels at which they are expressed. If this is the case, then any features pertaining to populations may also hold for populations of populations.

A dynamic aspect of recursion, in the context of functional segregation or specialisation, is the receptive field of a receptive field. We can construe the responses of primary sensory neurons, say, for example, in V1, as an interaction between sensory input and the receptive fields of neurons. The receptive fields of V2 units are themselves determined by the receptive fields of V1 units from which they receive afferents and likewise for higher order extrastriate and further brain regions. In short, the response of any neuronal population can be understood as a recursive assembly of elemental receptive fields that are elaborated to an unimaginably complex receptive field in space and time. In an extreme version of this view the receptive fields of motor units may encompass nearly all sensory modalities and by virtue of attentional and mnemonic modulation of their component receptive fields may have a temporal domain spanning many years (*i.e.*, an event during motor learning in childhood can influence motor unit responses now). In other words, changing something in the sensorium in the distant past can result in different responses at the time of measurement. If the brain is a recursive collation of very high order receptive fields, the role of imaging neuroscience is simple and reduces to a characterisation of these receptive fields at each point in the brain. Indeed, one can look at most imaging experiments in terms of an experimental manipulation of the sensorium to evoke selective responses in exactly the same way as direction-selective responses in striate cortex were identified early in the modern history of visual neuroscience.

Note, however, that our receptive field metaphor for functional segregation or specialisation is an incomplete one. The brain is not a static array of converging and diverging connections that elaborate successively refined "receptive fields." The receptive field of a unit in V5 is not determined only by efferents from lower visual areas but also by inputs from higher areas. In other words, the receptive field of a particular point in the brain has, as one of its elements, a superordinate receptive field of which it is a component, so that many receptive fields in the brain contain transformed copies of themselves in an infinite regress. Perhaps this is an ultimate example of recursion. The nature of the transformation depends on nonlinear time and activity dependent interactions between neurons, commonly understood in terms of modulation. The dynamic modulation of receptive fields, and embedding of receptive fields within receptive fields, calls for a more comprehensive metaphor wherein the responses of one brain region configure or modulate the responses or receptive fields of other regions. This line of reasoning brings us to functional integration and the second theme we identify as important to our consideration of the future of neuroimaging science, namely, connectivity.

B. Dynamic Connections

A dominant characteristic of brain organisation is its connectivity (compare the brain to a forest), suggesting that the interactions and relationships between activity in different parts of the brain may be as important as regionally specific neuronal dynamics. In other words, the salient aspects of functional anatomy are not simply the things that are connected but the connections themselves. This is not to say that a bridge is more important than the river banks that it connects, but the development of and transactions between communities on both side of the river, facilitated by the bridge, rely fundamentally upon it. The ontology of great cities around the world centres on bridges. Imagine Paris without the Seine. The ancient craft of bridge building, disseminated throughout Europe by the Romans, was preserved through the Dark Ages by orders of monks and acquired an ecclesiastical status. Hence the Pope's title "Pontifex Maximus" (bridge builder in chief) or the role of an *Arch*bishop in relation to his Bishops. The bridges between functionally segregated systems in the brain are no less important and are identified in terms like cognitive *arch*itecture. Perhaps what we search for is a "functional architecture" as opposed to a "functional anatomy" where the architecture embodies the interactions and integration that bridge the dynamics of segregated areas. In what follows, we consider a number of possible developments in imaging neuroscience that relate to functional integration and "effective connectivity" among specialised areas.

We have devoted a whole chapter to the characterisation and assessment of effective connectivity and here comment upon the direction that this research is likely to take. The most obvious development is the adoption of nonlinear models of effective connectivity. Although some early work has been done in this field [16] it remains a very difficult area. One of the most problematic issues is that it is difficult to establish any construct validity for effective connectivity by virtue of the fact that there are so few existing approaches to its measurement. We have tried to overcome this problem by developing two parallel research programmes that have the same objective and yet use entirely different methods. The hope is that we will be able to establish the validity of one approach in terms of the other. The first approach involves an extension of the nonlinear model of haemodynamic responses that employs Volterra series (see above). In this case, instead of considering the nonlinear response to a stimulus, we replace the stimulus with activities measured in other parts of the brain. The Volterra kernels that mediate the influences of distant regions on the dynamics of the region in question provide a reasonably comprehensive model of effective connectivity. These estimates are measured in terms of kernel coefficients and inferences can be made about their significance using standard statistical techniques and other devices mentioned above. Although we will not go into details here, such analyses provide measurements of the direct and modulatory influences of one region on another and a P value can be associated with these inferences. A typical example of the connectivity that can be determined in this way is shown in Fig. 5. This analysis was based on an fMRI study of a single subject who viewed radially moving stimuli under different attentional conditions (*i.e.*, he was asked to attend or ignore changes in the speed of stimuli that did not actually occur during the scanning window).

A second parallel approach to the same biological problem, namely the nature of interactions in the visual stream that mediate attention to visual motion, involves a nonlinear extension of "structural equation modelling" [17], wherein second order terms are included explicitly in the model. The second order terms are simply the products of activities in two brain regions. These second order terms are sometimes referred to as "moderator variables" and in the context of imaging neuroscience can be interpreted as the effect on activity in a target region that is the result of a modulating influence of one area on the effect of another. There are a number of differences between a nonlinear system identification approach and a nonlinear structural equation modelling approach. Perhaps the most fundamental difference is that the first

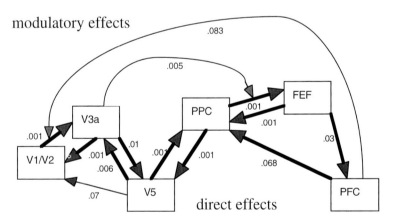

FIGURE 5 Connections among regions implicated in attention to visual motion. This analysis was based on a fMRI study of a single subject who watched radially moving stimuli under different attentional sets. The analysis started with one region and assessed the influence of activity in all the remaining regions by modeling these activities as inputs and the response, in the region chosen, as an output, with a multivariate Volterra series expansion. By using second order approximations and expanding in terms of temporal basis functions the system of equations was rendered linear. The General Linear Model was then employed to make statistical inferences about the significance of the connections (both direct and modulatory). This was repeated for each region in turn. The resulting P values are shown next to their respective connections. Only connections with $P < 0.01$ are shown. PFC—prefrontal cortex; FEF—frontal eye fields; PPC—posterior parietal cortex; V1, V2, V3a, V5—cortical visual areas.

identifies parameters of the model that allow it to emulate an observed imaging time series. In structural equation modelling one minimises the difference between the implied covariances over time and those actually observed.

These new approaches to functional integration have been greatly facilitated by fMRI and represent an ambitious, but important way forward. The importance of these models is that they are on the one hand unconstrained, in the sense that they allow for nonlinear effects, yet on the other hand they allow for the possibility of building into them prior anatomical and physiological knowledge. In structural equation modelling the anatomical constraints are embodied by a specification of the structural or anatomical model within which connection strengths are estimated. Although an ability to incorporate anatomical knowledge into models of functional integration may appear to be an advantage, it is also a disadvantage in that we have so little precise information about how areas are connected to each other. The future may see a convergence of nonlinear structural equation modelling and anatomically based models of connectivity to comprehensively characterise interactions amongst different cortical areas. There is growing interest, although not much work, on using diffusion-weighted MRI to provide such anatomical constraints. Diffusion-weighted MRI can be used to measure anisotropic diffusion of water down myelin sheaths of white matter tracts. Although there is much work to be done, one can imagine the day when a structural equation model, based on functional data, is solved using weighted least squares where the weights are based on probabilistic estimates of the anatomical connectivity from diffusion-weighted MRI. This approach would represent a pleasing integration of functional and structural MRI.

At the beginning of this section we mentioned that dynamic modulation of receptive fields and responsiveness are key features of functional integration in the brain. Phrases like *"the classical receptive field is dead!"* are usually inspired by an appreciation that receptive fields are dynamic and plastic and reflect many more influences than the sensory input to which they are responding. The classical receptive field is not dead and functional segregation has not been a portent of a "dark age" for integration. Modulation and context-sensitive changes of effective connectivity are two vitally important aspects of functional integration that place functional specialisation in a more proper context. We now present an example that also serves to show that not all advances in imaging neuroscience depend upon clever mathematical models. The example illustrates an experiment examining a psychophysiological interaction. By psychophysiological interaction we refer to an interaction between some psychological or experimental parameter and physiological activity measured somewhere else in the brain. The idea here is to try and explain the responses observed at one locus in the brain in terms of an interaction between the afferent input from another region and some experimentally designed, stimulus-specific, or cognitive variable. Generally, interactions are expressed in terms of the effect of one factor on the effect of another. Psychophysiological interactions can therefore be looked at from two points of view. First, a psychological or sensory factor can affect or modulate the physiological influence of one brain area upon another. Second, the same interaction can be construed as a modulation of responses in a target area to sensory or cognitive changes, by activity from the source area. The empirical example we have chosen involves the same fMRI study, mentioned above, of attention to visual motion. In this study subjects were asked to view radially moving dots that gave the impression of "optic flow." In between these stimuli subjects simply viewed a fixation point. On alternate presentations of the moving stimulus subjects were asked to attend to changes in the speed of the stimuli (these changes in speed did not actually occur during scanning). We were interested in whether attention could be shown to modulate the efferent influence from the V1/V2 complex to area V5. We addressed this issue by regressing the activity at every voxel on that in V1/V2 under each attentional state, separately. We tested the significance of the difference in the resulting regression slopes (*i.e.*, the psychophysiological interaction between V1/V2 complex activity and attentional set) in the usual way to give an SPM reflecting the significance of this putative modulatory effect. Significant regions are shown in temporo-occipital cortices on a structural T1-weighted MRI in Fig. 6 (top) in a region in the vicinity of V5. The bottom panel of the figure shows the regression plot for the most significant voxel in this region and demonstrates that when subjects expected changes in the motion of the visual stimulus the regression slope was markedly steeper. In other words, the influence of V1 on V5 was positively modulated by attention to this aspect of visual motion.

Consider again the two regression slopes in Fig. 6. Recall that there are two interpretations of psychophysiological interactions: (i) a context-specific change in the influence or connectivity between two regions or (ii) a modulation of responsiveness by this influence. The first interpretation is more intuitive in explaining the results of our illustrative experiment in the sense that attention can be thought of as modulating the influence that V1/V2 exerts over V5. However, the complementary perspective is equally valid. In this instance attention-dependent responses in V5 are realised only in the presence of stimulus-dependent afferent input from V1/V2. The second perspective can be appreciated more clearly by noting that the dark and grey dots on the right-hand side of Fig. 6 (bottom) segregate only when V1/V2 activity is high. In other words, V5 discriminates between situations associated with changes in attentional set when, and only when, V1/V2 input is present. This example of psychophysiological interactions shows how imaging neuroscience can be used to make inferences about the modulation of regionally specific responses in a fairly simple way. This approach can be extended to include nonlinear effects and to embrace more complex interactions; the principles remain the same.

C. Connections and Plasticity

The functional architecture of the brain would be completely specified if we knew every connection strength of all the intrinsic and extrinsic connections in the brain and the operational characteristics of these connections. Clearly this is an unreasonable functional map to aspire to. However, there may be principles behind the formation and organisation of such connections that can be derived. Can imaging neuroscience be used to elucidate these principles or confirm theoretical predictions about them? We will review an example that suggests that, in principle, it can. This example pertains to theories about how the brain's connectivity develops and adapts with experience. There are many large scale theories of how the brain is organised [18]. Theoretical neurobiology can generate compelling ideas about the ontology and maintenance of connections, for example, "*value-dependent selection*" in the context of "*neuronal Darwinism*" [14,15]. The idea is very simple and potentially powerful. It suggests that, after a crude infrastructure of connections has

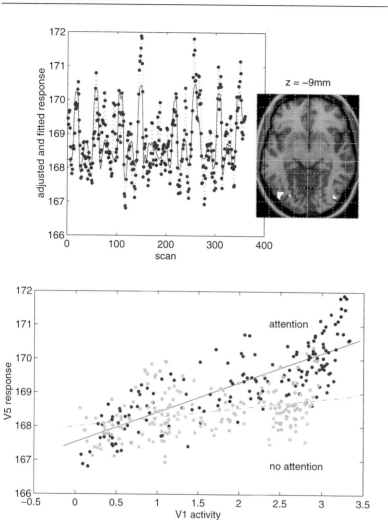

FIGURE 6 (Top) SPM thresholded at $P = 0.001$ (height - uncorrected) and $P = 0.05$ (volume - corrected) superimposed on a structural T_1-weighted image. This SPM was testing for a significant psychophysiological interaction between activity in V1 and attention to visual motion. The most significant effects are seen in the vicinity of V5 (white region on the lower right) and the associated time-series of the most significant ($Z = 4.46$) voxel in this region is shown in the top panel (fitted data, line; adjusted data, dots). (Bottom) Regression of V5 activity (at 42, −78, −9 mm) on V1 activity when the subject was asked to attend to changes in the speed of radially moving dots and when she was not. The lines correspond to the regressions. The dots correspond to the observed data adjusted for confounds other than the main effects of V1 activity (dark grey dots, attention; light grey dots, no attention). Attention can be seen to augment the influence of V1 on V5.

been established by epigenetic mechanisms, synaptic efficacies are selectively consolidated whenever something "good" happens that elicits an adaptive or valuable response. An adaptive response is one that elicits activity in neuronal systems capable of consolidating changes in synaptic efficacy. This description is deliberately circular or tautological by analogy with the tautology implicit in definitions of adaptive fitness in evolutionary selection. We can escape the tautology by considering the types of event that elicit activity in systems capable of consolidating plastic changes of connectivity (referred to as "value systems"). Initially responses are limited to any changes in the internal milieu that maintain adaptive homeostasis. Such responses are mediated by genetically determined pathways, from interoceptors to the value system. To recap, connections are consolidated when anything of adaptive value occurs. An event with adaptive value, by definition, activates systems responsible for this consolidation. Initially, the only events that can activate such systems are changes in the state of the organism that are of innate value. Innate value is determined by evolutionary selection (in simple terms, those phenotypes with the wrong connections to the system mediating value will die, those with the right connections will not and will pass on the genetically specified connections to subsequent generations). As organisms grow and adapt to their environment, events which precede a valuable response gain access to value systems. If this happens these events themselves now have adaptive value (by definition) and are capable of reinforcing their precedents. The capacity of antecedent events to excite activity in value systems is a natural consequence of the value system consolidating afferents from the cortex to itself. This is yet another example of recursion. This theory is reasonably complete mechanistically, has a plausible biological basis, and makes itself accountable to many other theories of brain and behaviour, ranging from high-order reinforcement schedules in conditioning paradigms [19] to temporal difference models in computational neurobiology [20]. A key mechanistic aspect of this theory is the presence of neurotransmitter systems that are capable of consolidating or modulating associative plasticity. In principle this is where imaging neuroscience could be used to look at such mechanisms *in vivo*. There are several candidates for neurotransmitter systems capable of consolidating synaptic efficacy (*e.g.*, the ascending cholinergic system from the nucleus basalis [21] or the dopaminergic system arising in the ventral tegmental area [22]). Nearly all of them can be manipulated pharmacologically. By combining established techniques such as psychopharmacological designs (as described in Chapter 16) and using time dependent measures of effective connectivity, we are very nearly in a position to examine which neurotransmitter systems are capable of modulating plasticity in the way suggested by theory.

VII. BRAIN STATES, EVENTS, AND INTERACTIONS

A. Event-Related and State-Related Neuroimaging

Since the advent of fMRI a new distinction has emerged in imaging neuroscience, that between event-related methods and state-associated methods. By virtue of the half-life of the radioactive tracers used, PET imaging has been largely restricted to studying differences in brain states engendered by the repeated presentation of stimuli or the enduring performance of some task. With fMRI new techniques are being developed that allow evoked haemodynamic responses to single stimuli or events to be characterised and compared. This technical advance is of fundamental importance for experimental design because the ability to present experimental trials in isolation frees one from the potentially confounding effects of states like attentional set. For example, we can now examine directly brain responses to novel events in "odd ball paradigms" and more generally, separate the effects of a particular stimulus from the context in which that stimulus is presented (see below). Figure 7 makes a distinction between state and event related brain responses with an fMRI study in which a subject was asked to listen passively to words presented at a fixed rate over an extended period of time or to single words presented in isolation. These analyses represent a simple version of the Volterra series approach described above and rely upon the use of temporal basis functions. Event related fMRI presents an opportunity to adopt similar experimental designs to those that have proved to be so useful in neurophysiological evoked potential work. The advantage of event related fMRI is its high spatial resolu-

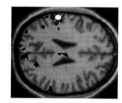

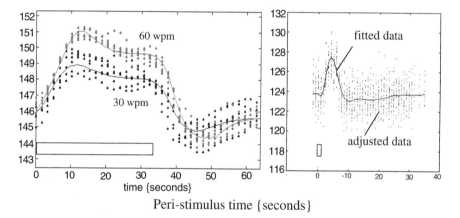

Peri-stimulus time {seconds}

FIGURE 7 Although there is a great overlap between PET and fMRI, there are some fundamental constraints on an experimental design imposed by the different techniques: Consider the distinction between state-related responses and event-related responses. By virtue of the relatively long half-life of the tracers used, PET can measure only responses summed over fairly long periods of time. Consequently PET can be used only to measure differences between brain states. In contrast, fMRI can be used in two ways. Epochs of repeated stimuli or continuous task performance can be presented and the ensuing signal interpreted as a brain-state dependent measure (left). Alternatively, event-related responses to a single stimulus can be measured by analogy to evoked potentials in electrophysiology (right). The data above were acquired from a single subject using echo planar imaging (EPI) fMRI at a rate of one volume image every 1.7 sec. The subject listened to words in epochs of 34 sec at a variety of different frequencies. The fitted peri-auditory responses (lines) and adjusted data (dots) are shown for two rates (30 and 60 words per minute) on the left. The solid bar denotes the presentation of words. By removing confounds and specifying the appropriate design matrix one can show that fMRI is exquisitely sensitive to single events. The data shown on the right were acquired from the same subject whilst simply listening to single words presented every 34 sec. Event-related responses were modeled using a small set of temporal basis [gamma] functions of the peristimulus time. The SPM{F} reflecting the significance of these event-related responses shown has been thresholded at $P = 0.001$ (uncorrected) and displayed on a T_1 weighted structural MRI.

tion. The main disadvantage, of course, is that elicited responses are smoothed with a haemodynamic response function whose time constants are in the order of 5–8 sec. Other advantages of event-related fMRI include the ability to randomise stimuli and hence to avoid confounds due to processes such as maintenance of a particular attentional set. Event-related fMRI can be used directly to map events or stimuli that are not under experimental control, for example hallucinations. Finally, one can, potentially, make inferences about temporal components of an evoked haemodynamic response. Undoubtedly, event-related fMRI offers an opportunity for some interesting experiments and clever applications. We have already successfully demonstrated significant event-related differential fMRI responses to semantically coherent and incoherent sentences.

The advantage of state-associated fMRI relative to event-related techniques is that many more stimuli can be presented, thereby providing a much more potent compound stimulus and hence response. In event-related fMRI the events have to be spaced by at least 16 sec, limiting the total number of stimuli per session. A second advantage of state-related techniques is that parametric variations of the way in which stimuli relate to each other can be explored in a fashion that it is not possible with event-related fMRI. A simple example is the experimental variation that can be induced by differing frequencies of stimulus presentation.

Perhaps it is worth considering here event-related PET. Of course it is not necessary to measure individual responses to stimuli to make inferences about them. We will briefly review two examples where PET has been used to examine the transient dynamics evoked by words. In the first example words were presented visually, at a fixed rate, during PET scanning. The only variable was the exposure duration of the stimuli which varied between 150 and 750 msec. Responses in the extrastriate cortex showed a monotonic increase with exposure duration. By using a parametric design, in conjunction with a nonlinear regression analysis, we were able to show that the evoked responses deviated from a linear relationship with relatively attenuated responses at longer durations (see Fig. 8). These observations have two potential explanations. First, extrastriate responses to visually presented stimuli are preferentially enhanced by attentional mechanisms when the stimuli are very brief. This interpretation is supported by the observation that activity in anterior cingulate cortex was maximal at the shortest exposure durations. A second explanation is that there is intrinsic adaptation during prolonged visual presentations resulting in a progressive fall in the average response, per millisecond of exposure, with increasing exposure duration. These alternative explanations provide a nice example where event-related fMRI could be used to adjudicate between them. By repeating the experiment with event-related fMRI one can remove the attentional influences and determine whether adaption does indeed occur. Note, however, if we had just performed the event-related fMRI study, and the responses showed a linear dependency on exposure duration, we would have completely missed the selective enhancement of responses to short stimuli. This putative context-sensitive effect could be revealed only by a state-related approach that allowed one to establish the "context."

In the second example we asked subjects to produce words at a variety of rates. This was a factorial design in that the words were either produced, in response to a heard letter (intrinsically), or by simply repeating a heard word (extrinsically). By examining the imaging data for an interaction between the nature of word production and word production rate we identified a region

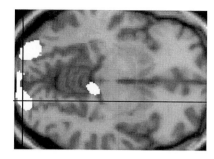

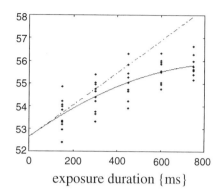

exposure duration {ms}

Figure 8 (Left) SPM{F} testing for the significance of a second order polynomial regression of activity on the duration of visually presented words as measured in five normal subjects using PET. Bilateral extrastriate regions are shown as white regions surviving a threshold of $P = 0.05$ (uncorrected) on a structural T_1-weighted MRI. (Right) An example of this regression for the voxel under the cross hairs on the left. It can be seen that the observed deviates from the linear relationship that would be expected if the amount of neural activity elicited was proportional to the duration over which it was elicited.

in the posterior temporal cortex in which activity correlated positively with extrinsically generated word rate and negatively with intrinsically generated word rate. The latter observation is remarkable and suggests that activity is reduced when more of these word production events occur. The only explanation for this observation is that it represents a true deactivation, or a reduction in brain activity, associated with the intrinsic production of each word (Fig. 9). The existence of transient decreases in BOLD signal, mediated by increases in deoxyhaemoglobin concentration that may themselves be associated with a decrease in perfusion and an increased oxygen extraction fraction, can, of course, be confirmed with event-related fMRI. An example of this is shown in Fig. 10 where a region with an initial biphasic decrease in BOLD signal was found in the posterior superior temporal region with passive listening to single words.

B. Interactions: Another Approach to Functional Integration

In the previous section we consider the distinction between event- and state-related brain responses. In this section we look at interactions between various factors that determine responses. Many of the more compelling experiments described in this book have employed factorial designs, wherein the interaction between experimental factors has been as interesting, if not more so, than the main effects of the factors themselves. In terms of future trends we anticipate that factorial designs will become standard for brain mapping. We have already alluded, both in this chapter and in previous chapters, to the importance of regionally specific interactions as distinct from regionally specific activations. We think this idea is important for future research for the following reasons. If it is the case that activations are always context-sensitive then many effects that have hitherto been ascribed to simple activations by cognitive or sensory processes may, in fact, reflect interactions between one factor and another. However, if the second factor is not explicitly included in an experiment, any interaction will reduce to a simple main effect

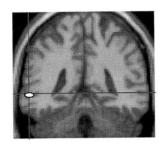

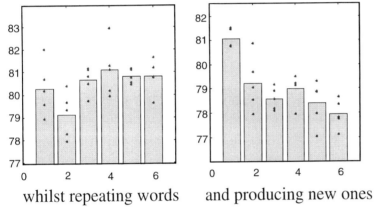

whilst repeating words   and producing new ones

FIGURE 9 Adjusted activity from a voxel in the posterior superior temporal region is shown as a function of word-production rate under the two conditions of extrinsic and intrinsic word generation. The change in slope is obvious. The voxel from which these data derived is shown on the SPM{t} (top). These data come from a PET study of six normal subjects.

of the single factor used. This simple main effect will be interpreted as an activation. Consider the following example. Imagine that we have discovered extrastriate activations when subjects view words as opposed to false font letter strings. We might ascribe this activation to the difference between the stimuli and label the region as a "word-form area." However, this regionally specific effect could arise as a result of an interaction between implicit phonological retrieval and the presentation of letter strings. To test this hypothesis one would need a factorial design in which the presence of letter strings was crossed with implicit phonological retrieval (see Chapter 13). On the basis of this experiment we might find that the region responded to the presence of letter strings relative to single characters and that this activation was enhanced by implicit phonological retrieval (when implicitly naming the word or letter). In other words, we could also interpret this regionally specific effect as a modulation of letter string specific responses by implicit phonological retrieval. In the absence of phonological retrieval there may be no differences in the response of the area to words or nonword letter strings. This distinction between word-specific responses in an extrastriate region and word recognition-dependent modulation of extrastriate responses to any letter string is not a specious one. Consider it in the light of the receptive field metaphor we use above. The difference between the two interpretations is that (i) there are

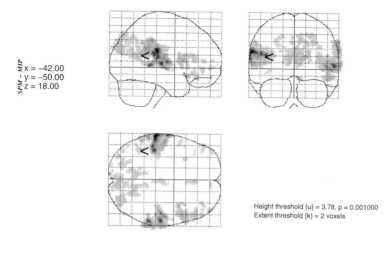

Height threshold {u} = 3.78, p = 0.001000
Extent threshold {k} = 2 voxels

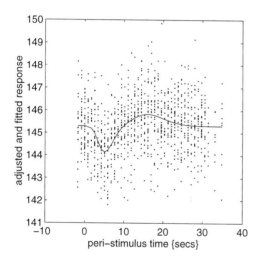

FIGURE 10 Event-related deactivation. (Top) SPM{F} relating to an event-related single-word presentation fMRI experiment in a single subject. The SPM{F} has been thresholded at $P < 0.001$ (uncorrected). The arrowheads point to a voxel in the right superior temporal region at -42, -50, 18 mm. (Bottom) The event-related response based on the zeroth and first order Volterra kernel estimates (solid line) for the voxel identified above. The dots correspond to the adjusted data.

receptive fields for words in extrastriate regions and (ii) there is a selective modulation of receptive fields for any letter-string by higher cortical areas with receptive fields for the phonology of a stimulus. If we were able to inhibit the activity of these higher order receptive fields (using, for example, transcranial magnetic stimulation of infero-temporal regions) the extrastriate responses might no longer differentiate between word-like and non-word-like letter strings. If this were the case should the extrastriate area be designated a word-form area? Clearly not in a simple way; however, it would constitute a necessary component of a distributed system involved in the perception of visually presented words. It would be implicated in this system by virtue of the interaction effect. In this way interactions can be thought of as reflecting the integration or dynamic modulation of receptive fields that embodies transactions among the functionally segregated components of distributed brain systems. (An interesting corollary of this arguement is to consider the behavioural and clinical effects of brain lesions. If a lesion occurs in a modulating brain area it could conceivably alter functions normally attributable to brain regions that the lesion has not affected structurally.) From a psychological perspective one could postulate an "extra" psychological processing component that was responsible for the integration of phonological retrieval and visual analysis. The interaction would then represent an activation on comparing brain activity in states that did and did not require this integration.

In summary, our example highlights the importance of regionally specific interactions and factorial experimental designs. An interpretation of interactions is that they represent the integration of different processes (*e.g.*, visual processing of letter strings and phonological retrieval). One can envisage a whole class of brain mapping experiments dedicated purely to mapping the effects of integrating two or more processes. Imagine an imaging neuroscience unit devoted to studying single-word processing. Eight components of interest are identified (these may include phonological retrieval, structural identification, early visual processing, semantic analysis, and so on). Using a simple subtraction design, eight experiments are sufficient to characterise completely the simple differences between them. Such a programme runs and is completed. Imagine now that a new head of the language group is appointed who realises that such a characterisation of language processing is incomplete. Furthermore she holds the deep conviction that a proper understanding of functional architectures will come about only by explicitly measuring the integration of all the language processing components. She works out that on the basis of the eight original experiments, there are 28 unique two by two factorial designs. Each of these factorial experiments will identify regionally specific interactions that reflect a pair-wise integration of the eight cardinal components. Although this scenario may sound contrived it is actually far from hypothetical.

In the previous paragraph we consider interactions in terms of integration of two or more cognitive or sensorimotor processes. Another important example of interactions are time by condition interactions. These are generally interpretable in terms of plasticity or adaptation. Such experiments have evolved considerably since the first demonstration of adaptation in the motor system using interactions (see Chapter 12). By using single-subject fMRI and modeling time-dependent changes in evoked responses with temporal basis functions, we can now look in some detail at the reorganisation of physiological responses during learning. Figure 11 shows the results of an experiment designed by Paul Fletcher, in which subjects learned an artificial grammar. The learning implicit in this design occurred across sessions of explicit learning of exemplars that conformed to a hidden set of orthographic rules (grammar). Using this design we were able to differentiate between time-dependent changes in evoked responses due to learning simple associations and to those due to rule learning. The results, shown in Fig. 11, illustrate both these within-session and between-session effects in the dorsolateral prefrontal cortex.

VIII. CONCLUSION

In conclusion, this chapter has focused on the distinction between the empiricism of imaging neuroscience, which lends itself naturally to map making, and

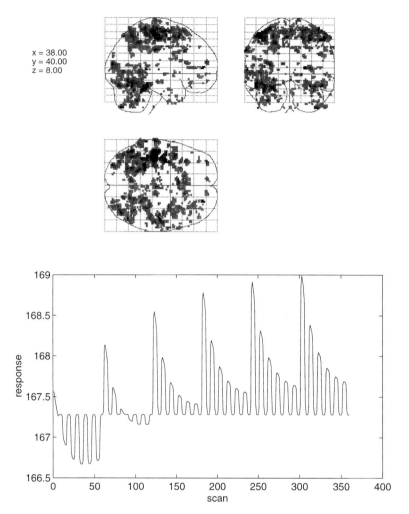

x = 38.00
y = 40.00
z = 8.00

FIGURE 11   (Top) SPM{*t*} reflecting the significance of time × condition interactions (*P* < 0.01, uncorrected). The subject learnt an artificial grammar with specific exemplars within-session and different sets of exemplars (but the same rules) between sessions. (Bottom) Fitted activity of a voxel in the right dorsolateral prefrontal cortex showing adaptation within-session but a progressive increase in responsiveness during strategic learning over sessions. These data were fitted using exponential temporal basis functions to model the interactions.

the search for principles that underlie the organisation and dynamics of the maps produced. The "BIG atlas" idea (Chapter 17) is an important one and is an essential precursor for extracting more general principles that bring order and parsimony to neuroimaging observations. We think that a "BIG atlas" should not only encompass many modalities (*e.g.*, histochemistry, connectivity, cytoarchitectonics), but could also be extended conceptually to embrace interactions and integration of measured brain responses. We have tried to emphasise the importance of continually reevaluating assumptions and progressively refining (or elaborating) the conceptual and mathematical models that are used to make sense of the neuroimaging data acquired. Imaging neuroscience, like any other science, develops in a broader context. Advances in understanding neuronal codes, progress in nonlinear system identification and dynamic systems theory, the molecular biology of synaptic plasticity, developments in computational neurobiology, and a dialogue between cognitive science and theoretical neuroscience will all have an effect on what happens to imaging neuroscience in the future. Many of the examples provided above speak to this conclusion.

For those readers who are dismayed not to have found one sentence in this final chapter containing the word "consciousness," here it is!

References

1. E. Mayr. "The Growth of Biological Thought," pp. 147–300. The Belknap Press of Harvard Univ. Cambridge, MA, 1982.
2. E. Kraepelin. "Dementia Praecox and Paraphrenia." Livingston, Edinburgh, UK, 1919.
3. P. F. Liddle. The symptoms of chronic schizophrenia: A re-examination of the positive-negative dichotomy. *Br. J. Psychiatry* **151,** 145–151 (1987).
4. S. A. Kauffman. "Origins of Order: Self Organization and Selection in Evolution." OUP, Oxford, UK, 1994.
5. K. J. Friston, G. Tononi, O. Sporns, and G. M. Edelman. Characterising the complexity of neuronal interactions. *Hum. Brain Mapping* **3,** 302–314 (1995).
6. D. Malonek and A. Grinvald. Interactions between electrical activity and cortical microcirulation revealed by imaging spectroscopy: Implications for functional brain mapping. *Science* **272,** 551–554 (1995).
7. M. N. Shadlen and W. T. Newsome. Noise, neural codes and cortical organization. *Curr. Opin. Neurobiol.* **4,** 569–579 (1995).
8. C. Von der Malsburg. Nervous structures with dynamical links. *Ber Bunsenges. Phys. Chem.* **89,** 703–710 (1985).
9. C. M. Gray and W. Singer. Stimulus specific neuronal oscillations in orientation columns of cat visual cortex *Proc. Natl. Acad. Sci. USA* **86,** 1698–1702 (1989).
10. M. Abeles, Y. Prut, H. Bergman, and E. Vaadia. Synchronisation in neuronal transmission and its importance for information processing. *In* "Temporal Coding in the Brain" (E. Buzsaki, R. Llinas, W. Singer, A. Berthoz, and Y. Christen, Eds.), pp. 39–50. Springer Verlag, Berlin, 1995.
11. K. J. Friston. Neuronal transients. *Proc. R. Soc. London B* **261,** 401–405 (1995).
12. E. D. Lumer, G. M. Edelman, and G. Tononi. Neural dynamics in a model of the thalamocortical system. II. The role of neural synchrony tested through perturbations of spike timing. *Cereb. Cortex* **7,** 228–236 (1997).
13. J. Talairach and P. Tournoux. "A Co-planar Stereotaxic Atlas of a Human Brain." Thieme, Stuttgart, 1988.
14. G. M. Edelman. Neural Darwinism: Selection and reentrant signalling in higher brain function. *Neuron* **10,** 115–125 (1993).
15. K. J. Friston, G. Tononi, G. H. Reeke, O. Sporns, and G. E. Edelman. Value-dependent selection in the brain: Simulation in a synthetic neural model. *Neuroscience* **39,** 229–243 (1994).
16. K. J. Friston, L. G. Ungerleider, P. Jezzard, and R. Turner. Characterizing modulatory interactions between V1 and V2 in human cortex with fMRI. *Hum. Brain Mapping* **2,** 211–224 (1995).
17. A. R. McIntosh and F. Gonzalez-Lima. Structural equation modelling and its application to network analysis in functional brain imaging. *Hum. Brain Mapping* **2,** 2–22 (1994).
18. C. Koch and J. L. Davis. "Large Scale Neuronal Theories of the Brain." MIT Press, London, UK, 1994.
19. D. Gaffan and S. Harrison. Amygdalectomy and disconnection in visual learning for auditory secondary reinforcement by monkeys. *J. Neurosci.* **7,** 2285–2292 (1987).
20. R. S. Sutton and A. G. Barto. Time derivative models of Pavlovian reinforcement. *In* "Learning and Computational Neuroscience: Foundations of Adaptive Net-

works'' (M. Gabriel and J. Moore, Eds.), pp. 497–538. MIT Press, Cambridge, MA, 1990.

21. N. W. Weinberger, J. H. Ashe, R. Metherate, T. M. McKenna, D. M. Diamond, J. S. Bakin, R. C. Lennartz, and J. M. Cassady. Neural adaptive information processing: A preliminary model of receptive field plasticity in auditory cortex during Pavlovian conditioning. *In "Learning and Computational Neuroscience: Foundations of Adaptive Networks"* (M. Gabriel and J. Moore, Eds.), pp. 91–138. MIT Press, Cambridge, MA, 1990.

22. J. McGaugh. Neuromodulatory systems and the regulation of memory storage. *In* "Neuropsychology of Memory" (L. Squire and N. Butters, Eds.), pp. 386–401. Guildford Press, New York, 1992.

INDEX